Craniofacial Development and Growth

Craniofacial Development and Growth

Editor: Mitch Pittman

AMERICAN
MEDICAL PUBLISHERS
www.americanmedicalpublishers.com

AMERICAN
MEDICAL PUBLISHERS
www.americanmedicalpublishers.com

Cataloging-in-Publication Data

Craniofacial development and growth / edited by Mitch Pittman.
p. cm.
Includes bibliographical references and index.
ISBN 979-8-88740-028-0
1. Skull--Growth. 2. Facial bones--Growth. 3. Head--Molecular aspects.
4. Face--Abnormalities. 5. Skull--Abnormalities. I. Pittman, Mitch.
RC936 .C73 2023
617.510 757 2--dc23

American Medical Publishers,
41 Flatbush Avenue,
1st Floor, New York,
NY 11217, USA

ISBN 979-8-88740-028-0 (Hardback)

Contents

Preface

This book has been an outcome of determined endeavour from a group of educationists in the field. The primary objective was to involve a broad spectrum of professionals from diverse cultural background involved in the field for developing new researches. The book not only targets students but also scholars pursuing higher research for further enhancement of the theoretical and practical applications of the subject.

Craniofacial growth is a complex phenomenon that involves the enlargement and differentiation of hard and soft tissues that are characterized by cephalocaudal and allometric designs. It involves the basic mechanisms underlying the post-natal growth of the cranium. There are two prominent ways in which the basic craniofacial bone pattern is laid during embryonic development. The first method of craniofacial development is a highly coordinated process under a tight genetic control and environmental influence. For managing the patients in the best possible manner, it is essential to understand the primary concepts related with the growth and development of the craniofacial skeleton. The craniofacial skeleton develops naturally as a result of different developmental events, which include brain growth and development, optic pathway development, speech and swallowing development, airway and pharyngeal development, muscle development, and tooth development and eruption. This book is a valuable compilation of topics, ranging from the basic to the most complex advancements in the study of craniofacial development and growth. It will serve as a reference to a broad spectrum of readers.

It was an honour to edit such a profound book and also a challenging task to compile and examine all the relevant data for accuracy and originality. I wish to acknowledge the efforts of the contributors for submitting such brilliant and diverse chapters in the field and for endlessly working for the completion of the book. Last, but not the least; I thank my family for being a constant source of support in all my research endeavours.

Editor

1

Diverse Fate of an Enigmatic Structure: 200 Years of Meckel's Cartilage

Eva Svandova[1], Neal Anthwal[2], Abigail S. Tucker[2] and Eva Matalova[1,3]*

[1] Institute of Animal Physiology and Genetics, Academy of Sciences, Brno, Czechia, [2] Centre for Craniofacial and Regenerative Biology, King's College London, Guy's Hospital, London, United Kingdom, [3] Department of Physiology, University of Veterinary and Pharmaceutical Sciences, Brno, Czechia

***Correspondence:**
Abigail S. Tucker
abigail.tucker@kcl.ac.uk

Meckel's cartilage was first described by the German anatomist Johann Friedrich Meckel the Younger in 1820 from his analysis of human embryos. Two hundred years after its discovery this paper follows the development and largely transient nature of the mammalian Meckel's cartilage, and its role in jaw development. Meckel's cartilage acts as a jaw support during early development, and a template for the later forming jaw bones. In mammals, its anterior domain links the two arms of the dentary together at the symphysis while the posterior domain ossifies to form two of the three ear ossicles of the middle ear. In between, Meckel's cartilage transforms to a ligament or disappears, subsumed by the growing dentary bone. Several human syndromes have been linked, directly or indirectly, to abnormal Meckel's cartilage formation. Herein, the evolution, development and fate of the cartilage and its impact on jaw development is mapped. The review focuses on developmental and cellular processes that shed light on the mechanisms behind the different fates of this cartilage, examining the control of Meckel's cartilage patterning, initiation and maturation. Importantly, human disorders and mouse models with disrupted Meckel's cartilage development are highlighted, in order to understand how changes in this cartilage impact on later development of the dentary and the craniofacial complex as a whole. Finally, the relative roles of tissue interactions, apoptosis, autophagy, macrophages and clast cells in the removal process are discussed. Meckel's cartilage is a unique and enigmatic structure, the development and function of which is starting to be understood but many interesting questions still remain.

Keywords: jaw development, craniofacial, mammal evolution, congenital birth defects, chondrogenesis

INTRODUCTION

The developing face is created by a fusion of a number of facial processes, with the lower jaw created by cells largely from the first pharyngeal arch. The structure of the face is first outlined by the cartilaginous chondrocranium, with a single cartilage defining the lower jaw, known as Meckel's cartilage (MC). MC was first described in mammals by the German anatomist Johann Friedrich Meckel the Younger in the Handbuch der menschlichen Anatomie (Meckel, 1820), 200 years ago. Here Meckel described the relationship between a cartilage rod that ran along the jaw and the forming malleus, and compared this rod to similar structures previously described in fish, amphibians and birds (Meckel, 1820). The cartilage was later named Meckel's cartilage by his followers (Amano et al., 2010). During development, MC begins life as two rods of cartilage, which meet in the midline to form a V-structure outlining the forming lower jaw (**Figures 1A,B**). After the first wave of chondrogenesis, the membranous bones form around the cartilaginous templates to create the dermatocranium, with secondary cartilages capping the bones at key points of articulation and mechanical force (Depew et al., 2002). Meckel's cartilage forms the lower jaw strut in all jawed vertebrates during embryonic development, and as such plays a key conserved role in vertebrate jaw development and evolution (Anthwal et al., 2013). In mammals, the main body of Meckel's cartilage is largely transient but acts as a template for later formation of the bones of the lower jaw, with defects leading to anomalies in the pattern and size of the jaw in mouse mutants and in human embryos (Bhaskar et al., 1953; Amano et al., 2010). In addition to its role as a jaw support, MC also forms two of the three mammalian middle ear bones (malleus and incus), which sit in the middle ear cavity and, along with the stapes, form a chain of ossicles to transfer sound from the outer to the inner ear. MC function therefore spans both roles in feeding and hearing.

In this review the development of the mammalian MC is followed from initiation to final function, highlighting the molecular mechanisms involved in its creation, remodelling and loss, as documented in the research literature. In particular we aim to put into context the recent discoveries in MC development since the last review on this subject (Amano et al., 2010), and highlight the gaps that call for further study of this important cartilage. Over the last ten years, the use of conditional transgenic mice has revealed many of the molecular aspects of MC, providing an understanding of the spatial and temporal dynamics of lower jaw development, and highlighting roles for processes such as autophagy. Likewise the recent use of mammalian models outside mice has shed light on the level of conservation of many of these processes, and the relevance to human development and congenital defects. The fate of different parts of MC in mammals, however, is still unclear, along with the stimuli, both mechanical or molecular, that trigger the changes during ossification, resorption and transformation.

MECKEL'S CARTILAGE: A KEY FEATURE OF JAWED VERTEBRATES

Meckel's cartilage is present in all jawed vertebrates (gnathostomes), and has been hypothesised to have evolved from the ventral gill support structures of the first pharyngeal arch of jawless fish (agnathians) (Mallat, 2008). However, MC may alternatively have formed *de novo* from first arch derived crest in jawed vertebrates. The specialisation of the first arch was a key process in the evolution of jaws, and as such the specification of MC was necessary for the emergence of jawed vertebrates (see Donoghue et al., 2006; Brazeau and Friedman, 2015; Maier and Ruf, 2016; Miyashita, 2016; DeLaurier, 2019; Woronowicz and Schneider, 2019 for further information on the history and evolutionary origins of MC and the jaw). Among non-mammalian jawed vertebrates, MC remains largely cartilaginous in the adult, and acts as a permanent scaffold around which the membranous bones of the mandible are positioned. In these non-mammalian jawed vertebrates, the proximal portion of MC ossifies to form the bones that articulate the upper and lower jaw, with the articular and the quadrate part of the palatoquadrate forming from the same type II collagen expressing condensation in the chick (Wilson and Tucker, 2004). The joint marker *Bapx1* turns on between the quadrate and articular in the chick, creating distinct alcian blue expressing skeletal elements (Wilson and Tucker, 2004).

Uniquely in extant mammals, instead of forming the bones of the jaw joint, the proximal portion of MC ossifies and forms the malleus and incus, two bones of the mammalian three ossicle middle ear (**Figure 1C**). The malleus is homologous to the articular, while the incus is homologous to the quadrate, with a *Bapx1*-expressing joint forming between the two (Tucker et al., 2004). The incus, malleus and MC are initially united as a single type II collagen expressing condensation, with the incus and malleus dividing into two due to the upregulation of joint markers, creating two distinct cartilages, in a similar manner to the situation observed in the chick (Amin and Tucker, 2006; Amin et al., 2007). In the mouse this occurs at E14.5, while the incus and malleus do not fully separate until after birth in some mammals (platypus, echidna, opossum) (Anthwal et al., 2020).

Fossil evidence indicates that Mesozoic mammal-like reptiles had a persistent ossified MCs (Meng et al., 2003, 2011; Luo, 2011; Luo et al., 2015; Anthwal et al., 2017; Mao et al., 2020). Ossification of Meckel's in these extinct mammaliforms is likely to have provided a support for the malleus and incus as they became integrated in the middle ear while still being physically attached to the mandibular apparatus (Luo, 2011). The loss of the proximal part of MC during mammal evolution allowed for the complete detachment of the middle ear and mandibular units, resulting in enhanced function of the middle ear ossicles, which would then have been able to freely vibrate (Luo, 2011). Loss of MC, therefore, played a key part in the separation of the ear bones from the jaw during the transition from reptiles to mammals (Anthwal et al., 2013).

EARLY DEVELOPMENT OF MAMMALIAN MECKEL'S CARTILAGE

The mandible forms from the first pharyngeal arch and is specified early in development by an absence of Hox gene expression (Hunt et al., 1991). MC forms from within the mandibular mesenchyme, and grafting experiments have indicated it is primarily derived from cranial neural crest cells in birds (CNCCs)(Le Douarin and Dupin, 1993). From mouse lineage labelling studies using the Wnt1cre driver, not all chondrocytes in MC are labelled (Chai et al., 2000; Ito et al., 2002), however, its unclear whether this is due to a substantial non-crest contribution in the mouse or due to the fact that this Cre appears to have different activity in midbrain and hindbrain crest (Chen et al., 2017). Labelling with Mesp1cre, a

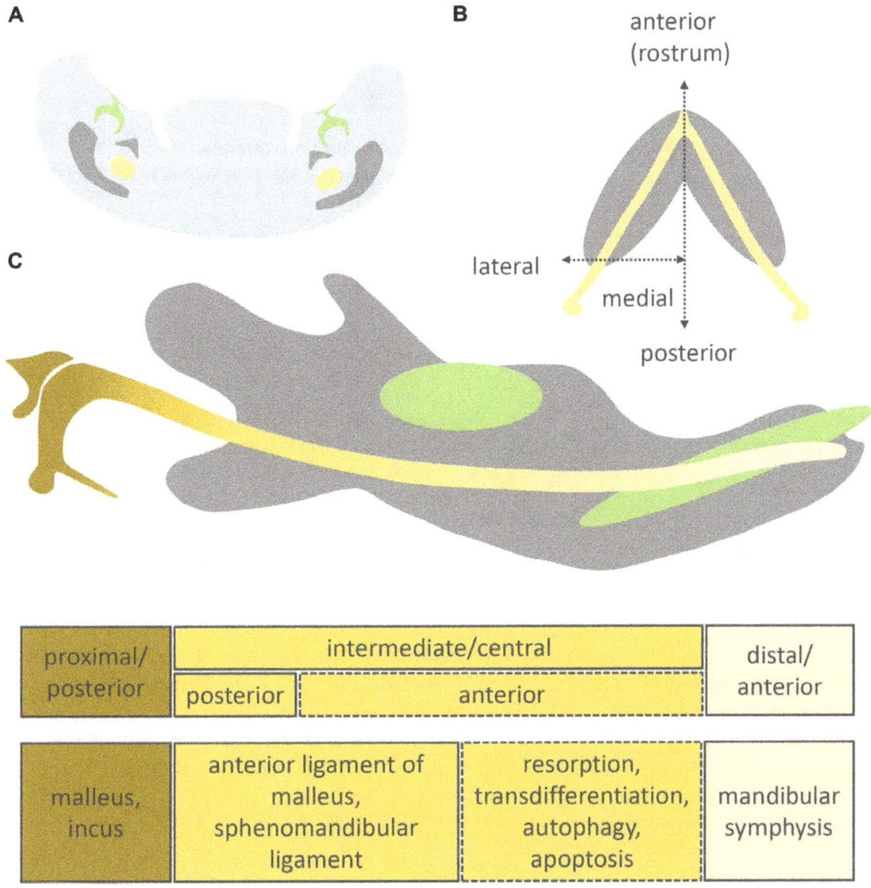

FIGURE 1 | Position of Meckel's cartilage in the mandible and its different developmental fates. Original schematic showing a frontal section of the intermediate part of the murine mandible **(A)**, longitudinal section of the murine mandible **(B)**, sagittal section of the murine mandible **(C)**. Molar/incisor (green), mandibular bone (grey), Meckel's cartilage (yellow).

mesoderm marker, does not label MC or the malleus (Bildsoe et al., 2013). MC has been proposed to be pre-patterned very early on in jaw development, around embryonic day (E) 10 in mice (Ramaesh and Bard, 2003), and initally condenses in the region of the first molar tooth germ at around E11 (Frommer and Margolies, 1971). MC then proceeds to extend anteriorly and posteriorly from this site of initiation (Chai et al., 2000). Formation of MC during mouse development is summarised in **Table 1**. In human development, condensing mesenchyme cells in the mandible are evident from 32 days (stage 13), with muscular attachments associated with MC observed at 44 days (stage 18) (Wyganowska and Przystanska, 2011). In mice the two rods of MC fuse to create a rostral process (**Figure 1B**), while in humans the two rods come in close contact but do not appear to fuse (Rodriguez-Vazquez et al., 1997).

At E13.5, the mouse MC is composed of small, round and densely packed pre-chondroblasts (**Figure 2C**). Earlier stages (E12 or E11) are characterised by condensed mesenchymal cells lacking secreted cartilage matrix (**Figures 2A,B**). Upon differentiation, the chondroblasts become more loosely packed (**Figures 2D,D_1**) and reside in cartilage lacuna embedded in extracellular matrix, rich in type II collagen (Frommer and Margolies, 1971). Transverselly orientated clones introduce new cells in columns into MC, controlling the diameter of the rod (Kaucka et al., 2017). This transverse addition of cells from the periphery of the cartilage cannot explain the longitudinal extension of MC, which is therefore presumably due to differentiation of chondrogenic mesenchyme on either end of the cartilage, which is then in turn expanded via the transverse proliferation of chondrocytes (Kaucka et al., 2017). Elongation of MC has been proposed to be driven in part by paracrine factors signalling from the vascular network of the mandibular mesenchyme (Wiszniak et al., 2015). Here it appears that insulin growth factor (IGF), secreted by blood vessels, plays a role in directing growth of MC, with loss of IGF from blood vessels leading to a shorter MC and mandible (Marchant et al., 2020).

At E13 the dentary starts to form (**Figure 2C**), with MC proposed to have a role in initiating and regulating the growth of the primary ossification centre of the mandible (Frommer and Margolies, 1971). The mandibular dentary bone develops around MC and gradually encases the cartilaginous rod as shown in **Figures 3A–C** (Anthwal et al., 2008). In other mammalian species, such as the marsupial opossum, MC sits within a groove on the medial surface of the mandible bone and

TABLE 1 | Time schedule of MC development in the mouse (as the most common model of MC investigation).

	What happens	How it looks like	References
E8	migration of CNCCs into the 1st pharyngeal arch	undifferentiated ecto-mesenchyme	Chai et al., 1998
E10	clonal expansion of CNCs	undifferentiated ecto-mesenchyme	Takahashi et al., 2001
E11-12	chondroblastic commitment/differentiation	primordium of condensed ecto-mesenchyme	Frommer and Margolies, 1971
E13	chondroblastic differentiation and proliferation, anterio-posterior elongation, fusion of two cartilaginous bars anteriorly	V-shaped structure consisting of chondroblasts and fibrous tissue, formation of malleal-incudo part posteriorly	Frommer and Margolies, 1971 Amin and Tucker, 2006
E14	rapid growth, anterio-posterior elongation	MC consists of chondroblasts and perichondrium	Sakakura et al., 2007 Ricks et al., 2002
E15	initial hypertrophy of chondrocytes attracts angiogenic cells and precursors of osteoclasts	pre-hypertrophic chondrocytes in intermediate part, TRAP-positive cells apparent on lateral side of intermediate part of MC, malleus separated from incus	Frommer and Margolies, 1971 Sakakura et al., 2005 Amin and Tucker, 2006 Sakakura et al., 2007
E16	binding of Ca^{2+} in hypertrophic region, MC degradation by TRAP-positive cells starts near to mental foramen, blood capillaries penetrate into MC	calcified MC matrix in the intermediate part, TRAP-positive cells and apoptotic bodies cumulate in the area of degradation (apoptotic bodies present also in perichondrium with low frequency)	Ishizeki et al., 1999 Ramaesh and Bard, 2003 Amano et al., 2010
E17	intermediate part of MC disappears	ossification is apparent in the lateral part of the cartilage medially to the mandible	Yang et al., 2012
E18	resorbed area is occupied by osteoblasts, TRAP positive cells and blood capillaries	disconnected anterior and posterior ends of MC, persisting hypertrophic chondrocytes in the posterior portion	Ishizeki et al., 1999
P0	degradation of MC culminates, ossification of middle ear ossicles	chondroblastic cells apparent in the rostral area and posterior region with malleus	Amin and Tucker, 2006 Amano et al., 2010 Anthwal et al., 2013
P3	ossification of middle ear ossicles continues	malleus separates from MC	Anthwal et al., 2013

is only encased at the rostral most portion (Anthwal et al., 2017). From E15 onwards the different parts of the cartilage undergo divergent fates.

DIVERSE FATES WITHIN ONE CARTILAGE

In mammals, Meckel's cartilage can be separated into 3 parts according to the fate of each region: anterior/distal, intermediate/central, and posterior/proximal (**Figure 1C**). The intermediate part is largely surrounded by the forming dentary bone and is further subdivided into anterior and posterior zones (Bhaskar et al., 1953; Ito et al., 2002; Shimo et al., 2004; **Figure 1C**).

From E15, the cartilage cells in the intermediate region continue to mature, having acquired a perichondrium, enlarged lacunae, and a thin matrix in the central part of MC. From this point, chondrocytes adjacent to the ossification centres of the mandibular bone show focal hypertrophy, while the rostral process remains less differentiated (**Figure 2E**). One day later, the process of hypertrophy culminates (**Figure 2F**), and is accompanied by type X collagen expression in the intermediate region, while expression of ALP (alkaline phosphatase) is detected in the perichondrium, matrix vesicles and hypertrophic chondrocytes of MC (Ishizeki et al., 1999; Shimo et al., 2004). From E16, calcification of the perichondrium and hypertrophic chondrocytes initiates, with subsequent invasion of the calcified matrix by capillaries (Ishizeki et al., 1999). This blood flow provides bone marrow-derived precursors of multinuclear chondroclasts/osteoclasts that can resorb the calcified cartilaginous matrix (Savostin-Asling and Asling, 1975). New osseous islands are evident at E17 (**Figure 2G**), which express both type I and type II collagens, and Opn (osteopontin), suggesting a potential contribution of MC to the bone of the mandible (Ishizeki et al., 1999).

Degradation of the cartilage matrix starts around the incisors between E15 and 16 in mice (**Figures 2F,G**), moving posteriorly toward the molar region and beyond but leaving the most rostral cartilage in place (**Figures 2I,J, 3A,B**). By E19, the more posterior parts of MC are completely disconnected from the most anterior/distal region (**Figures 2H, 3C**). This rostral part of MC then either undergoes endochondral ossification to form the mandibular symphysis, or remains cartilaginous in a species dependent manner (Bhaskar et al., 1953). In humans, the rostral region remains cartilaginous,

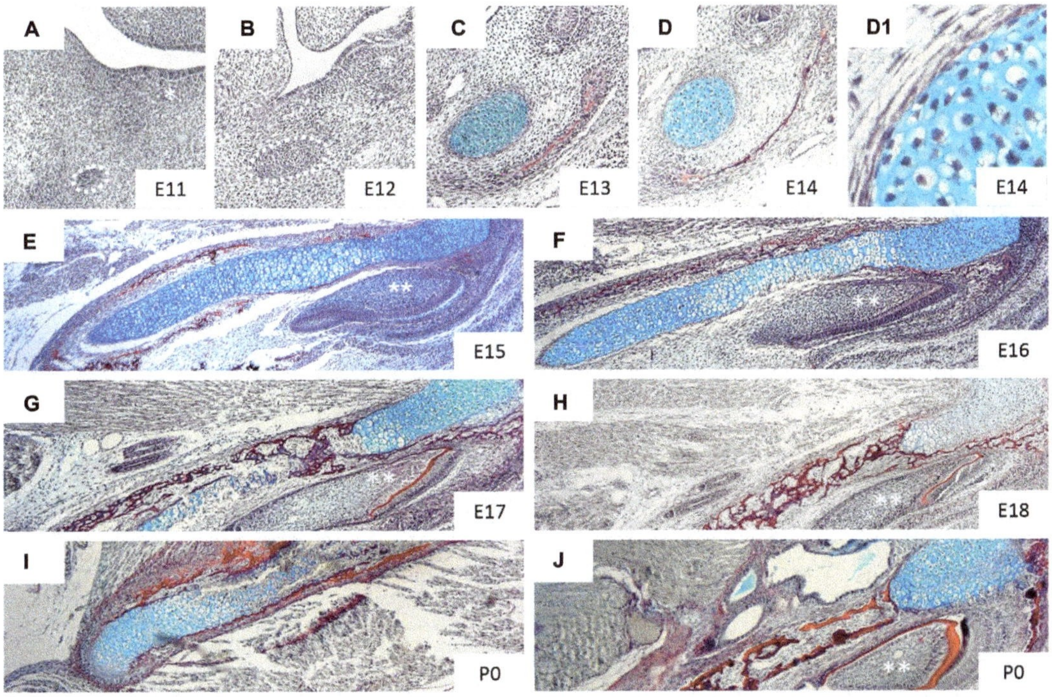

FIGURE 2 | Histological appearance of Meckel's cartilage during development. Histological sections of mandible stained with trichrome: sirius red (bone), alcian blue (cartilage), haematoxylin (nuclei). Figures show: frontal section of mandible at E11 **(A)**, 12 **(B)**, 13 **(C)**, 14 **(D,D$_1$)** and transversal section of mandible at E15 **(E)**, 16 **(F)**, 17 **(G)**, 18 **(H)**, P0 **(I,J)**. * (molar region), ** (incisor). Taken from slides available in Svandova lab.

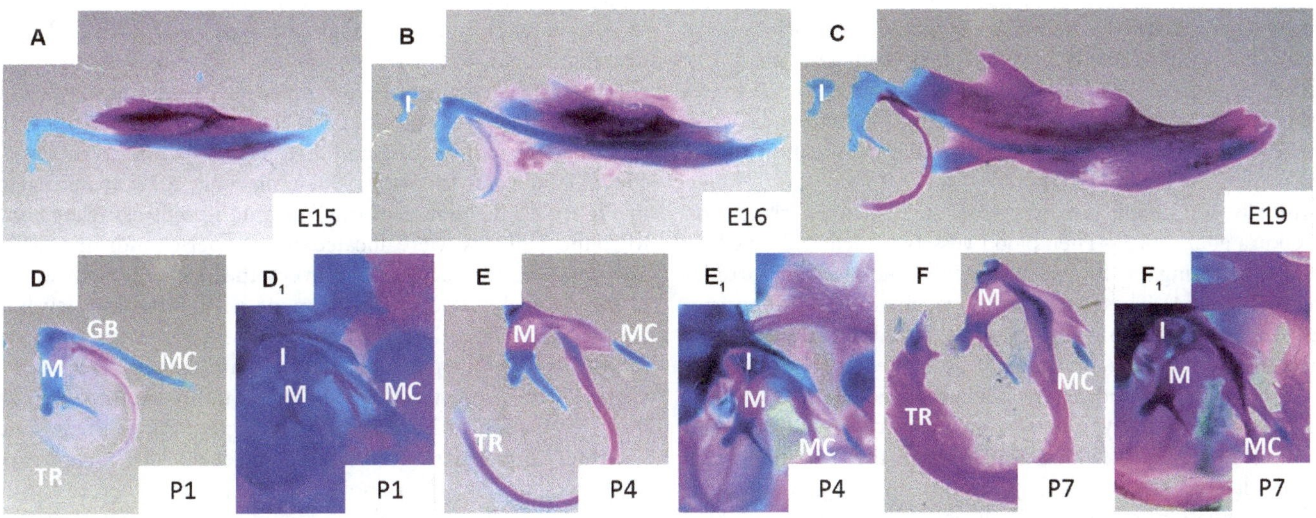

FIGURE 3 | Disappearance of Meckel's cartilage during development. Murine skeletal elements stained with alizarin red (bone) and alcian blue (cartilage) at stages: E15 **(A)**, 16 **(B)**, 19 **(C)**, P1 **(D,D$_1$)**, P4 **(E,E$_1$)**, P7 **(F,F$_1$)**. In figures **(D,E,F)** MC has been dissected away from the surrounding tissues, in figures **(D$_1$,E$_1$,F$_1$)** MC remains *in situ* surrounded by the cranial skeletal elements of the ear and jaw. Gonial bone (GB), incus (I), malleus (M), Meckel's cartilage (MC), tympanic ring (TR). Taken from skeletal preps available in Svandova lab.

forming nodules on the dorsal surface of the symphysis (Rodriguez-Vazquez et al., 1997).

From the perinatal stage, the most posterior part of MC undergoes endochondral ossification (**Figures 3D$_1$–F$_1$**) to form the middle ear ossicles – malleus (**Figures 3D–F**) and incus (Bhaskar et al., 1953; Frommer and Margolies, 1971; Amin and Tucker, 2006). In mice, the cartilage connection between the mandible and middle ear is still apparent at birth (**Figure 3D**), but is disconnected by a second site of resportion next to the malleus, resulting in seperation of the ear from the jaw by P4

(**Figure 3E**; Anthwal et al., 2013). At P7, other than the rostral region and ear ossicles, MC is almost entirely degraded, except for a small nodule next to the dentary (**Figures 3F, F$_1$**). The part of MC adjacent to the ossicles, outside of the dentary, is thought to transdifferentiate to become the anterior ligament of the malleus and the sphenomandibular ligament (Anthwal et al., 2013). In this case, it is proposed that the cartilage matrix is removed and the chondrocytes change to a ligamentous fate. This transformation may involve epidermal growth factor (EGF) signalling, as in the absence of EGF *in vitro* no transformation of MC occured (Ishizeki et al., 2001). From posterior to anterior MC therefore has diverse fates: middle ear bones, ligament, subsumed by the dentary, cartilage.

THE REMOVAL OF THE INTERMEDIATE DOMAIN OF MECKEL'S CARTILAGE

The fate of the intermediate part of MC is unclear. The cells of MC are thought either to contribute to the ossification of the mandible bone, or to undergo cell death (Bhaskar et al., 1953; Richman and Diewert, 1988; Harada and Ishizeki, 1998; Rodriguez-Vazquez et al., 1997; Ishizeki et al., 1999). In either scenario, the matrix of MC is first removed. Meckel's cartilage extracellular matrix is characteristic of hyaline/hypertrophic cartilage, including the presence of components such as type II and X collagens, aggrecan, versican, decorin, and biglycan (Silbermann and von der Mark, 1990; Shimo et al., 2004; Ababneh and Al-Khateeb, 2009; Tsuzurahara et al., 2011), which provide the mechanical characteristics of cartilage (Shibata et al., 2013). During degeneration of Meckel's cartilage, metalloproteinases (MMP) Mmp2, Mmp9, Mmp13, and Mmp14 have been detected, with crosstalk among them regulating the degradation of the matrix (Sakakura et al., 2007).

Initially Rank/Opg are expressed at the site of resorption (Sakakura et al., 2005). Then blood vessels, as detected by CD31 expression, bring precursors cells to breakdown the cartilage matrix (**Figure 4**). These include the precursors of TRAP positive clast cells, as well as macrophages that are observed in the MC perichondrium at E16 and might play a role via stimulation of IL-1β secreted by chondrocytes (Tsuzurahara et al., 2011).

The ossification hypothesis is supported by the apparent calcification of MC, which starts from the perichondrium on the lateral side, with hypertrophy of the chondrocytes and upregulation of type X collagen (Shimo et al., 2004). Transdifferentiation of chondroblasts into osteoblasts/-cytes has previously been identified during endochondral ossification in other skeletal elements (Yang et al., 2014). Importantly, in cell culture experiments, MC chondrocytes have been shown to be able to transdifferentiate into type I collagen, Alp, Ocn (Osteocalcin) or Osx (Osterix) expressing osteogenic cells (Ishizeki et al., 1996, 1999, 2009; Harada and Ishizeki, 1998; Eames et al., 2004; Ishizeki, 2012). However, the evidence for ossification of the main body of MC through transdifferentiation *in vivo* during normal development is currently limited (Ishizeki et al., 1999). Furthermore, there is no evidence of an ossified MC

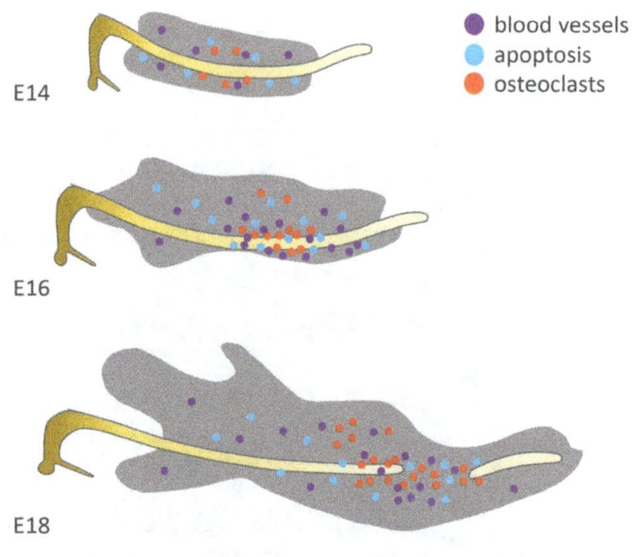

FIGURE 4 | Distribution of factors suspected to be involved in Meckel's cartilage degradation. Original schematic showing localisation of osteoclasts/osteoclastic precursors (red = TRAP+), endothelial cells (purple = CD31+) and apoptotic cells (blue = TUNEL+) in the mouse at E14, 16 and 18. Based on the published literature (see Harada and Ishizeki, 1998; Sakakura et al., 2005; Yang et al., 2012).

in species, such as the opossum, where the cartilage is not fully encased by the dentary bone (Urban et al., 2017).

Alternatively MC cells may undergo cell death following degradation of the cartilage matrix. Apoptosis is the most common mechanism of programmed cell death, however, only a few scattered apoptotic cells have been reported in the intermediate part at E16 and E18 (Trichilis and Wroblewski, 1997; Harada and Ishizeki, 1998; Yang et al., 2012) (summarised in **Figure 4**). Moreover, of those apoptotic cells associated with MC, the majority were located in the perichondrium, where apoptosis may be acting to prevent the lateral growth of MC (Amano et al., 2010). In agreement with these low levels of apoptosis, the heat shock protein (HSP) 25 is strongly expressed in MC in hypertrophic, proliferative and resting cells and is suggested to protect cells from apoptotic death. Interestingly, down-regulation of Hsp25 results in hypoplasia of the anterior and intermediate parts of MC (Shimada et al., 2003). If apoptosis is not responsible for removal of cells, then other cell death processes might be involved, including autophagy, which is supported by the presence of major autophagic markers Beclin1 and LC3 in the central part of MC (Yang et al., 2012). Beclin1 and LC3, were immunolocalised mostly in prehypertrophic and hypertrophic regions of MC. However, in addition to their engagement in cell death (Bohensky et al., 2014), autophagy has been identified also as a survival mechanism in MC (Song et al., 2017; Luo et al., 2019). Notably, caspase-2 and -8 were found to be activated in the Beclin1 positive regions suggesting a role of these two regulators in autophagy (Bilikova et al., 2019) and indicating that these pro-apoptotic caspases may be acting in a non-canonical manner in MC.

In addition to the intermediate zone, MC also breaks down next to the malleus, separating the ear and the jaw. Like the initial breakdown in the rostal MC, this proximal breakdown point is dependent on chondroclast activity (Anthwal et al., 2017). Interestingly, in the absence of removal of this part of MC by clast cells, in the *cFos* mouse mutant, MC starts to ossify, similar to the situation observed in the mammalian fossil record (Anthwal et al., 2017). Here, ossification appears to be a default state if the cartilage matrix can not be degraded. The loss of Meckel's cartilage at this point has been recently suggested to be linked to the development of the neighbouring gonial bone, with cartilage cells potentially contributing to the periosteum of this bone (Shibata et al., 2019). No apoptotic cell death has been detected in this region in mice, similar to the situation in the intermediate section, however, there is evidence for apoptosis acting in the disconnection of the middle ear and MC in marsupial opossums (Urban et al., 2017). The exact mechanism for breakdown may therefore be species specific.

HOW DO MECKEL'S CARTILAGE CHONDROCYTES COMPARE WITH THOSE OF OTHER CARTILAGES?

There are conflicting opinions as to the characterisation of MC chondroblasts/-cytes when compared to chondrocytes in other cartilages. MC chondroblasts/-cytes are compared most often to those in the growth plate (GP) of the endochondral bone, in particular the limbs. However, mesenchymal precursors of GP and MC chondroblasts are often of different origin, with the cells of MC being mostly derived from the cranial neural crest (CNC), while limb GP cells are derived from mesoderm (Chai et al., 2000). Despite this, several markers, such as Ihh (Indian hedgehog) (Koyama et al., 1996; Nakamura et al., 1997; Shimo et al., 2004), Vegf (Vascular endothelial growth factor) (Carlevaro et al., 2000; Shimo et al., 2004; Zelzer et al., 2004), Sox9, Bmps (Bone morphogenetic proteins) etc. (Mori-Akiyama et al., 2003; Wang et al., 2013; Michigami, 2014) play an important role in differentiation of both MC and GP chondrocytes. Furthermore, metalloproteinases such as Mmp9, 13, and 14, which are known to play important roles in degradation of the extracellular matrix, are found in both endochondral ossification and MC (Vu et al., 1998; Malemud, 2006; Sakakura et al., 2007).

Moreover, MC was found to be affected by a deficiency in trangenic mice of factors known to play a role in GP growth and maturation, including *Fgf3* (Fibroblast growth factor) and Ctgf (Connective tissue growth factor), where proliferation or hypertrophy of MC and GP chondroblasts was disrupted (Shimo et al., 2004).

Molecular signalling proteins do not, however, always have the same distribution and or function in MC and GP cells. For example, Hsp25 (Heat shock protein) is expressed in the GP cartilage in hypertrophic chondrocytes but not in resting and proliferating chondrocytes, however, in MC it was detected from early stage of development in proliferating chondroblasts (Shimada et al., 2003). Specific patterns were observed also for

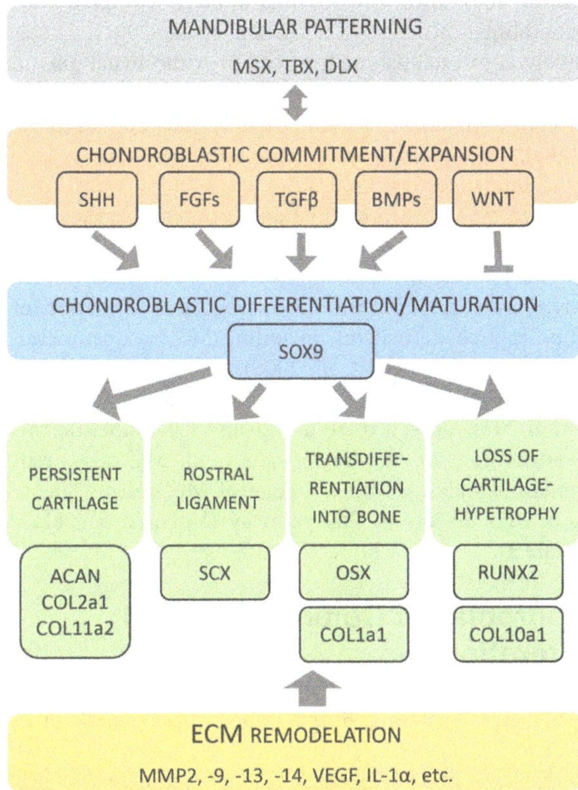

FIGURE 5 | Molecular factors involved in development of Meckel's cartilage. Original schematic shows key factors identified during formation and disappearance of MC. Factors are clustered according to different developmental events.

Rankl (Receptor activator of nuclear factor kappa-B ligand), which is expressed exclusively in hypertrophic chondrocytes of GP but is constitutively present in immature and mature MC chondrocytes (Sakakura et al., 2005).

THE MOLECULAR BIOLOGY OF MECKEL'S CARTILAGE

The signalling networks within MC are not yet completely understood. Nevertheless, several molecular networks acting in MC patterning, chondroblastic commitment, expansion, differentiation and survival have been identified (Jeong et al., 2004; Liu et al., 2005; Reid et al., 2011; Bonilla-Claudio et al., 2012; Zhang et al., 2013; Billmyre and Klingensmith, 2015) and are summarised here (**Figure 5**).

Patterning of the Mandibular Arch

Patterning of the mandibular arch is regulated by several homeobox containing transcription factors including members of the Msx (Msh homeobox), Dlx (Drosophila distal-less), and Tbx (T-box) families. Msx2 is expressed in CNC progenitors, including those that give rise to MC (Davideau et al., 1999). Msx2 was shown to inhibit the chondrogenic differentiation of progenitor cells until CNCCs migration is completed within the mandibular processes (Takahashi et al., 2001). Dlx genes are involved in establishment of the proximo-distal axis in the mandible and maxilla (Depew et al., 2005), coordinated by the Endothelin signalling pathway (Sato et al., 2008; Ruest and Clouthier, 2009). Tbx1 is expressed in the early pharyngeal arch and influences Fgf8 and Bmp4 expression, with its absence resulting in truncated mandible development (Aggarwal et al., 2010). Signalling molecules also play a role in MC patterning. Shh (Sonic hedgehog), although expressed in epithelial domains (Billmyre and Klingensmith, 2015), regulates formation of the mandibular arch derivatives, including MC, as documented in *Shh*-null mice (Melnick et al., 2005). In these mice, increased mesenchymal cell death in the first pharyngeal arch after CNCCs migration was observed resulting in a hypoplastic/missing MC. Formation of the lower jaw and MC also requires endothelin signalling, with a "range of MC defects" in mouse mutants with defects in this pathway (Yanagisawa et al., 1998) (see **Table 3**).

Chondroblastic Commitment and Proliferation

Chondroblastic commitment and proliferation are regulated by secreted factors, including Bmps (Bone morphogenetic proteins) (Denker et al., 1999; Zehentner et al., 1999; Yoon et al., 2005) that appears to be strictly time/site regulated during MC development (Wang et al., 2013). Bmp2 and Bmp7 (but not Bmp4) were expressed in MC at E11.5-12.5 (Wang et al., 2013). Noggin, a negative regulator of Bmp signalling (Zimmerman et al., 1996; Groppe et al., 2002), was expressed in MC during the entire gestation period. In the absence of Noggin, enhanced proliferation was detected with an increased size of MC and a persisting intermediate part (Wang et al., 2013). Proliferation of MC precursors is also regulated by Fgfs (Mina and Havens, 2007; Terao et al., 2011). Fgfr3 is implemented in both, the elongation of MC and the expression of *Sox9* during chondrogenic differentiation (Duplan et al., 2016).

Tgfβ (Transforming growth factor beta) stimulates proliferation of CNC–derived chondrocytes and production of chondroblastic extracellular matrix (Chai et al., 1994; Ito et al., 2002; Oka et al., 2007). Tgfβ signalling acts through intracellular SMADs in a dose–dependent manner, with Smad2 and 3 acting positively, and Smad7 acting negatively (Ito et al., 2002). Tgfβ induces the expression of Ctgf, which is expressed along the entire length of MC (and the perichondrium) from E12.5 to E15.5, playing a role in cell condensation followed by chondroblast differentiation and maturation at later stages (Shimo et al., 2004; Parada et al., 2013). The effect of Ctgf was suggested to result from cell-cell interactions and expression of condensation-associated genes (Ivkovic et al., 2003; Arnott et al., 2011).

Differentiation and Maturation of Chondroblasts

Differentiation and maturation of chondroblasts is regulated by three master transcription factors Sox9 (SRY-box 9), Runx2 (Runt-related transcription factor 2), and Osx (Osterix) (Zou et al., 2006; Kaback et al., 2008; Nishimura et al., 2012; Zhang et al., 2013). Sox9 (highlighted in **Figure 5**) is a crucial factor for determination of the chondrogenic lineage in CNCCs population (Mori-Akiyama et al., 2003), promoting the early stage of chondrocyte differentiation (Mori-Akiyama et al., 2003; Yamashita et al., 2009). When *Sox9* was conditionally deleted in CNC-derived cells, differentiation into chondrocytes was blocked, leading to an absence of MC, and instead cells produced osteoblast markers, suggesting their re-specification into an osteoblast lineage (Mori-Akiyama et al., 2003).

Runx2 is a positive regulator (highlighted in **Figure 5**) of hypertrophic differentiation (Mikasa et al., 2011; Ding et al., 2012), which acts downstream of IHH (Amano et al., 2014). In MC, Runx2 was found in the zone of hypertrophy (Zhang et al., 2013). *Runx2*-null mice lack all bone and hypertrophic cartilage (Shibata et al., 2004). MC initiates as normal, but has two ectopic cartilaginous processes, which may results from a change in the normal muscle attachment patterns caused by loss of the bone (Shibata et al., 2004). Hypertrophy is also regulated by BMPs (Valcourt et al., 2002; Kobayashi et al., 2005).

Osx plays essential role in osteoblastic differentiation. In MC, Osx was abundantly expressed by hypertrophic chondrocytes and was suggested to be important for conversion of MC chondrocytes into osteoblasts/-cytes (Zhang et al., 2013). In *Osx* null mice, mandibular bone was absent (except for initial condensations), however, the development of Meckel's cartilage was undistinguishable from the wild type (Nakashima et al., 2002). Since Osx regulates expression of osteoblastic genes, the enhanced expression of osterix in mature chondrocytes might explain the upregulation of type I collagen in these tissues (Nakashima et al., 2002; Zhang et al., 2013). Molecular expression patterns during MC development are detailed in **Table 2.**

CONSEQUENCES OF DEFECTS IN MECKEL'S CARTILAGE DEVELOPMENT

The more posterior parts of the mammalian MC contribute to the formation of two of the three mammalian ear bones (malleus and incus) and associated ligaments (anterior ligament of malleus, sphenomandibular ligament) of the ear and jaw (Ogutcen-Toller, 1995). Defects in the development of these elements lead to hearing loss, as observed in Treacher Collins syndrome and Branchio-oto-renal syndrome (Pron et al., 1993). The very rostral part of MC, remains cartilaginous and contributes to the symphysis. Although a transient structure, the main body of MC supports the development of the mandibular skeleton that forms around it (Ramaesh and Bard, 2003). A number of different mouse mutants that cause reduction or absence of MC consequently develop a shortening of the mandibular bone. For example in $Sox9^{fl/fl}$;Wnt1-Cre mouse mutants, the mandibular bones form but are severerly shortened, suggesting that the primary role for the main strut of MC's is to regulate the length of the mandible (Mori-Akiyama et al., 2003). Other mouse mutants with a reduced MC and shortened mandible include the *Fuz−/−* mice (Zhang et al., 2011) and

TABLE 2 | Factors engaged in MC development.

Gene	When	Where	References
Dlx5	8.25 – 10.5 (R)	mandible: proximo-distal axis	Depew et al., 1999, 2005
Msx2	E8, 10 (R)	condensed mesenchyme	Takahashi et al., 2001
Msx1	E13.5, 14.5 (R)	perichondrium	Oka et al., 2007
Ednra	E8.5-10.5	mandible CNC	Ruest and Clouthier, 2009
Tbx1	E16.5 (P)	transient expression in NC	Funato et al., 2015
Bmp2, -7	E11.5 – 12.5 (R)	intermediate part of MC	Wang et al., 2013
Noggin	E11.5 – 18.5 (R, A)	intermediate part of MC	Wang et al., 2013
Tgfβ1	E12 (R)	condensed mesenchyme	Shimo et al., 2004
	E18 (R)	post-HC zone of anterior and intermediate part of MC	
Fuz	E12.5 (A)	condensed mesenchyme,	Zhang et al., 2011
	E14.5 (A)	chondroblasts and perichondrium of MC	
Cd47	E13, 15 (P)	intermediate part of MC	Shimada et al., 2011
Ctgf	E12 (R)	anterior, central, and posterior part of MC	Shimo et al., 2004
	E18 (R)	HC in anterior region and most-rostral half of central region of MC	Parada et al., 2013
	E12.5 (R)	perichondrium	
Sox9	E8 (R)	migratory CNC cells	Takahashi et al., 2001
	E11.5 (R)	condensation of mesenchymal cells	Li et al., 2017
	E12, E15 (R)	chondroblasts of MC	Shimo et al., 2004
	P0 (P)	weak expression in uncalcified cartilage	Zhang et al., 2013
Runx2	E11.5 (R)	condensation of mesenchymal cells	Li et al., 2017
	P0 (P)	weak expression in uncalcified cartilage	Zhang et al., 2013
Osx	P0 (P)	hypertrophic chondrocytes in the centre of the uncalcified MC	Zhang et al., 2013
Ihh	E18	intermediate part of MC	Shimo et al., 2004
Fibronectin	E12 (R)	condensed mesenchyme	Shimo et al., 2004
	E15 (R)	peripheral chondrocytes and perichondrium	
	E18 (R)	mature chondrocytes	
Type I col	E19 (P)	matrix of MC	Tsuzurahara et al., 2011
Type II col	E15, E18 (R)	condensed mesenchyme (decreased in HC)	Shimo et al., 2004
	18 (P)	matrix of MC	Tsuzurahara et al., 2011
Type X col	E18	hypertrophic zones	Shimo et al., 2004
Il-1α	E14, E17 (R)	chondrocytes	Tsuzurahara et al., 2011
Mmp2	E16 (P)	faint detection in HC	Sakakura et al., 2007
Mmp9	E15/E16 (P)	hypertrophic chondrocytes/ chondroclasts	Sakakura et al., 2007
	E18 (R)	post-hypertrophic chondrocytes	Shimo et al., 2004
Mmp13	E16 (P)	chondroclasts in resorption area on the lateral side of the cartilage	Sakakura et al., 2007
Mmp14	E15/E16 (P)	peripheral cells/pre-hypertrophic chondrocytes	Sakakura et al., 2007
Vegf	E18 (R)	post-HC zone of anterior and intermediate part of MC	Shimo et al., 2004
	E9.5-15.5 (R, P)	MC chondroblasts	Wiszniak et al., 2015
Hsp25	E12 – 15 (P)	resting and proliferating chondrocytes in anterior and intermediate part of MC	Shimada et al., 2003
Hsp70	E14 – 15 (P)	throughout of MC	Shimada et al., 2003
Caspase-2, -8	E15 (P)	chondrocytes in intermediate part	Bilikova et al., 2019
Caspase-3	E15 (P)	few cells of perichondrium	Bilikova et al., 2019
Beclin-1	E15 (P)	chondrocytes in intermediate part	Bilikova et al., 2019
	E16-17(P)	pre-hypertrophic/hypertrophic chondrocytes	Yang et al., 2012
LC3b	E16-17(P)	pre-hypertrophic/hypertrophic chondrocytes	Yang et al., 2012

R (examination at RNA level), P (examination at protein level), A (activity). Patterning of the mandibular arch – grey, proliferation of precursors and chondroblastic commitment – pink, chondroblastic differentiation and hypertrophy – purple, factors of extracellular matrix – green, factors involved in matrix degradation – yellow, factors of cells death – light blue.

mice with a first pharyngeal arch deletion of *Shh* (Billmyre and Klingensmith, 2015). Activating mutations in *Fgfr3* lead to abnormal differentiation of chondrocytes and a reduced zone of hypertrophy resulting in shortened skeletal elements, including a truncated MC (Duplan et al., 2016). In this case the activating mutation mimics patients with achondroplasia.

TABLE 3 | Phenotypic abnormalities of Meckel's cartilage connected with abnormal gene expression.

Genotype	Impact	References
Alk2$^{fl/fl}$; *Wnt1-Cre* (Bc-MP type I receptor)	missing distal extremity of MC	Dudas et al., 2004
c-Fos$^{-/-}$	persistence of MC beyond juvenile stage	Anthwal et al., 2017
Ctgf$^{-/-}$	MC deformations	Ivkovic et al., 2003
Dlx2$^{-/-}$	abnormal posterior MC, malformed middle ear ossicles	Depew et al., 2005
Dlx5$^{-/-}$	MC is shortened and its path back toward the middle ear is disrupted	Depew et al., 2005
Dlx5/6$^{-/-}$	complete loss of MC	Robledo et al., 2002
Dmm/Dmm (semi-dominant Col2a1 mutation)	growth retardation of MC, osteoarthritis	Ricks et al., 2002
Ednra constituative activation	transformed upper jaw, with duplication MC	Sato et al., 2008
Ednta $^{fl/fl}$; *Wnt1-Cre*	duplicated maxilla, loss MC	Ruest and Clouthier, 2009
Egfr$^{-/-}$	MC deformations	Miettinen et al., 1999
Endothelin –/–	defect lower jaw, vestigial MC	Ozeki et al., 2004
Fgfr3$^{Y367C/+}$	shortened hypertrophic zone of MC, achondroplasia	Duplan et al., 2016
Fgf8$^{neo/-}$	absent or hypoplastic MC	Abu-Issa et al., 2002
Fuz$^{-/-}$	hyperplastic malformed MC	Zhang et al., 2011
Hand 2 $^{fl/fl}$; *Wnt1-Cre*	duplicated mandible and MC	Funato et al., 2016
Isl1$^{fl/fl}$; *Shh-Cre*	smaller MC (E13.5), lack of cartilage at the distal tip resulting in fused growth of two ossifying elements	Li et al., 2017
Nog$^{-/-}$	increased size of MC (due to proliferation) endochondral-like ossification of intermediate part	Wang et al., 2013
Runx2$^{-/-}$	two ectopic cartilaginous processes in MC (indirect effect of missing bone)	Shibata et al., 2004
Setdb1$^{fl/fl}$; *Wnt1-Cre*	enlarged MC resulting from increased proliferation and hyperplasia, increased hypertrophy	Yahiro et al., 2017
Shh^{fx}/–; *Nkx2.5-Cre*	no apparent MC from E14.5	Billmyre and Klingensmith, 2015
Shh$^{-/-}$	hypoplastic mesenchymal condensation, no apparent MC	Melnick et al., 2005
Snai1$^{flox/-}$ *Snai2*$^{-/-}$; *Wnt1-Cre*	overall shorter length, missing rostral MC and midline fusion	Murray et al., 2007
Sox9$^{fl/fl}$; *Wnt1-Cre*	total absence of MC	Mori-Akiyama et al., 2003
Sox9 $^{+/-}$	MC interrupted and bent toward the body appearing as shortened, campomelic dysplasia	Bi et al., 2001
Tgfbr2$^{fl/fl}$; *Wnt1-Cre* (E14.5)	curvy shape of MC, un-uniform thickness, disrupted perichondrium	Oka et al., 2007
Tgfβ2 $^{-/-}$	abnormal shape of MC	Sanford et al., 1997
Vegfa$^{fl/fl}$;*Wnt1-Cre* (E17.5)	mandibular hypoplasia, decreased size of MC resulting from abnormal vascularisation	Wiszniak et al., 2015

A list of transgenic mouse mutants with defects in MC is shown in **Table 3**.

Several human disorders that are directly or indirectly connected with abnormal MC formation have also been described. Similar to the mouse, defects in MC result in the formation of a smaller, malformed dentary bone, resulting in agnathia, micrognathia, or mandibular hypoplasia. Such mandibular defects are fairly common birth defects, with small jaws leading to additional problems associated with airway obstruction and feeding difficulties (Manocha et al., 2019). Mandible defects can be observed in various syndromes including hemifacial microsomia, campomelic dysplasia, Pierre Robin syndrome/sequence, Treacher Collins syndrome, DiGeorge syndrome, and Goldenhar syndrome (Mckenzie, 1958; Bi et al., 2001; Ricks et al., 2002; Wiszniak et al., 2015; Duplan et al., 2016), or be nonsyndromic (see Manocha et al., 2019 for a systematic review). In the case of campomelic dysplasia, causative mutations have been identified in *SOX9*, the master cartilage gene, again highlighing that the microagnathia observed in these patients is due to a defect in MC rather than the later developing dentary (Mansour et al., 2002). In such cases, if the primary jaw defects are due to abnormal development of MC, then the problems could be traced back very early in embryonic development (5–7 weeks), prior to development of the dentary. In the case of Pierre-Robin syndrome/sequence, the formation of a small jaw is thought to have knockon consequences for elevation of the palate, leading to a cleft (Ricks et al., 2002). Similarly, the cleft palate observed in transferrin receptor knockout mice, has been attributed to a failure of Meckel's cartilage to extend (Lei et al., 2016). As MC contributes both to the jaw and to the middle ear during development, it is perhaps unsuprising that many syndromes, such as Treacher Collins syndrome, combine defects in the jaw and in the ear. In rare cases Meckel's cartilage fails to breakdown, with the consequence that the jaw and ear remain in physical contact and MC can ossify (Keith, 1910; Herring, 1993). The manifestations of these syndromes are devastating in physical but also psychological aspects and highlight the clinical importance of investigating MC. In addition, understanding the developmental origins of the MC derived anterior malleolar ligament helps to explain why temporomandibular joint (TMJ) trauma can be associated with dislocation of the ear bones (Cheynet et al., 2003). The anatomy only makes sense in the light of an understanding of the development and evolution of the structures.

WHAT IS KNOWN AND WHAT REMAINS?

Meckel's cartilage is an crucial yet transient structure required for the proper formation of the mammalian mandible. The differences in its persistence across jawed animals, and the different fates of the anterior, intermediate, and posterior parts in mammals mean that in understanding the MC we can learn lessons about evolution, skeletal biology, and tissue fate decisions (e.g., Bhaskar et al., 1953; Goret-Nicaise et al., 1984; Ramaesh and Bard, 2003; Amano et al., 2010). Although two hundred years have passed since the discovery of MC, there are still many open questions regarding developmental, cellular and molecular events related to its formation and final fate.

In the mouse model, the timing of the appearance of MC and its propagation and degradation (see **Table 1**) has been described, the temporospatial pattern of a number genes connected to MC development has been established (see **Table 2**), and genetic manipulations have pointed to several factors essential for its formation (Sox9, Dlx5/6, Fgf8 or Shh), growth (Alk2, Snail1/2, VegfA) and patterning (Fuz, Noggin, Setdb1) (see **Table 3**). Both Fgf and Bmp signalling, for example, have been highlighted as involved in non-syndromic lower jaw defects (Manocha et al., 2019).

However, there remain many questions connected with MC. We do not fully understand what induces the formation of MC itself? It is likely that paracrine signals from surrounding tissues play a role, and in line with this a role for Fgf10 has been suggested in early control of MC development (Terao et al., 2011). MC still forms in Fgf10 null mutants (Teshima et al., 2016), however, genetic polymorphisms in Fgf10 have been linked to mandibular prognathism in humans (Cruz et al., 2017). More information is therefore required to understand the identity and location of the signals and how the initiation point for MC is determined. In murine lineage labelling studies the Wnt1cre labelled neural crest cells have been shown to only contribute to a subset of chondrocytes, with the ratios of neural crest and non-neural crest cells changing over time as the cartilage grows (Chai et al., 2000). Whether neural crest cells only form a subset of MC could be tested using a variety of other Cre lines to trace the lineage of cells.

We also do not fully understand the processes by which MC is removed, in particular the intermediate part. In murine culture, isolated MC persists when dissected out at E14 but degrades when dissected out at E17, suggesting that a cue comes from the surrounding tissue in between these time points (Tsuzurahara et al., 2011). This cue might be molecular or mechanical. For example, it has been suggested that tissue interactions between teeth and MC may induce the breakdown of MC (Sakakura et al., 2005), or that muscle interaction might provide the stimulus for break down (Wyganowska and Przystanska, 2011). A signal might arrive from the surrounding tissue, but equally the signal could be generated from MC itself, stimulating the arrival of macrophages and clast cells to initiate matrix removal (Sakakura et al., 2005, 2007; Tsuzurahara et al., 2011).

Although ample evidence, from *in vitro* studies and mouse mutants, points to MC chondrocytes being able to mineralise (Ishizeki et al., 1999; Anthwal et al., 2017), whether MC ossifies and contributes to the dentary *in vivo* is debated. Novel lineage tracing experiments following the fate of MC cells will be able to address this in future. Such lineage studies would also help to aid our understanding of the transformation of MC into a ligament, shedding light on which cells are involved (perichondrium, chondrocytes) and the nature of the triggers that confine this transformation to just a small subset of the cartilage.

In addition, a number of questions linked to the evolution of MC remain. For example, while the advantage in auditory function gained from removal of the proximal portion of MC during mammal evolution is apparent, the reason for the resorption of the intermediate portion within the mandible is not as obvious. The tapering seen in the ossified MCs of mammal ancestor fossils such as Liaoconodon (Meng et al., 2011) suggests that the anterior MC either degenerated, similar to modern mammals, or may have been present as a cartilage (which did not fossilize). The former might indicate that the resorption of the intermediate MC is more ancient than the breakdown allowing for the separation of the middle ear from the mandible. Interestingly, a late cretaceous mammal has recently been discovered with a tapered ossified MC alongside a decoupled middle ear (Mao et al., 2020). Therefore, perhaps the separation of the middle ear from the MC evolved before the destruction of the intermediate MC. These and other topics remain open and are challenging for further investigations of this transient organ important for evolutionary, clinical and basic research.

CONCLUDING REMARKS

Here we have charted the evolution, development and clinical aspects of Meckel's cartilage, highlighting the important role this cartilage plays in the lower jaw. We have detailed the current knowledge but also emphasised the areas where we only have a very basic understanding of the processes involved. With the advent of new lineage tracing techniques, and the availability of conditional mouse mutants, many of these questions are just waiting to be answered.

AUTHOR CONTRIBUTIONS

ES wrote the first draft of the manuscript and constructed the figures and tables. NA wrote sections of the manuscript. AT and EM planned the review and finalised the manuscript. All authors contributed to the article and approved the submitted version.

REFERENCES

Ababneh, K. T., and Al-Khateeb, T. H. (2009). Immunolocalization of proteoglycans in Meckel's cartilage of the rat. *Open Dent. J.* 3, 177–183. doi: 10.2174/1874210600903010177

Abu-Issa, R., Smyth, G., Smoak, I., Yamamura, K., and Meyers, E. N. (2002). Fgf8 is required for pharyngeal arch and cardiovascular development in the mouse. *Development* 129, 4613–4625.

Aggarwal, V. S., Carpenter, C., Freyer, L., Liao, J., Petti, M., and Morrow, B. E. (2010). Mesodermal Tbx1 is required for patterning the proximal mandible in mice. *Dev. Biol.* 344, 669–681. doi: 10.1016/j.ydbio.2010.05.496

Amano, K., Densmore, M., Nishimura, R., and Lanske, B. (2014). Indian hedgehog signaling regulates transcription and expression of collagen type X via Runx2/Smads interactions. *J. Biol. Chem.* 289, 24898–24910. doi: 10.1074/jbc.m114.570507

Amano, O., Doi, T., Yamada, T., Sasaki, A., Sakiyama, K., Kanegae, H., et al. (2010). Meckel's cartilage: discovery, embryology and evolution. *J. Oral Biosci.* 52, 125–135. doi: 10.2330/joralbiosci.52.125

Amin, S., Matalova, E., Simpson, C., Yoshida, H., and Tucker, A. S. (2007). Incudomalleal joint formation: the roles of apoptosis, migration and downregulation. *BMC Dev. Biol.* 7:134–146. doi: 10.1186/1471-213X-7-134

Amin, S., and Tucker, A. S. (2006). Joint formation in the middle ear: lessons from the mouse and guinea pig. *Dev. Dyn.* 235, 1326–1333. doi: 10.1002/dvdy.20666

Anthwal, N., Chai, Y., and Tucker, A. S. (2008). The role of transforming growth factor B signalling in the patterning of the proximal processes of the murine dentary. *Dev. Dyn.* 237, 1604–1613. doi: 10.1002/dvdy.21567

Anthwal, N., Fenelon, J. C., Johnston, S. D., Renfree, M. B., and Tucker, A. S. (2020). Transient role of the middle ear as a jaw support in mammals. *eLife* 9:e57860.

Anthwal, N., Joshi, L., and Tucker, A. S. (2013). Evolution of the mammalian middle ear and jaw: adaptations and novel structures. *J. Anat.* 222, 147–160. doi: 10.1111/j.1469-7580.2012.01526.x

Anthwal, N., Urban, D. J., Luo, Z.-X., Sears, K. E., and Tucker, A. S. (2017). Meckel's cartilage breakdown offers clues to mammalian middle ear evolution. *Nat. Ecol. Evol.* 1:93. doi: 10.1038/s41559-017-0093

Arnott, J. A., Lambi, A. G., Mundy, C., Hendesi, H., Pixley, R. A., Owen, T. A., et al. (2011). The role of connective tissue growth factor (CTGF/CCN2) in skeletogenesis. *Crit. Rev. Eukary. Gene Exp.* 21, 43–69. doi: 10.1615/critreveukargeneexpr.v21.i1.40

Bhaskar, S. N., Weinmann, J. P., and Schour, I. (1953). Role of Meckel's cartilage in the development and growth of the rat mandible. *J. Dent. Res.* 32, 398–410. doi: 10.1177/00220345530320031401

Bi, W., Huang, W., Whitworth, D. J., Deng, J. M., Zhang, Z., Behringer, R. R., et al. (2001). Haploinsufficiency of Sox9 results in defective cartilage primordia and premature skeletal mineralization. *Proc. Natl. Acad. Sci.* 98, 6698–6703. doi: 10.1073/pnas.111092198

Bildsoe, H., Loebel, D. A. F., Jones, V. J., Hor, A. C. C., Braithwaite, A. W., Chen, Y.-T., et al. (2013). The mesenchymal architecture of the cranial mesoderm of mouse embryos is disrupted by the loss of Twist1 function. *Dev. Biol.* 374, 295–307. doi: 10.1016/j.ydbio.2012.12.004

Bilikova, P., Svandova, E., Vesela, B., Doubek, J., Poliard, A., and Matalova, E. (2019). Coupling activation of pro-apoptotic caspases with autophagy in the Meckel's cartilage. *Physiol. Res.* 68, 135–140. doi: 10.33549/physiolres.933947

Billmyre, K. K., and Klingensmith, J. (2015). Sonic hedgehog from pharyngeal arch 1 epithelium is necessary for early mandibular arch cell survival and later cartilage condensation differentiation. *Dev. Dyn.* 244, 564–576. doi: 10.1002/dvdy.24256

Bohensky, J., Shapiro, I. M., Leshinsky, S., Terkhorn, S. P., Adams, C. S., and Srinivas, V. (2014). HIF-1 regulation of chondrocyte apoptosis: induction of the autophagic pathway. *Autophagy* 3, 207–214. doi: 10.4161/auto.3708

Bonilla-Claudio, M., Wang, J., Bai, Y., Klysik, E., Selever, J., and Martin, J. F. (2012). Bmp signaling regulates a dose-dependent transcriptional program to control facial skeletal development. *Development* 139, 709–719. doi: 10.1242/dev.073197

Brazeau, M. D., and Friedman, M. (2015). The origin and early phylogenetic history of jawed vertebrates. *Nature* 520, 490–497. doi: 10.1038/nature14438

Carlevaro, M. F., Cermelli, S., Cancedda, R., and Descalzi Cancedda, F. (2000). Vascular endothelial growth factor (VEGF) in cartilage neovascularization and chondrocyte differentiation: auto-paracrine role during endochondral bone formation. *J. Cell Sci.* 113, 59–69.

Chai, Y., Jiang, X., Ito, Y., Han, J., Rowitch, D. H., Soriano, P., et al. (2000). Fate of the mammalian cranial neural crest during tooth and mandibular morphogenesis. *Development* 127, 1671–1679.

Chai, Y., Mah, A., Crohin, C., Groff, S., Bringas, P., Le, T., et al. (1994). Specific transforming growth Factor-β subtypes regulate embryonic mouse Meckel's cartilage and tooth development. *Dev. Biol.* 162, 85–103. doi: 10.1006/dbio.1994.1069

Chai, Y., Shuler, C., Devaney, E., Grosschedl, R., and Slavkin, H. C. (1998). A mouse mandibular culture model permits the study of neural crest cell migration and tooth development. *Int. J. Dev. Biol.* 42, 87–94.

Chen, G., Isham, M., Yang, J., Kishigami, S., Fukada, T., Scott, G., et al. (2017). Specific and spatial labelling of P0-cre versus Wnt-1Cre in cranial neural crest in early mouse embryos. *Genesis* 55:10.1002/dvg.23034. doi: 10.1002/dvg.23034

Cheynet, F., Guyot, L., Richard, O., Layoun, W., and Gola, R. (2003). Discomallear and malleomandibular ligaments: anatomical study and clinical applications. *Surg. Radiol. Anat.* 25, 152–157. doi: 10.1007/s00276-003-0097-y

Cruz, C. V., Mattos, C. T., Maia, J. C., Granjeiro, J. M., Reis, M. F., Mucha, J. N., et al. (2017). Genetics polymorphisms underlying the skeletal Class III phenotype. *Am. J. Orthod. Dentofacial Orthop.* 151, 700–707. doi: 10.1016/j.ajodo.2016.09.013

Davideau, J.-L., Demri, P., Hotton, D., Gu, T.-T., MacDougall, M., Sharpe, P., et al. (1999). Comparative study of MSX-2, DLX-5, and DLX-7 gene expression during early human tooth development. *Pediatr. Res.* 46, 650–650. doi: 10.1203/00006450-199912000-00015

DeLaurier, A. (2019). Evolution and development of the fish jaw skeleton. *Wiley Interdiscip. Rev. Dev. Biol.* 8:e337. doi: 10.1002/wdev.337

Denker, A. E., Haas, A. R., Nicoll, S. B., and Tuan, R. S. (1999). Chondrogenic differentiation of murine C3H10T1/2 multipotential mesenchymal cells: I. Stimulation by bone morphogenetic protein-2 in high-density micromass cultures. *Differentiation* 64, 67–76. doi: 10.1046/j.1432-0436.1999.6420067.x

Depew, M. J., Liu, J. K., Long, J. E., Presley, R., Meneses, J. J., Pedersen, R. A., et al. (1999). Dlx5 regulates regional development of the branchial arches and sensory capsules. *Development* 126, 3831–3846.

Depew, M. J., Simpson, C. A., Morasso, M., and Rubenstein, J. L. R. (2005). Reassessing the Dlx code: the genetic regulation of branchial arch skeletal pattern and development. *J. Anat.* 207, 501–561. doi: 10.1111/j.1469-7580.2005.00487.x

Depew, M. J., Tucker, A. S., and Sharpe, P. T. (2002). "Craniofacial development," in *Mouse Development: Patterning, Morphogenesis and Organogenesis*, eds J. Rossant and P. P. L. Tam (London: Academic Press), 421–498.

Ding, M., Lu, Y., Abbassi, S., Li, F., Li, X., Song, Y., et al. (2012). Targeting Runx2 expression in hypertrophic chondrocytes impairs endochondral ossification during early skeletal development. *J. Cell. Physiol.* 227, 3446–3456. doi: 10.1002/jcp.24045

Donoghue, P. C. J., Sansom, I. J., and Downs, J. P. (2006). Early evolution of vertebrate skeletal tissues and cellular interactions, and the Canalization of skeletal development. *J. Exp. Zool. Part B Mol. Dev. Evol.* 306B, 278–296.

Dudas, M., Sridurongrit, S., Nagy, A., Okazaki, K., and Kaartinen, V. (2004). Craniofacial defects in mice lacking BMP type I receptor Alk2 in neural crest cells. *Mechan. Dev.* 121, 173–182. doi: 10.1016/j.mod.2003.12.003

Duplan, M., Komla-Ebri, D., Heuzé, Y., Estibals, V., Gaudas, E., Kaci, N., et al. (2016). Meckel's and condylar cartilages anomalies in achondroplasia result in defective development and growth of the mandible. *Hum. Mol. Genet.* 25, 2997–3010.

Eames, B. F., Sharpe, P. T., and Helms, J. A. (2004). Hierarchy revealed in the specification of three skeletal fates by Sox9 and Runx2. *Dev. Biol.* 274, 188–200. doi: 10.1016/j.ydbio.2004.07.006

Frommer, J., and Margolies, M. R. (1971). Contribution of Meckel's cartilage to ossification of the mandible in mice. *J. Dent. Res.* 50, 1260–1267. doi: 10.1177/00220345710500052801

Funato, N., Kokubo, H., Nakamura, M., Yanagisawa, H., and Saga, Y. (2016). Specification of jaw identity by the Hand2 transcription factor. *Sci. Rep.* 22:28405.

Funato, N., Nakamura, M., Richardson, J. A., Srivastava, D., and Yanagisawa, H. (2015). Loss of Tbx1 induces bone phenotypes similar to cleidocranial dysplasia. *Hum. Mol. Genet.* 24, 424–435. doi: 10.1093/hmg/ddu458

Goret-Nicaise, M., Lengele, B., and Dhem, A. (1984). The function of Meckel's and secondary cartilages in the histomorphogenesis of the cat mandibular symphysis. *Arch. Anat. Microsc. Morphol. Exp.* 73, 291–303.

Groppe, J., Greenwald, J., Wiater, E., Rodriguez-Leon, J., Economides, A. N., Kwiatkowski, W., et al. (2002). Structural basis of BMP signalling inhibition by the cystine knot protein Noggin. *Nature* 420, 636–642. doi: 10.1038/nature01245

Harada, Y., and Ishizeki, K. (1998). Evidence for transformation of chondrocytes and site-specific resorption during the degradation of Meckel's cartilage. *Anat. Embryol.* 197, 439–450. doi: 10.1007/s004290050155

Herring, S. W. (1993). Formation of the vertebrate face: epigenetic and functional influences. *Am. Zool.* 33, 472–483. doi: 10.1093/icb/33.4.472

Hunt, P., Gulisano, M., Cook, M., Sham, M.-H., Faiella, A., Wilkinson, D., et al. (1991). A distinct Hox code for the branchial region of the vertebrate head. *Nature* 353, 861–864. doi: 10.1038/353861a0

Ishizeki, K. (2012). Imaging analysis of osteogenic transformation of Meckel's chondrocytes from green fluorescent protein-transgenic mice during intrasplenic transplantation. *Acta Histochem.* 114, 608–619. doi: 10.1016/j.acthis.2011.11.008

Ishizeki, K., Kagiya, T., Fujiwara, N., Otsu, K., and Harada, H. (2009). Expression of osteogenic proteins during the intrasplenic transplantation of Meckel's chondrocytes: a histochemical and immunohistochemical study. *Arch. Histol. Cytol.* 72, 1–12. doi: 10.1679/aohc.72.1

Ishizeki, K., Nawa, T., Takigawa, M., and Suzuki, F. (1996). Mouse Meckel's cartilage chondrocytes evoke bone-like matrix and further transform into osteocyte-like cells in culture. *Anat. Rec.* 245, 25–35. doi: 10.1002/(sici)1097-0185(199605)245:1<25::aid-ar5>3.0.co;2-e

Ishizeki, K., Saito, H., Shinagawa, T., Fujiwara, N., and Nawa, T. (1999). Histochemical and immunohistochemical analysis of the mechanism of calcification of Meckel's cartilage during mandible development in rodents. *J. Anat.* 194, 265–277. doi: 10.1046/j.1469-7580.1999.19420265.x

Ishizeki, K., Takahashi, N., and Nawa, T. (2001). Formation of the sphenomandibular ligament by Meckel's cartilage in the mouse: possible involvement of epidermal growth factor as revealed by studies in vivo and in vitro. *Cell Tiss. Res.* 304, 67–80. doi: 10.1007/s004410100354

Ito, Y., Bringas, P., Mogharei, A., Zhao, J., Deng, C., and Chai, Y. (2002). Receptor-regulated and inhibitory Smads are critical in regulating transforming growth factor β-mediated Meckel's cartilage development. *Dev. Dyn.* 224, 69–78. doi: 10.1002/dvdy.10088

Ivkovic, S., Yoon, B. S., Popoff, S. N., Safadi, F. F., Libuda, D. E., Stephenson, R. C., et al. (2003). Connective tissue growth factor coordinates chondrogenesis and angiogenesis during skeletal development. *Development* 130, 2779–2791. doi: 10.1242/dev.00505

Jeong, J., Mao, J., Tenzen, T., Kottmann, A. H., and McMahon,. A. P. (2004). Hedgehog signaling in the neural crest cells regulates the patterning and growth of facial primordia. *Genes Dev.* 18, 937–951 doi: 10.1101/gad.1190304

Kaback, L. A., Soung, D. Y., Naik, A., Smith, N., Schwarz, E. M., O'Keefe, R. J., et al. (2008). Osterix/Sp7 regulates mesenchymal stem cell mediated endochondral ossification. *J. Cell. Physiol.* 214, 173–182. doi: 10.1002/jcp.21176

Kaucka, M., Zikmund, T., Tesarova, M., Gyllborg, D., Hellander, A., Jaros, J., et al. (2017). Orientated clinal cell dynamics enables accurate growth and shaping of vertebrate cartilage. *eLife* 6:e25902.

Keith, A. (1910). Abnormal ossification of Meckel's cartilage. *J. Anat. Physiol.* 44, 151–152.

Kobayashi, T., Lyons, K. M., McMahon, A. P., and Kronenberg, H. M. (2005). BMP signaling stimulates cellular differentiation at multiple steps during cartilage development. *Proc. Natl. Acad. Sci. U.S.A.* 102, 18023–18027. doi: 10.1073/pnas.0503617102

Koyama, E., Leatherman, J. L., Noji, S., and Pacifici, M. (1996). Early chick limb cartilaginous elements possess polarizing activity and express hedgehog-related morphogenetic factors. *Dev. Dyn.* 207, 344–354.

Le Douarin, N. M., and Dupin, E. (1993). Cell lineage analysis in neural crest ontogeny. *J. Neurobiol.* 24, 146–161. doi: 10.1002/neu.480240203

Lei, R., Zhang, K., Liu, K., Shao, X., Ding, Z., Wang, F., et al. (2016). Transferrin receptor facilitates TGFb and BMP signaling activation to control craniofacial morphogenesis. *Cell Death Dis.* 7:e2282. doi: 10.1038/cddis.2016.170

Li, F., Fu, G., Liu, Y., Miao, X., Li, Y., Yang, X., et al. (2017). ISLET1-dependent β-Catenin/Hedgehog signaling is required for outgrowth of the lower jaw. *Mol. Cell. Biol.* 37:e00590-16. doi: 10.1128/MCB.00590-16

Liu, W., Selever, J., Murali, D., Sun, X., Brugger, S. M., Ma, L., et al. (2005). Threshold-specific requirements for Bmp4 in mandibular development. *Dev. Biol.* 283, 282–293. doi: 10.1016/j.ydbio.2005.04.019

Luo, P., Gao, F., Niu, D., Sun, X., Song, Q., Guo, C., et al. (2019). The role of autophagy in chondrocyte metabolism and osteoarthritis: a comprehensive research review. *Biomed. Res. Int.* 2019:5171602. doi: 10.1155/2019/5171602

Luo, Z.-X. (2011). Developmental patterns in Mesozoic evolution of mammal ears. *Annu. Rev. Ecol. Evol. Syst.* 42, 355–380. doi: 10.1146/annurev-ecolsys-032511-142302

Luo, Z.-X., Gatesy, S. M., Jenkins, F. A., Amaral, W. W., and Shubin, N. H. (2015). Mandibular and dental characteristics of Late Triassic mammaliaform Haramiyavia and their ramifications for basal mammal evolution. *Proc. Natl Acad. Sci. U.S.A.* 112, E7101–E7109.

Maier, W., and Ruf, I. (2016). Evolution of the mammalian middle ear: a historical review. *J. Anat.* 228, 270–283. doi: 10.1111/joa.12379

Malemud, C. J. (2006). Matrix metalloproteinases: role in skeletal development and growth plate disorders. *Front. Biosci.* 11:1702–1715. doi: 10.2741/1916

Mallat, J. (2008). The evolution of the vertebrate Jaw: neoclassical ideas verses newer, development-based ideas. *Zool. Sci.* 25, 990–998. doi: 10.2108/zsj.25.990

Manocha, S., Farokhnia, N., Khosropanah, S., Bertol, J. W., Santiago Junior, J., and Fakhouri, W. D. (2019). Systematic review of hormonal and genetic factors involved in the non-syndromic disorders of the lower jaw. *Dev. Dyn.* 248, 162–172. doi: 10.1002/dvdy.8

Mansour, S., Offiah, A. C., McDowall, S., Sim, P., Tolmie, J., and Hall, C. (2002). The phenotype of survivors of campomelic dysplasia. *J. Med. Genet.* 39, 597–602. doi: 10.1136/jmg.39.8.597

Mao, F., Hu, Y., Li, C., Wang, Y., Chase, M. H., Smith, A. K., et al. (2020). Integrated hearing and chewing modules decoupled in a Cretaceous stem therian mammal. *Science* 367, 305–308. doi: 10.1126/science.aay9220

Marchant, C., Anderson, P., Schwarz, Q., and Wisziak, S. (2020). Vessel-derived angiocrine IGF1 promotes Meckel's cartilage proliferation to drive jaw growth during embryogenesis. *Development* 147:dev190488. doi: 10.1242/dev.190488

Mckenzie, J. (1958). The first arch syndrome. *Arch. Dis. Child* 33, 477–486.

Meckel, J. F. (1820). *Handbuch der menschlichen Anatomie. IV.* Berlin: Lehre und Geschichte des Foetud.

Melnick, M., Witcher, D., Bringas, P. Jr., Carlsson, P., and Jaskoll, T. (2005). Meckel's cartilage differentiation is dependent on hedgehog signaling. *Cells Tissues Organs* 179, 146–157. doi: 10.1159/000085950

Meng, J., Hu, Y., Wang, Y., and Li, C. (2003). The ossified Meckel's cartilage and internal groove in Mesozoic mammaliaforms: implications to origin of the definitive mammalian middle ear. *Zool. J. Linn. Soc.* 138, 431–448. doi: 10.1046/j.1096-3642.2003.00064.x

Meng, J., Wang, Y., and Li, C. (2011). Transitional mammalian middle ear from a new Cretaceous Jehol eutriconodont. *Nature* 472, 181–185. doi: 10.1038/nature09921

Michigami, T. (2014). Current understanding on the molecular basis of chondrogenesis. *Clin. Pediatr. Endocrinol.* 23, 1–8.

Miettinen, P. J., Chin, J. R., Shum, L., Slavkin, H. C., Shuler, C. F., Derynck, R., et al. (1999). Epidermal growth factor receptor function is necessary for normal craniofacial development and palate closure. *Nat. Genet.* 22, 69–73. doi: 10.1038/8773

Mikasa, M., Rokutanda, S., Komori, H., Ito, K., Tsang, Y. S., Date, Y., et al. (2011). Regulation of Tcf7 by Runx2 in chondrocyte maturation and proliferation. *J. Bone Miner. Metab.* 29, 291–299. doi: 10.1007/s00774-010-0222-z

Mina, M., and Havens, B. (2007). FGF signaling in mandibular skeletogenesis. *Orthodont. Craniofac. Res.* 10, 59–66. doi: 10.1111/j.1601-6343.2007.00385.x

Miyashita, T. (2016). Fishing for jaws in early vertebrate evolution: a new hypothesis of mandibular confinement. *Biol. Rev.* 91, 611–657. doi: 10.1111/brv.12187

Mori-Akiyama, Y., Akiyama, H., Rowitch, D. H., and de Crombrugghe, B. (2003). Sox9 is required for determination of the chondrogenic cell lineage in the cranial neural crest. *Proc. Natl. Acad. Sci. U.S.A.* 100, 9360–9365. doi: 10.1073/pnas.1631288100

Murray, S. A., Oram, K. F., and Gridley, T. (2007). Multiple functions of Snail family genes during palate development in mice. *Development* 134, 1789–1797. doi: 10.1242/dev.02837

Nakamura, T., Aikawa, T., Iwamoto-Enomoto, M., Iwamoto, M., Higuchi, Y., Maurizio, P., et al. (1997). Induction of osteogenic differentiation by hedgehog proteins. *Biochem. Biophys. Res. Commun.* 237, 465–469. doi: 10.1006/bbrc.1997.7156

Nakashima, K., Zhou, X., Kunkel, G., Zhang, Z., Deng, J. M., Behringer, R. R., et al. (2002). The novel zinc finger-containing transcription factor osterix is required for osteoblast differentiation and bone formation. *Cell* 108, 17–29. doi: 10.1016/s0092-8674(01)00622-5

Nishimura, R., Wakabayashi, M., Hata, K., Matsubara, T., Honma, S., Wakisaka, S., et al. (2012). Osterix regulates calcification and degradation of chondrogenic matrices through matrix metalloproteinase 13 (MMP13) expression in association with transcription factor Runx2 during endochondral ossification. *J. Biol. Chem.* 287, 33179–33190. doi: 10.1074/jbc.m111.337063

Ogutcen-Toller, M. (1995). The morphogenesis of the human discomalleolar and sphenomandibular ligaments. *J. Craniomaxillofac. Surg.* 23, 42–46. doi: 10.1016/s1010-5182(05)80254-9

Oka, K., Oka, S., Sasaki, T., Ito, Y., Bringas, P., Nonaka, K., et al. (2007). The role of TGF-β signaling in regulating chondrogenesis and osteogenesis during mandibular development. *Dev. Biol.* 303, 391–404. doi: 10.1016/j.ydbio.2006.11.025

Ozeki, H., Kurihara, Y., Tonami, K., Watatani, S., and Kurihara, H. (2004). Endothelin-1 regulates the dorsoventral branchial arch patterning in mice. *Mech. Dev.* 121, 387–395. doi: 10.1016/j.mod.2004.02.002

Parada, C., Li, J., Iwata, J., Suzuki, A., and Chai, Y. (2013). CTGF mediates smad-dependent transforming growth Factor β signalingto regulate mesenchymal cell proliferation during palate development. *Mol. Cell. Biol.* 33, 3482–3493. doi: 10.1128/mcb.00615-13

Pron, G., Galloway, C., Armstrong, D., and Posnick, J. (1993). Ear malformation and hearing loss in patients with treacher collins syndrome. *Cleft Palate Craniofac. J.* 30, 97–103. doi: 10.1597/1545-1569_1993_030_0097_emahli_2.3.co_2

Ramaesh, T., and Bard, J. B. L. (2003). The growth and morphogenesis of the early mouse mandible: a quantitative analysis. *J. Anat.* 203, 213–222. doi: 10.1046/j.1469-7580.2003.00210.x

Reid, B. S., Yang, H., Melvin, V. S., Taketo, M. M., and Williams, T. (2011). Ectodermal WNT/β-catenin signaling shapes the mouse face. *Dev. Biol.* 349, 261–269. doi: 10.1016/j.ydbio.2010.11.012

Richman, J. M., and Diewert, V. M. (1988). The fate of Meckel's cartilage chondrocytes in ocular culture. *Dev. Biol.* 129, 48–60. doi: 10.1016/0012-1606(88)90160-1

Ricks, J. E., Ryder, V. M., Bridgewater, L. C., Schaalje, B., and Seegmiller, R. E. (2002). Altered mandibular development precedes the time of palate closure in mice homozygous for disproportionate micromelia: an oral clefting model supporting the Pierre-Robin sequence. *Teratology* 65, 116–120. doi: 10.1002/tera.10022

Robledo, R. F., Rajan, L., Li, X., and Lufkin, T. (2002). The Dlx5 and Dlx6 homeobox genes are essential for craniofacial, axial, and appendicular skeletal development. *Genes Dev.* 16, 1089–1101. doi: 10.1101/gad.988402

Rodriguez-Vazquez, J. F., Merida-Velasco, J. R., Merida-Velasco, J. A., Sanchez-Montesinos, I., Espin-Ferra, J., and Jimenez-Collado, J. (1997). Development of Meckel's cartilage in the symphyseal region in man. *Anat. Rec.* 249, 249–254. doi: 10.1002/(sici)1097-0185(199710)249:2<249::aid-ar12>3.0.co;2-o

Ruest, L. B., and Clouthier, D. E. (2009). Elucidating timing and function of endothelin-A receptor signaling during craniofacial development using neural crest cell-specific gene deletion and receptor antagonism. *Dev. Biol.* 328, 94–108. doi: 10.1016/j.ydbio.2009.01.005

Sakakura, Y., Hosokawa, Y., Tsuruga, E., Irie, K., and Yajima, T. (2007). In situ localization of gelatinolytic activity during development and resorption of Meckel's cartilage in mice. *Eur. J. Oral Sci.* 115, 212–223. doi: 10.1111/j.1600-0722.2007.00447.x

Sakakura, Y., Tsuruga, E., Irie, K., Hosokawa, Y., Nakamura, H., and Yajima, T. (2005). Immunolocalization of receptor activator of nuclear factor-kappaB ligand (RANKL) and osteoprotegerin (OPG) in Meckel's cartilage compared with developing endochondral bones in mice. *J. Anat.* 207, 325–337. doi: 10.1111/j.1469-7580.2005.00466.x

Sanford, L. P., Ormsby, I., Sariola, H., Friedman, R., Boivin, G. P., Cardell, E. L., et al. (1997). TGFbeta2 knockout mice have multiple developmental defects that are non-overlapping with other TGFbeta knockout phenotypes. *Development* 124, 2659–2670.

Sato, T., Kurihara, Y., Asai, R., Kawamura, Y., Tonami, K., Uchijima, Y., et al. (2008). An endothelin-1 switch specifies maxillomandibular identity. *Proc. Natl. Acad. Sci. U.S.A.* 105, 18806–18811. doi: 10.1073/pnas.0807345105

Savostin-Asling, I., and Asling, C. W. (1975). Transmission and scanning electron microscope studies of calcified cartilage resorption. *Anat. Rec.* 183, 373–391. doi: 10.1002/ar.1091830303

Shibata, S., Sakamoto, Y., Baba, O., Qin, C., Murakami, G., and Cho, B. H. (2013). An immunohistochemical study of matrix proteins in the craniofacial cartilage in midterm human fetuses. *Eur. J. Histochem.* 57:e39. doi: 10.4081/ejh.2013.e39

Shibata, S., Suda, N., Yoda, S., Fukuoka, H., Ohyama, K., Yamashita, Y., et al. (2004). Runx2-deficient mice lack mandibular condylar cartilage and have deformed Meckel's cartilage. *Anat. Embryol.* 208, 273–280.

Shibata, S., Takahashi, M., and Fujikawa, K. (2019). Histochemical and ultrastructural study of the developing gonial bone with evidence to intial ossification of the malleus and reduction of Meckel's cartilage in mice. *Anat. Rec.* 302, 1916–1933. doi: 10.1002/ar.24201

Shimada, K., Nakajima, A., Ikeda, K., Ishibashi, K., Shimizu, N., and Ito, K. (2011). CD47 regulates the TGF-β signaling pathway in osteoblasts and is distributed in Meckel's cartilage. *J. Oral Sci.* 53, 169–175. doi: 10.2334/josnusd.53.169

Shimada, M., Yamamoto, M., Wakayama, T., Iseki, S., and Amano, O. (2003). Different expression of 25-kDa heat-shock protein (Hsp25) in Meckel's cartilage compared with other cartilages in the mouse. *Anat. Embryol.* 206, 163–173. doi: 10.1007/s00429-002-0297-y

Shimo, T., Kanyama, M., Wu, C., Sugito, H., Billings, P. C., Abrams, W. R., et al. (2004). Expression and roles of connective tissue growth factor in Meckel's cartilage development. *Dev. Dyn.* 231, 136–147. doi: 10.1002/dvdy.20109

Silbermann, M., and von der Mark, K. (1990). An immunohistochemical study of the distribution of matrical proteins in the mandibular condyle of neonatal mice. I. Collagens. *J. Anat.* 170, 11–22.

Song, B., Song, H., Wang, W., Wang, H., Peng, H., Cui, J., et al. (2017). Beclin 1 overexpression inhibits chondrocyte apoptosis and downregulates extracellular matrix metabolism in osteoarthritis. *Mol. Med. Rep.* 16, 3958–3964. doi: 10.3892/mmr.2017.7064

Takahashi, K., Nuckolls, G. H., Takahashi, I., Nonaka, K., Nagata, M., Ikura, T., et al. (2001). Msx2 is a repressor of chondrogenic differentiation in migratory cranial neural crest cells. *Dev. Dyn.* 222, 252–262.

Terao, F., Takahashi, I., Mitani, H., Haruyama, N., Sasano, Y., Suzuki, O., et al. (2011). Fibroblast growth factor 10 regulates Meckel's cartilage formation during early mandibular morphogenesis in rats. *Dev. Biol.* 350, 337–347.

Teshima, T. H. N., Lourenco, S. V., and Tucker, A. S. (2016). Multiple cranial organ defects after conditionally knocking out Fgf10 in the neural crest. *Front. Physiol.* 7:488. doi: 10.3389/fphys.2016.00488

Trichilis, A., and Wroblewski, J. (1997). Expression of p53 and hsp70 in relation to apoptosis during Meckel's cartilage development in the mouse. *Anat. Embryol.* 196, 107–113.

Tsuzurahara, F., Soeta, S., Kawawa, T., Baba, K., and Nakamura, M. (2011). The role of macrophages in the disappearance of Meckel's cartilage during mandibular development in mice. *ActaHistochemica* 113, 194–200.

Tucker, A. S., Watson, R. P., Lettice, L. A., Yamada, G., and Hill, R. E. (2004). Bapx1 regulates patterning in the middle ear: altered regulatory role in the transition from the proxial jaw during vertebrate evolution. *Development* 131, 1235–1245.

Urban, D. J., Anthwal, N., Luo, Z.-X., Maier, J. A., Sadier, A., Tucker, A. S., et al. (2017). A new developmental mechanism for the separation of the mammalian middle ear ossicles from the jaw. *Proc. R. Soc. B Biol. Sci.* 284:20162416. doi: 10.1098/rspb.2016.2416

Valcourt, U., Gouttenoire, J., Moustakas, A., Herbage, D., and Mallein-Gerin, F. (2002). Functions of transforming growth factor-β family Type I receptors and smad proteins in the hypertrophic maturation and osteoblastic differentiation of chondrocytes. *J. Biol. Chem.* 277, 33545–33558.

Vu, T. H., Shipley, J. M., Bergers, G., Berger, J. E., Helms, J. A., Hanahan, D., et al. (1998). MMP-9/Gelatinase B is a key regulator of growth plate angiogenesis and apoptosis of hypertrophic chondrocytes. *Cell* 93, 411–422.

Wang, Y., Zheng, Y., Chen, D., and Chen, Y. P. (2013). Enhanced BMP signaling prevents degeneration and leads to endochondral ossification of Meckel's cartilage in mice. *Dev. Biol.* 381, 301–311.

Wilson, J., and Tucker, A. S. (2004). Fgf and Bmp signals repress the expression of Bapx1 in the mandibular mesenchyme and control the position of the developing jaw joint. *Dev. Biol.* 266, 138–150.

Wiszniak, S., Mackenzie, F. E., Anderson, P., Kabbara, S., Ruhrberg, C., and Schwarz, Q. (2015). Neural crest cell-derived VEGF promotes embryonic jaw extension. *Proc. Natl. Acad. Sci. U.S.A.* 112, 6086–6091.

Woronowicz, K. C., and Schneider, R. A. (2019). Molecular and cellular mechanisms underlying the evolution of form and function in the amniote jaw. *Evodevo* 10:17. doi: 10.1186/s13227-019-0131-8

Wyganowska-Świątkowska, M., and Przystanska, A. (2011). The Meckel's cartilage in human embryonic and early fetal periods. *Anat. Sci. Int.* 86, 98–107.

Yahiro, K., Higashihori, N., and Moriyama, K. (2017). Histone methyltransferase Setdb1 is indispensable for Meckel's cartilage development. *Biochem. Biophys. Res. Commun.* 482, 883–888.

Yamashita, S., Andoh, M., Ueno-Kudoh, H., Sato, T., Miyaki, S., and Asahara, H. (2009). Sox9 directly promotes Bapx1 gene expression to repress Runx2 in chondrocytes. *Exp. Cell Res.* 315, 2231–2240.

Yanagisawa, H., Kapur, R. P., Richardson, J. A., Williams, S. C., Clouthier, D. E., Wit, D., et al. (1998). Dual genetic pathways of endothelin-mediated intercellular signaling revealed by targeted disruption of endothelin converting enzyme-1 gene. *Development* 125, 825–836.

Yang, L., Tsang, K. Y., Tang, H. C., Chan, D., and Cheah, K. S. (2014). Hypertrophic chondrocytes can become osteoblasts and osteocytes in endochondral bone formation. *Proc. Natl. Acad. Sci. U.S.A.* 111, 12097–12102.

Yang, R.-T., Zhang, C., Liu, Y., Zhou, H.-H., and Li, Z.-B. (2012). Autophagy prior to chondrocyte cell death during the degeneration of Meckel's cartilage. *Anat. Rec.* 295, 734–741.

Yoon, B. S., Ovchinnikov, D. A., Yoshii, I., Mishina, Y., Behringer, R. R., and Lyons, K. M. (2005). Bmpr1a and Bmpr1b have overlapping functions and are essential for chondrogenesis in vivo. *Proc. Natl. Acad. Sci.* 102, 5062–5067.

Zehentner, B. K., Dony, C., and Burtscher, H. (1999). The transcription factor Sox9 is involved in BMP-2 signaling. *J. Bone Mineral Res.* 14, 1734–1741.

Zelzer, E., Mamluk, R., Ferrara, N., Johnson, R. S., Schipani, E., and Olsen, B. R. (2004). VEGFA is necessary for chondrocyte survival during bone development. *Development* 131, 2161–2171.

Zhang, H., Zhao, X., Zhang, Z., Chen, W., and Zhang, X. (2013). An Immunohistochemistry Study of Sox9, Runx2, and osterix expression in the mandibular cartilages of newborn mouse. *BioMed. Res. Int.* 2013, 1–11.

Zhang, Z., Wlodarczyk, B. J., Niederreither, K., Venugopalan, S., Florez, S., Finnell, R. H., et al. (2011). Fuz regulates craniofacial development through tissue specific responses to signaling factors. *PLoS One* 6:e24608. doi: 10.1371/journal.pone.0024608

Zimmerman, L. B., De Jesús-Escobar, J. M., and Harland, R. M. (1996). The spemann organizer signal noggin binds and inactivates bone morphogenetic protein 4. *Cell* 86, 599–606.

Zou, L., Zou, X., Li, H., Mygind, T., Zeng, Y., Lü, N., et al. (2006). Molecular mechanism of osteochondroprogenitor fate determination during bone formation. *Adv. Exp. Med. Biol.* 585, 431–441.

2

Non-syndromic Cleft Palate: An Overview on Human Genetic and Environmental Risk Factors

Marcella Martinelli[1], Annalisa Palmieri[1], Francesco Carinci[2] and Luca Scapoli[1]*

[1] Department of Experimental, Diagnostic and Specialty Medicine, Alma Mater Studiorum – University of Bologna, Bologna, Italy,

[2] Department of Morphology, Surgery and Experimental Medicine, University of Ferrara, Ferrara, Italy

***Correspondence:**
Marcella Martinelli
marcella.martinelli@unibo.it

The epithelial and mesenchymal cells involved in early embryonic facial development are guided by complex regulatory mechanisms. Any factor perturbing the growth, approach and fusion of the frontonasal and maxillary processes could result in orofacial clefts that represent the most common craniofacial malformations in humans. The rarest and, probably for this reason, the least studied form of cleft involves only the secondary palate, which is posterior to the incisive foramen. The etiology of cleft palate only is multifactorial and involves both genetic and environmental risk factors. The intention of this review is to give the reader an overview of the efforts made by researchers to shed light on the underlying causes of this birth defect. Most of the scientific papers suggesting potential environmental and genetic causes of non-syndromic cleft palate are summarized in this review, including genome-wide association and gene–environment interaction studies.

Keywords: non-syndromic cleft palate, NSCPO, risk factors, etiology, *GRHL3*, *FOXE1*, *PAX7*

INTRODUCTION

Orofacial clefts are the most common orofacial malformations in humans and include cleft lip (CL), cleft lip with or without cleft palate (CL/P), and cleft palate only (CPO). CPO (MIM 119540) is a birth defect that occurs when only the secondary palate is involved and can affect the hard palate and/or the soft palate, sometimes limited to one cleft uvula. It represents one third of all oral clefts and affects about 1 to 25 per 10.000 newborns worldwide (Mossey et al., 2009). The incidence of CPO is highly influenced by ethnicity and race, with the highest rates observed in non-Hispanic Whites and the lowest in Africans (Mossey and Modell, 2012). Besides, females are more prone to the defect than males (1:1.075) (Mossey and Catilla, 2003).

Cleft palate only is a multifactorial disorder influenced by both genetic and environmental factors that act during palatogenesis (Meng et al., 2009; Dixon et al., 2011). Moreover, the local changes in growth factors, extracellular matrix (ECM), and cell adhesion molecules may also play a part in CPO onset. A variety of signaling pathways are involved in palate development and several mutations on developmental genes that have been found to contribute to CPO will be discussed.

Furthermore, the environmental contribution to CPO by tobacco, alcohol and multivitamin supplementation has been highlighted by epidemiological studies hereinafter detailed.

Classification

Cleft lip with or without cleft palate and CPO are considered as different congenital malformations, having distinct embryologic origins and recurrence risks. Hence, CPO refers to any cleft of the palate which is posterior to the palatine foramen, and which does not involve the alveolar process or lip. A number of different classifications have been proposed since Veau's version in 1931 (Veau, 1931; Danescu et al., 2015). In **Figure 1**, a collection of different types of CPO, including the recently introduced submucous microform (Danescu et al., 2015).

Another kind of classification divides CPO into two major groups: (i) isolated CPO or non-syndromic CPO (NSCPO), when clefting is an isolated defect unassociated with any other additional anomalies, representing 54.8% of the total CPO cases; (ii) syndromic CPO, when clefting is associated with other anomalies in a recognizable (27.2%), or unrecognizable syndrome (18%) (Calzolari et al., 2004).

Although the presence of an evident pattern of anomalies makes the diagnosis easier, some features may not be fully expressed or could represent subclinical phenotypes more difficult to diagnose. Most frequently, the defects associated with CPO affect the heart (31.1%), the encephalon (hydrocephaly 11.2%), the urinary tract (9.7%), or digits (polydactyly 9.2%) (Mossey and Catilla, 2003). The number of syndromes involving cleft palate, among orofacial clefts, is subject to progressive implementation but already in 1978 it was quoted as 77 (Cohen, 1978).

The most common syndromes in which cleft palate deformity represents one of the features are: Apert Syndrome, Crouzon Syndrome, DiGeorge Syndrome, Loeys-Dietz Syndrome, Treacher Collins Syndrome, X-linked cleft palate Syndrome, Ankyloglossia, Bamforth-Lazarus Syndrome[1]. An exhaustive overview of the syndromes that count cleft palate among their features, as well as the responsible genes, can be found in a paper by Burg et al. (2016).

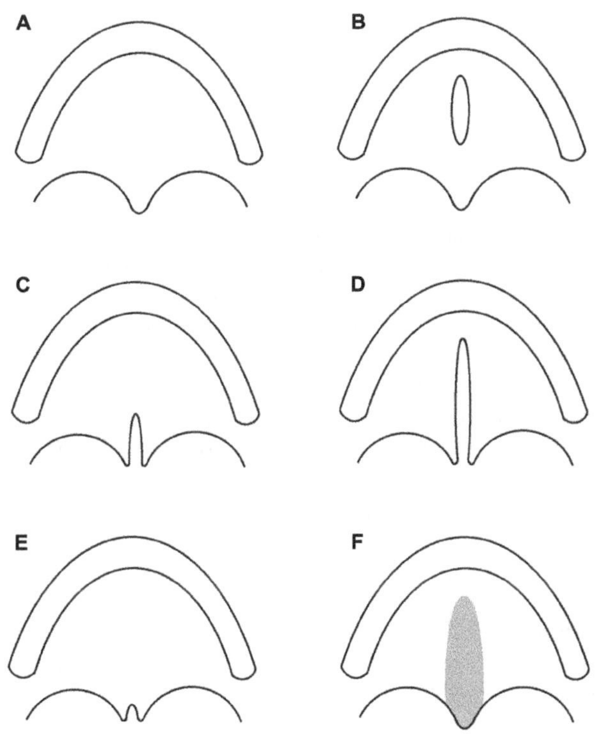

FIGURE 1 | Subtypes of cleft palate only. Each sketch illustrates the alveolar process and the palatal rim. **(A)** Normal palate. **(B)** Cleft of the hard palate. **(C)** Cleft of the soft palate. **(D)** Cleft of the hard and soft palate. **(E)** Cleft uvula. **(F)** Submucous cleft palate.

Palatogenesis

The human palate separates the nasal and oral cavities and consists of a bony *hard palate* (the anterior two thirds) and a fibromuscular *soft palate* (the posterior one third). The incisive foramen divides the *hard palate* into primary and secondary portions. The secondary portion separates the nasal passage from the pharynx and is marked by a median palatine raphe. The *soft palate*, or velum, is a mobile muscular fold forming a curtain posterior to the hard palate, ending with a conical mass called the *uvula*. The soft palate separates the nasopharynx from the oropharynx.

Palatal development takes place between the fifth and twelfth embryonic weeks, with the most critical period occurring during the sixth to ninth weeks (Merritt, 2005), when the lateral palatine processes fuse, after the fusion of the secondary palate to the primary palate with a junction marked by the incisive foramen. The palate body is composed by mesenchymal cells, mainly derived from migrating neural crest cells, layered by epithelial cells that surround the mesenchyme (Ito et al., 2003). The correct growth, migration, transition, differentiation, and apoptosis of these cells form the basis of a regular development of the palate. Palatal shelves, initially grown in a vertical position, have to rotate from the sides to the top of the tongue in order to acquire a horizontal position. Then, shelves approach and fuse with each other in an antero-posterior direction in the transient midline epithelial seam (Ferguson, 1988; Meng et al., 2009).

Conceivably, there are several molecular, mechanical and morphological steps, including the key step of epithelial to mesenchymal transition, involved in the orchestra of palate development which could go wrong (Diewert and Lozanoff, 2002). Clefting of the secondary palate may then arise in any one of these critical steps, and may be caused by failure in growth, elevation, adhesion or fusion of the palatal shelves.

Epidemiology

Cleft palate affects newborns with a world prevalence of about 3.1/10,000, which significantly varies depending on the geographical location. According to the Global Burden of Disease (GBD) study, the highest rates of CPO are found in the Oceanic continent, and the lowest in Sub-Saharan Africa, with overall values ranging from 0.4 to 11.3 every 10,000 births (Mossey and Modell, 2012). Nevertheless, there are very few epidemiological studies about OFC in African populations and estimated values of CPO incidence may not be accurate. Moreover, even inside the same continent, CPO prevalence values vary among different geographical areas, as in Europe. In fact, according to the EUROCAT registries Finland and Malta show the highest rates while Portugal and Romania the lowest, with more than three-times difference in rates (EUROCAT).

[1] https://www.ncbi.nlm.nih.gov/omim

Besides geographical differences, there is also a disparity in the CPO incidence between genders. In fact, while for isolated CL/P cases the sex ratio was estimated at 1.81 (95% CI, 1.75–1.86), isolated CPO counts more females than males, with a sex ratio of 0.93 (95% CI, 0.89–0.96) in the world (Mossey and Catilla, 2003) and reported as 0.78 in Europe (Calzolari et al., 2004). This discrepancy is probably due to the delay of 1 week in the fusion of the palatal shelves in female embryos compared to males (Burdi and Faist, 1967). Possibly, in this period of time the morphogenesis could be more influenced by teratogens, thus justifying the higher CPO rate in girls.

ETIOLOGY

Environmental Factors

The complex etiology of NSCPO can be explained, beside genetic factors, by the intervention of unmodifiable (e.g., race/ethnicity, sex, family history of clefts) and modifiable factors, acting in the period from 1 month before through 2 months after conception. Fundamentally, maternal factors such as health/disease status, lifestyle, medication, exposure to environmental teratogens can affect/influence the intrauterine environment, more heavily during embryo development, and have been the topic of a number of studies looking at their association with NSCPO risk.

Surprisingly, it is the older age of the father that has been reported to increase the risk of NSCPO in the offspring, rather than that of the mother (Savitz et al., 1991; Bille et al., 2005) as confirmed by a meta-analysis (Herkrath et al., 2012).

Among the maternal behavioral factors, alcohol consumption during the first trimester of pregnancy has been suggested to have a correlation with oral cleft onset (Romitti et al., 2007; DeRoo et al., 2008). However, there are few evidences supporting a role in the CP etiology (DeRoo et al., 2008; Sabbagh et al., 2015). A recent meta-analysis (Yin et al., 2019) concluded that there is no evidence of a correlation between moderate periconceptional alcohol consumption and the risk of both non-syndromic CL/P and CP in infants. However, authors suggest that the potential risk of binge-drinking cannot be excluded, because of the heterogeneity of the threshold level for alcohol consumption in the different investigations and of the limited sample sizes of heavy drinker mother cohorts.

Also maternal tobacco smoking has been deeply investigated as an NSCPO risk factor. The studies were recently considered in two meta-analyses, which concluded by supporting a role for both maternal tobacco smoking (Little et al., 2004) and passive smoking (Sabbagh et al., 2015) in NSCPO etiology. Nevertheless, it should be taken into account that the results of meta-analyses could be biased because the sample size, ethnicity, and consumption levels vary widely from one study to another. Moreover, the alcohol and tobacco teratogenic dose-response effect is still a matter of debate.

A recent study examined the effect of maternal exposure to water disinfection by-products (DBP), a heterogeneous group of compounds that can originate from a combination of chemical disinfectants (e.g., chlorine, chloramine) and organic matter present in water (Kaufman et al., 2018). Studying the association between DBP and the risk of craniofacial malformation, the authors obtained evidence that some DBPs (specifically: DBP9, HAA5, trichloroacetic acid, and dichloroacetic acid) can increase the risk of NSCPO. Similarly, a previous study suggested an increased risk of NSCPO as a result of maternal exposure to total trihalomethanes, but at lower ranges than those of the above-mentioned work (Hwang et al., 2008). Moreover, nitrate intake from drinking water was seen to increase the risk of NSCPO in a large cohort study (OR, 1.9; 95% CI, 1.17–3.09) (Brender et al., 2013).

Since the nutritional status of the embryo is fully dependent on maternal food intake and metabolism, unbalanced maternal nutrition during the first trimester of pregnancy can lead to birth defects. Several essential micronutrients, substances that cannot be synthesized by our body in sufficient amount, are needed for health maintenance, pregnancy progression and normal embryonic development. In case of maternal nutrition deficiencies, supplementation during pregnancy is strongly advised. It is commonly accepted that folic acid-fortified multivitamin supplementation before conception and continuing through the first trimester reduces the overall occurrence of several congenital anomalies. However, only few systematic reviews or meta-analyses regarding orofacial clefts have been conducted and findings on cleft palate are inconclusive. A systematic review analyzed data from five clinical trials in order to evaluate if supplementation with folic acid, alone or in combination with vitamins and minerals, can prevent the occurrence of neural tube defects (NTD) and other birth defects. No evidence of any preventive or negative effects on cleft palate by periconceptional oral folate supplementation was detected (RR, 0.73; 95% CI, 0.05–10.89) (De-Regil et al., 2015). A reduced risk of NSCPO resulted in a meta-analysis of case–control studies for mothers who took multivitamin supplementation starting from before pregnancy (OR, 0.76; 95% CI, 0.62–0.93) (Ingrid Goh et al., 2006). An observational study reported that after food grain fortification with folic acid, the prevalence of NSCPO in United States had a significant 12% reduction (Canfield et al., 2005). On the other hand, Sutton et al. (2011) measured levels of red cell folate (RCF), vitamin B12 and homocysteine (tHcy) in the blood of women who were pregnant with a malformed baby at a time when multivitamin supplementation or food fortification was still rare. They found that the level of B12, which plays a critical role in folate metabolism, was surprisingly higher in mothers expecting a baby with cleft palate than in mothers of unmalformed offspring, with no differences in levels of RCF and tHcy (Sutton et al., 2011).

Retinoic acid (RA), a derivate of Vitamin A, is an important regulator of processes that occur during embryogenesis, such as proliferation, differentiation, and apoptosis (Finnell et al., 2004). Only few epidemiological studies on human maternal intake of Vitamin A are available (Ackermans et al., 2011). Nevertheless, an excess of Vitamin A is considered teratogenic, causing congenital malformations, including cleft palate. On the other hand, Johansen et al. (2008) evidenced a substantial protective association between high (1.91–9.64 mg) maternal intake of Vitamin A and risk of NSCPO (adjusted OR [aOR], 0.47;

95% CI, 0.24–0.94), indicating that a deficit of Vitamin A is also to be considered a risk factor for NSCPO. The need for maternal zinc supplementation during pregnancy is still an unresolved issue with conflicting results from observational data. Higher maternal plasma zinc concentration was seen to be protective against NSCPO in a sample study of Filipino women (Tamura et al., 2005), whereas the same authors did not confirm the association in a sample study from Utah (Munger et al., 2009), probably attributable to the fact that zinc status in US mothers is not compromised to a certain severity as commonly seen in the Philippines.

Medicament intake during the periconceptional/first trimester period has long been generally ascertained to be correlated with an increased risk of adverse maternal outcomes. On the spectrum of congenital anomalies considered, cleft palate showed a significant increase in odd ratio with several treatments, including the use of inhaled β2-agonists as a medical treatment for asthma (OR, 1.63; 95% CI, 1.05–2.52) (Garne et al., 2015); use of valproic acid (OR, 5.8; 95% CI, 3.3–9.5) and carbamazepine (OR, 2.4; 95% CI, 1.1–4.5) as antiepileptic drugs (in the United States) (Gilboa et al., 2011); use of aspirin as analgesic (OR, 1.7; 95% CI, 1.0–2.9) (Hernandez et al., 2012); use of corticosteroids (OR, 5.3; 95% CI, 1.1–26.5) (Carmichael and Shaw, 1999); use of ondansetron to treat hyperemesis gravidarum (RR, 1.29; 95% CI, 1.00–1.65) (Huybrechts et al., 2018); and the use of nitrosatable amides as anti-infectives (aOR, 1.27, 95% CI, 1.00–1.62) (Brender et al., 2012).

Maternal sickness could influence the pregnancy outcome, as hypothesized for influenza, common cold and cystitis by Metneki et al. (2005). These authors highlighted the teratogenic effect of hyperthermia, which was confirmed the following year by Acs et al. (2006), who reported that the fever associated with acute respiratory infections seemed to increase the risk for posterior cleft palate in their Hungarian sample study. In 2020, in a Caucasian population-based case-control study with 751 NSCPO cases, again by Acs et al. (2020), analyzed the role of maternal diseases in the increased risk for developing NSCPO. Specifically, the authors evidenced significantly altered odd ratios for CP when mothers where affected by acute inflammatory diseases such as: influenza (OR, 1.8; 95% CI, 1.3–2.5), acute upper respiratory infections (OR, 2.5; 95% CI, 1.9–3.1), acute lower respiratory infections (OR, 2.4; 95% CI, 1.4–4.2), urogenital infections (OR, 2.0; 95% CI, 1.4–2.8), and unspecified high temperature (OR, 8.1; 95% CI, 2.9–22.6). Besides, they found a strong association with herpes simplex infection (OR, 14.8; CI, 5.7–38.5). The association between chronic maternal diseases and an increased risk for NSCPO in the offspring was observed for: Graves' disease (OR, 4.3; 95% CI, 1.7–10.6), epilepsy (OR, 4.6; 95% CI, 2.4–8.8), migraine (OR, 2.8; 95% CI, 1.2–6.8), essential hypertension (OR, 1.7; 95% CI, 1.2–2.4) and neuro-musculoskeletal pain syndromes. However, these findings have to be considered along with the teratogenic effect of medicament assumption to alleviate the symptoms of such conditions (Acs et al., 2020). According to Acs et al. (2020) the significantly higher risk observed for anemic mothers to have an NSCPO child (OR, 1.84; 95% CI, 1.25–2.71) could be a consequence of embryonic hypoxia during the critical morphogenetic period.

A meta-analysis carried out to assess the association between maternal obesity and congenital anomalies, evidenced a barely but significantly increased risk of cleft palate (Stothard et al., 2009), a datum that was later confirmed by Block et al. (2013).

Gestational diabetes mellitus has been associated with an increased risk of cleft palate in the offspring (OR, 1.54; 95% CI, 1.01–2.37) of women with a pre-pregnancy BMI $\geq$ 25 kg/m^2, but the authors stress the need to consider the possibility of undiagnosed type 2 diabetes mellitus and the subsequent hyperglycemia as a real cause of the embryo malformation (Correa et al., 2008). With regard to pregestational diabetes, a very large population-based birth defect case-control study, carried out this year in the United States, evidenced an association with cleft palate alone (OR, 4.3; 95% CI, 2.9–6.5), while a smaller increased risk was observed in association with gestational diabetes (OR, 1.4; 95% CI, 1.1–1.8) (Tinker et al., 2020).

Genetic Factors

Increased recurrence risk in relatives indicates a high level of heritability for NSCPO (Grosen et al., 2010). Hence, the evidence of a genetic component in the etiology of this birth defect and the challenge taken up by researchers to obtain a better understanding of the NSCPO molecular bases.

During secondary palate formation, the palatal shelves grow, approach and fuse. The cells need to activate a series of biological mechanisms, including cell migration, epithelial–mesenchymal transition, and apoptosis, necessary to remove epithelial cells from the palatal epithelia medial edge, leading to the continuity of the mesenchyme and to palatal formation. For this reason, it has been hypothesized that many genes that code for proteins involved in the formation of cytoskeleton filaments, for cell adhesion molecules, or for ECM components, may contribute, if altered, to the clefted palate phenotype (Gibbins et al., 1999; Tudela et al., 2002). Here, we browse through the association studies on genes involved in mechanisms crucial for palatal development (**Table 1**).

Cell–Cell Adhesion

The epithelial adhesion molecule cadherin (CDH1) participates actively in the epithelial–mesenchymal transition, the developmental step when the epithelial cells at the palatal midline disappear, allowing mesenchymal continuity and palatal fusion. Alterations in the *CDH1* gene contribute to the complex events that drive orofacial cleft, as demonstrated for the onset of non-syndromic cleft lip with or without cleft palate (NSCL/P) (Letra et al., 2009). Some studies have recently hypothesized that this gene may also represent a risk factor for NSCPO (Song and Zhang, 2011; Rafighdoost et al., 2013; Song et al., 2017).

Another gene involved in cell adhesion and motility that is crucial for craniofacial development is *CRISPLD2*. It contains an LCCL domain, common to other proteins involved in cellular migration (Chiquet et al., 2007). *CRISPLD2* product has also been shown to be important for normal migration and differentiation of neural crest cells during early palate formation (Swindell et al., 2015). A significant association between allelic variants at rs1546124 and rs4783099 in the *CRISPLD2* gene and the risk for

TABLE 1 | Published association studies between gene polymorphisms and NSCPO.

Gene[#]	Locus	SNP information	Country	Sample size	*P*-value[†]	OR (95% CI)	References
CDH1	16q22.1	rs16260	China	26 cases – 107 controls	0.004	6.90 (1.47–32.40)[‡]	Song and Zhang (2011)
		rs11642413	Iran	31 cases – 100 controls	0.019	3.70 (1.26–10.87)	Rafighdoost et al. (2013)
		rs16260		31 cases – 100 controls	NS		
		rs9929218	Latvia	10 cases – 190 controls	NS		Krasone et al. (2014)
		rs16260; rs11642413	Africa	163 cases – 1078 controls	NS		Gowans et al. (2016)
		rs1801552	China	115 cases – 271 controls	0.036	0.62 (0.40–0.97)	Song et al. (2017)
		rs16260; rs9929218			NS		
COL2A1	12q13.11	rs1793949	Baltic regions	104 cases – 606 controls	7.26×10^{-4}	1.659 (1.235–2.229)	Nikopensius et al. (2010)
		rs6823			0.0058	1.517 (1.270–2.041)	
		rs12228854			0.0067	1.663 (1.148–2.409)	
		rs12368284			0.0093	0.661 (0.483–0.904)	
		rs10875713			0.0197	1.596 (1.074–2.370)	
		rs11168359			0.0203	0.544 (0.323–0.916)	
		rs1793949	Brazil	107 triads	NS		Machado et al. (2016)
CRISPLD2	16q24.1	rs12051468; rs8061351; rs721005; rs1546124; rs16974880; rs4783099	Ireland	293 cases – 902 controls	NS		Carter et al. (2010)
		rs1546124	China	118 cases – 463 controls	5.4×10^{-4}	2.93 (1.69–5.07)[‡]	Shen et al. (2011)
		rs4783099			1.1×10^{-3}	0.48 (0.30–0.77)	
		rs16974880			NS		
		rs4783099	Africa	163 cases – 1078 controls	0.02	0.74	Gowans et al. (2016)
		rs1546124			NS		
		rs4783099	Brazil	236 cases – 693 controls	0.01	1.31 (1.05–1.62)	Messetti et al. (2017)
		rs1546124; rs8061351; rs2326398			NS		
FOXE1	9q22.33	rs1867278	Denmark, Norway, United States, Philippines	524 triads	4.1×10^{-4}		Moreno et al. (2009)
		Other 14 SNPs genotyped			NS		
		rs111846096	Thailand	77 cases – 90 controls	NS		Srichomthong et al. (2013)
		rs4460498	Germany, The Netherlands, Maya	165 cases – 1500 controls	0.017	0.81 (0.56–1.17)	Ludwig et al. (2014)
			Europe	156 triads	0.043	0.913 (0.51–1.65)	Ludwig et al. (2014)
		rs4460498; rs3758249	China	51 triads	NS		Liu et al. (2015)
		rs894673; rs3758249	Africa	163 cases – 1078 controls	NS		Gowans et al. (2016)
		rs6586	California (Hispanic)	66 cases – 476 controls		0.34 (0.13–0.90)[‡]	Lammer et al. (2016)
		rs4618817				0.34 (0.15–0.80)	
		other 11 SNPs genotyped			NS		
GRHL3	1p36.11	rs2486668; rs545809	China	297 cases – 377 controls	NS		He and Bian (2016)
		rs41268753	Norway, Denmark, United States	246 cases – 1685 controls	2.81×10^{-4}	2.16 (1.43–3.27)	Leslie et al. (2016)
		rs113965554			6.82×10^{-4}	1.97 (1.33–2.91)	
		rs41268753	Europe, Yemen	288 cases – 725 controls	2.63×10^{-5}	2.46 (1.62–3.74)	Mangold et al. (2016)
			Germany	116 cases[§] – 267 controls	0.94		Mangold et al. (2016)

(Continued)

TABLE 1 | Continued

Gene[#]	Locus	SNP information	Country	Sample size	*P*-value[†]	OR (95% CI)	References
IRF6	1q32.2	rs4844880; rs669694; rs2235371; rs2235375; rs2013162; rs126280	Norway	117 triads	NS		Jugessur et al. (2008)
		rs2235371	China	25 cases – 96 controls		0.25 (0.061–0.57)	Tang et al. (2009)
		rs2235371; rs2013162; rs7552506; rs2235377	Ireland	293 cases – 902 controls	NS		Carter et al. (2010)
		rs17389541	Baltic regions	104 cases – 606 controls	5.45×10^{-4}	1.726 (1.263–2.358)	Nikopensius et al. (2010)
		rs9430018			0.0454	1.351 (1.006–1.814)	
		rs4844880; rs2235371; rs2013162; rs861019; rs2073487; rs658860	Brazil	53 cases – 285 controls	NS		Letra et al. (2012)
		rs34743335; rs642961	Africa	163 cases – 1078 controls	NS		Gowans et al. (2016)
		rs642961; rs77542756; rs2235371	Thailand	83 triads	NS		Wu-Chou et al. (2019)
		rs2235371	Brazil	38 cases – 182 controls	0.004	3.01 (0.97–8.97)	Bezerra et al. (2019)
		rs642961; rs2236907; rs861019; rs1044516			NS		
JAG2	14q32.33	rs11624283	Estonia	53 cases – 205 controls	0.0016		Jagomagi et al. (2010)
		rs10134946	Baltic regions	104 cases – 606 controls	0.0318	1.384 (1.028–1.864)	Nikopensius et al. (2010)
		rs1057744	Brazil	81 cases – 413 controls	NS		Paranaiba et al. (2013)
MSX1	4p16.2	rs1106514	Estonia	53 cases – 205 controls	0.0037		Jagomagi et al. (2010)
			Baltic regions	104 cases – 606 controls	0.0095	1.482 (1.100–1.998)	Nikopensius et al. (2010)
		rs3821949; rs12532; rs104893854 – P147Q	China	42 triads	NS		Huang et al. (2011)
		rs62636562	Brazil	81 cases – 413 controls	NS		Paranaiba et al. (2013)
		rs12532	Iran	31 cases – 100 controls	0.008	10.83 (2.38–49.38)[‡]	Rafighdoost et al. (2013)
		rs3775261			NS		
		rs12532; rs3821949	China	56 cases – 605 controls	NS		Ma et al. (2014)
		rs2073242	Brazil	75 cases – 823 controls	NS		Kuchler et al. (2014)
		rs1106514	Brazil	107 triads	NS		Machado et al. (2016)
		rs115200552	Africa	163 cases – 1078 controls	0.01	1.81	Gowans et al. (2016)
		rs12532			NS		
		pCA	Europe	180 triads	NS		Mossey et al. (2017)
PAX7	1p36.13	rs742071	Europe	266 triads	NS		Bohmer et al. (2013)
		rs4920520; rs766325	Iowa, Asia	94 triads	NS		Butali et al. (2013)
		rs742071	China	56 cases – 605 controls	NS		Pan et al. (2013)
		rs766325; rs742071	Africa	163 cases – 1078 controls	NS		Gowans et al. (2016)
		rs742071	China	144 triads	0.025	3 (1.09–8.25)	Duan et al. (2017)
		rs4920522; rs766325; rs6695765			NS		

(Continued)

TABLE 1 | Continued

Gene[#]	Locus	SNP information	Country	Sample size	*P*-value[†]	OR (95% CI)	References
ROCK1	18q11.1	rs35996865	Italy, Iran	189 triads	0.006	0.63 (0.45–0.88)	Palmieri et al. (2020)
SUMO1	2q33.1	rs3769817	Ireland	293 cases – 902 controls	0.038	1.45 (1.06–1.99)	Carter et al. (2010)
		rs12470401			NS		
TBX22	Xq21.1	rs6523677; rs6621541; rs7055763; rs58147590; rs6621542; rs41307258; rs6621543	Brazil, Europe, North America	126 cases – 295 controls	NS		Pauws et al. (2009)
TCOF1	5q32-q33.1	rs2255796	Taiwan, Singapore, United States	81 triads	0.033	2.08	Sull et al. (2008)
		rs2748222			0.096	1.77	
		rs1864957			0.077	1.91	
		rs15251			0.007	2.88	
		rs15251; rs28372960; rs2569062	Brazil	107 triads	NS		Machado et al. (2016)
TGFA	2p13.3	*Taq* I polymorphism*; GGAA4D07	Iowa	62 cases – 251 controls	NS		Lidral et al. (1998)
		rs2166975	Lithuania	18 triads	0.045		Morkuniene et al. (2007)
			Ireland	293 cases – 902 controls	0.041	1.42 (1.05–1.42)	Carter et al. (2010)
		rs6743202	Baltic regions	104 cases – 606 controls	0.0467	1.356 (1.004–1.831)	Nikopensius et al. (2010)
		rs1058213; rs2166975; rs930655; rs1523305; rs2902345; rs377122	Brazil	53 cases – 285 controls	NS		Letra et al. (2012)
		Taq I polymorphism*	Brazil	28 triads	NS		Souza et al. (2012)
		rs2166975	Ireland	296 triads – 62 dyads – 15 NSCPO	0.047		Fan et al. (2013)
		c.3851T>C; c.3822G>A	China	62 cases – 150 controls	NS		Xu et al. (2014)

[#]*Further information about the molecular function, biological process and relative pathway is given in* ***Supplementary Table S1****.*
[†]*NS, not significant.*
[‡]*OR for homozygous variant genotype.*
[§]*Submucous cleft palate only.*
**Deletion of 4 bp in intron V, creating a Taq I site.*

NSCPO, has been reported in case–control studies (Shen et al., 2011; Gowans et al., 2016; Messetti et al., 2017).

One of the genes that participate in the signaling mechanism required for normal palate development is *JAG2*, which encodes a ligand for Notch family transmembrane receptors. *JAG2* and *NOTCH1* are spatio-temporally activated in the oral epithelia during palate development for the correct cell adhesion of the elevated palatal shelves, preventing their premature adhesion to other oral tissues (Casey et al., 2006). Nevertheless, only few studies investigated a possible involvement of *JAG2* in the onset of NSCPO, with controversial results. *JAG2* collaborates with *IRF6* on the same molecular pathway during oral epithelial differentiation. This coordination is essential for the control of palatal adhesion and fusion competence (Richardson et al., 2009). *IRF6* plays an important role in the formation and maintenance of the oral periderm, the spatiotemporal regulation of which is essential to ensure appropriate palatal adhesion (Richardson et al., 2009). Mutations in *IRF6* cause two common forms of syndromic cleft, known as Van der Woude Syndrome (VWS) and popliteal pterygium syndrome (Kondo et al., 2002). The crucial role of *IRF6* in the genesis of NSCL/P has been widely demonstrated in several studies. Zucchero et al. (2004), in a vast NSCL/P sample study from different countries, first demonstrated that genetic variants in *IRF6*, underlying VWS, might also be involved in the etiology of isolated clefts. However, although a strong association between genetic variants at *IRF6* and NSCL/P risk was successively confirmed by independent studies (Blanton et al., 2005; Ghassibe et al., 2005; Scapoli et al., 2005; Srichomthong et al., 2005), the existing results regarding NSCPO are contradictory (**Table 1**). This could be due to the low power of the studies because of small sample sizes, but also to the widely demonstrated different etiology of NSCPO with respect to NSCL/P.

A number of scientific evidences suggest that *FOXE1* is one of the most consistent genetic factors in the NSCPO etiology. Mutations of *FOXE1* cause Bamforth-Lazarus, a recessive syndrome characterized by cleft palate and congenital hypothyroidism (Castanet et al., 2002). Mice lacking *Foxe1* express a similar phenotype (De Felice et al., 1998). The FOXE1 is a transcription factor expressed in the shelf epithelium of the secondary palate during the fusion and regulates both *MSX1* and *TGFB3*, which are required for proper palate formation (Venza et al., 2011). Various studies reported a strong association between *FOXE1* and both NSCL/P or NSCPO (Moreno et al., 2009; Nikopensius et al., 2011; Lammer et al., 2016). No common missense mutations in *FOXE1* can explain the association signal evidenced by different authors, suggesting the hypothesis of a common variant in a regulatory region (Lidral et al., 2015). Sequence analysis identified a novel non-coding polymorphism c.-1204C>G in the promoter of *FOXE1* in 11 Italian NSCPOs (Venza et al., 2009), while Srichomthong et al. (2013) identified five non-synonymous mutations, none of which was present in the control population.

In craniofacial development, *TGFA* is expressed during the fusion of the palatine shelves at the level of the medial edge epithelium. Evidence of the involvement of *TGFA* in NSCPO etiology was found by several authors investigating different populations, but not by others, as detailed in **Table 1**.

Cell Proliferation

TCOF1 actively participates in the formation of neural crests. Alterations of this gene cause development anomalies that lead to craniofacial malformations (Dixon et al., 2006). Indeed, *TCOF1* is a causative gene for Treacher Collins syndrome, characterized by hypoplasia of the facial bones, cleft palate, and middle and external ear defects. Sull et al. (2008) identified the SNP rs15251 variant as a possible risk factor for NSCPO.

The homeobox gene *MSX1* actively participates in cell proliferation, differentiation, and apoptosis, all crucial processes for normal embryonic development. This gene plays a critical role in the epithelial–mesenchymal interaction during the formation of craniofacial bones (Satokata and Maas, 1994). Many studies on animal models have amply demonstrated *MSX1* involvement in palatal, facial and dental development (Satokata and Maas, 1994; Jumlongras et al., 2001). Genetic studies conducted on humans have ascertained a specific role for *MSX1* in the orofacial cleft (Jezewski et al., 2003; Modesto et al., 2006; Tasanarong et al., 2019). However, the association studies specifically dedicated to NSCPO cohorts obtained conflicting evidence, possibly due to the small sample sizes and the different ethnic groups considered (**Table 1**). A recent meta-analysis performed by Gu et al. (2018) of investigations published till 2017, indicated the SNP rs12532, able to affect mRNA expression and stability of *MSX1*, as a possible risk factor for NSCPO but not for NSCL/P.

TBX22 encodes a transcription factor important for the mesenchymal proliferation and elevation of palatal shelves before their fusion. Its normal expression is related to a correct development of the palate, while *TBX22* mutations cause the hereditary X-linked disorder, cleft palate with ankyloglossia (CPX, OMIM 303400) (Marcano et al., 2004; Stanier and Moore, 2004). Marcano et al. (2004) screened for *TBX22* mutations in 238 NSCPOs from the Philippines, North America, and Brazil, and found 15 different variants: five mutations affecting the coding region, as well as several putative splice site mutations. Suphapeetiporn et al. (2007) by sequencing the *TBX22* gene in 53 NSCPO cases in the Thai population, found three missense mutations and a deletion in four affected individuals. Fu et al. (2015) reported a functional -73G>A mutation in the promoter of *TBX22*, in all five affected males of a six-generation Chinese family of NSCPO (Fu et al., 2015). Both *TBX22* and *MSX1* are post-translationally modified by SUMO1, a regulating factor that participates in the modulation of many other genes, with evidence of a role in human oral clefts (Dobreva et al., 2003; Ghioni et al., 2005; Lee et al., 2006; Andreou et al., 2007).

Shi et al. (2009) identified a *de novo* deletion on chromosome 2 in a Danish child affected by NSCPO. The estimated size of the deletion is 124.2 kb and contains *SUMO1* (Shi et al., 2009). In a large Irish study population composed by 383 NSCPO patients, the SNP rs3769817 located in *SUMO1* intron 2 was associated with an increased risk for cleft palate (Carter et al., 2010).

The PAX transcription factors are critical for neural crest induction (Monsoro-Burq, 2015). In particular, Pax7 regulates the cell cycle of embryonic stem cells and mouse embryonic fibroblasts (Czerwinska et al., 2016). The intronic rs742071 *PAX7* polymorphism, previously proposed as a risk factor for NSCL/P (Ludwig et al., 2012), was also found significantly associated with NSCPO in a family-based association study carried out with 266 European triads (Bohmer et al., 2013). The association with NSCPO was then confirmed in the Chinese and sub-Saharan African populations (Duan et al., 2017; Butali et al., 2019).

Another transcriptional factor widely involved in the processes of closure of the neural tube and craniofacial development is encoded by *GRHL3*. In families that do not show mutations at the *IRF6* locus, *GRHL3* seems to be the second candidate gene in VWS (Peyrard-Janvid et al., 2014). Functional analyses demonstrate that *GRHL3* is a target of IRF6 in the processes of periderm differentiation (de la Garza et al., 2013). In a genome-wide association study, Leslie et al. (2016) identified an association between the rs41268753 SNP and NSCPO in two independent populations. The importance of *GRHL3* in NSCPO etiology was independently confirmed by Mangold et al. (2016), who collected evidences supporting the non-synonymous polymorphism rs41268753 as a susceptibility factor for NSCPO and described rare mutations of this gene in patients. *COL2A1* is a cartilage-specific marker involved in cranial neural crest differentiation by complex mechanisms that involve epithelial–mesenchymal transition, migration, and differentiation (Ghassibe-Sabbagh et al., 2011). Mutations in genes coding for cartilage collagens II cause syndromes that are often associated with cleft palate or micrognathia, such as Pierre-Robin sequence and Stickler syndrome (Kannu et al., 2012). Evidence of an association between *COL2A1* alleles and NSCPO risk was found (Nikopensius et al., 2010), though not confirmed by others (Machado et al., 2016).

Cell Migration

The two Rho kinase isoforms (ROCK1 and ROCK2) play essential roles in fundamental cellular processes such as contraction, adhesion, migration, apoptosis, and proliferation. ROCK regulates stress fiber and focal adhesion assembly (Phillips et al., 2012) and modulates cytoskeleton organization by phosphorylating different substrates, mainly myosin light chain and myosin phosphatase, involved in the contractility pathway that leads to normal palate development. A recent family-based association study carried out in two cohorts from Italy and Iran, showed a significant level of association between *ROCK1* rs35996865-G and NSCPO (Palmieri et al., 2020). Currently, there are no reports demonstrating the involvement of *ROCK2* in the onset of orofacial cleft, however, some studies show that the loss of both chromosome 18q and 2p (where *ROCK1* and *ROCK2* reside, respectively) determines a series of anomalies including defects of the palate and micrognathia (Suzuki et al., 2016).

FLNB belongs to a family of actin-binding proteins. Filamins are also able to interact with receptors and intracellular proteins involved in cytoskeleton-dependent cell proliferation, differentiation, and migration (Hu et al., 2014). Mutations in this gene cause malformations that include cleft palate as a feature, as reported by Jugessur et al. (2010) who suggest a maternal effect for variants mapping in this gene, in their NSCPO cohort (Jugessur et al., 2010).

Genes Involved in Folate and Homocysteine Metabolism

Vitamin B9 or folate is not synthesized by our organism but is present, for example, in legumes, leafy green vegetables, some fruits, and eggs. Folic acid is the most stable form of folate, synthetically produced and usually used in vitamin supplements and fortified foods (Bailey et al., 2015). Adequate folate intake is essential for cell division and homeostasis. Indeed, the folate pathway plays a crucial role in several strategic biochemical processes such as DNA biosynthesis, methionine regeneration, amino acid metabolism, mitochondrial protein translation, and DNA methylation. Folate deficiency and/or aberrant folate metabolism during embryogenesis were therefore assumed to cause congenital malformations because of the alteration of the precise interplay of cell proliferation and death, migration, and differentiation needed in this delicate moment of development. However, as above documented, there is no strong association between folate supplementation during the periconceptional period and a decreased risk of having an NSCPO baby (Johnson and Little, 2008). Nevertheless, the folate pathway, with its enzymes and substrates, was suspected to have a role in the NSCPO etiology and several studies investigated associations between polymorphisms in genes related to one-carbon metabolism and cleft palate risk. The most investigated gene is *MTHFR*, with its C677T polymorphism. However, in a meta-analysis based on five studies, with a total of 576 CP cases and 2587 controls, no statistical significances were observed for the risk of NSCPO for heterozygotes, neither for homozygotes (Luo et al., 2012).

Table 2 reports information on folate and homocysteine metabolism gene polymorphisms investigated for their potential association with cleft palate, published until June 2020 in PubMed. Only single studies with data from a cohort or a subset of non-syndromic cleft palate cases have been considered in the table.

Genes Responsible for Syndromic Forms as Candidate for NSCPO

As mentioned above, referring to Burg et al.'s (2016) work, the responsible genes have been identified in a number of syndromes that include cleft palate among their features. Based on the assumption that genes implicated in syndromic forms of cleft could also have a role in non-syndromic phenotypes, the variant association of such genes has been questioned in case control and family based studies on different NSCPO worldwide cohorts.

The attempts of researchers to confirm this hypothesis are summarized in **Table 3**, where genes already mentioned in a previous section (*FLNB*) or in **Table 1** (*TBX22*, *FOXE1 COL2A1*, *IRF6*, *TCOF1*) are omitted.

Genome-Wide Analysis

The rapid improvement, in recent years, of technological tools for genotyping and sequencing has allowed researchers

TABLE 2 | Association studies between polymorphisms of one-carbon metabolism genes and NSCPO.

Gene[#]	Locus	SNP information	Country	Sample size[†]	*P*-value[‡]	OR (95% CI)	References
AHCY	20q11.22	rs819142; rs819133	Norway	93 triads	NS		Boyles et al. (2009)
BHMT	5q14.1	rs3733890 – G742A – R239Q	Norway	191 triads	NS		Boyles et al. (2008)
			Norway	93 triads	0.022[§]		Boyles et al. (2009)
		rs567754; rs585800	Norway	93 triads	NS		Boyles et al. (2009)
BHMT2	5q14.1	rs626105	Caucasians, Hispanics, others	236 cases – 201 controls		0.9 (0.6–1.3)	Zhu et al. (2005)
		rs542721; rs10944	Norway	93 triads	NS		Boyles et al. (2009)
CBS	21q22.3	844ins68	Norway	191 triads	NS		Boyles et al. (2008)
			Norway	93 triads	NS		Boyles et al. (2009)
		rs234706 – C699T	Norway	191 triads	NS		Boyles et al. (2008)
			Norway	93 triads	NS		Boyles et al. (2009)
		rs234705; rs234709; rs4920037	Norway	93 triads	NS		Boyles et al. (2009)
		rs2124459	France	125 cases – 145 controls	0.02	0.61 (0.40–0.93)	Goffinet et al. (2016)
			Belgium	79 cases – 225 controls	0.02	0.64 (0.44–0.93)	Goffinet et al. (2016)
		rs4920037	Italy	129 triads	NS	1.18 (0.74–1.88)	Carinci et al. (2019)
			Iran – Tibet – Bangladesh	65 triads	NS	1.00 (0.48–2.10)	Carinci et al. (2019)
CTH	1p31.1	rs681475; rs1145920; rs515064; rs1021737	Norway	93 triads	NS		Boyles et al. (2009)
		rs663649	Norway	93 triads	0.047[§]		Boyles et al. (2009)
DHFR	5q14.1	rs2618372; rs380691	Norway	93 triads	NS		Boyles et al. (2009)
DMGDH	5q14.1	rs250513; rs479405; rs642013; rs2034899; rs1805074; rs248386; rs185077; rs532964	Norway	93 triads	NS		Boyles et al. (2009)
FOLH1	11p11.12	rs6485963; rs11040270; rs7113251; rs202720; rs10839236; rs202676	Norway	93 triads	NS		Boyles et al. (2009)
FOLR1	11q13.4	rs3016432; rs11235468	Norway	93 triads	NS		Boyles et al. (2009)
FOLR2	11q13.4	rs514933	Norway	93 triads	NS		Boyles et al. (2009)
		rs2298444			0.003		
FOLR3	11q13.4	rs533207; rs555306; rs575341	Norway	93 triads	NS		Boyles et al. (2009)
FTCD	21q22.3	rs1980983; rs9978174; rs4819208; rs2277820	Norway	93 triads	NS		Boyles et al. (2009)
FTHFD	3q21.3	rs1127717; rs3772430; rs2290053; rs2365004; rs2886059; rs1823213	Norway	93 triads	NS		Boyles et al. (2009)
GNMT	6p21.1	rs2296805; rs2274514	Norway	93 triads	NS		Boyles et al. (2009)
MAT1A	10q22.3	rs1556894; rs2993763; rs9285726	Norway	93 triads	NS		Boyles et al. (2009)

(Continued)

TABLE 2 | Continued

Gene[#]	Locus	SNP information	Country	Sample size[†]	*P*-value[‡]	OR (95% CI)	References
MAT2A	2p11.2	rs6739015; rs2028900; rs2028898; rs7568458	Norway	93 triads	NS		Boyles et al. (2009)
MAT2B	5q34	rs10515861; rs4869087; rs4869089; rs729352	Norway	93 triads	NS		Boyles et al. (2009)
MTHFD1	14q23.3	rs2236225 – G1958A – R653Q	Norway	191 triads	NS		Boyles et al. (2008)
			Ireland	321 triads	NS	1.31 (0.94–1.82)	Mills et al. (2008)
			Ireland	321 mothers – 1599 controls	0.02[§]	1.41 (1.05–1.09)	Mills et al. (2008)
			Norway	93 triads	NS		Boyles et al. (2009)
			Europe	242 triads	NS	0.93 (0.55–1.57)*	Mossey et al. (2017)
		rs3783731; rs8003379; rs1950902; rs2236224; rs1256146	Norway	93 triads	NS		Boyles et al. (2009)
MTHFD2	2p13.1	rs1667627; rs702462	Norway	93 triads	NS		Boyles et al. (2009)
MTHFR	1p36.3	rs1801133 – C677T – A222V	California	117 cases – 383 control	NS	0.8 (0.5–1.2)	Shaw et al. (1999)
			Norway	63 triads		2.4 (1.2–4.6)	Jugessur et al. (2003b)
			France	56 triads	NS	1.31 (0.6–3.0)	Chevrier et al. (2007)
			Norway	191 triads	NS		Boyles et al. (2008)
			UK	47 triads + 19 dyads[¥]		0.9 (0.44–1.77)	Little et al. (2008)
			Ireland	321 triads	NS	0.96 (0.64–1.43)	Mills et al. (2008)
			Ireland	321 mothers – 1599 controls	0.03[§]	1.5 (1.05–2.16)	Mills et al. (2008)
			Norway	93 triads	NS		Boyles et al. (2009)
			Africa	163 cases – 1078 controls	NS		Gowans et al. (2016)
			Europe	292 triads	NS	0.53 (0.31–0.92)*	Mossey et al. (2017)
			Italy	129 triads	NS	0.98 (0.68–1.42)	Carinci et al. (2019)
			Iran – Tibet – Bangladesh	65 triads	NS	1.17 (0.54–2.52)	Carinci et al. (2019)
		rs1801131 – A1298C – A429E	Norway	191 triads	NS		Boyles et al. (2008)
			Ireland	321 triads	NS	0.83 (0.49–1.40)	Mills et al. (2008)
			Norway	93 triads	NS		Boyles et al. (2009)
			Africa	163 cases – 1078 controls	NS		Gowans et al. (2016)
		rs4845877; rs1476413; rs3737964; rs12404124	Norway	93 triads	NS		Boyles et al. (2009)
MTHFS	15q25.1	rs685487; rs6495452; rs2562744	Norway	93 triads	NS		Boyles et al. (2009)
MTR	1q43	rs1805087 – A2756G	Norway	191 triads	NS		Boyles et al. (2008)
			Norway	93 triads	NS		Boyles et al. (2009)
		rs10925235; rs16834521	Norway	93 triads	NS		Boyles et al. (2009)
MTRR	5p15.31	rs1801394 – A66G	Norway	191 triads	NS		Boyles et al. (2008)
			Norway	93 triads	NS		Boyles et al. (2009)

(Continued)

TABLE 2 | Continued

Gene[#]	Locus	SNP information	Country	Sample size[†]	*P*-value[‡]	OR (95% CI)	References
		rs1532268	Norway	93 triads	0.021[§]		Boyles et al. (2009)
		rs3776455			0.038[§]		
		rs162031; rs162036; rs10380			NS		
NOS3	7q36.1	rs1800779 – A(-922G)	California	99 cases – 588 controls		0.9 (0.6–1.4)	Shaw et al. (2005)
		rs1799983 – G894T – E298D				1.1 (0.7–1.7)	
PON1	7q21.3	rs662 – A575G	Norway	191 triads	NS		Boyles et al. (2008)
			Norway	93 triads	NS		Boyles et al. (2009)
		rs854547; rs8491; rs854549; rs2237582; rs3917498; rs2074351; rs854565; rs2299261; rs705382	Norway	93 triads	NS		Boyles et al. (2009)
SHMT1	17p11.2	rs2168781	Norway	93 triads	0.015		Boyles et al. (2009)
		rs7207306			NS		
SHMT2	12q13.3	rs7311958	Norway	93 triads	NS		Boyles et al. (2009)
SLC19A1/RFC1	21q22.3	rs1051266 – A80G	California	123 cases – 364 controls		0.8 (0.5–1.3)	Shaw et al. (2003)
			Norway	191 triads	NS		Boyles et al. (2008)
			Norway	93 triads	NS		Boyles et al. (2009)
SLC46A1	17q11.2	rs9894260	Utah	109 triads	NS	0.75 (0.32–1.78)	VanderMeer et al. (2016)
		rs739439			NS	1.40 (0.62–3.15)	
		rs2239907			NS	0.73 (0.42–1.27)	
TCN2	22q12.2	rs1801198 – C776G – P259R	Norway	191 triads	NS		Boyles et al. (2008)
			Ireland	321 triads	NS	1.05 (0.73–1.52)	Mills et al. (2008)
			Norway	93 triads	NS		Boyles et al. (2009)
			Italy	129 triads	NS	0.98 (0.69–1.40)	Carinci et al. (2019)
			Iran – Tibet – Bangladesh	65 triads	NS	1.10 (0.60–2.02)	Carinci et al. (2019)
		rs9606756 – A67G	Norway	191 triads	NS		Boyles et al. (2008)
			Norway	93 triads	NS		Boyles et al. (2009)
TYMS	18p11.32	rs502396; rs2244500; rs10502290; rs10502289	Norway	93 triads	NS		Boyles et al. (2009)
		rs16430 – 1494del6	California	123 cases – 581 controls		1.3 (0.8–2.0)	Shaw et al. (2013)
		rs45445694 – 28-bp VNTR	California	123 cases – 581 controls	Significant	1.8 (1.1–3.1)*	Shaw et al. (2013)

[#] *Further information about the molecular function, biological process and relative pathway is given in* ***Supplementary Table S2****.*
[†] *Studies with a cohort bigger than 50 cases are reported.*
[‡] *NS, not significant.*
[§] *When the maternal association is considered.*
**OR for homozygous variant genotype.*
[¥] *In the sample study are included 11 cases of Pierre Robin sequence.*

TABLE 3 | Genes responsible for syndromic cleft palate, studied in NSCPO cohorts.

Gene[#]	Locus	Syndrome with cleft palate	SNP information	Country	Sample size	*P* value[†]	OR (95% CI)	References
BCOR	Xp11.4	Oculofaciocardiodental	Haplotype rs4076107-rs6520620-rs5963158-rs4308866	Asia	253 triads	$<10^{-4}$[‡]		Skare et al. (2017)
			rs6609051; rs12687359	Norway – Denmark	114 + 69 triads	NS		Jugessur et al. (2012)
COL11A1	1p21.1	Pierre Robin Sequence and Stickler	42 genotyped SNPs	Baltic regions	104 cases – 182 controls	NS		Nikopensius et al. (2010)
COL11A2	6p21.32	Pierre Robin Sequence and Stickler	rs213209	Baltic regions	104 cases – 182 controls	0.0138	0.63 (0.435–0.912)	Nikopensius et al. (2010)
			rs9277928			0.0451	0.637 (0.408–0.993)	
EFNB1	Xq13.1	Craniofrontonasal	rs877818	Norway – Denmark	114 + 69 triads	NS		Jugessur et al. (2012)
FGFR1	8p11.23	Kallman type 2	rs2978083	Baltic regions	104 cases – 606 controls	0.014	0.3 (0.109–0.829)	Nikopensius et al. (2010)
			rs7829058			0.0049	1.789 (1.189–2.720)	
				Brazil	41 triads	NS		Machado et al. (2016)
FGFR2	10q26.13	Apert and Crouzon	rs1047100	Ireland	293 cases – 902 controls	NS	0.85 (0.64–1.14)	Carter et al. (2010)
FLNA	Xq28	Otopalatodigital spectrum disorders	rs766419; rs2070822; rs2070816	Norway – Denmark	114 + 69 triads	NS		Jugessur et al. (2012)
OFD1/CXORF5	Xp22.2	Oral-facial-digital syndrome 1	rs2285635; rs2283707	Norway – Denmark	114 + 69 triads	NS		Jugessur et al. (2012)
PHF8	Xp11.22	Siderius type	rs6521788; rs12115965; rs7876951; rs5960612	Norway – Denmark	114 + 69 triads	NS		Jugessur et al. (2012)
PQBP1	Xp11.23	Renpenning	rs4824733; rs2016813; rs741932	Norway – Denmark	114 + 69 triads	NS		Jugessur et al. (2012)
SMS	Xp22.11	Snyder-Robinson	rs2040357; rs5951678	Norway – Denmark	114 + 69 triads	NS		Jugessur et al. (2012)
SOX9	17q24.3	Pierre Robin sequence and Campomelic dysplasia	rs12941170	China	46 triads	0.03	0.56 (0.3–0.96)	Jia et al. (2017)
			rs2229989			0.06	0.57 (0.3–1.03)	
TGFB2	1q41	Loeys-Dietz	pPC-27 probe	Philippines	48 cases – 214 controls	NS		Lidral et al. (1997)

[#] *Further information about the molecular function, biological process and relative pathway is given in* ***Supplementary Table S3****.*
[†] *NS, not significant.*
[‡] *Association among 100 males.*

to approach whole genome studies. The aim is to identify as many susceptibility genes as possible, while the challenge is to collect and analyze dataset large enough to deliver the required statistical power. The genome-wide association studies (GWAS) approach is an indirect mapping technique, able to identify associated polymorphisms, while exome/genome sequencing (WES/WGS) studies are more focused on rare genetic mutations. **Table 4** reports genes and polymorphisms associated with NSCPO detected by GWAS. Besides *IRF6*, an already known genetic risk factor for orofacial clefts, the list includes several new candidate genes. Among these *GRHL3*, whose involvement in NSCPO etiology was confirmed in an independent European cohort (Leslie et al., 2016) and by Mangold et al. (2016) in a subsequent investigation in which they evidenced common and rare causative mutations.

Whole exome sequencing (WES) searching for NSCPO mutations was performed in affected individuals from multiplex families with NSCPO (Hoebel et al., 2017). A probable deleterious mutation in *ARHGAP29*, a gene expressed in developing palate, was found in four individuals of a single family affected by cleft of the soft palate (Liu et al., 2017). The WES of 16 individuals from 8 multiplex families allowed Hoebel et al. (2017) to select 26 candidate genes that were sequenced in additional 132 NSCPO cases. The investigation failed to identify genes with recurrent deleterious mutations but produced data that may be useful for subsequent investigations.

The potential role of epigenetic regulation in NSCPO has been recently explored by two groups (Sharp et al., 2017; Xu et al., 2019). In these investigations, epigenome-wide association studies (EWAS) were conducted to test whether DNA methylation of blood, or other relevant tissues, was associated with orofacial clefting. These preliminary investigations suggest differences in methylation profiles of patients and unaffected controls, as well as between different types of clefts. However, future result replications may be difficult because methylation status may consistently vary as a function of kind of investigated tissue, and of patient age at the moment of sampling.

Gene × Gene Interaction

Gene–gene epistatic interaction (GxG) analysis has been successfully adopted for other diseases in order to narrow a critical region (Cox et al., 1999) or to identify additional loci (Pankratz et al., 2003). A small number of researchers tested for GxG in cohorts that do not include syndromic forms of CPO nor patients with CL. In detail, Jugessur et al. (2003a) found a significant 6.3-fold increased risk of NSCPO in patients carrying the *TGFA Taq* I A2A2 genotype in combination with one or two copies of the T-allele at *MTHFR* C677T polymorphism. This same gene–gene interaction was investigated by Mossey et al. (2017), evidencing an opposite effect when considering the combination *Taq* I A2 and one or two copies of *MTHFR* variant for the child genotype, with a 6 and 12.5-fold reduced risk, respectively. Lastly, Duan et al. (2017) evidenced an epistatic interaction between rs4844913

TABLE 4 | Genome wide association studies in NSCPO cohorts.

SNP information	Locus	Gene[#]	Country	Sample size	P-value[†]	OR (95% CI)	References
			49% Europe – 47% Asia – 3% Africa	550 triads	NS		Beaty et al. (2011), Shi et al. (2012), and Ludwig et al. (2017)
rs41268753	1p36.11	*GRHL3*	Europe	38 cases – 93 – triads – 835 controls	4.08×10^{-9}	8.3 (1.17–59.15)	Leslie et al. (2016)
rs117496742	11q22.1	*YAP1*	Europe	38 cases – 93 – triads – 835 controls	3.13×10^{-8}	11.2 (1.04–121.8)	Leslie et al. (2016)
rs12175475	6p26	*PARK2*	Multiethnic	78 cases – 165 triads – 1700 controls	8.66×10^{-9}	6.6 (1.12–39.58)	Leslie et al. (2016)
rs80004662	2p12	*CTNNA2*	Sub-Saharan Africa	205 cases – 2159 controls	7.41×10^{-9}	7.5 (3.45–16.28)	Butali et al. (2019)
rs730570	14q32.2	*DLK1*	China	2071 cases – 10145 controls	6.59×10^{-10}	1.28	Huang et al. (2019)
rs4646211	13q32.3	*DOCK9*	China	2071 cases – 10145 controls	4.78×10^{-12}	1.28	Huang et al. (2019)
rs8061677	16q24.2	*FOXC2-FOXL1*	China	2071 cases – 10145 controls	9.11×10^{-11}	1.29	Huang et al. (2019)
rs72741048	1q32.2	*IRF6*	China	2071 cases – 10145 controls	3.07×10^{-15}	1.314	Huang et al. (2019)
rs1009136	19p13.11	*MAU2*	China	2071 cases – 10145 controls	2.66×10^{-9}	1.25	Huang et al. (2019)
rs730643	14q13.3	*PAX9*	China	2071 cases – 10145 controls	2.92×10^{-16}	0.74	Huang et al. (2019)
rs6791526	3p22.1	*POMGNT2*	China	2071 cases – 10145 controls	1.62×10^{-10}	1.46	Huang et al. (2019)
rs3468	4p16.3	*WHSC1*	China	2071 cases – 10145 controls	5.4×10^{-11}	1.256	Huang et al. (2019)

[#] *Further information about the molecular function, biological process and relative pathway is given in* ***Supplementary Table S4****.*
[†] *NS, not significant SNP detected.*

(43 kb 3′ of *DIEXF*) and rs11119388 (*SYT14*) and between rs6072081 (53 kb 3′ of *MAFB*) and rs6102085 (33 kb 3′ of *MAFB*).

Gene x Environment Interactions

Orofacial clefts, including NSCPO, are considered as typical complex diseases caused by several genetic and environmental factors. Although many candidate gene studies and GWAS have been performed to reveal genetic factors of NSCPO, the genetic variants identified so far can explain only a small fraction of heritability of this common malformation. This has opened the hypothesis that the effect of genetic factors on a disorder can be modulated by environmental factors and *vice versa*. Several different models of gene–environment interactions (GxE) were postulated; in some cases it could be easier to detect the effect of genetic factors if the effect of environmental factors is also considered (Ottman, 1996).

The first attempts to investigate GxE interaction in OFC were reviewed by Murray (2002). Most of these studies included NSCL/P cases only, or NSCL/P cases together with a small fraction of NSCPO cases. Some possible GxE interactions were suggested but not confirmed (Murray, 2002).

An interaction between the rs7205289 polymorphism and passive smoking in NSCPO was observed in the Chinese population (Li et al., 2011). The rs7205289 lies in the microRNA-140 gene and can reduce its expression (Li et al., 2011). Interestingly, tobacco smoke had the same effect in cultured mouse palatal mesenchymal cells (Li et al., 2011). This data is particularly relevant because dysregulation of miRNA-140 was found to cause palatal malformations in zebrafish by targeting *Pdgfra* (Eberhart et al., 2008; Li et al., 2011). The *Pdgfra* has a critical role in neural crest development, mesenchymal cell migration, and palatogenesis also in mice (McCarthy et al., 2016). Finally, mutations in *PDGFRA* were found in NSCPO patients (Rattanasopha et al., 2012).

In a GxE study on OFC cases, Shi et al. (2007) investigated the interaction between maternal smoking and 16 candidate genes involved in detoxification. An interaction was found with *GSTT1* among OFC, with a higher effect in the NSCPO subgroup. In particular, the combination of fetal *GSTT1*-null genotype and maternal smoking provided the highest risk of cleft. This finding was important, because it confirmed a previous study involving an OFC sample from The Netherlands (van Rooij et al., 2001).

A GWAS conducted with 550 patient-parents triads supported the importance of a GxE interaction investigation. Indeed, while no individual gene reached the statistical threshold of significance in the test of association with NSCPO, several genes demonstrated an association when their interaction was considered. In particular, polymorphisms of *MLLT3* and *SMC2* interacted with maternal alcohol consumption; *TBK1* and *ZNF236* with maternal smoking; and *BAALC* with multivitamin supplementation (Beaty et al., 2011). Data were further examined by stratifying the sample by European and Asian ancestry (Wu et al., 2014). Several polymorphisms of a chromosome 4 region that includes *SLC2A9* and *WDR1* genes were associated with NSCPO in Asians when the interaction with environmental tobacco smoke exposure was tested.

The same dataset was investigated with an alternative model that includes the parent of origin (PoO) effect, i.e., the risk in the child varies on whether the allele is inherited from the mother or the father. The hypothesis of interaction between PoO and maternal exposure (PoOxE) provided the evidence for new genes involved in NSCPO etiology. Indeed, several polymorphisms in *ICE2* and *NAALADL2* showed PoOxSmoke interaction in European families (Haaland et al., 2017).

DISCUSSION

Defects of the closure of the secondary palate only are, among orofacial clefts, the rarest, the least studied, and those with the least obvious nature. CPO can occur as a feature of Mendelian single gene disorders or of several chromosomal syndromes. On the other hand, the isolated form of CPO is considered to have a multifactorial etiology, and in the last decades researchers have attempted to elucidate all the teratogenic and genetic factors causing this common malformation. The identification of causal factors and understanding of the molecular mechanisms of cleft formation would be an invaluable aid for clinicians in optimizing prevention approaches, providing genetic counseling, and planning personalized surgical and medical treatments.

Several evidences have highlighted the fact that NSCPO and NSCL/P are different malformations with different, or slightly overlapping, causes. Scientific research has been mainly focused on NSCL/P, while NSCPO study has been marginal, maybe owing to the lower incidence that makes harder to collect cohorts of comparable size. In recent years, this gap has been reducing, but new insights on CPO are accumulating more slowly than expected, especially with regards GWAS. A possible explanation is a limited contribution of common genetic variants in NSCPO etiology, which lower the success rate of association analyses. Genetic investigations have provided convincing evidences for a limited number of heritable factors that do not account for the high level of hereditability of NSCPO. These include *FOXE1*, *GRHL3*, and *PAX7*, while a number of investigations provided support for transcription and regulatory factors necessary for the normal development of neural crests. If rare variants play a major role in CPO etiology, future large-scale sequencing efforts may represent a promising approach to detect genetic factors. Emerging trends of research regard more complex models, including gene–gene interaction, gene–environment interaction, and epigenetic analyses, which could be more powerful to explain missing heritability, but all of these require larger sample sizes. However, such approaches need a deeper investigation, in order to earlier predict NSCPO risk and to plan healthcare strategies aimed at improving environmental conditions and reducing exposure to potential epigenetic factors.

Considering the long, but not exhaustive, list of potential susceptibility factors for NSCPO, a wide range prevention could appear unrealistic, also because palate closure occurs during a gestation period in which the mother is often unaware she is pregnant. It is in any case crucial to identify exposure risks acting around the conception time (1 month before, 3 months after) that may impact embryonic development. A consistent bulk of data supports an epidemiological role for both active and passive tobacco smoking, while contrasting evidences have been collected for moderate alcohol consumption. On the contrary, folate fortification and multivitamin supplementation seem to decrease the risk of NSCPO.

AUTHOR CONTRIBUTIONS

MM conceived the idea and design of the manuscript, acquired most of the references and data, and contributed to the drafting, revision, and final approval of the manuscript. AP and FC contributed to the manuscript design and critical revisions and final approval of the manuscript. LS contributed to the design, drafting, acquisition of statistical data, revision, and final approval of the manuscript. All authors contributed to the article and approved the submitted version.

REFERENCES

Ackermans, M. M., Zhou, H., Carels, C. E., Wagener, F. A., and Von den Hoff, J. W. (2011). Vitamin A and clefting: putative biological mechanisms. *Nutr. Rev.* 69(10), 613–624. doi: 10.1111/j.1753-4887.2011.00425.x

Acs, L., Banyai, D., Nemes, B., Nagy, K., Acs, N., Banhidy, F., et al. (2020). Maternal-related factors in the origin of isolated cleft palate-A population-based case-control study. *Orthod. Craniofac. Res.* 23(2), 174–180. doi: 10.1111/ocr.12361

Acs, N., Banhidy, F., Puho, E. H., and Czeizel, A. E. (2006). Acute respiratory infections during pregnancy and congenital abnormalities: a population-based case-control study. *Cong. Anom* 46(2), 86–96. doi: 10.1111/j.1741-4520.2006.00108.x

Andreou, A. M., Pauws, E., Jones, M. C., Singh, M. K., Bussen, M., Doudney, K., et al. (2007). TBX22 missense mutations found in patients with X-linked cleft palate affect DNA binding, sumoylation, and transcriptional repression. *Am. J. Hum. Genet* 81(4), 700–712. doi: 10.1086/521033

Bailey, L. B., Stover, P. J., McNulty, H., Fenech, M. F., Gregory, J. F., 3rd, Mills, J. L., et al. (2015). Biomarkers of Nutrition for Development-Folate Review. *J. Nutr.* 145(7), 1636S–1680S. doi: 10.3945/jn.114.206599

Beaty, T. H., Ruczinski, I., Murray, J. C., Marazita, M. L., Munger, R. G., Hetmanski, J. B., et al. (2011). Evidence for gene-environment interaction in a genome wide study of nonsyndromic cleft palate. *Genet Epidemiol.* 35(6), 469–478. doi: 10.1002/gepi.20595

Bezerra, J. F., Silva, H., Bortolin, R. H., Luchessi, A. D., Ururahy, M. A. G., Loureiro, M. B., et al. (2019). IRF6 polymorphisms in Brazilian patients with non-syndromic cleft lip with or without palate. *Braz J. Otorhinolaryngol.* 18, S1808-8694. doi: 10.1016/j.bjorl.2019.04.011

Bille, C., Skytthe, A., Vach, W., Knudsen, L. B., Andersen, A. M., Murray, J. C., et al. (2005). Parent's age and the risk of oral clefts. *Epidemiology* 16(3), 311–316. doi: 10.1097/01.ede.0000158745.84019.c2

Blanton, S. H., Cortez, A., Stal, S., Mulliken, J. B., Finnell, R. H., and Hecht, J. T. (2005). Variation in IRF6 contributes to nonsyndromic cleft lip and palate. *Am. J. Med. Genet A* 137A(3), 259–262. doi: 10.1002/ajmg.a.30887

Block, S. R., Watkins, S. M., Salemi, J. L., Rutkowski, R., Tanner, J. P., Correia, J. A., et al. (2013). Maternal pre-pregnancy body mass index and risk of selected birth defects: evidence of a dose-response relationship. *Paediatr. Peri. Epidemiol.* 27(6), 521–531. doi: 10.1111/ppe.12084

Bohmer, A. C., Mangold, E., Tessmann, P., Mossey, P. A., Steegers-Theunissen, R. P., Lindemans, J., et al. (2013). Analysis of susceptibility loci for nonsyndromic orofacial clefting in a European trio sample. *Am. J. Med. Genet A* 161A(10), 2545–2549. doi: 10.1002/ajmg.a.36141

Boyles, A. L., Wilcox, A. J., Taylor, J. A., Meyer, K., Fredriksen, A., Ueland, P. M., et al. (2008). Folate and one-carbon metabolism gene polymorphisms and their associations with oral facial clefts. *Am. J. Med. Genet A* 146A(4), 440–449. doi: 10.1002/ajmg.a.32162

Boyles, A. L., Wilcox, A. J., Taylor, J. A., Shi, M., Weinberg, C. R., Meyer, K., et al. (2009). Oral facial clefts and gene polymorphisms in metabolism of folate/one-carbon and vitamin A: a pathway-wide association study. *Genet Epidemiol.* 33(3), 247–255. doi: 10.1002/gepi.20376

Brender, J. D., Werler, M. M., Shinde, M. U., Vuong, A. M., Kelley, K. E., Huber, J. C. Jr., et al. (2012). Nitrosatable drug exposure during the first trimester of pregnancy and selected congenital malformations. *Bir. Def. Res. A Clin. Mol. Teratol.* 94(9), 701–713. doi: 10.1002/bdra.23060

Brender, J. D., Weyer, P. J., Romitti, P. A., Mohanty, B. P., Shinde, M. U., Vuong, A. M., et al. (2013). Prenatal nitrate intake from drinking water and selected birth defects in offspring of participants in the national birth defects prevention study. *Environ. Health Perspect.* 121(9), 1083–1089. doi: 10.1289/ehp.1206249

Burdi, A.R., and Faist, K. (1967). Morphogenesis of the palate in normal human embryos with special emphasis on the mechanisms involved. *Am. J. Anat.* 120, 149–159

Burg, M. L., Chai, Y., Yao, C. A., Magee, W., 3rd., and Figueiredo, J. C. (2016). Epidemiology, Etiology, and Treatment of Isolated Cleft Palate. *Front. Physiol.* 7:67. doi: 10.3389/fphys.2016.00067

Butali, A., Mossey, P. A., Adeyemo, W. L., Eshete, M. A., Gowans, L. J. J., Busch, T. D., et al. (2019). Genomic analyses in African populations identify novel risk loci for cleft palate. *Hum. Mol. Genet.* 28(6), 1038–1051. doi: 10.1093/hmg/ddy402

Butali, A., Suzuki, S., Cooper, M. E., Mansilla, A. M., Cuenco, K., Leslie, E. J., et al. (2013). Replication of genome wide association identified candidate genes confirm the role of common and rare variants in PAX7 and VAX1 in the etiology of nonsyndromic CL(P). *Am. J. Med. Genet. A* 161A(5), 965–972. doi: 10.1002/ajmg.a.35749

Calzolari, E., Bianchi, F., Rubini, M., Ritvanen, A., Neville, A. J., and Group, E. W. (2004). Epidemiology of cleft palate in Europe: implications for genetic research. *Cleft. Palate Craniofac. J.* 41(3), 244–249. doi: 10.1597/02-074.1

Canfield, M. A., Collins, J. S., Botto, L. D., Williams, L. J., Mai, C. T., Kirby, R. S., et al. (2005). Changes in the birth prevalence of selected birth defects after grain fortification with folic acid in the United States: findings from a multi-state population-based study. *Birt. Def. Res. A Clin. Mol. Teratol.* 73(10), 679–689. doi: 10.1002/bdra.20210

Carinci, F., Palmieri, A., Scapoli, L., Cura, F., Borelli, F., Morselli, P. G., et al. (2019). Non-syndromic cleft palate: association analysis on three gene polymorphisms of the folate pathway in Asian and Italian populations. *Int, J. Immunopathol. Pharmacol.* 33:2058738419858572. doi: 10.1177/2058738419858572

Carmichael, S. L., and Shaw, G. M. (1999). Maternal corticosteroid use and risk of selected congenital anomalies. *Am. J. Med. Genet* 86(3), 242–244.

Carter, T. C., Molloy, A. M., Pangilinan, F., Troendle, J. F., Kirke, P. N., Conley, M. R., et al. (2010). Testing reported associations of genetic risk factors for oral clefts in a large Irish study population. *Bir. Def. Res. A. Clin. Mol. Teratol.* 88(2), 84–93. doi: 10.1002/bdra.20639

Casey, L. M., Lan, Y., Cho, E. S., Maltby, K. M., Gridley, T., and Jiang, R. (2006). Jag2-Notch1 signaling regulates oral epithelial differentiation and palate development. *Dev. Dyn.* 235(7), 1830–1844. doi: 10.1002/dvdy.20821

Castanet, M., Park, S. M., Smith, A., Bost, M., Leger, J., Lyonnet, S., et al. (2002). A novel loss-of-function mutation in TTF-2 is associated with congenital hypothyroidism, thyroid agenesis and cleft palate. *Hum. Mol. Genet* 11(17), 2051–2059. doi: 10.1093/hmg/11.17.2051

Chevrier, C., Perret, C., Bahuau, M., Zhu, H., Nelva, A., Herman, C., et al. (2007). Fetal and maternal MTHFR C677T genotype, maternal folate intake and the risk of nonsyndromic oral clefts. *Am. J. Med. Genet A* 143, 248–257.

Chiquet, B. T., Lidral, A. C., Stal, S., Mulliken, J. B., Moreno, L. M., Arcos-Burgos, M., et al. (2007). CRISPLD2: a novel NSCLP candidate gene. *Hum. Mol. Genet* 16(18), 2241–2248. doi: 10.1093/hmg/ddm176

Cohen, M. M. Jr. (1978). Syndromes with cleft lip and cleft palate. *Cleft. Palate J.* 15, 306–328.

Correa, A., Gilboa, S. M., Besser, L. M., Botto, L. D., Moore, C. A., Hobbs, C. A., et al. (2008). Diabetes mellitus and birth defects. *Am. J. Obstet. Gynecol.* 199(3), e231–239. doi: 10.1016/j.ajog.2008.06.028

Cox, N. J., Frigge, M., Nicolae, D. L., Concannon, P., Hanis, C. L., Bell, G. I., et al. (1999). Loci on chromosomes 2 (NIDDM1) and 15 interact to increase susceptibility to diabetes in Mexican Americans. *Nat. Genet* 21(2), 213–215. doi: 10.1038/6002

Czerwinska, A. M., Nowacka, J., Aszer, M., Gawrzak, S., Archacka, K., Fogtman, A., et al. (2016). Cell cycle regulation of embryonic stem cells and mouse embryonic fibroblasts lacking functional Pax7. *Cell Cycle* 15(21), 2931–2942. doi: 10.1080/15384101.2016.1231260

Danescu, A., Mattson, M., Dool, C., Diewert, V. M., and Richman, J. M. (2015). Analysis of human soft palate morphogenesis supports regional regulation of palatal fusion. *J. Anat.* 227(4), 474–486. doi: 10.1111/joa.12365

De Felice, M., Ovitt, C., Biffali, E., Rodriguez-Mallon, A., Arra, C., Anastassiadis, K., et al. (1998). A mouse model for hereditary thyroid dysgenesis and cleft palate. *Nat. Genet.* 19(4), 395–398. doi: 10.1038/1289

de la Garza, G., Schleiffarth, J. R., Dunnwald, M., Mankad, A., Weirather, J. L., Bonde, G., et al. (2013). Interferon regulatory factor 6 promotes differentiation of the periderm by activating expression of Grainyhead-like 3. *J. Invest. Dermatol.* 133(1), 68–77. doi: 10.1038/jid.2012.269

De-Regil, L. M., Pena-Rosas, J. P., Fernandez-Gaxiola, A. C., and Rayco-Solon, P. (2015). Effects and safety of periconceptional oral folate supplementation for preventing birth defects. *Cochrane. Datab. Syst. Rev.* 12:CD007950. doi: 10.1002/14651858.CD007950.pub3

DeRoo, L. A., Wilcox, A. J., Drevon, C. A., and Lie, R. T. (2008). First-trimester maternal alcohol consumption and the risk of infant oral clefts in Norway: a population-based case-control study. *Am. J. Epidemiol.* 168(6), 638–646. doi: 10.1093/aje/kwn186

Diewert, V.M., and Lozanoff, S. (2002). "Animal models of facial clefting: experimental, congenital,and transgenic," in *Understanding Craniofacial Anomalies: The Etiopathogenesis of Craniosynostoses and Facial Clefting*, eds. M.P. Mooney & M.I. Siegel. (New York, NY: Wiley-Liss), 251–272.

Dixon, J., Jones, N. C., Sandell, L. L., Jayasinghe, S. M., Crane, J., Rey, J. P., et al. (2006). Tcof1/Treacle is required for neural crest cell formation and proliferation deficiencies that cause craniofacial abnormalities. *Proc. Natl. Acad. Sci. U S A.* 103(36), 13403–13408. doi: 10.1073/pnas.0603730103

Dixon, M. J., Marazita, M. L., Beaty, T. H., and Murray, J. C. (2011). Cleft lip and palate: understanding genetic and environmental influences. *Nat. Rev. Genet.* 12, 167–178.

Dobreva, G., Dambacher, J., and Grosschedl, R. (2003). SUMO modification of a novel MAR-binding protein, SATB2, modulates immunoglobulin mu gene expression. *Genes. Dev.* 17(24), 3048–3061. doi: 10.1101/gad.1153003

Duan, S. J., Huang, N., Zhang, B. H., Shi, J. Y., He, S., Ma, J., et al. (2017). New insights from GWAS for the cleft palate among han Chinese population. *Med. Oral. Patol. Oral. Cir. Bucal.* 22(2), e219–e227. doi: 10.4317/medoral.21439

Eberhart, J. K., He, X., Swartz, M. E., Yan, Y. L., Song, H., Boling, T. C., et al. (2008). MicroRNA Mirn140 modulates Pdgf signaling during palatogenesis. *Nat. Genet.* 40(3), 290–298. doi: 10.1038/ng.82

Fan, R., Lee, A., Lu, Z., Liu, A., Troendle, J. F., and Mills, J. L. (2013). Association analysis of complex diseases using triads, parent-child dyads and singleton monads. *BMC Genet.* 14:78. doi: 10.1186/1471-2156-1478

Ferguson, M. W. (1988). Palate development. *Development* 103, 41–60.

Finnell, R. H., Shaw, G. M., Lammer, E. J., Brandl, K. L., Carmichael, S. L., and Rosenquist, T. H. (2004). Gene-nutrient interactions: importance of folates and retinoids during early embryogenesis. *Toxicol. Appl. Pharmacol.* 198(2), 75–85. doi: 10.1016/j.taap.2003.09.031

Fu, X., Cheng, Y., Yuan, J., Huang, C., Cheng, H., and Zhou, R. (2015). Loss-of-function mutation in the X-linked TBX22 promoter disrupts an ETS-1 binding site and leads to cleft palate. *Hum. Genet.* 134(2), 147–158. doi: 10.1007/s00439-014-15031508

Garne, E., Hansen, A. V., Morris, J., Zaupper, L., Addor, M. C., Barisic, I., et al. (2015). Use of asthma medication during pregnancy and risk of specific congenital anomalies: a European case-malformed control study. *J. Allerg. Clin. Immunol.* 136(6), 1496–1502 e. doi: 10.1016/j.jaci.2015.05.043

Ghassibe, M., Bayet, B., Revencu, N., Verellen-Dumoulin, C., Gillerot, Y., Vanwijck, R., et al. (2005). Interferon regulatory factor-6: a gene predisposing to isolated cleft lip with or without cleft palate in the Belgian population. *Eur. J. Hum. Genet.* 13(11), 1239–1242. doi: 10.1038/sj.ejhg.5201486

Ghassibe-Sabbagh, M., Desmyter, L., Langenberg, T., Claes, F., Boute, O., Bayet, B., et al. (2011). FAF1, a gene that is disrupted in cleft palate and has conserved function in zebrafish. *Am. J. Hum. Genet.* 88(2), 150–161. doi: 10.1016/j.ajhg.2011.01.003

Ghioni, P., D'Alessandra, Y., Mansueto, G., Jaffray, E., Hay, R. T., La Mantia, G., et al. (2005). The protein stability and transcriptional activity of p63alpha are regulated by SUMO-1 conjugation. *Cell. Cycle* 4(1), 183–190. doi: 10.4161/cc.4.1.1359

Gibbins, J. R., Manthey, A., Tazawa, Y. M., Scott, B., Bloch-Zupan, A., and Hunter, N. (1999). Midline fusion in the formation of the secondary palate anticipated by upregulation of keratin K5/6 and localized expression of vimentin mRNA in medial edge epithelium. *Int. J. Dev. Biol.* 43, 237–244.

Gilboa, S. M., Broussard, C. S., Devine, O. J., Duwe, K. N., Flak, A. L., Boulet, S. L., et al. (2011). Influencing clinical practice regarding the use of antiepileptic medications during pregnancy: modeling the potential impact on the prevalences of spina bifida and cleft palate in the United States. *Am. J. Med. Genet. C Semin. Med. Genet.* 157C(3), 234–246. doi: 10.1002/ajmg.c.30306

Goffinet, L., Oussalah, A., Gueant-Rodriguez, R. M., Chery, C., Basha, M., Avogbe, P. H., et al. (2016). Cystathionine beta-synthase genetic variant rs2124459 is associated with a reduced risk of cleft palate in French and Belgian populations. *J. Med. Genet* 53(12), 828–834. doi: 10.1136/jmedgenet-2016104111

Gowans, L. J., Adeyemo, W. L., Eshete, M., Mossey, P. A., Busch, T., Aregbesola, B., et al. (2016). Association Studies and Direct DNA Sequencing Implicate Genetic Susceptibility Loci in the Etiology of Nonsyndromic Orofacial Clefts in Sub-Saharan African Populations. *J. Dent. Res.* 95(11), 1245–1256. doi: 10.1177/0022034516657003

Grosen, D., Chevrier, C., Skytthe, A., Bille, C., Molsted, K., Sivertsen, A., et al. (2010). A cohort study of recurrence patterns among more than 54,000 relatives of oral cleft cases in Denmark: support for the multifactorial threshold model of inheritance. *J. Med. Genet* 47(3), 162–168. doi: 10.1136/jmg.2009.069385

Gu, M., Zhang, Y., Liu, H., Liu, J., Zhu, D., and Yang, X. (2018). MSH homeobox 1 polymorphisms and the risk of non-syndromic orofacial clefts: a meta-analysis. *Eur. J. Oral. Sci.* 126(3), 180–185. doi: 10.1111/eos.12414

Haaland, O. A., Jugessur, A., Gjerdevik, M., Romanowska, J., Shi, M., Beaty, T. H., et al. (2017). Genome-wide analysis of parent-of-origin interaction effects with environmental exposure (PoOxE): an application to European and Asian cleft palate trios. *PLoS One* 12(9):e0184358. doi: 10.1371/journal.pone.0184358

He, M., and Bian, Z. (2016). Lack of Association between Missense Variants in GRHL3 (rs2486668 and rs545809) and Susceptibility to Non-Syndromic Orofacial Clefts in a Han Chinese Population. *PLoS One* 11(7):e0159940. doi: 10.1371/journal.pone.0159940

Herkrath, A. P., Herkrath, F. J., Rebelo, M. A., and Vettore, M. V. (2012). Parental age as a risk factor for non-syndromic oral clefts: a meta-analysis. *J. Dent.* 40(1), 3–14. doi: 10.1016/j.jdent.2011.10.002

Hernandez, R. K., Werler, M. M., Romitti, P., Sun, L., Anderka, M., and National Birth Defects Prevention, S. (2012). Nonsteroidal antiinflammatory drug use among women and the risk of birth defects. *Am. J. Obstet. Gynecol.* 206(3), e221–228. doi: 10.1016/j.ajog.2011.11.019

Hoebel, A. K., Drichel, D., van de Vorst, M., Bohmer, A. C., Sivalingam, S., Ishorst, N., et al. (2017). Candidate Genes for Nonsyndromic Cleft Palate Detected by Exome Sequencing. *J. Dent. Res.* 96(11), 1314–1321. doi: 10.1177/0022034517722761

Hu, J., Lu, J., Lian, G., Ferland, R. J., Dettenhofer, M., and Sheen, V. L. (2014). Formin 1 and filamin B physically interact to coordinate chondrocyte proliferation and differentiation in the growth plate. *Hum. Mol. Genet.* 23(17), 4663–4673. doi: 10.1093/hmg/ddu186

Huang, L., Jia, Z., Shi, Y., Du, Q., Shi, J., Wang, Z., et al. (2019). Genetic factors define CPO and CLO subtypes of nonsyndromicorofacial cleft. *PLoS Genet.* 15(10):e1008357. doi: 10.1371/journal.pgen.1008357

Huang, Y. Q., Ma, J., Ma, M., Deng, Y., Li, Y. D., Ren, H. W., et al. (2011). Association between MSX1 variants and oral clefts in Han Chinese in western China. *DNA Cell Biol.* 30(12), 1057–1061. doi: 10.1089/dna.2010.1208

Huybrechts, K. F., Hernandez-Diaz, S., Straub, L., Gray, K. J., Zhu, Y., Patorno, E., et al. (2018). Association of Maternal First-Trimester Ondansetron Use With Cardiac Malformations and Oral Clefts in Offspring. *JAMA* 320(23), 2429–2437. doi: 10.1001/jama.2018.18307

Hwang, B. F., Jaakkola, J. J., and Guo, H. R. (2008). Water disinfection by-products and the risk of specific birth defects: a population-based cross-sectional study in Taiwan. *Environ. Health* 7:23. doi: 10.1186/1476-069X-723

Ingrid Goh, Y., Bollano, E., Einarson, T. R., and Koren, G. (2006). Prenatal multivitamin supplementation and rates of congenital anomalies: a meta-analysis. *J. Obstet. Gynaecol. Can.* 28(8), 680–689. doi: 10.1016/S1701-2163(16) 3222732227

Ito, Y., Yeo, J. Y., Chytil, A., Han, J., Bringas, P. Jr., et al. (2003). Conditional inactivation of Tgfbr2 in cranial neural crest causes cleft palate and calvaria defects. *Development* 130(21), 5269–5280. doi: 10.1242/dev.00708

Jagomagi, T., Nikopensius, T., Krjutskov, K., Tammekivi, V., Viltrop, T., Saag, M., et al. (2010). MTHFR and MSX1 contribute to the risk of nonsyndromic cleft lip/palate. *Eur. J. Oral. Sci.* 118(3), 213–220. doi: 10.1111/j.1600-0722.2010. 00729.x

Jezewski, P. A., Vieira, A. R., Nishimura, C., Ludwig, B., Johnson, M., O'Brien, S. E., et al. (2003). Complete sequencing shows a role for MSX1 in non-syndromic cleft lip and palate. *J. Med. Genet.* 40(6), 399–407. doi: 10.1136/jmg.40.6.399

Jia, Z. L., He, S., Jiang, S. Y., Zhang, B. H., Duan, S. J., Shi, J. Y., et al. (2017). Rs12941170 at SOX9 gene associated with orofacial clefts in Chinese. *Arch. Oral. Biol.* 76, 14–19. doi: 10.1016/j.archoralbio.2016.12.010

Johansen, A. M., Lie, R. T., Wilcox, A. J., Andersen, L. F., and Drevon, C. A. (2008). Maternal dietary intake of vitamin A and risk of orofacial clefts: a population-based case-control study in Norway. *Am. J. Epidemiol.* 167(10), 1164–1170. doi: 10.1093/aje/kwn035

Johnson, C. Y., and Little, J. (2008). Folate intake, markers of folate status and oral clefts: is the evidence converging? *Int. J. Epidemiol.* 37(5), 1041–1058. doi: 10.1093/ije/dyn098

Jugessur, A., Lie, R. T., Wilcox, A. J., Murray, J. C., Taylor, J. A., Saugstad, O. D., et al. (2003a). Cleft palate, transforming growth factor alpha gene variants, and maternal exposures: assessing gene-environment interactions in case-parent triads. *Genet Epidemiol.* 25(4), 367–374. doi: 10.1002/gepi.10268

Jugessur, A., Rahimov, F., Lie, R. T., Wilcox, A. J., Gjessing, H. K., Nilsen, R. M., et al. (2008). Genetic variants in IRF6 and the risk of facial clefts: single-marker and haplotype-based analyses in a population-based case-control study of facial clefts in Norway. *Genet Epidemiol.* 32(5), 413–424. doi: 10.1002/gepi.20314

Jugessur, A., Shi, M., Gjessing, H. K., Lie, R. T., Wilcox, A. J., Weinberg, C. R., et al. (2010). Maternal genes and facial clefts in offspring: a comprehensive search for genetic associations in two population-based cleft studies from Scandinavia. *PLoS One* 5(7):e11493. doi: 10.1371/journal.pone.0011493

Jugessur, A., Skare, O., Lie, R. T., Wilcox, A. J., Christensen, K., Christiansen, L., et al. (2012). X-linked genes and risk of orofacial clefts: evidence from two population-based studies in Scandinavia. *PLoS One* 7(6):e39240. doi: 10.1371/journal.pone.0039240

Jugessur, A., Wilcox, A. J., Lie, R. T., Murray, J. C., Taylor, J. A., Ulvik, A., et al. (2003b). Exploring the effects of methylenetetrahydrofolate reductase gene variants C677T and A1298C on the risk of orofacial clefts in 261 Norwegian case-parent triads. *Am. J. Epidemiol.* 157(12), 1083–1091. doi: 10.1093/aje/kwg097

Jumlongras, D., Bei, M., Stimson, J. M., Wang, W. F., DePalma, S. R., Seidman, C. E., et al. (2001). A nonsense mutation in MSX1 causes Witkop syndrome. *Am. J. Hum. Genet* 69(1), 67–74. doi: 10.1086/321271

Kannu, P., Bateman, J., and Savarirayan, R. (2012). Clinical phenotypes associated with type II collagen mutations. *J. Paediatr. Child. Health* 48(2), E38–43. doi: 10.1111/j.1440-1754.2010.01979.x

Kaufman, J. A., Wright, J. M., Evans, A., Rivera-Nunez, Z., Meyer, A., and Narotsky, M. G. (2018). Associations Between Disinfection By-Product Exposures and Craniofacial Birth Defects. *J. Occup. Environ. Med.* 60(2), 109–119. doi: 10. 1097/JOM.0000000000001191

Kondo, S., Schutte, B. C., Richardson, R. J., Bjork, B. C., Knight, A. S., Watanabe, Y., et al. (2002). Mutations in IRF6 cause Van der Woude and popliteal pterygium syndromes. *Nat. Genet* 32(2), 285–289. doi: 10.1038/ng985

Krasone, K., Lace, B., Akota, I., Care, R., Deeley, K., Kuchler, E. C., et al. (2014). IRF6 AP-2a binding site promoter polymorphism is associated with oral clefts in Latvia. *Stomatologija* 16, 132–136.

Kuchler, E. C., Saboia, T. M., Vieira, T. C., Lips, A., Tannure, P. N., Deeley, K., et al. (2014). Studies of genes involved in craniofacial development and tumorigenesis: FGF3 contributes to isolated oral clefts and may interact with PAX9. *Acta Odontol. Scand.* 72(8), 1070–1078. doi: 10.3109/00016357.2014. 903514

Lammer, E. J., Mohammed, N., Iovannisci, D. M., Ma, C., Lidral, A. C., and Shaw, G. M. (2016). Genetic variation of FOXE1 and risk for orofacial clefts in a California population. *Am. J. Med. Genet A* 170(11), 2770–2776. doi: 10.1002/ajmg.a.37871

Lee, H., Quinn, J. C., Prasanth, K. V., Swiss, V. A., Economides, K. D., Camacho, M. M., et al. (2006). PIAS1 confers DNA-binding specificity on the Msx1 homeoprotein. *Genes Dev.* 20(7), 784–794. doi: 10.1101/gad.1392006

Leslie, E. J., Liu, H., Carlson, J. C., Shaffer, J. R., Feingold, E., Wehby, G., et al. (2016). A Genome-wide Association Study of Nonsyndromic Cleft Palate Identifies an Etiologic Missense Variant in GRHL3. *Am. J. Hum. Genet* 98(4), 744–754. doi: 10.1016/j.ajhg.2016.02.014

Letra, A., Fakhouri, W., Fonseca, R. F., Menezes, R., Kempa, I., Prasad, J. L., et al. (2012). Interaction between IRF6 and TGFA genes contribute to the risk of nonsyndromic cleft lip/palate. *PLoS One* 7(9):e45441. doi: 10.1371/journal. pone.0045441

Letra, A., Menezes, R., Granjeiro, J. M., and Vieira, A. R. (2009). AXIN2 and CDH1 polymorphisms, tooth agenesis, and oral clefts. *Birt. Defects. Res. A Clin. Mol. Teratol.* 85(2), 169–173. doi: 10.1002/bdra.20489

Li, L., Zhu, G. Q., Meng, T., Shi, J. Y., Wu, J., Xu, X., et al. (2011). Biological and epidemiological evidence of interaction of infant genotypes at Rs7205289 and maternal passive smoking in cleft palate. *Am. J. Med. Genet A* 155A(12), 2940–2948. doi: 10.1002/ajmg.a.34254

Lidral, A. C., Liu, H., Bullard, S. A., Bonde, G., Machida, J., Visel, A., et al. (2015). A single nucleotide polymorphism associated with isolated cleft lip and palate, thyroid cancer and hypothyroidism alters the activity of an oral epithelium and thyroid enhancer near FOXE1. *Hum. Mol. Genet* 24(14), 3895–3907. doi: 10.1093/hmg/ddv047

Lidral, A. C., Murray, J. C., Buetow, K. H., Basart, A. M., Schearer, H., Shiang, R., et al. (1997). Studies of the candidate genes TGFB2, MSX1, TGFA, and TGFB3 in the etiology of cleft lip and palate in the Philippines. *Cleft Palate Craniofac. J.* 34, 1–6.

Lidral, A. C., Romitti, P. A., Basart, A. M., Doetschman, T., Leysens, N. J., Daack-Hirsch, S., et al. (1998). Association of MSX1 and TGFB3 with nonsyndromic clefting in humans. *Am. J. Hum. Genet* 63(2), 557–568. doi: 10.1086/301956

Little, J., Cardy, A., and Munger, R. G. (2004). Tobacco smoking and oral clefts: a meta-analysis. *Bull. World Health Organ.* 82, 213–218.

Little, J., Gilmour, M., Mossey, P. A., Fitzpatrick, D., Cardy, A., Clayton-Smith, J., et al. (2008). Folate and clefts of the lip and palate–a U.K.*-based case-control study: Part II: Biochemical and genetic analysis. Cleft. Palate Craniofac. J.* 45(4), 428–438. doi: 10.1597/06-151.1

Liu, H., Busch, T., Eliason, S., Anand, D., Bullard, S., Gowans, L. J. J., et al. (2017). Exome sequencing provides additional evidence for the involvement of ARHGAP29 in Mendelian orofacial clefting and extends the phenotypic spectrum to isolated cleft palate. *Bir. Defects. Res.* 109(1), 27–37. doi: 10.1002/bdra.23596

Liu, K., Lu, Y., Ai, L., Jiao, B., Yu, J., Zhang, B., et al. (2015). Association between FOXE1 and non-syndromic orofacial clefts in a northeastern Chinese population. *Br. J. Oral. Maxillofac. Surg.* 53(8), 705–710. doi: 10.1016/j.bjoms. 2015.05.021

Ludwig, K. U., Bohmer, A. C., Bowes, J., Nikolic, M., Ishorst, N., Wyatt, N., et al. (2017). Imputation of orofacial clefting data identifies novel risk loci and sheds light on the genetic background of cleft lip +/- cleft palate and cleft palate only. *Hum. Mol. Genet* 26(4), 829–842. doi: 10.1093/hmg/ddx012

Ludwig, K. U., Bohmer, A. C., Rubini, M., Mossey, P. A., Herms, S., Nowak, S., et al. (2014). Strong association of variants around FOXE1 and orofacial clefting. *J. Dent. Res.* 93(4), 376–381. doi: 10.1177/0022034514523987

Ludwig, K. U., Mangold, E., Herms, S., Nowak, S., Reutter, H., Paul, A., et al. (2012). Genome-wide meta-analyses of nonsyndromic cleft lip with or without cleft palate identify six new risk loci. *Nat. Genet* 44(9), 968–971. doi: 10.1038/ng.2360

Luo, Y. L., Cheng, Y. L., Ye, P., Wang, W., Gao, X. H., and Chen, Q. (2012). Association between MTHFR polymorphisms and orofacial clefts risk: a meta-analysis. *Bir. Defects. Res. A Clin. Mol. Teratol.* 94(4), 237–244. doi: 10.1002/bdra.23005

Ma, L., Xu, M., Li, D., Han, Y., Wang, Z., Yuan, H., et al. (2014). A miRNA-binding-site SNP of MSX1 is Associated with NSOC Susceptibility. *J. Dent. Res.* 93(6), 559–564. doi: 10.1177/0022034514527617

Machado, R. A., Messetti, A. C., de Aquino, S. N., Martelli-Junior, H., Swerts, M. S., de Almeida Reis, S. R., et al. (2016). Association Between Genes Involved in Craniofacial Development and Nonsyndromic Cleft Lip and/or Palate in the Brazilian Population. *Cleft. Palate Craniofac. J.* 53(5), 550–556. doi: 10.1597/15107

Mangold, E., Bohmer, A. C., Ishorst, N., Hoebel, A. K., Gultepe, P., Schuenke, H., et al. (2016). Sequencing the GRHL3 Coding Region Reveals Rare Truncating Mutations and a Common Susceptibility Variant for Nonsyndromic Cleft Palate. *Am. J. Hum. Genet* 98(4), 755–762. doi: 10.1016/j.ajhg.2016.02.013

Marcano, A. C., Doudney, K., Braybrook, C., Squires, R., Patton, M. A., Lees, M. M., et al. (2004). TBX22 mutations are a frequent cause of cleft palate. *J. Med. Genet* 41(1), 68–74. doi: 10.1136/jmg.2003.010868

McCarthy, N., Liu, J. S., Richarte, A. M., Eskiocak, B., Lovely, C. B., Tallquist, M. D., et al. (2016). Pdgfra and Pdgfrb genetically interact during craniofacial development. *Dev. Dyn.* 245(6), 641–652. doi: 10.1002/dvdy.24403

Meng, L., Bian, Z., Torensma, R., and Von den Hoff, J. W. (2009). Biological mechanisms in palatogenesis and cleft palate. *J. Dent. Res.* 88(1), 22–33. doi: 10.1177/0022034508327868

Merritt, L. (2005). Part 1. *Understanding the embryology and genetics of cleft lip and palate. Adv. Neonatal. Care* 5(2), 64–71. doi: 10.1016/j.adnc.2004.12.006

Messetti, A. C., Machado, R. A., de Oliveira, C. E., Martelli-Junior, H., de Almeida Reis, S. R., Moreira, H. S., et al. (2017). Brazilian multicenter study of association between polymorphisms in CRISPLD2 and JARID2 and non-syndromic oral clefts. *J. Oral. Pathol. Med.* 46(3), 232–239. doi: 10.1111/jop.12470

Metneki, J., Puho, E., and Czeizel, A. E. (2005). Maternal diseases and isolated orofacial clefts in Hungary. *Bir. Defec. Res. A Clin. Mol. Teratol.* 73(9), 617–623. doi: 10.1002/bdra.20177

Mills, J. L., Molloy, A. M., Parle-McDermott, A., Troendle, J. F., Brody, L. C., Conley, M. R., et al. (2008). Folate-related gene polymorphisms as risk factors for cleft lip and cleft palate. *Bir. Defec. Res. A Clin. Mol. Teratol.* 82(9), 636–643. doi: 10.1002/bdra.20491

Modesto, A., Moreno, L. M., Krahn, K., King, S., and Lidral, A. C. (2006). MSX1 and orofacial clefting with and without tooth agenesis. *J. Dent. Res.* 85(6), 542–546. doi: 10.1177/154405910608500612

Monsoro-Burq, A. H. (2015). PAX transcription factors in neural crest development. *Semin. Cell Dev. Biol.* 44, 87–96. doi: 10.1016/j.semcdb.2015.09.015

Moreno, L. M., Mansilla, M. A., Bullard, S. A., Cooper, M. E., Busch, T. D., Machida, J., et al. (2009). FOXE1 association with both isolated cleft lip with or without cleft palate, and isolated cleft palate. *Hum. Mol. Genet* 18(24), 4879–4896. doi: 10.1093/hmg/ddp444

Morkuniene, A., Steponaviciut, D., Utkus, A., and Kucinskas, V. (2007). Few associations of candidate genes with nonsyndromic orofacial clefts in the population of Lithuania. *J. Appl. Genet* 48(1), 89–91. doi: 10.1007/BF03194663

Mossey, P. A., and Modell, B. (2012). Epidemiology of oral clefts 2012: an international perspective. *Front. Oral. Biol.* 16, 1–18. doi: 10.1159/000337464

Mossey, P. A., Little, J., Munger, R. G., Dixon, M. J., and Shaw, W. C. (2009). Cleft lip and palate. *Lancet* 374(9703), 1773–1785. doi: 10.1016/S0140-6736(09)6069560694

Mossey, P. A., Little, J., Steegers-Theunissen, R., Molloy, A., Peterlin, B., Shaw, W. C., et al. (2017). Genetic Interactions in Nonsyndromic Orofacial Clefts in Europe-EUROCRAN Study. *Cleft. Palate Craniofac. J.* 54(6), 623–630. doi: 10.1597/16037

Mossey, P.A., and Catilla, E.E. (2003). *Global registry and database on craniofacial anomalies: report of a WHO Registry Meeting on Craniofacial Anomalies.* Geneva: World Health Organization.

Munger, R. G., Tamura, T., Johnston, K. E., Feldkamp, M. L., Pfister, R., and Carey, J. C. (2009). Plasma zinc concentrations of mothers and the risk of oral clefts in their children in Utah. *Bir. Defects. Res. A Clin. Mol. Teratol.* 85(2), 151–155. doi: 10.1002/bdra.20516

Murray, J. C. (2002). Gene/environment causes of cleft lip and/or palate. *Clin. Genet* 61(4), 248–256. doi: 10.1034/j.1399-0004.2002.610402.x

Nikopensius, T., Jagomagi, T., Krjutskov, K., Tammekivi, V., Saag, M., Prane, I., et al. (2010). Genetic variants in COL2A1, COL11A2, and IRF6 contribute risk to nonsyndromic cleft palate. *Bir. Defects. Res. A Clin. Mol. Teratol.* 88(9), 748–756. doi: 10.1002/bdra.20700

Nikopensius, T., Kempa, I., Ambrozaityte, L., Jagomagi, T., Saag, M., Matuleviciene, A., et al. (2011). Variation in FGF1, FOXE1, and TIMP2 genes is associated with nonsyndromic cleft lip with or without cleft palate. *Bir. Def. Res. A Clin. Mol. Teratol.* 91(4), 218–225. doi: 10.1002/bdra.20791

Ottman, R. (1996). Gene-environment interaction: definitions and study designs. *Prev. Med.* 25(6), 764–770. doi: 10.1006/pmed.1996.0117

Palmieri, A., Scapoli, L., Carrozzo, M., Cura, F., Morselli, P. G., Pannuto, L., et al. (2020). ROCK1 is associated with non-syndromic cleft palate. *J. Oral. Pathol. Med.* 49(2), 164–168. doi: 10.1111/jop.12973

Pan, Y., Han, Y., Zhang, H., Zhou, L., Li, D., Cai, Q., et al. (2013). Association and cumulative effects of GWAS-identified genetic variants for nonsyndromic orofacial clefts in a Chinese population. *Environ. Mol. Mutagen.* 54(4), 261–267. doi: 10.1002/em.21773

Pankratz, N., Nichols, W. C., Uniacke, S. K., Halter, C., Murrell, J., Rudolph, A., et al. (2003). Genome-wide linkage analysis and evidence of gene-by-gene interactions in a sample of 362 multiplex Parkinson disease families. *Hum. Mol. Genet* 12(20), 2599–2608. doi: 10.1093/hmg/ddg270

Paranaiba, L. M., de Aquino, S. N., Bufalino, A., Martelli-Junior, H., Graner, E., Brito, L. A., et al. (2013). Contribution of polymorphisms in genes associated with craniofacial development to the risk of nonsyndromic cleft lip and/or palate in the Brazilian population. *Med. Oral. Patol. Oral. Cir. Bucal.* 18(3), e414–420. doi: 10.4317/medoral.18357

Pauws, E., Moore, G. E., and Stanier, P. (2009). A functional haplotype variant in the TBX22 promoter is associated with cleft palate and ankyloglossia. *J. Med. Genet* 46(8), 555–561. doi: 10.1136/jmg.2009.066902

Peyrard-Janvid, M., Leslie, E. J., Kousa, Y. A., Smith, T. L., Dunnwald, M., Magnusson, M., et al. (2014). Dominant mutations in GRHL3 cause Van der Woude Syndrome and disrupt oral periderm development. *Am. J. Hum. Genet* 94(1), 23–32. doi: 10.1016/j.ajhg.2013.11.009

Phillips, H. M., Papoutsi, T., Soenen, H., Ybot-Gonzalez, P., Henderson, D. J., and Chaudhry, B. (2012). Neural crest cell survival is dependent on Rho kinase and is required for development of the mid face in mouse embryos. *PLoS One* 7(5), e37685. doi: 10.1371/journal.pone.0037685

Rafighdoost, H., Hashemi, M., Narouei, A., Eskanadri-Nasab, E., Dashti-Khadivaki, G., and Taheri, M. (2013). Association between CDH1 and MSX1 gene polymorphisms and the risk of nonsyndromic cleft lip and/or cleft palate in a southeast Iranian population. *Cleft. Palate Craniofac. J.* 50(5), e98–e104. doi: 10.1597/12144

Rattanasopha, S., Tongkobpetch, S., Srichomthong, C., Siriwan, P., Suphapeetiporn, K., and Shotelersuk, V. (2012). PDGFRa mutations in humans with isolated cleft palate. *Eur. J. Hum. Genet* 20(10), 1058–1062. doi: 10.1038/ejhg.2012.55

Richardson, R. J., Dixon, J., Jiang, R., and Dixon, M. J. (2009). Integration of IRF6 and Jagged2 signalling is essential for controlling palatal adhesion and fusion competence. *Hum. Mol. Genet* 18(14), 2632–2642. doi: 10.1093/hmg/ddp201

Romitti, P. A., Sun, L., Honein, M. A., Reefhuis, J., Correa, A., and Rasmussen, S. A. (2007). Maternal periconceptional alcohol consumption and risk of orofacial clefts. *Am. J. Epidemiol.* 166(7), 775–785. doi: 10.1093/aje/kwm146

Sabbagh, H. J., Hassan, M. H., Innes, N. P., Elkodary, H. M., Little, J., and Mossey, P. A. (2015). Passive smoking in the etiology of non-syndromic orofacial clefts: a systematic review and meta-analysis. *PLoS One* 10(3):e0116963. doi: 10.1371/journal.pone.0116963

Satokata, I., and Maas, R. (1994). Msxl deficient mice exhibit cleft palate and abnormalities of craniofacial and tooth development. *Nat. Genet* 6(4), 348–356. doi: 10.1038/ng0494-348

Savitz, D. A., Schwingl, P. J., and Keels, M. A. (1991). Influence of paternal age, smoking, and alcohol consumption on congenital anomalies. *Teratology* 44(4), 429–440. doi: 10.1002/tera.1420440409

Scapoli, L., Palmieri, A., Martinelli, M., Pezzetti, F., Carinci, P., Tognon, M., et al. (2005). Strong evidence of linkage disequilibrium between polymorphisms at the IRF6 locus and nonsyndromic cleft lip with or without cleft palate, in an Italian population. *Am. J. Hum. Genet.* 76(1), 180–183. doi: 10.1086/427344

Sharp, G. C., Ho, K., Davies, A., Stergiakouli, E., Humphries, K., McArdle, W., et al. (2017). Distinct DNA methylation profiles in subtypes of orofacial cleft. *Clin. Epigenet.* 9:63. doi: 10.1186/s13148-017-0362362

Shaw, G. M., Iovannisci, D. M., Yang, W., Finnell, R. H., Carmichael, S. L., Cheng, S., et al. (2005). Endothelial nitric oxide synthase (NOS3) genetic variants, maternal smoking, vitamin use, and risk of human orofacial clefts. *Am. J. Epidemiol.* 162(12), 1207–1214. doi: 10.1093/aje/kwi336

Shaw, G. M., Todoroff, K., Finnell, R. H., Rozen, R., and Lammer, E. J. (1999). Maternal vitamin use, infant C677T mutation in MTHFR, and isolated cleft palate risk. *Am. J. Med. Genet* 85, 84–85.

Shaw, G. M., Yang, W., Perloff, S., Shaw, N. M., Carmichael, S. L., Zhu, H., et al. (2013). Thymidylate synthase polymorphisms and risks of human orofacial clefts. *Bir. Def. Res. A. Clin. Mol. Teratol.* 97(2), 95–100. doi: 10.1002/bdra.23114

Shaw, G. M., Zhu, H., Lammer, E. J., Yang, W., and Finnell, R. H. (2003). Genetic variation of infant reduced folate carrier (A80G) and risk of orofacial and conotruncal heart defects. *Am. J. Epidemiol.* 158(8), 747–752. doi: 10.1093/aje/kwg189

Shen, X., Liu, R. M., Yang, L., Wu, H., Li, P. Q., Liang, Y. L., et al. (2011). The CRISPLD2 gene is involved in cleft lip and/or cleft palate in a Chinese population. *Bir. Def. Res. A. Clin. Mol. Teratol.* 91(10), 918–924. doi: 10.1002/bdra.20840

Shi, M., Christensen, K., Weinberg, C. R., Romitti, P., Bathum, L., Lozada, A., et al. (2007). Orofacial cleft risk is increased with maternal smoking and specific detoxification-gene variants. *Am. J. Hum. Genet* 80, 76–90.

Shi, M., Mostowska, A., Jugessur, A., Johnson, M. K., Mansilla, M. A., Christensen, K., et al. (2009). Identification of microdeletions in candidate genes for cleft lip and/or palate. *Bir. Def. Res. A. Clin. Mol. Teratol.* 85(1), 42–51. doi: 10.1002/bdra.20571

Shi, M., Murray, J. C., Marazita, M. L., Munger, R. G., Ruczinski, I., Hetmanski, J. B., et al. (2012). Genome wide study of maternal and parent-of-origin effects on the etiology of orofacial clefts. *Am. J. Med. Genet A* 158A(4), 784–794. doi: 10.1002/ajmg.a.35257.

Skare, O., Gjessing, H. K., Gjerdevik, M., Haaland, O. A., Romanowska, J., Lie, R. T., et al. (2017). A new approach to chromosome-wide analysis of X-linked markers identifies new associations in Asian and European case-parent triads of orofacial clefts. *PLoS One* 12(9):e0183772. doi: 10.1371/journal.pone.0183772

Song, H., Wang, X., Yan, J., Mi, N., Jiao, X., Hao, Y., et al. (2017). Association of single-nucleotide polymorphisms of CDH1 with nonsyndromic cleft lip with or without cleft palate in a northern Chinese Han population. *Medicine* 96(5):e5574. doi: 10.1097/MD.0000000000005574

Song, Y., and Zhang, S. (2011). Association of CDH1 promoter polymorphism and the risk of non-syndromic orofacial clefts in a Chinese Han population. *Arch. Oral. Biol.* 56(1), 68–72. doi: 10.1016/j.archoralbio.2010.08.019

Souza, L. T., Kowalski, T. W., Vanz, A. P., Giugliani, R., and Felix, T. M. (2012). TGFA/Taq I polymorphism and environmental factors in non-syndromic oral clefts in Southern Brazil. *Braz. Oral. Res.* 26(5), 431–435. doi: 10.1590/s1806-83242012005000016

Srichomthong, C., Ittiwut, R., Siriwan, P., Suphapeetiporn, K., and Shotelersuk, V. (2013). FOXE1 mutations in Thai patients with oral clefts. *Genet Res.* 95(5), 133–137. doi: 10.1017/S0016672313000177

Srichomthong, C., Siriwan, P., and Shotelersuk, V. (2005). Significant association between IRF6 820G-A and non-syndromic cleft lip with or without cleft palate in the Thai population. *J. Med. Genet* 42(7):e46. doi: 10.1136/jmg.2005.032235

Stanier, P., and Moore, G. E. (2004). Genetics of cleft lip and palate: syndromic genes contribute to the incidence of non-syndromic clefts. *Hum. Mol. Genet* 13, R73–81. doi: 10.1093/hmg/ddh052

Stothard, K. J., Tennant, P. W., Bell, R., and Rankin, J. (2009). Maternal overweight and obesity and the risk of congenital anomalies: a systematic review and meta-analysis. *JAMA* 301(6), 636–650. doi: 10.1001/jama.2009.113

Sull, J. W., Liang, K. Y., Hetmanski, J. B., Fallin, M. D., Ingersoll, R. G., Park, J. W., et al. (2008). Excess maternal transmission of markers in TCOF1 among cleft palate case-parent trios from three populations. *Am. J. Med. Genet A* 146A(18), 2327–2331. doi: 10.1002/ajmg.a.32302

Suphapeetiporn, K., Tongkobpetch, S., Siriwan, P., and Shotelersuk, V. (2007). TBX22 mutations are a frequent cause of non-syndromic cleft palate in the Thai population. *Clin. Genet* 72(5), 478–483. doi: 10.1111/j.1399-0004.2007.00891.x

Sutton, M., Mills, J. L., Molloy, A. M., Troendle, J. F., Brody, L. C., Conley, M., et al. (2011). Maternal folate, vitamin B12 and homocysteine levels in pregnancies affected by congenital malformations other than neural tube defects. *Bir. Def. Res. A Clin. Mol. Teratol.* 91(7), 610–615. doi: 10.1002/bdra.20817

Suzuki, A., Sangani, D. R., Ansari, A., and Iwata, J. (2016). Molecular mechanisms of midfacial developmental defects. *Dev. Dyn.* 245(3), 276–293. doi: 10.1002/dvdy.24368

Swindell, E. C., Yuan, Q., Maili, L. E., Tandon, B., Wagner, D. S., and Hecht, J. T. (2015). Crispld2 is required for neural crest cell migration and cell viability during zebrafish craniofacial development. *Genesis* 53(10), 660–667. doi: 10.1002/dvg.22897

Tamura, T., Munger, R. G., Corcoran, C., Bacayao, J. Y., Nepomuceno, B., and Solon, F. (2005). Plasma zinc concentrations of mothers and the risk of nonsyndromic oral clefts in their children: a case-control study in the Philippines. *Bir. Def. Res. A Clin. Mol. Teratol.* 73(9), 612–616. doi: 10.1002/bdra.20179

Tang, W., Du, X., Feng, F., Long, J., Lin, Y., Li, P., et al. (2009). Association analysis between the IRF6 G820A polymorphism and nonsyndromic cleft lip and/or cleft palate in a Chinese population. *Cleft. Palate Craniofac. J.* 46(1), 89–92. doi: 10.1597/07-131.1

Tasanarong, P., Pabalan, N., Tharabenjasin, P., and Jarjanazi, H. (2019). MSX1 gene polymorphisms and non-syndromic cleft lip with or without palate (NSCL/P): A meta-analysis. *Oral. Dis.* 25(6), 1492–1501. doi: 10.1111/odi.13127

Tinker, S. C., Gilboa, S. M., Moore, C. A., Waller, D. K., Simeone, R. M., Kim, S. Y., et al. (2020). Specific birth defects in pregnancies of women with diabetes: National Birth Defects Prevention Study, 1997-2011. *Am. J. Obstet. Gynecol.* 222(2), 171–176 e. doi: 10.1016/j.ajog.2019.08.028

Tudela, C., Formoso, M. A., Martinez, T., Perez, R., Aparicio, M., Maestro, C., et al. (2002). TGF-beta3 is required for the adhesion and intercalation of medial edge epithelial cells during palate fusion. *Int. J. Dev. Biol.* 46, 333–336.

van Rooij, I. A., Wegerif, M. J., Roelofs, H. M., Peters, W. H., Kuijpers-Jagtman, A. M., Zielhuis, G. A., et al. (2001). Smoking, genetic polymorphisms in biotransformation enzymes, and nonsyndromic oral clefting: a gene-environment interaction. *Epidemiology* 12(5), 502–507. doi: 10.1097/00001648-200109000200109007

VanderMeer, J. E., Carter, T. C., Pangilinan, F., Mitchell, A., Kurnat-Thoma, E., Kirke, P. N., et al. (2016). Evaluation of proton-coupled folate transporter (SLC46A1) polymorphisms as risk factors for neural tube defects and oral clefts. *Am. J. Med. Genet A* 170A(4), 1007–1016. doi: 10.1002/ajmg.a.37539

Veau, V. (1931). *Division palatine: Anatomie—chirurgie phonétique*. Paris: Masson.

Venza, I., Visalli, M., Parrillo, L., De Felice, M., Teti, D., and Venza, M. (2011). MSX1 and TGF-beta3 are novel target genes functionally regulated by FOXE1. *Hum. Mol. Genet* 20(5), 1016–1025. doi: 10.1093/hmg/ddq547

Venza, M., Visalli, M., Venza, I., Torino, C., Tripodo, B., Melita, R., et al. (2009). Altered binding of MYF-5 to FOXE1 promoter in non-syndromic and CHARGE-associated cleft palate. *J. Oral. Pathol. Med.* 38(1), 18–23. doi: 10.1111/j.1600-0714.2008.00726.x

Wu, T., Schwender, H., Ruczinski, I., Murray, J. C., Marazita, M. L., Munger, R. G., et al. (2014). Evidence of gene-environment interaction for two genes on chromosome 4 and environmental tobacco smoke in controlling the risk of nonsyndromic cleft palate. *PLoS One* 9(2):e88088. doi: 10.1371/journal.pone.0088088

Wu-Chou, Y. H., Lu, Y. C., Chen, K. P., Chang, H. F., Lin, Y. T., and Lo, L. J. (2019). Association Studies Between Regulatory Regions of IRF6/TP63 Genes and Nonsyndromic Oral Clefts. *Cleft. Palate Craniofac. J.* 56(6), 778–785. doi: 10.1177/1055665618809244

Xu, W., Han, W., Lu, Y., Yao, W., Li, Z., Fang, K., et al. (2014). Microarray analysis of two single-nucleotide polymorphisms of transforming growth factor alpha in patients with nonsyndromic cleft of north china. *Cleft. Palate Craniofac. J.* 51(4), 486–492. doi: 10.1597/12145

Xu, Z., Lie, R. T., Wilcox, A. J., Saugstad, O. D., and Taylor, J. A. (2019). A comparison of DNA methylation in newborn blood samples from infants with and without orofacial clefts. *Clin. Epigenet.* 11(1):40. doi: 10.1186/s13148-019-0638639

Yin, X., Li, J., Li, Y., and Zou, S. (2019). Maternal alcohol consumption and oral clefts: a meta-analysis. *Br. J. Oral. Maxillofac. Surg.* 57(9), 839–846. doi: 10.1016/j.bjoms.2019.08.013

Zhu, H., Curry, S., Wen, S., Wicker, N. J., Shaw, G. M., Lammer, E. J., et al. (2005). Are the betaine-homocysteine methyltransferase (BHMT and BHMT2) genes risk factors for spina bifida and orofacial clefts? *Am. J. Med. Genet. A* 135(3), 274–277. doi: 10.1002/ajmg.a.30739

Zucchero, T. M., Cooper, M. E., Maher, B. S., Daack-Hirsch, S., Nepomuceno, B., Ribeiro, L., et al. (2004). Interferon regulatory factor 6 (IRF6) gene variants and the risk of isolated cleft lip or palate. *N. Engl. J. Med.* 351(8), 769–780. doi: 10.1056/NEJMoa032909

3

MicroRNA-135a Protects Against Ethanol-Induced Apoptosis in Neural Crest Cells and Craniofacial Defects in Zebrafish by Modulating the Siah1/p38/p53 Pathway

*Fuqiang Yuan[1,2], Yang Yun[1,2,3], Huadong Fan[1,2], Yihong Li[1,2], Lanhai Lu[1,2], Jie Liu[1,2], Wenke Feng[1,2,4] and Shao-yu Chen[1,2]**

[1] *Department of Pharmacology and Toxicology, University of Louisville Health Sciences Center, Louisville, KY, United States,* [2] *University of Louisville Alcohol Research Center, Louisville, KY, United States,* [3] *College of Environment and Resource, Research Center of Environment and Health, Shanxi University, Taiyuan, China,* [4] *Department of Medicine, University of Louisville, Louisville, KY, United States*

***Correspondence:**
Shao-yu Chen
shaoyu.chen@louisville.edu

MicroRNAs (miRNAs) are small non-coding RNAs that are involved in various biological processes, including apoptosis, by regulating gene expression. This study was designed to test the hypothesis that ethanol-induced downregulation of miR-135a contributes to ethanol-induced apoptosis in neural crest cells (NCCs) by upregulating Siah1 and activating the p38 mitogen-activated protein kinase (MAPK)/p53 pathway. We found that treatment with ethanol resulted in a significant decrease in miR-135a expression in both NCCs and zebrafish embryos. Ethanol-induced downregulation of miR-135a resulted in the upregulation of Siah1 and the activation of the p38 MAPK/p53 pathway and increased apoptosis in NCCs and zebrafish embryos. Ethanol exposure also resulted in growth retardation and developmental defects that are characteristic of fetal alcohol spectrum disorders (FASD) in zebrafish. Overexpression of miRNA-135a significantly reduced ethanol-induced upregulation of Siah1 and the activation of the p38 MAPK/p53 pathway and decreased ethanol-induced apoptosis in NCCs and zebrafish embryos. In addition, ethanol-induced growth retardation and craniofacial defects in zebrafish larvae were dramatically diminished by the microinjection of miRNA-135a mimics. These results demonstrated that ethanol-induced downregulation of miR-135a contributes to ethanol-induced apoptosis in NCCs by upregulating Siah1 and activating the p38 MAPK/p53 pathway and that the overexpression of miRNA-135a can protect against ethanol-induced apoptosis in NCCs and craniofacial defects in a zebrafish model of FASD.

Keywords: miRNA-135a, ethanol, apoptosis, neural crest cells, Siah1, craniofacial defects, zebrafish

---

Abbreviations: miRNA, microRNA; FASD, fetal alcohol spectrum disorders; NCCs, neural crest cells; Siah1, seven *in absentia* homolog 1; Bcl-2, B-cell lymphoma 2; Nrf2, nuclear factor (erythroid-derived 2)-like 2; MAPK, mitogen-activated protein kinase; 3′-UTRs, 3′-untranslated region; hpf, hours post-fertilization; dpf, days post fertilization; TUNEL, terminal deoxynucleotidyl transferase dUTP nick end labeling; Bak, Bcl-2 homologous antagonist/killer; PUMA, p53 upregulated modulator of apoptosis; m, Meckel's cartilage; e, ethmoid plate; t, trabeculae cranii; pq, palatoquadrate; hs, hyosymplectic; ch, ceratohyal; cb, ceratobranchial; bh, basihyal.

INTRODUCTION

Fetal alcohol spectrum disorder (FASD) is an umbrella term used to describe the range of disorders that occur in an individual whose mother drinks alcohol during pregnancy. Individuals with FASD may have abnormal facial features, growth retardation, central nervous system dysfunction, and learning disabilities (Mukherjee et al., 2006; Mantha et al., 2014). Studies have shown that the ethanol-induced apoptosis in neural crest cells (NCCs), a multipotent progenitor cell population that can give rise to a diversity of cell types, including mesenchymal cells that form craniofacial cartilages, bones, and dermis (Smith, 1997; Dash and Trainor, 2020), is one of the major components of the pathogenesis of FASD (Cartwright and Smith, 1995a; Muralidharan et al., 2013). Multiple signaling pathways have been reported to be involved in ethanol-induced apoptosis, including B-cell lymphoma 2 (Bcl-2) (Hong et al., 2002), p53 (Jana et al., 2010), nuclear factor (erythroid-derived 2)-like 2 (Nrf2) (Chen et al., 2013a), p38 mitogen-activated protein kinase (MAPK), and seven *in absentia* homolog 1 (Siah1) (Yuan et al., 2017).

Seven *in absentia* homolog 1 is a member of a highly conserved family of E3 ubiquitin ligases (Carthew and Rubin, 1990) that is widely expressed in mouse embryos and adult tissues (Della et al., 1993). Siah plays a critical role in a variety of biological processes, including apoptosis (Nemani et al., 1996). Our previous study has demonstrated that ethanol treatment can significantly increase the expression and nuclear translocation of Siah1 in NCCs and that Siah1 signaling plays a critical role in ethanol-induced apoptosis in NCCs (Sun et al., 2014). We have also shown that ethanol-induced upregulation of Siah1 can induce apoptosis in NCCs through p38 MAPK-mediated activation of the p53 signaling pathway (Yuan et al., 2017). However, the mechanisms by which ethanol upregulates Siah1 in NCCs are not clear.

MicroRNAs are small non-coding RNAs that are involved in various physiological and pathological processes, including apoptosis, by regulating gene expression. MiR-135a, a member of the miR-135 superfamily, has been reported to be involved in the tumorigenesis and act as a tumor suppressor (Wu et al., 2012; Kroiss et al., 2015; Xu et al., 2016). MiR-135a expression in astrocytes has also been linked to brain inflammation and angiogenesis in Alzheimer's disease (Ko et al., 2015). Studies have also shown that miR-135a can promote proliferation and inhibit apoptosis of astrocytes in the bacterial meningitis rat models (Dong et al., 2019). Overexpression of miR-135a can also protect human umbilical vein endothelial cells against mechanical stretch-induced increases in apoptosis and ventilator-induced lung injury (Yan et al., 2018). In addition, Siah1 has been identified as a target of miR-135a in HeLa cells and mouse zygotes (Pang et al., 2011). It has been reported that miR-135a can upregulate β-catenin in cervical epithelial cells by targeting Siah1 (Leung et al., 2014).

Zebrafish is a well-established animal model for biomedical research, including FASD research (Bilotta et al., 2004) and an excellent animal model to study gene-ethanol interactions (McCarthy et al., 2013). The rapid external development of zebrafish embryos coupled with their transparency allows rapid analysis of structure and function in the intact embryos (Beis and Stainier, 2006). Studies have demonstrated that embryonic exposure to ethanol resulted in dysmorphology and behavioral deficits that parallel those of FASD in zebrafish (Bilotta et al., 2004; Carvan et al., 2004; Fernandes and Gerlai, 2009; Wang et al., 2018) and that the developmental defects induced by embryonic ethanol exposure can be examined in zebrafish larvae by measuring the eye diameter (Bilotta et al., 2004), body length, and craniofacial cartilage (Marrs et al., 2010).

In the present study, an *in vitro* model of NCCs and a zebrafish model of FASD were used to elucidate the mechanisms by which miR-135a modulates ethanol-induced apoptosis in NCCs and craniofacial defects in zebrafish embryos. We found that ethanol treatment decreased the expression of miR-135a and thereby increased the expression of its direct target, Siah1, which, in turn, activated the p38 MAPK/p53 pathway, increased apoptosis in NCCs and zebrafish embryos and resulted in growth retardation and developmental defects. Overexpression of miR-135a significantly reduced ethanol-induced upregulation of Siah1 and the activation of the p38 MAPK/p53 pathway, decreased ethanol-induced apoptosis in NCCs and zebrafish embryos, and diminished ethanol-induced growth retardation and dysmorphology in zebrafish larvae. These results demonstrate that ethanol-induced downregulation of miR-135a contributes to ethanol-induced apoptosis in NCCs and developmental defects in zebrafish embryos by upregulating Siah1 and activating the p38 MAPK/p53 pathway.

MATERIALS AND METHODS

Cell Culture and Ethanol Treatment

Neural crest cells (JoMa1.3 cells) were cultured as described previously (Maurer et al., 2007; Chen et al., 2013a). Cells were grown on cell culture plates/dishes coated with fibronectin and maintained in Dulbecco's modified Eagle's medium (DMEM): Ham's F12 (1:1) at 37°C in 5% CO_2. NCCs were exposed to medium containing 50 mM ethanol for 24 h. The stable ethanol levels were maintained by using the methods described previously (Yan et al., 2010).

Zebrafish Maintenance and Ethanol Treatment

Adult AB zebrafish (*Danio rerio*) were obtained from the Zebrafish International Resource Center (ZIRC) at the University of Oregon, Eugene, OR, United States and maintained in 14 h:10 h light: dark cycles at 28°C. Fertilized eggs were collected after natural spawning and used for this study. For ethanol treatment, the zebrafish embryos at 3 hours post-fertilization (hpf) were treated with 0, 1, or 1.5% ethanol. At 24 hpf, the embryos were either collected for molecular analysis or transferred to fresh system water. These embryos transferred to fresh system water were collected at 4 or 5 days post-fertilization (dpf) for morphological analysis. This study was approved by the Institutional Animal Care and Use Committee of the University of Louisville.

Microinjection of miRNA Mimics Into Zebrafish Embryos

Zebrafish embryos were microinjected at 1 hpf with 2 nl of synthetic miRNA-135a mimics and control mimics (10 μM) prepared with 1 × Danieau solution [58 mM NaCl, 0.7 mM KCl, 0.4 mM $MgSO_4$, 0.6 mM $Ca(NO_3)_2$, 5.0 mM HEPES, pH 7.6] by using a PLI-100A Plus Picoinjector (Harvard Apparatus, Holliston, MA, United States), as previously described (Pineda et al., 2005; Bill et al., 2009; Su et al., 2014). Successful injections were monitored via the co-injection with 0.1% Fast Green. After microinjection, embryos were transferred to a petri dish containing ethanol solution or system water for treatment from 3 to 24 hpf, as described above. Zebrafish embryos were collected at 24 hpf for analysis of the expression of miR-135a and Siah1, and the analysis of apoptosis. Zebrafish larvae were collected at 4 and 5 dpf for morphological analysis and craniofacial cartilage defect analysis, respectively.

Analysis of miRNA Expression

The expression of miRNA-135a in NCCs and zebrafish embryos was determined as previously described (Chen et al., 2015). Total RNA was isolated with mirVana miRNA Isolation Kit (Ambion, Austin, TX, United States), and quantitative RT-PCR was performed by using TaqMan MicroRNA assays (Ambion, Austin, TX, United States), following the manufacturer's instructions. All TaqMan microRNA assays were performed in triplicate. Data were normalized with snoRNA202 (NCCs) or U6 snRNA (zebrafish embryos) as endogenous controls. The relative expression of miR-135a was calculated using the comparative threshold cycle (Ct) method as described previously (Chen et al., 2015).

miRNA Mimics and Inhibitors Transfection

For transient transfection, miRNA-135a mimics, miRNA inhibitors, control mimics, or control inhibitors at a final concentration of 50 nM were transfected into NCCs using Lipofectamine 2000 (Life Technologies, Grand Island, NY, United States), following the manufacturer's instructions. The cells were harvested 48 h after transfection for additional treatments and analysis.

Construction of Luciferase Reporter Plasmids and Reporter Assays

MiRNA-135a target sites in the 3′-untranslated regions (3′-UTRs) of mouse Siahl mRNA were predicted by using Target Scan[1] and microRNA[2], and compared with the target sites reported in the previous study (Leung et al., 2014). The 3′-UTR of Siah1 containing putative miR-135a binding sites was amplified from mouse genomic DNA and cloned into the pMIR-REPORT™ (Ambion, Austin, TX, United States). Primers used to clone the DNA fragments containing the Siahl 3′-UTR were: 5′ gactACTAGTtttcttttaactgacaagccatctgcgtggtcatagAAGCTTgcta 3′; 5′ tagcAAGCTTctatgaccacgcagatggcttgtcagttaaaagaaaACTAGTagtc 3′. The reporter assays were performed as previously described (Chen et al., 2015). In brief, NCCs were co-transfected with 200 ng of constructed plasmids containing miR-135a binding sites, 20 ng Renilla luciferase pRL-TK control reporter vector (Promega, Madison, WI, United States) and 50 nM of miRNA-135a mimics or mimic control (Ambion, Austin, TX, United States) using Lipofectamine 2000 (Invitrogen, Carlsbad, CA, United States) according to the manufacturer's protocol. Luciferase activity was then measured at 48 h after the transfection using the Dual-Luciferase assay kit (Promega, Madison, WI, United States) with a Lumat LB 9507 Ultra Sensitive Tube Luminometer (Berthold Technologies, Bad Wildbad, Germany). The luciferase activity of each sample was normalized to the pRL/TK-driven Renilla luciferase activity.

Western Blotting

Western blotting was performed by standard protocols as described previously (Chen et al., 2013b; Sun et al., 2014). Proteins were probed with the following antibodies: SIAH1 rabbit pAb (Abcam, Cambridge, MA, United States), β-Actin mouse mAb (Santa Cruz, Santa Cruz, CA, United States), Phospho-p38 MAPK (Thr180/Tyr182) rabbit mAb (Cell Signaling Technology, Inc., Beverly, MA, United States), p38 MAPK rabbit pAb (Cell Signaling Technology, Inc., Beverly, MA, United States), Phospho-p53 (Ser15) rabbit pAb (Cell Signaling Technology, Inc., Beverly, MA, United States), p53 mouse mAb (Abcam, Cambridge, MA, United States), p53 upregulated modulator of apoptosis (PUMA) rabbit pAb (Abcam, Cambridge, MA, United States), Bcl-2 homologous antagonist/killer (Bak) rabbit pAb (Cell Signaling Technology, Inc., Beverly, MA, United States), and cleaved caspase-3 (Asp175) rabbit pAb (Cell Signaling Technology, Inc., Beverly, MA, United States). The membranes were developed on Molecular Imager ChemiDoc XRS + (Bio-Rad, Hercules, CA, United States), and the intensity of the protein band was analyzed by ImageJ software (1.48V, National Institutes of Health, United States). All Western blot analyses were performed in triplicate.

Analysis of Apoptosis

Apoptosis was determined by the analysis of caspase-3 cleavage and activity, as well as the terminal deoxynucleotidyl transferase dUTP nick end labeling (TUNEL) assay. Caspase-3 cleavage was determined by Western blot as described previously (Dong et al., 2008; Chen et al., 2013a). Caspase-3 activity was determined by using Caspase-Glo® 3/7 Assay Systems (Promega, Madison, WI, United States). TUNEL assay was performed by using a TiterTACS *In situ* Detection Kit (Trevigen, Inc., Gaithersburg, MD, United States), following the manufacturer's protocol.

Morphological Analysis and Whole-Mount Skeletal Staining

Morphological analysis of zebrafish larvae at 4 dpf was performed by using a stereoscopic microscope (Olympus SZX16, Tokyo, Japan). Whole-mount skeletal staining of zebrafish larvae at 5 dpf was conducted with Alcian blue staining (Sigma Chemical, Co.,

[1]http://www.targetscan.org/

[2]http://www.microrna.org/microrna/home/do

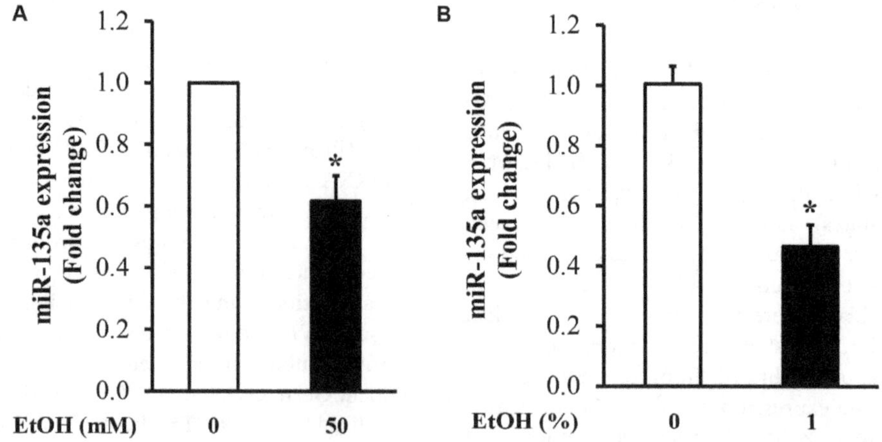

FIGURE 1 | Ethanol exposure decreased the expression of miR-135a in neural crest cells (NCCs) exposed to 50 mM ethanol for 24 h **(A)** and zebrafish embryos treated with 1% ethanol and collected at 24 h post-fertilization (hpf; **B**). The expression of miR-135a was determined by qRT-PCR, as described in the section "Materials and Methods". Data are expressed as fold change over control and represent the mean ± SD of three separate experiments. * $p < 0.05$ vs. control.

St Louis, MO, United States), as described by others (Neuhauss et al., 1996; Walker and Kimmel, 2007), and was visualized by a stereoscopic microscope (Olympus SZX16, Tokyo, Japan) as previously described (Carvan et al., 2004).

Statistical Analysis

Statistical analyses were performed as described previously (Chen et al., 2013b) using GraphPad Prism software (GraphPad Software, San Diego, CA, United States). All data were expressed as means ± SD of three separate experiments. One-way ANOVA was used to compare the difference between groups, and multiple comparison post-tests were conducted by using Bonferroni's test. Differences between groups were considered significant at $p < 0.05$.

RESULTS

Ethanol Treatment Significantly Decreased the Expression of miR-135a in NCCs and Zebrafish Embryos

To determine the effect of ethanol treatment on the expression of miRNA-135a in NCCs, NCCs were exposed to 50 mM ethanol for 24 h. MiR-135a expression level was examined by qRT-PCR. As shown in **Figure 1A**, exposure of NCCs to 50 mM ethanol for 24 h significantly decreased the expression of miR-135a in NCCs, indicating that ethanol treatment can downregulate the expression of miR-135a in NCCs. To determine whether ethanol exposure can also decrease the expression of miR-135a *in vivo*, zebrafish embryos at 3 hpf were treated with or without 1% ethanol and collected at 24 hpf for analysis of miR-135a expression using the qRT-PCR assay. As shown in **Figure 1B**, 1% ethanol treatment resulted in a significant reduction of miR-135a expression in zebrafish embryos. These results demonstrate that both *in vitro* and *in vivo* ethanol treatment can decrease the expression of miR-135a.

Siah1 Is the Direct Target of miR-135a in NCCs

Bioinformatics prediction indicated that Siah1 is a direct target of miR-135a (**Figure 2A**). Siah1 has also been validated to be a direct target of miRNA-135a in HeLa cells (Pang et al., 2011). To validate that Siah1 is also a direct target of miR-135a in NCCs, we cloned the 3′-UTR segments of Siah1 into the pMIR-Report vector to create a luciferase reporter system. NCCs were co-transfected with the vector containing pMIR reporter-luciferase fused with or without the 3′-UTR of Siah1 and miR135a mimic or miRNA control mimic. As shown in **Figure 2B**, co-transfected of the 3′-UTR of Siah1 mRNA and miR135a resulted in a significant reduction in luciferase activity as compared to the NCCs co-transfected with Siah1 3′-UTR and control miRNA mimic. In addition, overexpression of miR-135a by transfecting with miR-135a mimics greatly downregulated the protein expression of Siah1, while downregulation of endogenous miR-135a through transfecting with miR-135a inhibitors significantly elevated the protein expression of Siah1 (**Figure 2C**), demonstrating that Siah1 is a direct target of miR-135a in NCCs.

Over-Expression of miR-135a Diminished Ethanol-Induced Upregulation of Siah1 in NCCs and Zebrafish Embryos

To determine whether the downregulation of miR-135a contributes to ethanol-induced upregulation of Siah1, NCCs transfected with miR-135a mimics or control mimics were exposed to 50 mM ethanol, and the protein expression of Siah1 was analyzed. As shown in **Figure 3A**, ethanol exposure resulted in a significant increase in the protein expression of Siah1. Overexpression of miR-135a by transfection with miR-135a mimics diminished ethanol-induced upregulation of Siah1 in NCCs, demonstrating that downregulation of miR-135a contributes to ethanol-induced upregulation of Siah1 in NCCs. To determine whether overexpression of miR-135a can also

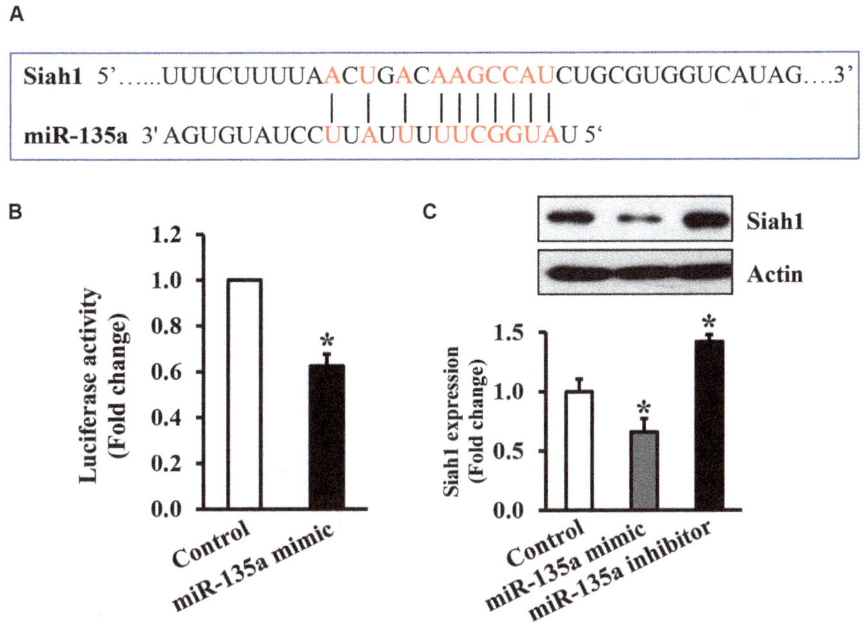

FIGURE 2 | Siah1 is the direct target of miR-135a in neural crest cells (NCCs). **(A)** The predicted binding sites of miR-135a in the 3′-UTR of Siah1 mRNA. **(B)** Luciferase reporter assays for the binding of miR-135a to the 3′-UTR of Siah1 in NCCs. **(C)** Western bolt analysis of the protein expression of Siah1 in NCCs transfected with miR-135a mimics or inhibitors for 48 h. Data are expressed as fold change over control and represent the mean ± SD of three separate experiments. * $p < 0.05$ vs. control.

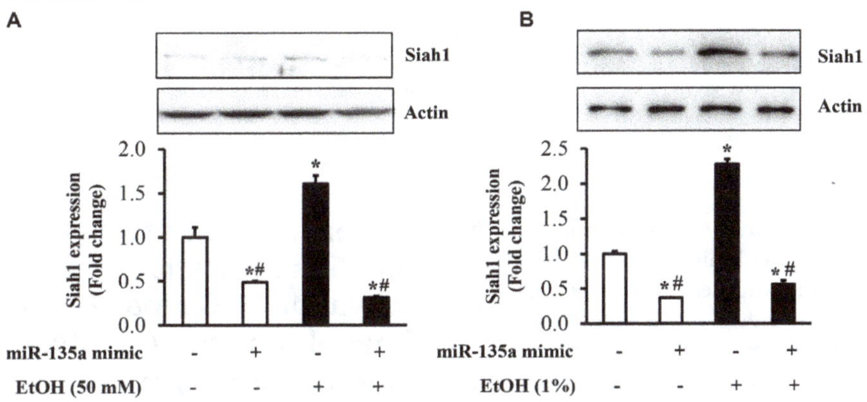

FIGURE 3 | Overexpression of miR-135a significantly decreased the ethanol-induced upregulation of Siah1 in neural crest cells (NCCs) and zebrafish embryos. NCCs transfected with control mimics or miR-135a mimics were treated with 50 mM ethanol for 24 h. Zebrafish embryos microinjected with control or miR-135a mimics were treated with 1% ethanol and collected at 24 h post-fertilization (hpf). The protein expression of Siah1 was examined in NCCs **(A)** and zebrafish embryos **(B)** by western blot. Data are expressed as fold change over control and represent the mean ± SD of three separate experiments. * $p < 0.05$ vs. control; # $p < 0.05$ vs. ethanol.

diminish ethanol-induced upregulation of Siah1 in zebrafish embryos, zebrafish embryos microinjected with miR-135a mimics and control mimics were exposed to 1% ethanol, and the protein expression of Siah1 was analyzed by western blot. As shown in **Figure 3B**, exposure to ethanol significantly increased the expression of Siah1. Microinjection of miR-135a mimics significantly diminished ethanol-induced upregulation of Siah1 in zebrafish embryos, indicating that overexpression of miR-135a can also prevent ethanol-induced upregulation of Siah1 in zebrafish embryos.

Overexpression of miR-135a Diminished Ethanol-Induced Activation of the p38 MAPK/p53 Pathway in NCCs

Our previous study has demonstrated that ethanol-induced upregulation of Siah1 triggered apoptosis in NCCs through promoting p38 MAPK-mediated activation of the p53 signaling pathway (Yuan et al., 2017). To determine whether the downregulation of miR-135a contributes to ethanol-induced apoptosis in NCCs through Siah1-mediated activation of the

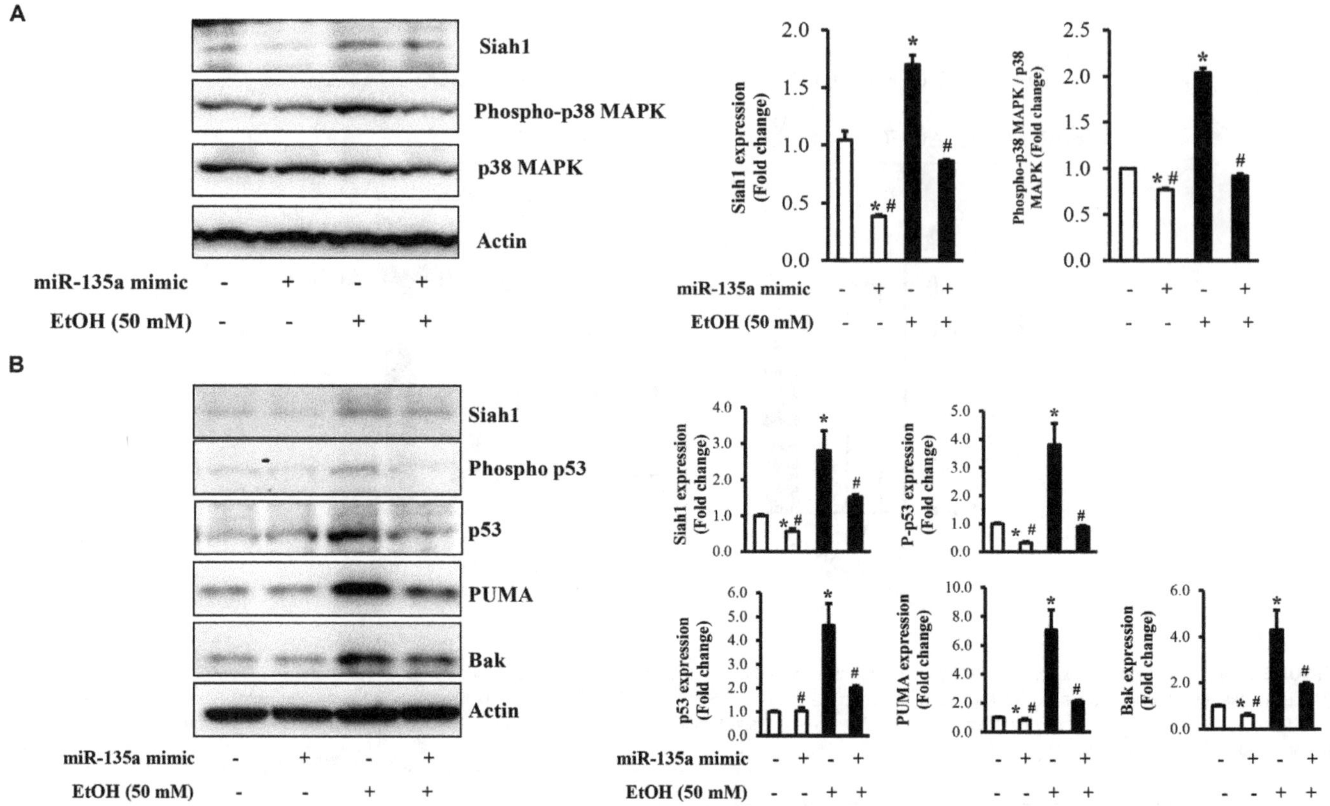

FIGURE 4 | Overexpression of miR-135a reduced the ethanol-induced activation of the p38 mitogen-activated protein kinase (MAPK)/p53 pathway in neural crest cells (NCCs). NCCs transfected with control mimics or miR-135a mimics were treated with 50 mM ethanol for 24 h. The expression of Siah1, total p38, and phosphorylated p38 **(A)**, and the expression of Siah1, phosphorylated p53, p53, p53 upregulated modulator of apoptosis (PUMA), and Bcl-2 homologous antagonist/killer (Bak; **B**) were determined by western blot. Data are expressed as fold change over control and represent the mean ± SD of three separate experiments. * $p < 0.05$ vs. control; # $p < 0.05$ vs. ethanol.

p38 MAPK/p53 pathway, we first examined whether the overexpression of miRNA-135a can inhibit the activation of the p38 MAPK pathway in ethanol-exposed NCCs. As shown in **Figure 4A**, ethanol treatment resulted in the activation of the p38 MAPK pathway, as indicated by enhanced phosphorylation of p38 MAPK, consisting with our previous studies (Yuan et al., 2017). Overexpression of miR-135a significantly diminished ethanol-induced expression of phosphor-p38 MAPK, indicating that miR-135a can inhibit the p38 MAPK pathway through downregulating Siah1. To determine the role of miRNA-135a on ethanol-induced apoptosis in NCCs, we next examined the p53 apoptotic pathway, which is the downstream targets of the p38 MAPK pathway that has been shown to be regulated tightly by Siah1 in NCCs (Yuan et al., 2017). We found that ethanol exposure increased the total protein levels of p53 and the levels of the phosphorylated p53. Ethanol treatment also significantly increased the expression of p53 downstream targets, PUMA and Bak. Overexpression of miRNA-135a significantly diminished ethanol-induced increases in the phosphorylation and total protein level of p53, and the expression of PUMA and Bak (**Figure 4B**), indicating that miRNA-135a can modulate the p38 MAPK/p53 apoptotic pathway in NCCs through targeting Siah1.

Overexpression of miR-135a Significantly Reduced Ethanol-Induced Activation of Caspase-3 and Diminished Ethanol-Induced Apoptosis in NCCs and Zebrafish Embryos

To determine whether overexpression of miR-135a can prevent ethanol-induced apoptosis in NCCs, NCCs transfected with miR-135a mimics were exposed to 50 mM ethanol for 24 h. As shown in **Figures 5A,B**, ethanol exposure resulted in a significant increase in caspase-3 cleavage and activity in NCCs, indicating that ethanol exposure can increase apoptosis in NCCs that was confirmed by the TUNEL assay (**Figure 5C**). Overexpression of miR-135a significantly diminished ethanol-induced increases in caspase-3 cleavage and activity and reduced apoptosis in ethanol-exposed NCCs (**Figures 5A–C**). These results demonstrate that overexpression of miR-135a can prevent ethanol-induced apoptosis in NCCs. To determine whether the upregulation of miR-135a can also prevent ethanol-induced apoptosis in zebrafish embryos, zebrafish embryos microinjected with miR-135a mimics and control mimics were exposed to ethanol from 3 to 24 hpf. As shown in **Figure 5D**, microinjection of miR-135a mimics significantly reduced ethanol-induced

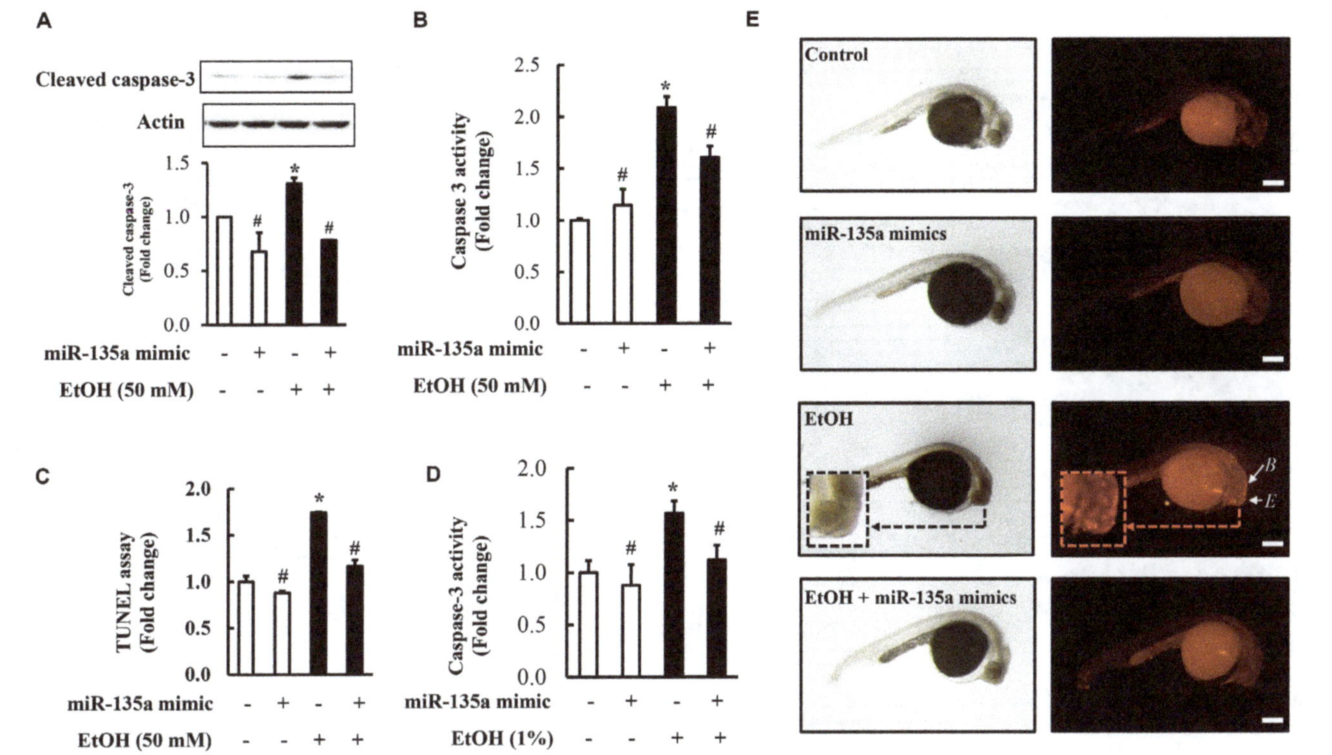

FIGURE 5 | Overexpression of miR-135a significantly decreased ethanol-induced caspase-3 activation and apoptosis in neural crest cells (NCCs) and zebrafish embryos. NCCs transfected with control mimics or miR-135a mimics were treated with 50 mM ethanol for 24 h. Zebrafish embryos microinjected with control or miR-135a mimics were treated with 1% ethanol and collected at 24 h post-fertilization (hpf). Ethanol-induced apoptosis in NCCs **(A-C)** and zebrafish embryos **(D,E)** was determined by analysis of caspase-3 cleavage **(A)**, caspase-3 activity **(B,D)**, and terminal deoxynucleotidyl transferase dUTP nick end labeling (TUNEL) analysis **(C,E)**. White arrows in **(E)** indicate brain **(B)** and eye **(E)** in zebrafish embryos. Data are expressed as fold change over control and represent the mean ± SD of three separate experiments. * $p < 0.05$ vs. control; # $p < 0.05$ vs. ethanol. Scale bar = 200 μm.

increase in caspase-3 activity in zebrafish embryos. Whole-mount TUNEL staining also shown that ethanol-induced apoptosis was significantly attenuated by the microinjection of miR-135a mimics in zebrafish embryos, especially in the brain and eye (**Figure 5E**).

Microinjection of miR-135a Mimics Attenuated Ethanol-Induced Growth Retardation and Dysmorphology in Zebrafish Larvae

It has been reported that ethanol-induced apoptosis in NCCs contributes heavily to the subsequent abnormalities that are characteristics of FASD (Kotch and Sulik, 1992a; Cartwright and Smith, 1995a). To determine whether microinjection of miR-135a mimics can attenuate ethanol-induced growth retardation and dysmorphology in zebrafish, zebrafish embryos microinjected with control or miR-135a mimics were treated with 1.5% ethanol from 3 to 24 hpf and then were allowed to grow in system water without ethanol. Zebrafish larvae from control and treated groups were collected at 4 dpf for morphological analysis. As shown in **Figure 6**, ethanol treatment resulted in significant growth retardation in zebrafish larvae, as indicated by the dramatically reduced body length. Ethanol exposure also resulted in significant developmental defects, including small eyes, microcephaly, and pericardial edema. Microinjection of miR-135a mimics significantly attenuated the ethanol-induced growth retardation and dysmorphology in zebrafish larvae.

Microinjection of miR-135a Mimics Significantly Diminished Ethanol-Induced Craniofacial Cartilage Defects in Zebrafish Larvae

To determine whether the microinjection of miR-135a mimics can attenuate the ethanol-induced craniofacial cartilage defects in zebrafish larvae, zebrafish embryos microinjected with control or miRNA-135a mimics were treated with 1.5% ethanol from 3 to 24 hpf. Zebrafish larvae were collected at 5 dpf and stained with Alcian blue. As shown in **Figure 7A**, ethanol exposure resulted in an overall reduction in head size and micrognathia due to reduced jaw outgrowth in zebrafish larvae. A closer examination of craniofacial cartilage at 5 dpf larvae revealed that the length of the mandibular arch cartilages (lower jaw), including the ventral Meckel's cartilage (m) and dorsal palatoquadrate (pq), were significantly reduced in ethanol-exposed zebrafish larvae, as compared to control. In addition, exposure to ethanol at the embryonic stage significantly reduced

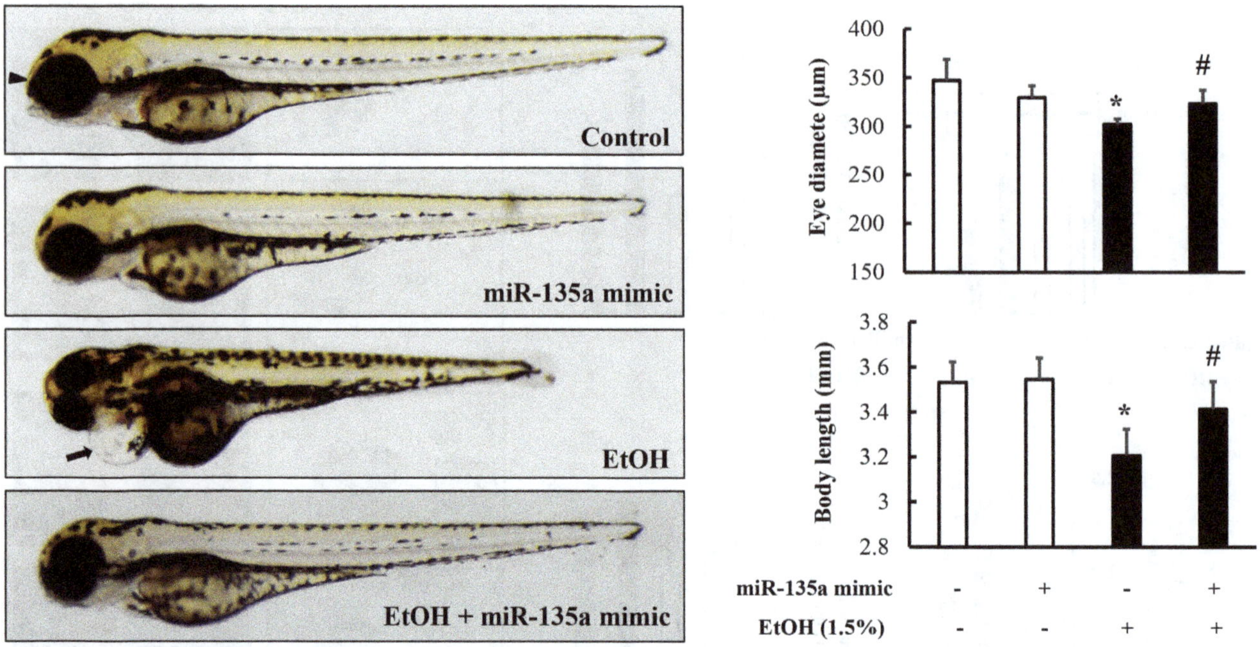

FIGURE 6 | Microinjection of miR-135a mimics diminished ethanol-induced growth retardation and dysmorphology in zebrafish larvae. Embryos microinjected with control or miR-135a mimics were treated with 1.5% ethanol from 3 to 24 h post-fertilization (hpf). Zebrafish larvae were collected at 4 days post-fertilization (dpf) for morphological analysis. Analysis of ethanol-induced growth retardation and dysmorphology was performed by using a stereoscopic microscope. The black arrows indicate the heart and the arrowheads indicate eye. Data represent the mean ± SD of three separate experiments. * $p < 0.05$ vs. control; # $p < 0.05$ vs. ethanol.

the length of hyosymplectic (hs) and ceratohyal (ch), and the distance between m and pq joint and between the arch of m and basihyal (bh; **Figure 7B**). Embryonic ethanol treatment also led to the abnormal angulation of the ch cartilage (**Figure 7C**). Overexpression of miR-135a significantly diminished ethanol-induced reduction in the length of m, pq, hs, and ch and the distance between m and pq joints and between m and bh. Microinjection of miR-135a also attenuated the ethanol-induced abnormal angulation of ch cartilage, indicating that the upregulation of miR-135a can attenuate ethanol-induced craniofacial cartilage defects in zebrafish larvae (**Figures 7A–C**).

DISCUSSION

Growing evidence suggests that impairment of differentiation, migration, and survival of NCCs is a major component of the pathogenesis of FASD and that dysregulation of gene expression is a key driver of the ethanol-induced impairment in NCCs (Kotch and Sulik, 1992b; Cartwright and Smith, 1995b; Rovasio and Battiato, 2002; Steventon et al., 2014; Zhang et al., 2017; Yuan et al., 2018; Fan et al., 2019; Li et al., 2019). MicroRNAs have been shown to be involved in the ethanol-induced impairment of NCCs. Our previous studies have shown that miR-125b can protect against ethanol-induced apoptosis in NCCs and mouse embryos by targeting Bak1 and PUMA and that microinjection of miR-125b mimics can prevent ethanol-induced embryotoxicity (Chen et al., 2015). We have also demonstrated that miR-34a can mediate ethanol-induced impairment of neural differentiation of NCCs by targeting autophagy-related gene 9a (Fan et al., 2019). In the present study, we found that ethanol exposure significantly reduced the expression of miR-135a, increased apoptosis in NCCs exposed to 50 mM ethanol and zebrafish embryos exposed to 1.0% ethanol, and resulted in growth retardation and developmental defects in zebrafish larvae exposed to 1.5% ethanol. There is a consensus that the ethanol levels in the zebrafish embryo tissue are approximately 25–35% of the levels of the medium (Flentke et al., 2014; Lovely et al., 2014). Therefore, 1.0 or 1.5% ethanol in the medium is ~ 300 or 450 mg/dL in the embryo tissue. These ethanol concentrations were chosen because studies have shown that a peak maternal blood alcohol concentration of 400–500 mg/dL (approximately 85–105 mM) is needed to produce major malformations with the characteristics of fetal alcohol syndrome in mouse embryos (Sulik et al., 1981; Kotch and Sulik, 1992a; Dunty et al., 2001). These ethanol concentrations are relatively high but are not beyond that which can be observed in chronic alcoholics (Adachi et al., 1991).

MiR-135a is a member of the miR-135 superfamily. A number of studies have reported that the downregulation of miR-135a was involved in tumorigenesis in a variety of cancers, in which miR-135a exerts tumor-suppressive effects (Yamada et al., 2013; Kroiss et al., 2015; Zhao et al., 2017). In contrast, other studies have shown that miR-135a is an oncogenic miRNA in colorectal carcinomas (Nagel et al., 2008) and that overexpression of miR-135a promoted tumorigenesis of portal vein tumor thrombus (Liu et al., 2012) and enhanced the growth of HeLa- and NC104-E6/E7-derived tumor (Leung et al., 2014). Studies have also shown that miR-135a is involved in

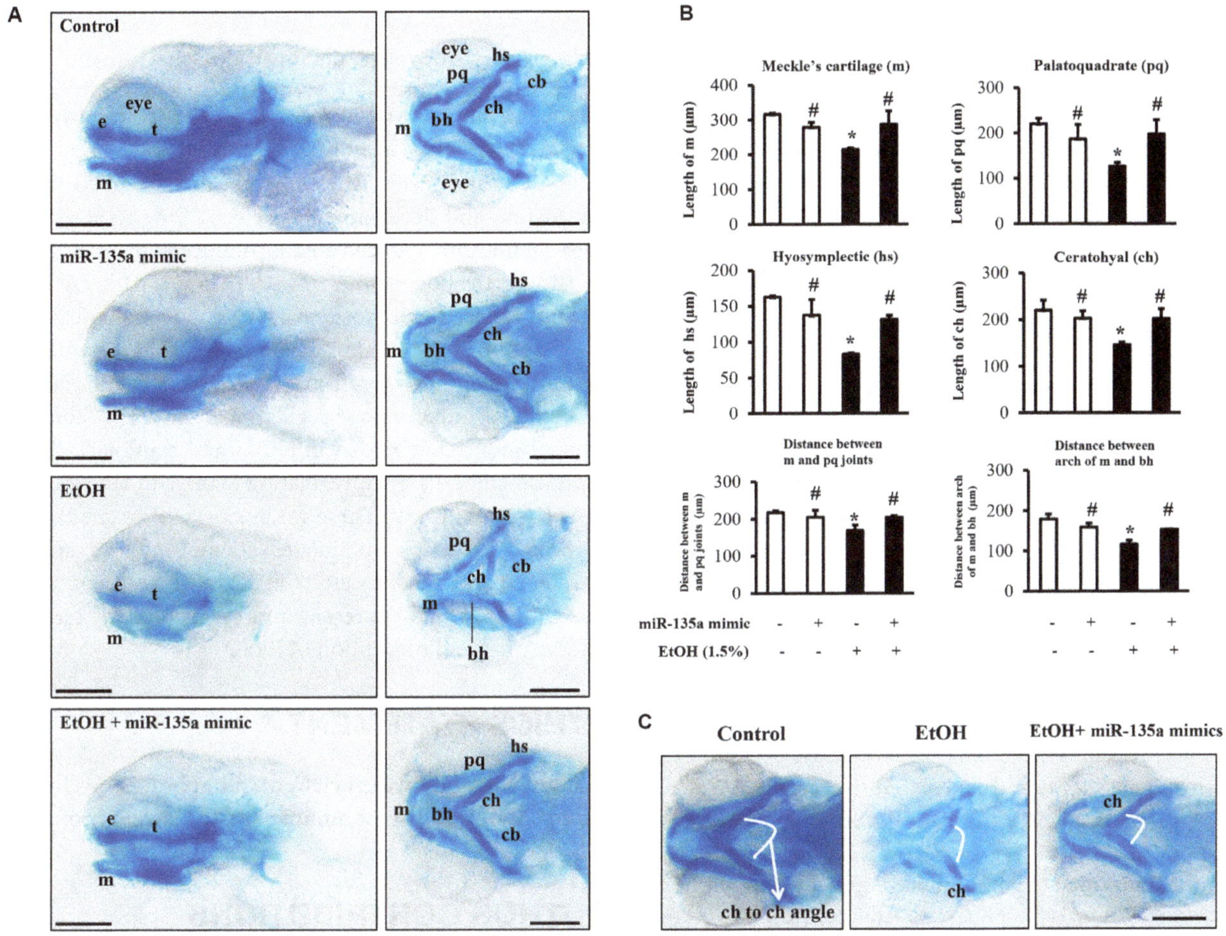

FIGURE 7 | Microinjection of miR-135a mimics attenuated ethanol-induced craniofacial cartilage defects in zebrafish larvae. Embryos microinjected with control or miR-135a mimics were treated with 1.5% ethanol from 3 h post-fertilization (hpf) to 24 hpf. Zebrafish larvae were collected at 5 days post-fertilization (dpf) for skeletal staining with Alcian blue. **(A)** Lateral and ventral view of Alcian blue-stained craniofacial cartilages in larvae from different treatment groups. **(B)** Morphometric analysis of the craniofacial cartilages in larvae from different treatment groups. The length of Meckel's cartilage (m), palatoquadrate (pq), hyosymplectic (hs), ceratohyal (ch), and the distance between m and pq joint, and between the arch of m and basihyal (bh) were measured. **(C)** Comparisons of ceratohyal cartilage (ch) angle between different treatment groups. Data represent the mean ± SD of three separate experiments. * $p < 0.05$ vs. control; # $p < 0.05$ vs. ethanol. e, ethmoid plate; t, trabeculae cranii; cb, ceratobranchial; bh, basihyal. Scale bar = 200 μm.

brain inflammation and angiogenesis in Alzheimer's disease (Ko et al., 2015). In addition, it has been reported that miR-135a can promote proliferation and prevent apoptosis. For example, a study by Dong et al., indicated that, by targeting HIF-1α, miR-135a downregulated pro-apoptotic genes Bax and Bad, upregulated anti-apoptotic gene Bcl-2, resulting in increased proliferation and reduced apoptosis of astrocytes in the bacterial meningitis rat models (Dong et al., 2019). Upregulation of miR-135a also protected human umbilical vein endothelial cells against mechanical stretch-induced increases in apoptosis and ventilator-induced lung injury through activating PI3K/Akt signaling pathway by targeting PH domain leucine-rich repeat-containing protein phosphatase 2 (PHLPP2) (Yan et al., 2018). In the present study, we have shown that ethanol-induced downregulation of miR-135a resulted in the upregulation of Siah1 and that overexpression of miR-135a significantly reduced ethanol-induced upregulation of Siah1, indicating that downregulation of miR-135a contributes to ethanol-induced upregulation of Siah1 in NCCs and zebrafish embryos.

Siah is a member of a highly conserved family of E3 ubiquitin ligases (Carthew and Rubin, 1990). Siah ligases are involved in the ubiquitination and proteasomal degradation of several proteins that are essential for a variety of signaling pathways, including membrane receptors (Liani et al., 2004; Winter et al., 2008), a microtubule-associated motor protein (Linares-Cruz et al., 1998) and transcriptional regulators (Zhang et al., 1998; Tiedt et al., 2001). The upregulation of Siah1 has also been found to induce cell-cycle arrest and the induction of apoptosis (Relaix et al., 2000; Matsuzawa and Reed, 2001). We have also demonstrated that ethanol treatment can significantly increase the expression and nuclear translocation of Siah1 in NCCs and that Siah1 signaling plays a critical role in ethanol-induced apoptosis in NCCs (Sun et al., 2014). In addition, we have shown that ethanol-induced up-regulation of Siah1 can induce apoptosis in NCCs through p38 MAPK-mediated activation of the p53 signaling pathway (Yuan et al., 2017). In this study, we found that, in addition to NCCs, ethanol exposure can also increase the expression of Siah1 in zebrafish embryos. We also found that ethanol-induced upregulation of Siah1 resulted in the activation of p38 MAPK/p53 pathway and that overexpression of miR-135a significantly diminished ethanol-induced activation of p38 MAPK/p53 pathway. These results consist of the findings from our previous study and demonstrate that the upregulation of miR-135a can inhibit p38 MAPK-mediated activation of the p53 signaling pathway through downregulating Siah1.

It is well known that p38 MAPK pathway can modulate apoptosis by regulating p53 pathway (Zheng et al., 2005; Gao et al., 2014) and that p53 is a transcription factor that regulates the expression of genes involved in apoptosis (Kho et al., 2004; Schuler and Green, 2005). Previous studies from our laboratory have shown that knockdown of Siah1 by siRNA significantly diminished the ethanol-induced increase in the phosphorylation of p38 MAPK, and significantly decreased ethanol-induced increases in p53 stability and its phosphorylation in NCCs, and that p38 MAPK activation is essential for ethanol-induced Siah1-mediated p53 activation, leading to apoptosis in ethanol-exposed NCCs (Yuan et al., 2017). In this study, we found that ethanol treatment significantly increased the expression of p53 downstream targets, PUMA and Bak, the activation of caspase-3 and apoptosis in NCCs. Overexpression of miRNA-135a significantly diminished ethanol-induced upregulation of PUMA and Bak and apoptosis in NCCs. In addition, microinjection of miR-135a mimics dramatically reduced the apoptosis in zebrafish embryos and diminished ethanol-induced growth retardation and dysmorphology in zebrafish larvae. These results demonstrate that the upregulation of miR-135a can prevent ethanol-induced apoptosis in NCCs and developmental defects in zebrafish embryos by modulating the Siah1-mediated p38 MAPK/p53 pathway.

CONCLUSION

The present study has demonstrated that ethanol treatment decreased the expression of miR-135a and thereby increased the expression of its direct target, Siah1, which, in turn, activated the p38 MAPK/p53 pathway, increased apoptosis in NCCs and zebrafish embryos and resulted in growth retardation and developmental defects. Overexpression of miR-135a significantly reduced ethanol-induced upregulation of Siah1 and the activation of the p38 MAPK/p53 pathway, decreased ethanol-induced apoptosis in NCCs and zebrafish embryos, and diminished ethanol-induced growth retardation and dysmorphology in zebrafish larvae. These results demonstrate that ethanol-induced downregulation of miR-135a contributes to ethanol-induced apoptosis in NCCs and craniofacical defects in zebrafish embryos by upregulating Siah1 and activating the p38 MAPK/p53 pathway. These findings elucidate the mechanisms by which miR-135a modulates ethanol-induced apoptosis in NCCs and craniofacial defects in zebrafish embryos and suggest that miR-135a may represent a novel therapeutic target for the intervention and prevention of FASD.

ETHICS STATEMENT

The animal study was reviewed and approved by Institutional Animal Care and Use Committee of the University of Louisville.

AUTHOR CONTRIBUTIONS

FY and SC conceptualized and designed the experiments and participated in data interpretation and manuscript preparation. FY, YY, and JL performed the experiments and participated in data analysis. HF, YL, LL, and WF participated in data interpretation and discussion. All authors reviewed the manuscript.

REFERENCES

Adachi, J., Mizoi, Y., Fukunaga, T., Ogawa, Y., Ueno, Y., and Imamichi, H. (1991). Degrees of alcohol intoxication in 117 hospitalized cases. *J. Stud. Alcohol* 52, 448–453. doi: 10.15288/jsa.1991.52.448

Beis, D., and Stainier, D. Y. (2006). *In vivo* cell biology: following the zebrafish trend. *Trends Cell Biol.* 16, 105–112. doi: 10.1016/j.tcb.2005.12.001

Bill, B. R., Petzold, A. M., Clark, K. J., Schimmenti, L. A., and Ekker, S. C. (2009). A primer for morpholino use in zebrafish. *Zebrafish* 6, 69–77. doi: 10.1089/zeb.2008.0555

Bilotta, J., Barnett, J. A., Hancock, L., and Saszik, S. (2004). Ethanol exposure alters zebrafish development: a novel model of fetal alcohol syndrome. *Neurotoxicol. Teratol.* 26, 737–743. doi: 10.1016/j.ntt.2004.06.011

Carthew, R. W., and Rubin, G. M. (1990). Seven in absentia, a gene required for specification of R7 cell fate in the Drosophila eye. *Cell* 63, 561–577. doi: 10.1016/0092-8674(90)90452-k

Cartwright, M. M., and Smith, S. M. (1995a). Increased cell death and reduced neural crest cell numbers in ethanol-exposed embryos: partial basis for the fetal alcohol syndrome phenotype. *Alcohol Clin. Exp. Res.* 19, 378–386.

Cartwright, M. M., and Smith, S. M. (1995b). Stage-dependent effects of ethanol on cranial neural crest cell development: partial basis for the phenotypic variations observed in fetal alcohol syndrome. *Alcohol Clin. Exp. Res.* 19, 1454–1462. doi: 10.1111/j.1530-0277.1995.tb01007.x

Carvan, M. J. III, Loucks, E., Weber, D. N., and Williams, F. E. (2004). Ethanol effects on the developing zebrafish: neurobehavior and skeletal morphogenesis. *Neurotoxicol. Teratol.* 26, 757–768. doi: 10.1016/j.ntt.2004.06.016

Chen, X., Liu, J., and Chen, S. Y. (2013a). Over-expression of Nrf2 diminishes ethanol-induced oxidative stress and apoptosis in neural crest cells by inducing an antioxidant response. *Reprod. Toxicol.* 42, 102–109. doi: 10.1016/j.reprotox.2013.08.003

Chen, X., Liu, J., and Chen, S. Y. (2013b). Sulforaphane protects against ethanol-induced oxidative stress and apoptosis in neural crest cells by the induction of Nrf2-mediated antioxidant response. *Br. J. Pharmacol.* 169, 437–448. doi: 10.1111/bph.12133

Chen, X., Liu, J., Feng, W. K., Wu, X., and Chen, S. Y. (2015). MiR-125b protects against ethanol-induced apoptosis in neural crest cells and mouse embryos by targeting Bak 1 and PUMA. *Exp. Neurol.* 271, 104–111. doi: 10.1016/j.expneurol.2015.04.026

Dash, S., and Trainor, P. A. (2020). The development, patterning and evolution of neural crest cell differentiation into cartilage and bone. *Bone* 137:115409. doi: 10.1016/j.bone.2020.115409

Della, N. G., Senior, P. V., and Bowtell, D. D. (1993). Isolation and characterisation of murine homologues of the Drosophila seven in absentia gene (sina). *Development* 117, 1333–1343.

Dong, J., Sulik, K. K., and Chen, S. Y. (2008). Nrf2-mediated transcriptional induction of antioxidant response in mouse embryos exposed to ethanol *in vivo*: implications for the prevention of fetal alcohol spectrum disorders. *Antioxid. Redox Signal.* 10, 2023–2033. doi: 10.1089/ars.2007.2019

Dong, Y., Wang, J., Du, K. X., Jia, T. M., Zhu, C. L., Zhang, Y., et al. (2019). MicroRNA-135a participates in the development of astrocytes derived from bacterial meningitis by downregulating HIF-1alpha. *Am. J. Physiol. Cell Physiol.* 316, C711–C721. doi: 10.1152/ajpcell.00440.2018

Dunty, W. C. Jr., Chen, S. Y., Zucker, R. M., Dehart, D. B., and Sulik, K. K. (2001). Selective vulnerability of embryonic cell populations to ethanol-induced apoptosis: implications for alcohol-related birth defects and neurodevelopmental disorder. *Alcohol Clin. Exp. Res.* 25, 1523–1535.

Fan, H., Yuan, F., Yun, Y., Wu, T., Lu, L., Liu, J., et al. (2019). MicroRNA-34a mediates ethanol-induced impairment of neural differentiation of neural crest cells by targeting autophagy-related gene 9a. *Exp. Neurol.* 320:112981. doi: 10.1016/j.expneurol.2019.112981

Fernandes, Y., and Gerlai, R. (2009). Long-term behavioral changes in response to early developmental exposure to ethanol in zebrafish. *Alcohol Clin. Exp. Res.* 33, 601–609. doi: 10.1111/j.1530-0277.2008.00874.x

Flentke, G. R., Klingler, R. H., Tanguay, R. L., Carvan, M. J. III, and Smith, S. M. (2014). An evolutionarily conserved mechanism of calcium-dependent neurotoxicity in a zebrafish model of fetal alcohol spectrum disorders. *Alcohol Clin. Exp. Res.* 38, 1255–1265. doi: 10.1111/acer.12360

Gao, J., Gao, J., Qian, L., Wang, X., Wu, M., Zhang, Y., et al. (2014). Activation of p38-MAPK by CXCL4/CXCR3 axis contributes to p53-dependent intestinal apoptosis initiated by 5-fluorouracil. *Cancer Biol. Ther.* 15, 982–991. doi: 10. 4161/cbt.29114

Hong, F., Kim, W. H., Tian, Z., Jaruga, B., Ishac, E., Shen, X., et al. (2002). Elevated interleukin-6 during ethanol consumption acts as a potential endogenous protective cytokine against ethanol-induced apoptosis in the liver: involvement of induction of Bcl-2 and Bcl-x(L) proteins. *Oncogene* 21, 32–43. doi: 10.1038/ sj.onc.1205016

Jana, K., Jana, N., De, D. K., and Guha, S. K. (2010). Ethanol induces mouse spermatogenic cell apoptosis in vivo through over-expression of Fas/Fas-L, p53, and caspase-3 along with cytochrome c translocation and glutathione depletion. *Mol. Reprod. Dev.* 77, 820–833. doi: 10.1002/mrd.21227

Kho, P. S., Wang, Z., Zhuang, L., Li, Y., Chew, J. L., Ng, H. H., et al. (2004). p53-regulated transcriptional program associated with genotoxic stress-induced apoptosis. *J. Biol. Chem.* 279, 21183–21192. doi: 10.1074/jbc.M311912200

Ko, C. Y., Chu, Y. Y., Narumiya, S., Chi, J. Y., Furuyashiki, T., Aoki, T., et al. (2015). CCAAT/enhancer-binding protein delta/miR135a/thrombospondin 1 axis mediates PGE2-induced angiogenesis in Alzheimer's disease. *Neurobiol. Aging* 36, 1356–1368. doi: 10.1016/j.neurobiolaging.2014.11.020

Kotch, L. E., and Sulik, K. K. (1992a). Experimental fetal alcohol syndrome: proposed pathogenic basis for a variety of associated facial and brain anomalies. *Am. J. Med. Genet.* 44, 168–176. doi: 10.1002/ajmg.1320440210

Kotch, L. E., and Sulik, K. K. (1992b). Patterns of ethanol-induced cell death in the developing nervous system of mice; neural fold states through the time of anterior neural tube closure. *Int. J. Dev. Neurosci.* 10, 273–279. doi: 10.1016/ 0736-5748(92)90016-s

Kroiss, A., Vincent, S., Decaussin-Petrucci, M., Meugnier, E., Viallet, J., Ruffion, A., et al. (2015). Androgen-regulated microRNA-135a decreases prostate cancer cell migration and invasion through downregulating ROCK1 and ROCK2. *Oncogene* 34, 2846–2855. doi: 10.1038/onc.2014.222

Leung, C. O., Deng, W., Ye, T. M., Ngan, H. Y., Tsao, S. W., Cheung, A. N., et al. (2014). miR-135a leads to cervical cancer cell transformation through regulation of beta-catenin via a SIAH1-dependent ubiquitin proteosomal pathway. *Carcinogenesis* 35, 1931–1940. doi: 10.1093/carcin/bgu032

Li, Y., Yuan, F., Wu, T., Lu, L., Liu, J., Feng, W., et al. (2019). Sulforaphane protects against ethanol-induced apoptosis in neural crest cells through restoring epithelial-mesenchymal transition by epigenetically modulating the expression of Snail1. *Biochim. Biophys. Acta Mol. Basis Dis.* 1865, 2586–2594. doi: 10.1016/ j.bbadis.2019.07.002

Liani, E., Eyal, A., Avraham, E., Shemer, R., Szargel, R., Berg, D., et al. (2004). Ubiquitylation of synphilin-1 and alpha-synuclein by SIAH and its presence in cellular inclusions and Lewy bodies imply a role in Parkinson's disease. *Proc. Natl. Acad. Sci. U.S.A.* 101, 5500–5505. doi: 10.1073/pnas.0401081101

Linares-Cruz, G., Bruzzoni-Giovanelli, H., Alvaro, V., Roperch, J. P., Tuynder, M., Schoevaert, D., et al. (1998). p21WAF-1 reorganizes the nucleus in tumor suppression. *Proc. Natl. Acad. Sci. U.S.A.* 95, 1131–1135. doi: 10.1073/pnas.95. 3.1131

Liu, S., Guo, W., Shi, J., Li, N., Yu, X., Xue, J., et al. (2012). MicroRNA-135a contributes to the development of portal vein tumor thrombus by promoting metastasis in hepatocellular carcinoma. *J. Hepatol.* 56, 389–396. doi: 10.1016/j. jhep.2011.08.008

Lovely, C. B., Nobles, R. D., and Eberhart, J. K. (2014). Developmental age strengthens barriers to ethanol accumulation in zebrafish. *Alcohol* 48, 595–602. doi: 10.1016/j.alcohol.2014.06.003

Mantha, K., Laufer, B. I., and Singh, S. M. (2014). Molecular changes during neurodevelopment following second-trimester binge ethanol exposure in a mouse model of fetal alcohol spectrum disorder: from immediate effects to long-term adaptation. *Dev. Neurosci.* 36, 29–43. doi: 10.1159/000357496

Marrs, J. A., Clendenon, S. G., Ratcliffe, D. R., Fielding, S. M., Liu, Q., and Bosron, W. F. (2010). Zebrafish fetal alcohol syndrome model: effects of ethanol are rescued by retinoic acid supplement. *Alcohol* 44, 707–715. doi: 10.1016/j. alcohol.2009.03.004

Matsuzawa, S. I., and Reed, J. C. (2001). Siah-1, SIP, and Ebi collaborate in a novel pathway for beta-catenin degradation linked to p53 responses. *Mol. Cell* 7, 915–926. doi: 10.1016/s1097-2765(01)00242-8

Maurer, J., Fuchs, S., Jager, R., Kurz, B., Sommer, L., and Schorle, H. (2007). Establishment and controlled differentiation of neural crest stem cell lines using conditional transgenesis. *Differentiation* 75, 580–591. doi: 10.1111/j.1432-0436. 2007.00164.x

McCarthy, N., Wetherill, L., Lovely, C. B., Swartz, M. E., Foroud, T. M., and Eberhart, J. K. (2013). Pdgfra protects against ethanol-induced craniofacial defects in a zebrafish model of FASD. *Development* 140, 3254–3265. doi: 10. 1242/dev.094938

Mukherjee, R. A., Hollins, S., and Turk, J. (2006). Fetal alcohol spectrum disorder: an overview. *J. R. Soc. Med.* 99, 298–302. doi: 10.1258/jrsm.99.6.298

Muralidharan, P., Sarmah, S., Zhou, F. C., and Marrs, J. A. (2013). Fetal alcohol spectrum disorder (FASD) associated neural defects: complex mechanisms and potential therapeutic targets. *Brain Sci.* 3, 964–991. doi: 10.3390/ brainsci3020964

Nagel, R., le Sage, C., Diosdado, B., van der Waal, M., Oude Vrielink, J. A., Bolijn, A., et al. (2008). Regulation of the adenomatous polyposis coli gene by the miR-135 family in colorectal cancer. *Cancer Res.* 68, 5795–5802. doi: 10.1158/0008-5472.CAN-08-0951

Nemani, M., Linares-Cruz, G., Bruzzoni-Giovanelli, H., Roperch, J. P., Tuynder, M., Bougueleret, L., et al. (1996). Activation of the human homologue of the Drosophila sina gene in apoptosis and tumor suppression. *Proc. Natl. Acad. Sci. U.S.A.* 93, 9039–9042. doi: 10.1073/pnas.93.17.9039

Neuhauss, S. C., Solnica-Krezel, L., Schier, A. F., Zwartkruis, F., Stemple, D. L., Malicki, J., et al. (1996). Mutations affecting craniofacial development in zebrafish. *Development* 123, 357–367.

Pang, R. T., Liu, W. M., Leung, C. O., Ye, T. M., Kwan, P. C., Lee, K. F., et al. (2011). miR-135A regulates preimplantation embryo development through down-regulation of E3 Ubiquitin Ligase Seven In Absentia Homolog 1A (SIAH1A) expression. *PLoS One* 6:e27878. doi: 10.1371/journal.pone.0027878

Pineda, R. H., Heiser, R. A., and Ribera, A. B. (2005). Developmental, molecular, and genetic dissection of INa in vivo in embryonic zebrafish sensory neurons. *J. Neurophysiol.* 93, 3582–3593. doi: 10.1152/jn.01070.2004

Relaix, F., Wei, X., Li, W., Pan, J., Lin, Y., Bowtell, D. D., et al. (2000). Pw1/Peg3 is a potential cell death mediator and cooperates with Siah1a in p53-mediated apoptosis. *Proc. Natl. Acad. Sci. U.S.A.* 97, 2105–2110. doi: 10.1073/pnas. 040378897

Rovasio, R. A., and Battiato, N. L. (2002). Ethanol induces morphological and dynamic changes on *in vivo* and *in vitro* neural crest cells. *Alcohol Clin. Exp. Res.* 26, 1286–1298. doi: 10.1097/01.ALC.0000026102.73486.65

Schuler, M., and Green, D. R. (2005). Transcription, apoptosis and p53: catch-22. *Trends Genet.* 21, 182–187. doi: 10.1016/j.tig.2005.01.001

Smith, S. M. (1997). Alcohol-induced cell death in the embryo. *Alcohol Health Res. World* 21, 287–297.

Steventon, B., Mayor, R., and Streit, A. (2014). Neural crest and placode interaction during the development of the cranial sensory system. *Dev. Biol.* 389, 28–38. doi: 10.1016/j.ydbio.2014.01.021

Su, Z., Si, W., Li, L., Zhou, B., Li, X., Xu, Y., et al. (2014). *MiR-144* regulates hematopoiesis and vascular development by targeting meis1 during zebrafish development. *Int. J. Biochem. Cell Biol.* 49, 53–63. doi: 10.1016/j.biocel.2014.01.005

Sulik, K. K., Johnston, M. C., and Webb, M. A. (1981). Fetal alcohol syndrome: embryogenesis in a mouse model. *Science* 214, 936–938. doi: 10.1126/science.6795717

Sun, H., Chen, X., Yuan, F., Liu, J., Zhao, Y., and Chen, S. Y. (2014). Involvement of seven in absentia homolog-1 in ethanol-induced apoptosis in neural crest cells. *Neurotoxicol. Teratol.* 46, 26–31. doi: 10.1016/j.ntt.2014.08.006

Tiedt, R., Bartholdy, B. A., Matthias, G., Newell, J. W., and Matthias, P. (2001). The RING finger protein Siah-1 regulates the level of the transcriptional coactivator OBF-1. *EMBO J.* 20, 4143–4152. doi: 10.1093/emboj/20.15.4143

Walker, M. B., and Kimmel, C. B. (2007). A two-color acid-free cartilage and bone stain for zebrafish larvae. *Biotech. Histochem.* 82, 23–28. doi: 10.1080/10520290701333558

Wang, K., Chen, X., Liu, J., Zou, L. P., Feng, W., Cai, L., et al. (2018). Embryonic exposure to ethanol increases the susceptibility of larval zebrafish to chemically induced seizures. *Sci. Rep.* 8:1845. doi: 10.1038/s41598-018-20288-2

Winter, M., Sombroek, D., Dauth, I., Moehlenbrink, J., Scheuermann, K., Crone, J., et al. (2008). Control of HIPK2 stability by ubiquitin ligase Siah-1 and checkpoint kinases ATM and ATR. *Nat. Cell Biol.* 10, 812–824. doi: 10.1038/ncb1743

Wu, S., Lin, Y., Xu, D., Chen, J., Shu, M., Zhou, Y., et al. (2012). MiR-135a functions as a selective killer of malignant glioma. *Oncogene* 31, 3866–3874. doi: 10.1038/onc.2011.551

Xu, B., Tao, T., Wang, Y., Fang, F., Huang, Y., Chen, S., et al. (2016). hsa-miR-135a-1 inhibits prostate cancer cell growth and migration by targeting EGFR. *Tumour Biol.* 37, 14141–14151. doi: 10.1007/s13277-016-5196-6

Yamada, Y., Hidaka, H., Seki, N., Yoshino, H., Yamasaki, T., Itesako, T., et al. (2013). Tumor-suppressive microRNA-135a inhibits cancer cell proliferation by targeting the c-MYC oncogene in renal cell carcinoma. *Cancer Sci.* 104, 304–312. doi: 10.1111/cas.12072

Yan, D., Dong, J., Sulik, K. K., and Chen, S. Y. (2010). Induction of the Nrf2-driven antioxidant response by tert-butylhydroquinone prevents ethanol-induced apoptosis in cranial neural crest cells. *Biochem. Pharmacol.* 80, 144–149. doi: 10.1016/j.bcp.2010.03.004

Yan, X., Li, W., Yang, L., Dong, W., Chen, W., Mao, Y., et al. (2018). MiR-135a protects vascular endothelial cells against ventilator-induced lung injury by inhibiting PHLPP2 to activate PI3K/Akt pathway. *Cell. Physiol. Biochem.* 48, 1245–1258. doi: 10.1159/000492010

Yuan, F., Chen, X., Liu, J., Feng, W., Cai, L., Wu, X., et al. (2018). Sulforaphane restores acetyl-histone H3 binding to Bcl-2 promoter and prevents apoptosis in ethanol-exposed neural crest cells and mouse embryos. *Exp. Neurol.* 300, 60–66. doi: 10.1016/j.expneurol.2017.10.020

Yuan, F., Chen, X., Liu, J., Feng, W., Wu, X., and Chen, S. Y. (2017). Up-regulation of Siah1 by ethanol triggers apoptosis in neural crest cells through p38 MAPK-mediated activation of p53 signaling pathway. *Arch. Toxicol.* 91, 775–784. doi: 10.1007/s00204-016-1746-3

Zhang, J., Guenther, M. G., Carthew, R. W., and Lazar, M. A. (1998). Proteasomal regulation of nuclear receptor corepressor-mediated repression. *Genes Dev.* 12, 1775–1780. doi: 10.1101/gad.12.12.1775

Zhang, P., Wang, G., Lin, Z., Wu, Y., Zhang, J., Liu, M., et al. (2017). Alcohol exposure induces chick craniofacial bone defects by negatively affecting cranial neural crest development. *Toxicol. Lett.* 281, 53–64. doi: 10.1016/j.toxlet.2017.09.010

Zhao, X., Sun, Z., Li, H., Jiang, F., Zhou, J., and Zhang, L. (2017). MiR-135a-5p modulates biological functions of thyroid carcinoma cells via targeting VCAN 3′-UTR. *Cancer Biomark.* 20, 207–216. doi: 10.3233/CBM-170566

Zheng, S. Y., Fu, X. B., Xu, J. G., Zhao, J. Y., Sun, T. Z., and Chen, W. (2005). Inhibition of p38 mitogen-activated protein kinase may decrease intestinal epithelial cell apoptosis and improve intestinal epithelial barrier function after ischemia- reperfusion injury. *World J. Gastroenterol.* 11, 656–660. doi: 10.3748/wjg.v11.i5.656

4

Zebrafish Models of Craniofacial Malformations: Interactions of Environmental Factors

S. T. Raterman[1,2,3], J. R. Metz[3], Frank A. D. T. G. Wagener[1,2] and Johannes W. Von den Hoff[1,2]*

[1] Radboud Institute of Molecular Life Sciences, Nijmegen, Netherlands, [2] Department of Dentistry-Orthodontics and Craniofacial Biology, Radboud University Medical Center, Nijmegen, Netherlands, [3] Department of Animal Ecology and Physiology, Institute for Water and Wetland Research, Radboud University, Nijmegen, Netherlands

***Correspondence:**
Johannes W. Von den Hoff
hans.vondenhoff@radboudumc.nl;
h.vondenhoff@dent.umcn.nl

The zebrafish is an appealing model organism for investigating the genetic (G) and environmental (E) factors, as well as their interactions (GxE), which contribute to craniofacial malformations. Here, we review zebrafish studies on environmental factors involved in the etiology of craniofacial malformations in humans including maternal smoking, alcohol consumption, nutrition and drug use. As an example, we focus on the (cleft) palate, for which the zebrafish ethmoid plate is a good model. This review highlights the importance of investigating ExE interactions and discusses the variable effects of exposure to environmental factors on craniofacial development depending on dosage, exposure time and developmental stage. Zebrafish also promise to be a good tool to study novel craniofacial teratogens and toxin mixtures. Lastly, we discuss the handful of studies on gene–alcohol interactions using mutant sensitivity screens and reverse genetic techniques. We expect that studies addressing complex interactions (ExE and GxE) in craniofacial malformations will increase in the coming years. These are likely to uncover currently unknown mechanisms with implications for the prevention of craniofacial malformations. The zebrafish appears to be an excellent complementary model with high translational value to study these complex interactions.

Keywords: zebrafish, craniofacial malformations, neural crest cells, environment, gene, interaction

INTRODUCTION

Craniofacial malformations are a heterogenic group of developmental defects of the skull and face, for which no preventive therapies exist. This broad group of over 700 disorders includes debilitating malformations of the skull (craniosynostosis), jaw (micrognathia), face (hemifacial microsomia, deformational plagiocephaly) and teeth (tooth agenesis), (Online Mendelian Inheritance in

---

Abbreviations: AhR, Aryl hydrocarbon receptor; BMP, Bone morphogenetic protein; BPA/AF/S/F, Bisphenol A/AF/S/F; CDC, Center for disease control; CLP, Cleft lip and/or palate; CNCC, Cranial neural crest cells; CYP1A, Cytochrome P450 1A; DHODH, Dihydroorotate dehydrogenase; dpf, Days post fertilization; E2, 17ß-estradiol; ENU, N-ethyl-n-nitrosourea; ER, Estrogen receptors; FA, Follic acid; FAS, Fetal alcohol syndrome; FASD, Fetal alcohol spectrum disorders; FDA, Food and drug administration; FGF, Fibroblast growth factor; FVSP, Fetal valproate spectrum disorder; GST, Glutathione-S-transferase; GWAS, Genome wide association studies; hpf, Hours post fertilization; M-PQ, Meckel's-palatoquadrate; OMIM, Online Mendelian Inheritance in Man; OR, Odds ratio; PAH, Polycyclic aromatic hydrocarbons; RA, Retinoic acid signaling; SHH, Sonic hedgehog; TGF, Transforming growth factor; TPM, Total particular matter; VPA, Valproic acid; WHO, World health organization; WNT, Wingless-Int-1 pathway.

Man) (OMIM). Heterogeneity is not only a principal feature of craniofacial phenotypes, but also contributes to their etiology, as malformations are often caused by complex interactions of genetic and environmental factors (Gardner et al., 1998; Dixon et al., 2011).

In this review, we focus on clefts of the palate, which oftentimes co-occur with cleft lip. Cleft lip and/or palate (CLP) is the most common congenital craniofacial birth defect. It affects the face uni- or bilaterally, as well as the hard and soft palate (Dixon et al., 2011). Extensive reconstructive surgery and dental treatment are often required until adulthood for the various forms of CLP (Acum et al., 2020; Martin et al., 2020). After surgery, CLP patients may still experience difficulties with speaking and hearing, leading to psychosocial problems (Martin et al., 2020). About 30% of CLP cases arise as part of a syndrome caused by a single genetic mutation. However, the majority of cases are non-syndromic and associated with both genetic (G) and environmental (E) risk factors (Beaty et al., 2011; Dixon et al., 2011; Stuppia et al., 2011).

Candidate genes for CLP are continually identified benefiting from genetic data from individuals, family-and-twin studies, and large-scale GWAS studies (Beaty et al., 2002; Mansilla et al., 2005; Leslie et al., 2015). Often, these genes relate to central regulatory pathways of development including sonic hedgehog (SHH), transforming growth factor (TGF), fibroblast growth factor (FGF), bone morphogenetic protein (BMP), retinoic acid signaling (RA) and Wingless-Int-1 pathway (WNT) signaling (Beaty et al., 2011; Dixon et al., 2011; Reynolds et al., 2019). For example, mutations of the BMP pathway gene *MSX1* and multiple canonical (WNT9B) and non-canonical (WNT5A) *WNT* pathway genes have been associated with non-syndromic CLP (Chiquet et al., 2008). In parallel, environmental factors such as smoking, drinking, drug use, diet and other lifestyle habits during pregnancy have been demonstrated to increase the risk of CLP (van Rooij et al., 2001; DeRoo et al., 2008; Jentink et al., 2010) and other craniofacial malformations (Gardner et al., 1998; Carmichael et al., 2008; Al-Ani et al., 2017). Due to the substantial number of factors involved in craniofacial malformations, the underlying etiology remains largely elusive. Moreover, interactions between genetic and environmental factors (GxE) further complicate the etiology. Since no single animal model can mimic all facets of genetic and environmental influences on craniofacial development in humans, the use of multiple model species is required to elucidate the etiology of craniofacial malformations.

Zebrafish are a promising model to study both genetic and environmental interactions in craniofacial malformations, such as palatal clefts. In the last decade, there has been a rapid increase in zebrafish genetic models for human disease-causing genes including CLP (reviewed by Duncan et al., 2017; Machado and Eames, 2017). Additionally, the growing zebrafish-based research field investigating the role of environmental factors in craniofacial malformations enhances the value of zebrafish in craniofacial research. Zebrafish studies have produced powerful mechanistic insights on both the genetic (variants) and environmental factors which disturb facial development. Up to now, investigations of GxE interactions are published less frequently. However, zebrafish studies in this field are upcoming since there is overwhelming evidence that GxE interactions are the crux of cleft etiology in humans (Wu et al., 2010; Beaty et al., 2011; Dixon et al., 2011; Stuppia et al., 2011).

We have outlined this review as follows: first we discuss zebrafish studies on the effects of maternal smoking, alcohol use, nutrition, drug use and household environmental factors on craniofacial development. We specifically focus on the molecular mechanisms and phenotypic outcomes. Environmental factors with the highest odds ratio (OR) for incidence of craniofacial malformations are discussed first. Secondly, we consider the limited but emerging field of GxE interactions in zebrafish models for craniofacial malformations, and propose strategies for future research.

ZEBRAFISH AS A CRANIOFACIAL MODEL SYSTEM

The teleost fish, the zebrafish has several advantages over the use of other vertebrate animal models for the study of congenital defects. In particular, zebrafish has a rapid, transparent early development and large brood sizes (Schilling and Kimmel, 1997). They develop a detailed and visible craniofacial skeleton as early as 5 days post fertilization (dpf) (Kimmel et al., 2001). Zebrafish embryos can also be directly exposed to environmental factors via the embryo medium. Zebrafish orthologous genes have been identified for 82% of disease-causing genes in humans as reported in OMIM (Howe et al., 2013). These assets make the zebrafish an attractive model for studying early craniofacial development alongside more traditional animal models such as mouse and chicken (Van Otterloo et al., 2016).

In zebrafish, craniofacial development commences with the migration of cells from the rhombomeres and mesencephalon of the neural crest. These cells migrate in tightly regulated lineages toward predetermined destinations in the head region (Dougherty et al., 2012; Rocha et al., 2020). The first lineage of cranial neural crest cells (CNCC) splits and one part migrates between the developing eyes making up the frontonasal CNCCs. The other part migrates ventrally to populate the first of seven pharyngeal arches (Wada et al., 2005; Swartz et al., 2011; Dougherty et al., 2012). Arches 2–7 are subsequently populated by other lineage of CNCCs, where, upon arrival, all CNCCs surround a mesoderm core (Mork and Crump, 2015). Orchestrated by evolutionary conserved intrinsic and extrinsic signaling, the CNCCs condense and undergo chondrogenic differentiation to form the head cartilages. Comprehensive data and resources on craniofacial development can be found at FaceBase[1], including "FishFace, an atlas of zebrafish craniofacial development" (Eames et al., 2013).

As mentioned, zebrafish develop a functional craniofacial skeleton within the first 5 days post fertilization (**Figure 1**). However, the zebrafish craniofacial skeleton is structurally more complex than that of most other vertebrates, and continues to grow throughout the fish's lifetime (Bruneel and Witten,

[1] www.facebase.org/

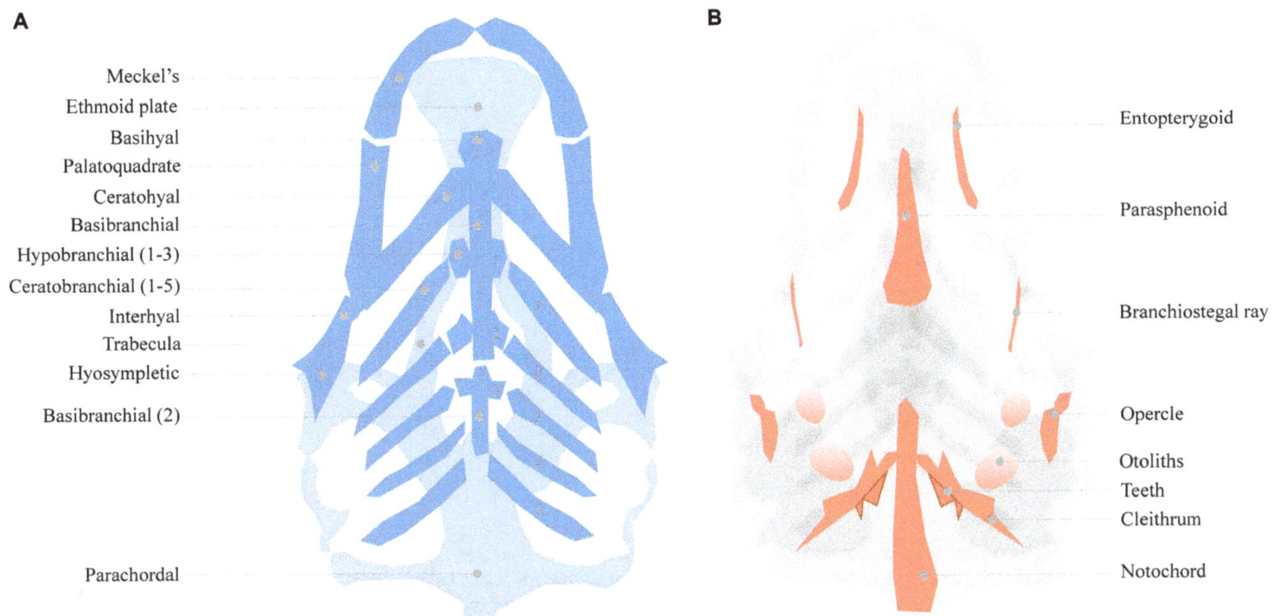

FIGURE 1 | (A) Cartilage structures of the zebrafish neuro- and viscerocranium at 5 dpf (light and dark blue, respectively), ventral perspective. A number of these structures is used as a homolog to human skeletal features: Meckel's cartilage for the lower jaw, the ethmoid plate for the hard palate and the palatoquadrate for the middle ear. **(B)** Intramembranous bones of the 5 dpf zebrafish head, dorsal view.

2015). The adult zebrafish head contains 73 bones, exceeding the number of bones in the mammalian skull at least three fold (Cubbage and Mabee, 1996). The early cartilage structures consist of only a few chondrocyte and perichondral cell layers (**Figure 1A**; Kimmel et al., 2001). The first cartilages can be detected as early as 3 dpf, while some intramembranous bone structures also start to form on the cartilage matrix (Aceto et al., 2015). At 5 dpf, a small number of bone structures are already present (detailed in **Figure 1B**). The cartilages are divided into the dorsally located neurocranial structures (CNCC- and mesoderm- derived) that support the developing brain, and the ventrally located pharyngeal arch-derived structures important for feeding and gill coverage (Kimmel et al., 2010). The cartilages are maintained during early larval stages and are progressively replaced by bone through endochondral ossification (Cubbage and Mabee, 1996; Bruneel and Witten, 2015; Weigele and Franz-Odendaal, 2016). Surprisingly, the zebrafish intramembranous bones are often disregarded in investigations of craniofacial development in the presence of environmental factors, resulting in significant knowledge gaps.

The zebrafish larval head can be used to study various craniofacial malformations. For instance, the cranial sutures of the juvenile (3–12 weeks) zebrafish skull can be manipulated to mimic craniosynostosis, while the Meckel's cartilage formation can be used study lower jaw defects (Miller et al., 2000; Andreeva et al., 2011; Laue et al., 2011; Cornille et al., 2019). To be concise, we focus on the ethmoid plate and the associated trabecula. These structures are part of the zebrafish neurocranium and are considered homologous to the mammalian palate (Bush and Jiang, 2012).

The ethmoid plate and the mammalian hard palate both derive from bilateral streams of anterior maxillary CNCC (Mork and Crump, 2015). In zebrafish, frontonasal CNCCs migrate below the eyes to the midline, while maxillary CNCCs from the first pharyngeal arch assemble laterally to the midline. Then, both lineages fuse to form the ethmoid plate (Dougherty et al., 2013). In humans, mice and, other mammals, the palate develops during gestational weeks 6–12 (humans) and E10–E16 (mice) (Bush and Jiang, 2012). The palate emanates from the outgrowth, vertical-to-horizontal reorientation and fusion of CNCC-derived maxillary prominences (Bush and Jiang, 2012). Mutations in PDGFRA and genes of the SHH pathway lead to inadequate midline fusion resulting in a cleft palate phenotype in mice, humans and zebrafish (Wada et al., 2005; Swartz et al., 2011; Dougherty et al., 2013; McCarthy et al., 2013). These shared disease etiologies confirm that similar molecular mechanisms are involved in the development of the palate and ethmoid plate. A commonly accepted interpretation hereof is that the ethmoid plate is homologous to the mammalian palate (Mork and Crump, 2015). In zebrafish, the cleft phenotype typically features aberrant chondrocyte morphology and stacking in the ethmoid plate. Also, the anterior border of the ethmoid plate can appear dented instead of smooth. More severe ethmoid phenotypes include two anteriorly unconnected outer rods or only a single rod. The spectrum of ethmoid plate disruptions is broad, but some representative examples taken from the literature on environmental factors are represented in **Figure 2**.

Additional morphological, cellular and molecular parallels between mammals and zebrafish are continually identified in craniofacial research. Virtually every new discovery further

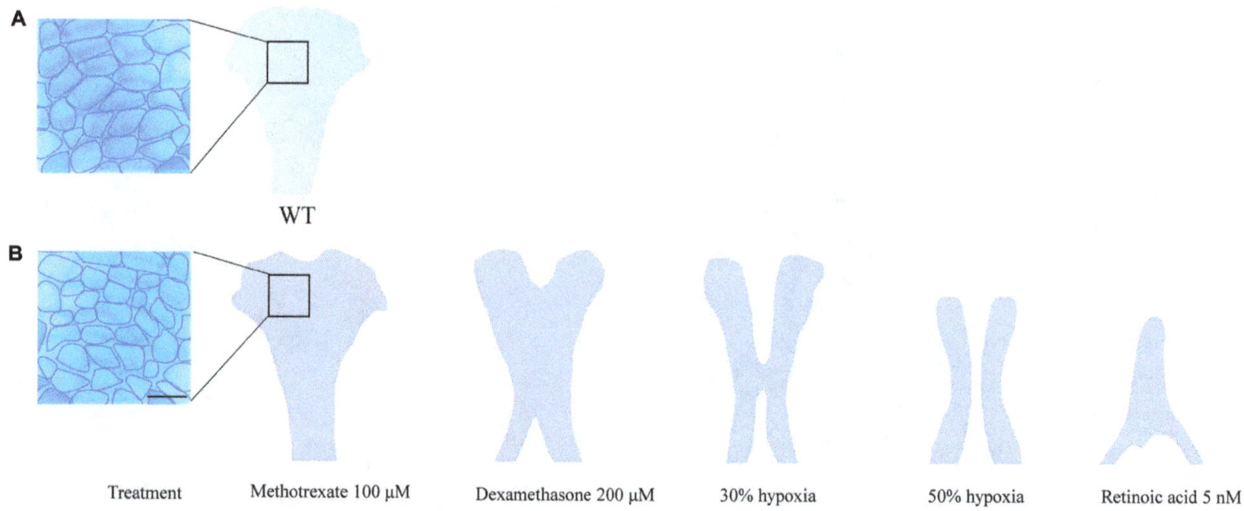

FIGURE 2 | (A) Wildtype ethmoid plate with associated stacking of chondrocytes. **(B)** Redrawn examples of ethmoid plate defects observed in zebrafish environmental factor exposure studies (Kuchler et al., 2018; Liu et al., 2020) (Methotrexate 100 μM, Dexamethasone 200 μM, retinoic acid 5 nM and hypoxia). A broad phenotypic range of ethmoid plate defects is observed, indicating that development of the ethmoid plate is affected variously by different compounds. Mild phenotypes include a rough edge to the anterior ethmoid plate, and differential cell morphology (round vs. elongated) and chondrocyte stacking is disordered, drawn from Liu et al. (2020) (scale bar 5 μm). At the other end of the spectrum, phenotypes are observed in which ethmoid plate structures are (partially) missing, indicating effects on migration, differentiation and survival CNCCs. Moreover, some factors affect early as well as late craniofacial development, and various effects can occur though differential exposure times during specific sensitivity windows.

supports the translational value of the zebrafish model. We advocate that zebrafish should be used more extensively as an additional tool complementary to established models such as the mouse. In the following sections, we discuss zebrafish models for investigating environmental factors in craniofacial malformations.

SMOKING

In epidemiological studies, maternal smoking before and during early pregnancy is consistently reported as an environmental risk factor for CLP (Stuppia et al., 2011; Sabbagh et al., 2015; Xuan et al., 2016). Despite decades of research, the mechanisms by which smoking affects development are still not fully understood. Since cigarette smoke consists of over 7,000 components, numerous mechanisms are involved (center for disease control) (CDC)[2]. Abundant components of smoke are polycyclic aromatic hydrocarbons (PAHs), carbon monoxide, tar and nicotine (Kennedy et al., 2017). These compounds can exert direct teratogenic effects when transported across the placenta to the amniotic fluid (Liszewski et al., 2012). Cigarette smoke contains inhibitors (nicotine) and inducers (PAH) of the aryl hydrocarbon receptor (AhR) pathway that activates cytochrome P450 1A (CYP1A). During xenobiotic metabolism, reactive products are formed from PAHs, mediated by CYP1A. These products can cause cell damage if they are not rapidly detoxified by metabolite glutathione-S-transferase (GST). Activity of this enzyme can be reduced by smoke itself or by genetic factors (van Rooij et al., 2001). For instance, a maternal GSTT1-null genotype in humans has been shown to increase the risk of clefting in the offspring of smoking mothers (odds ratio 3.2) (van Rooij et al., 2001). Thus, the toxicity of smoking can be further increased by genetic predisposition for suboptimal function of the enzymes for xenobiotic metabolism.

In studies on the effects of maternal smoking on development, zebrafish were traditionally used as a model to examine effects of single abundant compounds of cigarette smoke. Craniofacial malformations are consistently reported in zebrafish studies on smoke compounds such as PAHs, carbon monoxide (hypoxia) and nicotine (Billiard et al., 2006; Parker and Connaughton, 2007; Geier et al., 2018; Kuchler et al., 2018). Specifically, clefts in the ethmoid plate were observed when zebrafish are exposed to hypoxic conditions during early development. These clefts increased in severity as oxygen levels were reduced (Kuchler et al., 2018). Although single-factor investigations are interesting from a fundamental standpoint, they do not provide clinically relevant insights on the effects of maternal smoking on development, because the combined teratogenic effects of smoke compounds may be additive.

In recent years, there has been an increasing amount of literature on the effects of smoke on zebrafish development by exposure to the total particular matter (TPM) of cigarette smoke. TPM exposure lead to craniofacial malformations from above 6 μg/mL, but craniofacial malformations have not yet been evaluated in depth (Ellis et al., 2014; Massarsky et al., 2015; Palpant et al., 2015). Other reported effects of TPM are increased larval mortality, gross morphological deformities and distorted AhR pathway-related enzyme functions (CYP1A and GST). Cross-talk between the AhR pathway and Wnt/β-catenin

[2]https://www.cdc.gov/biomonitoring/tobacco.html

signaling in zebrafish embryos was also shown. Wnt/β-catenin signaling is a major pathway in craniofacial development (Zhang et al., 2016; Reynolds et al., 2019). Moreover, AhR activation down-regulated *sox9a* during cartilage formation in zebrafish (Xiong et al., 2008). Knockdown of the AhR pathway with simultaneous exposure to TPM reduced morphological defects, however knockdown of CYP1A or CYP1B1 increased defects (Massarsky et al., 2016). This confirms that the toxicity of TPM is partly dependent on the genetic factors controlling xenobiotic metabolism. Predictably, the overall teratogenic effects of TPM on zebrafish larvae were not mimicked by nicotine alone (Massarsky et al., 2015). This exemplifies the importance of evaluating compound interactions.

With the emergence of the e-cigarette, new risk factors for congenital malformations were introduced. Studies show that e-cigarettes are regarded by pregnant women as a safer alternative for tobacco during pregnancy (Wagner et al., 2017). The compounds in e-cigarette liquids differ considerably from regular cigarettes as the main components are nicotine, propylene glycerol and vegetable glycerin (the latter two account for ~90% of the content) (Schober et al., 2014). Upon partial combustion of propylene glycerol and vegetable glycerin, toxins such as formaldehyde, acrolein, benzene and reactive aldehydes form, that may pose a health risk (Schober et al., 2014). Zebrafish exposed to low levels of propylene glycerol (1.25, 2.5, or 5%, at 6–72 hpf) showed disrupted development, including cardiac defects and morphological malformations (Massarsky et al., 2017). It is concerning that such e-cigarette components are new widespread environmental factors that pregnant women are exposed to.

In e-cigarettes, a vast number of chemicals is also used to add optional flavors. Already, over 7,000 different flavors were on the market in 2014 (Zhu et al., 2014). Flavor ingredients are not listed by manufacturers, possibly because this is not required by law (Tierney et al., 2016). Zebrafish have previously been exposed to fruit flavored e-liquids containing the active compounds ethyl vanillin, maltol and vanillin. It was reported that this caused developmental defects including unspecified craniofacial malformations (Tierney et al., 2016; Holden et al., 2020). The combustion of "berry" and "cream" flavors appeared to cause craniofacial malformations more frequently, but the chemical composition of these (and most other) e-cigarette flavors is unknown. In *Xenopus*, e-cigarette flavors caused craniofacial defects, which were enhanced by co-exposure to nicotine. On its own, nicotine caused only minor malformations (Kennedy et al., 2017). These data confirm interactions between components of e-cigarette liquids and emphasize the need for combined TPM exposure studies. While some e-cigarette flavors have been studied in zebrafish and other animals, considerably more investigations are needed on their interactions and mechanisms of action.

ALCOHOL

Fetal alcohol syndrome (FAS) and fetal alcohol spectrum disorders (FASD) are pressing health conditions resulting from alcohol exposure during the first two trimesters of pregnancy. FAS (0.2–1.5 in 1,000 births) describes a multitude of congenital abnormalities of the nervous system, cardiovascular system and face. FASD (1–5 in 100 births) symptoms are less severe but also include central nervous system disorders and craniofacial malformations[3]. The variety in symptoms upon alcohol exposure can be attributed to factors including the timing of alcohol exposure, dosage, metabolism and epigenetics (McCarthy and Eberhart, 2014). Described craniofacial malformations include a flat midface (midface hypoplasia), short nose and smooth philtrum, a thin upper lip, microcephaly, micrognathia and, in 7% of FASD cases, cleft palate (Sampson et al., 1997; Li et al., 2007). Ethanol exposure and FAS/FASD etiology have received ample attention in zebrafish studies and other models, and studies are reviewed frequently (McCarthy and Eberhart, 2014; Facciol et al., 2019; Lovely, 2020).

Ethanol can be found in amniotic fluid after alcohol consumption by the mother and can thus impact the fetus directly. Within 1 h after consumption, fetal alcohol levels are equivalent to those in the maternal circulation (Burd et al., 2007). The known mechanisms of ethanol teratogenicity are many fold. Currently, they are known to include increased cell death, reactive oxygen species, altered growth factor signaling, altered retinoic acid signaling, disrupted cholesterol homeostasis and impaired cell adhesion (Li et al., 2007; Marrs et al., 2010; Soares et al., 2012; Sarmah et al., 2013; Muralidharan et al., 2015; Eason et al., 2017). The zebrafish is an established model to study the effects of ethanol on development. Importantly, the chorion, which surrounds the early zebrafish embryo, appears freely permeable for ethanol. Zebrafish embryonic ethanol levels reach approximately 25–35% of the embryo medium level (Blader and Strahle, 1998; Ali et al., 2011; Fernandes et al., 2019). In zebrafish, both short-term and chronic ethanol exposure increase the incidence of craniofacial malformations.

In search of ethanol sensitivity windows for craniofacial development, zebrafish embryos were exposed to a—rather extreme—regime of 10% ethanol during defined developmental stages (Ali et al., 2011). At 25 and 31 hpf (developmental stages prim-6 and prim-16, respectively) embryos were most susceptible to defects of the branchial arches and Meckel's cartilage (Ali et al., 2011). Furthermore, in the late blastula and early gastrula stages, embryos appeared to be specifically sensitive for the induction of cyclopia after exposure to 2.4% ethanol (Blader and Strahle, 1998). Upon chronic exposure, distinct craniofacial effects have been observed depending on ethanol dosage. Ethmoid plate development and head width were reduced at concentrations as low as 3 mM (0.01%), which can be reached in women upon drinking only one alcoholic beverage (Carvan et al., 2004; Ferdous et al., 2017). Interestingly, with rising concentrations, a sensitivity shift was reported. At 10 mM ethanol (0.04%), neurocranium structures were more severely affected than structures of the viscerocranium, while at 30 mM (0.13%) the opposite was observed (Carvan et al., 2004). Variations in sensitivity to ethanol exposure between zebrafish strains are also reported. Upon exposure, Ekkwill strain zebrafish presented with a severely affected viscerocranium

[3]www.cdc.gov/ncbddd/fasd/data.html

and increased apoptosis, whereas AB strain zebrafish had affected neurocranial cartilages such as the ethmoid plate. In Tübingen strain zebrafish larvae a high mortality rate was observed, but this strain was less prone to craniofacial defects (Loucks and Carvan, 2004). The strain specific sensitivity to ethanol implicates that predisposing genetic factors and GxE interactions are involved.

Most studies in which zebrafish were exposed to ethanol, used the timeframe between 6 and 24 hpf. This is equivalent to binge drinking (4–5 drinks) throughout the entire first trimester of pregnancy in humans. This poorly resembles a clinically relevant situation and, therefore, Zhang et al. transiently exposed zebrafish to alcohol, during early gastrulation (5.25–6.25 hpf) and neurulation (8–10 and 24–27 hpf) (Zhang et al., 2014). These larvae presented with FASD symptoms, including craniofacial malformations and differential expression of SHH pathway genes. Interaction with SHH signaling seems to be a central mechanism of ethanol teratogenicity (Li et al., 2007; Burton et al., 2017). Upon translation, Shh undergoes posttranslational modifications by cholesterol. This mechanism is crucial for craniofacial development, but ethanol (0.7–7 mM) treatment during gastrulation impaired modification of *shh* by cholesterol (Li et al., 2007). As previously mentioned, SHH pathway gene mutations are also implicated in craniofacial malformations in humans. Later in this review we will discuss evidence of interactions between genetic factors and ethanol, which further complicates the mechanism of action.

VITAMINS AND ExE INTERACTIONS

Proper development requires a delicate balance of micronutrients. Specifically, derivatives of vitamins A and B are crucial for craniofacial development in both fish and mammals. Zebrafish have been used to study the roles of vitamins A and B during development and in craniofacial malformations. Far less is currently known from the zebrafish model about other essential vitamins and trace elements implicated in craniofacial malformations.

Vitamin A

Retinoic acid (RA) is a vitamin A-derived retinol and an essential morphogen in embryonic development. Vitamin A is acquired through products such as meat, milk, eggs and carrots (Metzler and Sandell, 2016). Vitamin A deficiency (serum level < 0.70 μmol/L) is a public health concern in countries in Africa and South East Asia, and was associated with craniofacial malformations including CLP (WHO[4]) (Ackermans et al., 2011; Mammadova et al., 2014; Metzler and Sandell, 2016; Williams and Bohnsack, 2019). Supplementation with vitamin A was associated with a lower cleft risk (OR = 0.48) (Johansen et al., 2008). Use of acne medication that contains vitamin A derivatives during pregnancy may result in hypervitaminosis A. This increased the risk of craniofacial malformations including cleft lip, cleft palate, micrognathia and midface hypoplasia (Williams and Bohnsack, 2019).

In mammals, RA precursors are delivered to the fetus by the maternal circulation in the form of retinoids and carotenoids. In zebrafish, RA is synthesized by oxidation of all-trans-retinal derived from the yolk (Metzler and Sandell, 2016). RA subsequently acts through the nuclear retinoic acid receptors. These receptors belong to the steroid/thyroid superfamily (Joore et al., 1994; Metzler and Sandell, 2016). Zebrafish have two (α and γ) RA receptors while mammals have three (α, γ, and β). Retinoic acid receptors are widely expressed throughout the embryo and act by dimerization with retinoid x receptors. Active RA is degraded by CYP26A1 and CYP26B1, and a posterior-anterior increasing gradient of RA is maintained during early development (Williams and Bohnsack, 2019).

RA is a key regulator of Hox-family genes, which are essential for pharyngeal arch development (Williams and Bohnsack, 2019). RA targets the endoderm and ectoderm surrounding the CNCCs, which subsequently signal to CNCCs in the pharyngeal arches. In zebrafish, 1 nM of exogenous RA between 10.5 and 12.5 hpf increased expression of the *hoxa1* and *hoxb2* genes. This resulted in the fusion of structures of the first and second pharyngeal arches, such as fusion of the ceratohyal cartilage with Meckel's cartilage (Yan et al., 1998). Moreover, transient treatment with 1 μM RA during gastrulation (5.25–10 hpf) resulted in complete loss of expression of the neural crest cell marker *dlx* in the head at 24 hpf, and the absence of craniofacial cartilages. At 0.1 μM RA, *dlx* expression was detected in neurocranial structures, but not in the viscerocranium, suggesting specific sensitivity of these structures (Ellies et al., 1997). Embryos treated with 0.1 μM RA during neural crest migration (12–19 hpf) showed impaired Meckel's cartilage and palatoquadrate formation, which was also associated with reduced *dlx4* expression. RA treatment caused only mild effects on Meckel's cartilage upon treatment at 24 hpf, suggesting RA mainly affected CNCC migration (Ellies et al., 1997). In contrast to these findings, at a much lower concentration (5 nM) and using continual exposure between 4 and 96 hpf, exogenous RA had severe effects on the neurocranium. The ethmoid plate was reportedly severely shortened and resembled a single rod. Cells of the ethmoid plate were also disorderly stacked (Liu et al., 2020). After development, RA retains essential functions in regulating osteoblast and osteoclast activity, maintaining bone mineral density, and promoting cell survival (Williams and Bohnsack, 2019). Exogenous RA treatment (0.1 μM) in adult zebrafish during just 5 days resulted in an acute prognathic jaw. Inhibition of RA synthesis resulted in decreased head height (Chawla et al., 2018). Similarly, craniosynostosis phenotypes were observed in CYP26b (hypomorph)-deficient juvenile zebrafish as a result of disrupted RA degradation (Spoorendonk et al., 2008; Laue et al., 2011). These data support that a tight regulation of RA activity is necessary during and after craniofacial development.

Epidemiological studies showed that the risk of FASD and craniofacial malformation were higher in pregnancies with alcohol exposure in low socioeconomic environments. In these environments, maternal malnutrition and vitamin (A) deficiency

[4]www.who.int/elena/titles/vitamina_pregnancy/en/

are more frequent (Jiang et al., 2020). Ethanol competes with retinol for a dehydrogenase that converts retinol into RA and ethanol into acetaldehyde (Marrs et al., 2010). In zebrafish, RA and ethanol appear to exert opposing effects on ethmoid plate development. Zebrafish larvae treated with 100 mM (0.6%) ethanol showed a reduced ethmoid plate width, which was rescued by a low dose (1 nM) of exogenous RA. In the same study, RA addition without alcohol exposure resulted in a wider ethmoid plate (Marrs et al., 2010). Disruption of RA signaling appears to be a distinct mechanism of alcohol teratogenesis and is an example of an ExE interaction.

Folic Acid

Recommendations are given to pregnant women to commence vitamin B_9 or folic acid (FA) supplementation prior to conception (WHO)[5]. FA is converted to folate in the body and prevents neural tube defects such as spina bifida, anencephaly and craniorachischisis. FA was also shown to reduce CLP risk in a meta-analysis (Wilson et al., 2015; Millacura et al., 2017). Still, findings are contradictory as specific genetic predisposing factors combined with FA supplementation were reported to be detrimental to development (Marean et al., 2011). FA is required for nucleic acid synthesis and for histone and DNA methylation. Zebrafish embryos starved of folate showed defects early in development, which may be caused by cell cycle delay in the S-phase (Lee et al., 2012). Upon alcohol exposure during pregnancy, inefficient maternal-to-fetal FA transport leads to FA deficiency in the fetus. This is thought to result from reduced expression of folate binding and transport proteins under the influence of ethanol (Hutson et al., 2012). In zebrafish, FA supplementation rescued ethanol-induced craniofacial malformations most effectively when administered during early embryogenesis (6 hpf). Upon addition of FA, apoptosis in the embryos was reduced and *tbx-1* signaling was partially restored (Jiang et al., 2020). Notably, mutations of *TBX-1* have been associated with cleft palate in humans (Herman et al., 2012). The rescue by FA may be mediated by its antioxidant properties and epigenetic restoration of ethanol-induced effects (Muralidharan et al., 2015). The role of FA in birth defect prevention is well-characterized. However, future zebrafish studies may offer more insights into genetic predisposing factors that diminish the efficacy of FA to prevent congenital abnormalities (Marean et al., 2011).

PHARMACEUTICALS AND TERATOGENESIS IN ZEBRAFISH LARVAE

Use of pharmaceuticals during pregnancy can lead to craniofacial malformations. The FDA provides contraindications to pregnant women for the use of drugs associated with teratogenic effects. However, since pregnancies may be unplanned and/or undetected in the first months, it is not always possible to cease use of medication during early pregnancy (Finer and Zolna, 2016). Pharmaceuticals are a prime example of highly controllable environmental factors, as circulating doses in patients are standardized. By using equivalent doses in animal studies, direct comparisons of teratogenic effects can be made between species. In zebrafish, administration of drugs is relatively simple, but care should be taken to minimize effects of embryo medium conditions such as pH, salt concentration and temperature on drug uptake (Weigt et al., 2011).

For example, the widely used anti-epileptic drug and mood stabilizer VPA, prescribed to women of reproductive age, is frequently associated with craniofacial teratogenicity. VPA was reported to cause FVSP, with symptoms such as intellectual disability, facial abnormalities (including CLP) and cardiac defects (Clayton-Smith et al., 2019). VPA acts by inhibition of histone deacetylases, which results in changed expression of genes important for craniofacial development (Phiel et al., 2001; Gurvich et al., 2005). Altered WNT signaling is a known mechanism of VPA teratogenesis. Impaired WNT signaling by genetic or environmental causes is known to result in craniofacial malformations such as CLP in humans. For a comprehensive overview on the involvement of the WNT pathway in craniofacial development we refer to a previous review (Reynolds et al., 2019).

The reported phenotypic effects of VPA on zebrafish vary between studies. However, parallels between human FVSP and zebrafish phenotypes can be drawn. VPA exposure between 4 and 96 hpf (30 μM) resulted in microcephaly, a shortened ethmoid plate with rough anterior edge, and a hypoplastic Meckel's cartilage with disorganized chondrocyte stacking (Liu et al., 2020). These effects on the ethmoid plate parallel those of the cleft palate phenotype in FVSP. In our lab, early (1–13 hpf) and late (25–37 hpf) embryonic VPA exposure (50 and 100 μM VPA) resulted in a shortened head, reduced bone formation and smaller ceratohyals. Wnt marker *axin2* was downregulated, while the Wnt inhibitor *dkk1b* was upregulated at 5 dpf. This may account for the decreased ossification, as Wnt is essential in initiating ossification (Gebuijs et al., 2020). Martinez and colleagues reported on a dramatic decrease of survival and lack of development of the craniofacial cartilages in embryos exposed to 25, 50, and 100 μM at 4–96 hpf. The long exposure window used in this study may account for the phenotypic discrepancy with the results obtained in our lab.

In addition to VPA, many other drugs may affect craniofacial development. Obviously, the effects depend on the dose as well as on the exposure duration or corresponding developmental stage. A succinct, tabular overview of effects and mechanisms of selected teratogens from major drug classes is provided in **Table 1**. We systematically compared the effects reported in zebrafish with phenotypes described in humans (or if not available, in mouse models). Zebrafish models largely mimicked the phenotypic effects that were observed in mammals, and especially humans, in six out of eight selected teratogens from various drug classes. The target mechanisms implicated in craniofacial development largely varied, but in three cases

[5]www.who.int/elena/titles/guidance_summaries/daily_iron_pregnancy/en/

TABLE 1 | Reported effects of pharmaceuticals at various concentrations and exposure times on zebrafish craniofacial development and parallel craniofacial findings in humans or, if not available, in mice.

Compound	Concentration	Exposure time	Effects in zebrafish	References	Target mechanisms in craniofacial development	Effects on mammals
Phenytoin (Anti-epileptic)	200 μM	4–96 hpf	Irregular **anterior ethmoid** border and rounder cells, **shortened head**	Liu et al., 2020	Upregulated retinoic acid receptorsand growth factors IGF-2, TGFa, and TGFb1, (Gelineau-van Waes et al., 1999)	Causes fetal Hydantoinsyndrome with **microcephaly** cleft lip and/or **cleft palate** in humans (Gelineau-van Waes et al., 1999). In mice cleft lip and **palate** (Sulik et al., 1979; Mao and Tang, 2010)
Warfarin (Anticoagulant)	52.4 μM	2.5–72 hpf	Severe head malformations (unspecified), **eye and otolith defects**	Weigt et al., 2012	Upregulated Bmp antagonist *tsku*. Inhibited glutamyl to γ-carboxyglutamyl transition of vitamin K-dependent proteins such as osteocalcin and periostin (Hanumanthaiah et al., 2001; Fernandez et al., 2014)	Craniofacial malformations of the nose and airways, **eye/ear defects** and cleft lip in humans when taken during the first trimester of gestation (Hou, 2004)
	60 μM	4–96 hpf	Shortened head structures, a dent in the anterior ethmoid plate, which also showed altered cell morphology and disorganized cell stacking	Liu et al., 2020		
Methotrexate (Immunosuppressor)	100–200 μM	4–96 hpf	**Size reduction of the neurocranium, micro clefts in the anterior ethmoid plate.** Cells that make up the ethmoid plate appeared disorganized	Lee et al., 2013; Liu et al., 2020	Folic acid antagonist which inhibits DNA synthesis and cell proliferation by competitively inhibiting dihydrofolate reductase (Lee et al., 2012)	Craniosynostosis and **microcephaly and incomplete cleft palate** in humans (Granzow et al., 2003; Zarella et al., 2016)
Acetaminophen (Paracetamol)	2.5–13.4 mM	0–120/72–120 hpf	Palatoquadral length, ceratohyal length and head size reduced	Cedron et al., 2020	Activation cytochrome P450 and increased apoptosis (Cedron et al., 2020)	No affected phenotypes reported
Cyclosporin A (Immunmodulator)	10 μM	8–120 hpf	Hypoplasia of the ceratohyoids and ceratobranchials, and **reduced cartilage formation** in of the viscerocranium	Seda et al., 2019	Inhibitor of calcineurin, which dephosphorylates transcription factors Nuclear factor of activated T-cells, upon which these enter the cell nucleus and drive transcription (Winslow et al., 2006)	Cleft palate in mice (Gasser et al., 1992). Nfatc1-deficient mice exhibit reduced **reduced formation of mineralized bone** resulting in wider cranial sutures (Winslow et al., 2006)
Hydroxyurea (Sickle-cell anemia and psoriasis)	1 mM	4–96 hpf	Shortening of the head resembling micrognathia and **microcephaly**	Liu et al., 2020	Largely unknown. Ribonucleotide reductase inhibitor, by which DNA synthesis is inhibited (Woo et al., 2004)	In mice **microcephaly**, and hydrocephalus (Woo et al., 2004)
Leflunomide (Anit-rheumatic drug)	10 μM	8–120 hpf	Craniofacial cartilages did not form	Seda et al., 2019	Inhibitor of Dihydroorotate dehydrogenase (DHODH) (Pinto and Dougados, 2006)	Miller syndrome caused by DHODH gene defects micrognathia cleft palate cleft lip in humans (Ng et al., 2010)
	10 μM	8–24 hpf	Increase in the ceratohyal angle	Seda et al., 2019		
Dexamethasone (Corticosteroid)	200 μM	4–96 hpf	Shortening of the head region and **rough edge to the anterior ethmoid plate** and round, small chondrocytes	Liu et al., 2020	Increase of matrix metalloproteinase 2 and 9 expression and activity, trough the glucocorticoid receptor. Degradation of extracellular matrix components (Hillegass et al., 2008)	**Cleft palate** in mice via inhibiting Wnt/β-catenin signaling (Hu et al., 2013)
	254.81 μM	3–72/96 hpf	Shortened Meckel's cartilage	Hillegass et al., 2008		

Phenotypic parallels in bold.

a direct etiological link with major developmental pathways could be made. Other mechanisms involved direct effects on transcription or DNA synthesis. The translational value as well as the predictive value of the zebrafish model for the study of craniofacial malformations caused by teratogenic pharmaceuticals is demonstrated.

ESTROGENS AND CRANIOFACIAL MALFORMATIONS

Endocrine disruption in the embryo can occur by the intake of estrogen-resembling chemicals that disrupt estrogen signaling, such as oral contraceptives. Although no effects on craniofacial development have been reported on continued contraceptive pill use during pregnancy, abundant sources of exogenous estrogens in the (house/work) environment are present, for instance in food (Paterni et al., 2017). Estrogen-like compounds in household items can affect craniofacial development and analyzing such exposures in patients is complex. Zebrafish have been used to study the effects of supraphysiological doses of exogenous (xeno) estrogens on craniofacial development (Cohen et al., 2014).

Estrogens are crucial for development and act through nuclear estrogen receptors (ER) alpha and beta, that (hetero and homo) dimerize to form DNA binding domains (Tanko et al., 2008). Additionally, estrogens act by binding to transmembrane G-protein GPR-30, which induces signaling cascades via phospholipase C activation (Tanko et al., 2008). Endogenously, estrogens are synthesized from androgens by aromatase. Estrogens are pivotal for the maintenance of bone and cartilage. This is illustrated by the presence of ER on mesenchymal stem cells during chondrogenesis and the production of estrogens by chondrocytes to stimulate their proliferation (Chagin et al., 2006; Fushimi et al., 2009; Gao et al., 2013).

Zebrafish larvae exposed to exogenous 17ß-estradiol (E2), show dose and developmental stage-dependent craniofacial malformations with enhanced sensitivity during early chondrogenesis (1–2 dpf) (Fushimi et al., 2009). At E2 concentrations of 3–5 μM, craniofacial cartilages appeared flattened (Cohen et al., 2014). The angles of the Meckel's and ceratohyal cartilages were widened (Cohen et al., 2014). Below 3 μM, the length and width of craniofacial structures decreased with increasing concentrations (Cohen et al., 2014). Notably, the inhibition of estrogen biosynthesis with aromatase inhibitors phenocopied these results, exemplifying the requirement for tightly controlled estrogen biosynthesis during chondrogenesis (Cohen et al., 2014).

E2 effects on craniofacial development have been partially attributed to indirect inhibition of Shh signaling through estrogen receptor signaling (Fushimi et al., 2009). E2 impaired the migration of CNCCs into the median ethmoid plate, which resulted in a cleft phenotype (Dougherty et al., 2012). In addition to effects on Shh signaling, E2 resulted in differential expression of other skeletogenic pathway genes in an elaborate investigation of estrogen (2–5 μM) effects on zebrafish larval heads (3–7 dpf). Reduced expression of *bmp2a* was reported at 3 dpf. *Bmp2a* has a crucial function in cartilage and bone formation. Also, the osteoclast differentiation factor *rankl* was down-regulated at 3 and 4 dpf. Further, the inhibitor of the WNT pathway *sfrp1a* was down-regulated at 3 and 4 dpf, and the expression of hedgehog receptors *ptch1* and *ptch2* as well as the retinoic acid receptor *rarab* was decreased throughout development (3–7 dpf). Interestingly, many genes in these pathways were affected differently at 2 and 5 μM exposure, while the effects of 2 μM were often more dramatic (Pashay Ahi et al., 2016). When using much lower concentrations of E2 (0.8 μM) cartilage degradation was observed at 4 dpf and collagen genes were down-regulated at 6 and 7 dpf (He et al., 2018). In addition, E2 was reported to upregulate Wnt pathways genes such as *wdr62* (implicated in microcephaly: OMIM 613583) and *wnt11* which has been associated with non-syndromic CLP. The same study reported upregulation of *fstl1a*, a regulator of Bmp signaling, and upregulation of the Bmp inhibitor *nog1*, which is implicated in cleft lip etiology. Moreover, Tgfb receptor 1 expression was downregulated. Variations in this gene cause Loey-Dietz syndrome, which includes craniofacial malformations (He et al., 2018). Overall, exogenous E2 had effects on expression of multiple genes that are involved in craniofacial development.

Recently, a number of zebrafish studies have focused on the effects of bisphenols. Bisphenol A (BPA) is an environmental estrogen-like agent. BPA is found in humans in amniotic fluid, placental tissue and umbilical cord blood (Lee et al., 2018). Pregnant women are exposed to BPA via food packaging, dental fillings and inhalation of house dust (Rudel et al., 2003; Vandenberg et al., 2010; Lofroth et al., 2019). BPA binds to the ER, but it can also bind to the thyroid hormone receptor and to the estrogen-related receptor ERRγ (Saili et al., 2013). BPA is less potent than E2: similar morphological defects were found in zebrafish with 15 μM E2 and 80 μM BPA upon exposure between 8 and 120 hpf (Saili et al., 2013). It should be noted that the concentrations used in these studies exceed environmental concentrations. In zebrafish larvae, BPA induced craniofacial malformations by disrupting chondrocyte organization in the pharyngeal structures and inducing apoptosis (Huang et al., 2020). The BPA-based polymer Bis-GMA used in dental fillers decreased palatoquadral length in zebrafish larvae at 10 nM, while the palatoquadral-ceratohyal angle was decreased at 1 μM (Kramer et al., 2016). It was hypothesized that these effects are caused by ER-mediated altered expression of SHH and BMP pathway genes. Because of emerging evidence of health problems related to bisphenol, the use of BPA was restricted by the European Union.

Upon the reduction of BPA use, products containing alternative bisphenols including BPF, BPS and BPAF have spiked. Because of structural similarities to BPA, concerns also exist about the estrogenic properties of these compounds. BPF, BPS and BPAF are also identified in food products and house dust. In zebrafish, BPF reportedly resulted in severe craniofacial abnormalities at 20 mg/L. BPS caused malformations above 200 mg/L in zebrafish, while BPAF produced severe cardiac defects at 1 mg/L (Moreman et al., 2017). Indeed, the concentrations used in this study also exceed environmental

BPA concentrations. Future studies on bisphenols with detailed description of phenotypes and realistic exposure concentrations will provide more insight into the mode of action of various bisphenols on craniofacial development.

ExE INTERACTIONS IN HIGH-THROUGHPUT SCREENINGS

Craniofacial malformations often serve as outcome measures in zebrafish toxicological investigations. This is because the development of craniofacial structures is highly sensitive to perturbation. Many of the environmental factors discussed in this review have also been investigated in toxicological studies, but these studies lacked specific phenotypic and/or mechanistic information. In general, craniofacial abnormalities were regularly reported in compound studies in zebrafish, but without specifically analyzing the affected structures (Weigt et al., 2012; Ellis et al., 2014; Massarsky et al., 2015). Although purely toxicological investigations are beyond the scope of this review, the methodologies employed in this field can also be used in the study of craniofacial malformations.

For example, investigations of the cumulative effects of teratogens (i.e., ExE interactions) within the zebrafish model are increasing in number. Methods to assess the combinatorial effects of two compounds, synergistic or antagonistic, are currently being developed for toxins with effects on skeletal development (Staal et al., 2018; Heusinkveld et al., 2020; Zoupa et al., 2020). For instance, triazoles (fungicides) cause craniofacial malformations through inhibiting RA degradation by CYP26. These toxins with well-known mechanism of action have been used in co-exposure experiments with other agricultural fungicides that target different processes in craniofacial development. Thereby it was shown that binary mixture effects can be predicted using dose addition. This refers to adding up the toxicological effects of two chemicals to predict their effect in a mixture (Zoupa et al., 2020). This method may be helpful in further studies on multifactorial environmental exposures such as TPM of (e-cigarette) smoke.

To unify efforts in craniofacial toxicity screenings, standard outcome measures were optimized by Staal et al. (2018). The Meckel's-palatoquadrate (M-PQ) angle (**Figure 3**) offered a limited variability, proved applicable over wide concentration ranges, and was suitable to assess the effects of chemical mixtures (Cohen et al., 2014; Staal et al., 2018; Zoupa et al., 2020). The M-PQ angle can be translated as a measure for head and jaw deformations, which is affected in craniofacial malformations such as microcephaly and micrognathia. This relatively simple to obtain parameter is especially suitable for high-throughput screenings. It was also proposed to use in further studies in order to enhance inter-study data comparisons. Similarly, options for high-throughput phenotyping of craniofacial mutants by microcomputed tomography (microCT) are rapidly expanding, benefiting from improved resolution and software tools (Pardo-Martin et al., 2013; Charles et al., 2017). In pathophysiological investigations of craniofacial malformations using zebrafish, the techniques discussed above may be used to systematically assess, or even predict, the teratogenesis of novel environmental factors.

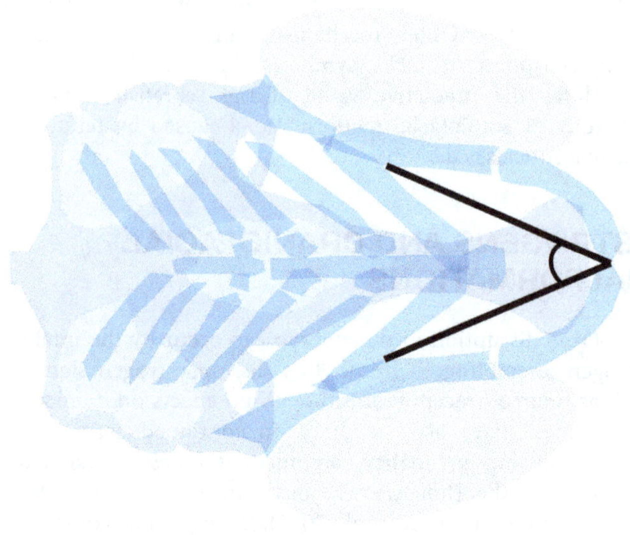

FIGURE 3 | Meckel's-palatoquadrate (M-PQ) angle is proposed as a reliable high-throughput standard parameter to assess craniofacial outcomes after single or mixed compound exposures. The measurements can be easily obtained by imaging of cartilage stained larvae and proved to be informative on a broad spectrum of craniofacial malformations. The M-PQ angle is especially affected in craniofacial malformations such as microcephaly and micrognathia.

GENE–ENVIRONMENT INTERACTIONS

It has become increasingly evident that the effects of environmental exposures during development may be different in individuals with different genotypes. Such interactions of genetic and environmental factors are poorly understood up to now (Lovely et al., 2017). A limited number of zebrafish studies have addressed the interactions between genetic risk factors and environmental factors in the etiology of craniofacial malformations. These studies focused on ethanol sensitivity of zebrafish mutants in FASD research. Screens of n-ethyl-n-nitrosourea (ENU)-induced mutants and unbiased screens for new candidate genes have been published. Mutants were generally exposed to 1% ethanol during development. This results in tissue levels between 41 and 51 mM, which correlates to blood-alcohol levels after binge drinking events in humans (Zhang et al., 2014). In search of GxE interactions, McCarthy et al. (2013) exposed *Pdgfra* zebrafish mutants to 1% ethanol. Loss of PDGFRA in humans has been associated with cleft palate, indicating a direct parallel with zebrafish studies (Rattanasopha et al., 2012). *Pdgfra*$^{+/-}$ zebrafish mutants only developed craniofacial malformations in the presence of ethanol (10–120 hpf) including clefts of the ethmoid plate and breaks in the trabeculae. Moreover, hypoplasia of Meckel's cartilage, the palatoquadrate and the hyosympletics were observed. *Pdgfra*$^{-/-}$ mutants showed enhanced sensitivity to ethanol as the ethmoid plate did not form at all, while the sensitivity window was determined at 10–24 hpf. Wildtype embryos exposed to ethanol developed mostly normal in this study with palatal defects only in less than 20% of the larvae. The protective effect of intact *pdgfra* against ethanol teratogenesis was shown to be PI3K/mTOR-mediated (McCarthy et al., 2013). This type of in-depth examinations of the mechanisms of action are needed to extrapolate models of gene–environment interactions in craniofacial disorders to clinical use.

Swartz et al. found that mutations of *foxi1, hinfp, mars, plk1* and *vangl2* also showed increased craniofacial malformations upon exposure to 1% ethanol compared to wildtypes (Swartz et al., 2014). In particular, ethmoid plate defects were observed in both *mars* and *vangl2* mutants exposed to ethanol. *Mars* is crucial for protein synthesis as it is involved in tRNA amino acylation. In *mars* mutants a gap in the posterior ethmoid palate was observed upon ethanol exposure. *Vangl2* is a regulator of the planar cell polarity Wnt pathway, and is expressed in the pharyngeal arches. In zebrafish mutants for this gene a narrow, single rod replacing the ethmoid plate was reported as a result of ethanol exposure (Swartz et al., 2014). In humans, VANGL2 is implicated in neural tube defects (Kibar et al., 2011). However, based on the zebrafish study, VANGL2 variations may also be a predisposing factor for cleft palate in case of alcohol use during pregnancy.

The screening of a library of unmapped (unknown alleles) ENU mutants recently identified six new ethanol-sensitive zebrafish mutants (Swartz et al., 2020). The observed malformations in these mutants were highly diverse, which suggests a variety of teratogenic effects of ethanol. One of the mutants was mapped by whole genome sequencing and was validated by targeting the same allele using CRISPR/Cas9 mutagenesis (Swartz et al., 2020). Other mutants of this study remain unmapped, but they seem to be new candidate genes for craniofacial malformations as the specific phenotypes were not previously observed (Swartz et al., 2020). This is a prominent example of why both candidate-based approaches and mutant-sensitivity screens are needed in research on GxE interactions. Candidate gene-driven research is focused whereas sensitivity screenings can lead to the discovery of new candidate genes.

The discovery of ethanol-sensitive gene variants in zebrafish shows that the effects of ethanol on craniofacial development may depend on the genetic background. It is highly conceivable this also applies to the teratogenic effect of other compounds. Yet, mechanistic insights into other GxE interactions are still scarce. CLP risks have been associated with genetic sensitivity for specific environmental factors. For instance, TGFA variations may interact with smoking and vitamin deficiency, TGFB3 variations with smoking and alcohol consumption, MTHFR variations with folate intake, RARA with vitamin A intake, and finally GSTT1 and CYP1A variations also with smoking (Stuppia et al., 2011). Zebrafish models are highly suitable to investigate the molecular mechanisms in these gene–environment interactions.

It is likely that zebrafish craniofacial mutants will be used increasingly to analyze the mechanisms of GxE interactions in the coming years. A number of strategies may be appropriate to approach this. The eminent availability of zebrafish mutants

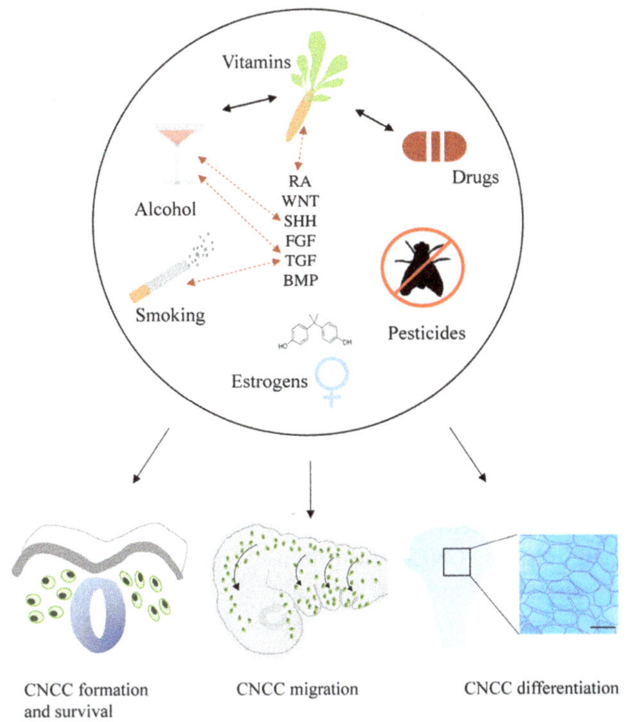

FIGURE 4 | General summary showing the environmental factors smoking, alcohol use, vitamin imbalance, drug use, (xeno) estrogens and pesticides. These factors (represented in the upper part of the figure) differentially affect critical developmental processes such as the formation, survival, delamination, migration, condensation, and differentiation of CNCCs (represented in the lower part of the figure). Evidence of interactions between environmental factors that result in craniofacial malformations has been reported as well, these are indicated by black arrows. Exposure to environmental factors often results in aberrant signaling of essential pathways in craniofacial development including SHH, TGF, FGF, BMP, RA, and WNT. Moreover, gene mutations in these pathways can also interact with environmental factors, complicating the etiology. Known GxE interactions are indicated in this figure with red dotted arrows.

from the zebrafish mutation project[6] and other sources, will facilitate high-throughput investigations of GxE interactions on craniofacial development. These efforts can be further optimized by using the broad range of available reporter lines for bone and cartilage formation (Hammond and Moro, 2012). Furthermore, advanced genome editing offers unprecedented opportunities for the investigation of GxE interactions of candidate genes. For instance, the first successful attempt to create loss-of-function alleles for all genes on zebrafish chromosome 1 was recently published, illustrating the astonishing strength of CRISPR/Cas9 techniques (Sun et al., 2019). Systematic gene editing to create zebrafish variants of those observed in human patients could be achieved in the future in view of the increasing success rates of knock-in zebrafish models. These models can be used for highly specific GxE interaction analyses, which may provide predictive data to clinicians.

[6]www.sanger.ac.uk/resources/zebrafish/zmp/

CONCLUDING NOTES

Craniofacial malformations are notorious for their multifactorial etiology including many genetic and environmental factors. CLP and other congenital traits in which GxE interactions play a prominent role, present a problem for the development of adequate preventive measures. Here, evidence from zebrafish studies on the phenotypic outcomes and mechanisms of action of a number of important environmental factors that pregnant women may encounter in daily life is reviewed. It stands out that the mechanisms of action for most of these factors remain incompletely understood, while the phenotypic descriptions vary widely in the amount of details given.

Craniofacial development is a highly sensitive process, which is regulated by major signaling pathways including WNT, BMP, FGF, SHH, and RA. This review substantiates that environmental factors may directly or indirectly affect these pathways and thereby disrupt CNCC formation, survival, migration and differentiation (**Figure 4**). It is not beyond imagination that multiple environmental factors can be present simultaneously during early pregnancy. Therefore, studies into ExE interactions are highly important.

Zebrafish prove to be a valuable translational model for a wide range of craniofacial malformations, and are also highly suited for identifying the mechanisms of action associated with environmental factors and GxE interactions. Moreover, zebrafish research will boost the identification and health risk assessment of new teratogens.

Although many health recommendations to prevent craniofacial and other congenital malformations have already been implemented by healthcare professionals for years, more research should be done to obtain a more extensive picture of the risks. After all, in the field of environmental exposures there is much to gain as—in theory—all of these factors can be eliminated if public health awareness is increased and risks are adequately identified. A better understanding of environmental teratogens and genetic risk factors will allow for routine screening and a personalized approach in the future. Evidence from zebrafish studies will help to translate preclinical data to practice and will support health recommendations to pregnant women to decrease the risks of CLP and other craniofacial malformations.

AUTHOR CONTRIBUTIONS

SR wrote the manuscript. JM, FW, and JV conceptualized and revised the manuscript. All authors contributed to the article and approved the submitted version.

ACKNOWLEDGMENTS

We would like to thank Tiffany Ernst for the constructive textual feedback.

REFERENCES

Aceto, J., Nourizadeh-Lillabadi, R., Maree, R., Dardenne, N., Jeanray, N., Wehenkel, L., et al. (2015). Zebrafish bone and general physiology are differently affected by hormones or changes in gravity. *PLoS One* 10:e0126928. doi: 10.1371/journal.pone.0126928

Ackermans, M. M., Zhou, H., Carels, C. E., Wagener, F. A., and Von den Hoff, J. W. (2011). Vitamin A and clefting: putative biological mechanisms. *Nutr. Rev.* 69, 613–624. doi: 10.1111/j.1753-4887.2011.00425.x

Acum, M., Mastroyannopoulou, K., O'Curry, S., and Young, J. (2020). The psychosocial patient-reported outcomes of end of pathway cleft surgery: a systematic review. *Cleft. Palate. Craniofac. J.* 57, 990–1007. doi: 10.1177/1055665620911328

Al-Ani, A. H., Antoun, J. S., Thomson, W. M., Merriman, T. R., and Farella, M. (2017). Hypodontia: an update on its etiology, classification, and clinical management. *Biomed. Res. Int.* 2017:9378325.

Ali, S., Champagne, D. L., Alia, A., and Richardson, M. K. (2011). Large-scale analysis of acute ethanol exposure in zebrafish development: a critical time window and resilience. *PLoS One* 6:e20037. doi: 10.1371/journal.pone.0020037

Andreeva, V., Connolly, M. H., Stewart-Swift, C., Fraher, D., Burt, J., Cardarelli, J., et al. (2011). Identification of adult mineralized tissue zebrafish mutants. *Genesis* 49, 360–366. doi: 10.1002/dvg.20712

Beaty, T. H., Hetmanski, J. B., Zeiger, J. S., Fan, Y. T., Liang, K. Y., VanderKolk, C. A., et al. (2002). Testing candidate genes for non-syndromic oral clefts using a case-parent trio design. *Genet. Epidemiol.* 22, 1–11. doi: 10.1002/gepi.1039

Beaty, T. H., Ruczinski, I., Murray, J. C., Marazita, M. L., Munger, R. G., Hetmanski, J. B., et al. (2011). Evidence for Gene-Environment Interaction in a Genome Wide Study of Nonsyndromic Cleft Palate. *Genet. Epidemiol.* 35, 469–478.

Billiard, S. M., Timme-Laragy, A. R., Wassenberg, D. M., Cockman, C., and Di Giulio, R. T. (2006). The role of the aryl hydrocarbon receptor pathway in mediating synergistic developmental toxicity of polycyclic aromatic hydrocarbons to zebrafish. *Toxicol. Sci.* 92, 526–536. doi: 10.1093/toxsci/kfl011

Blader, P., and Strahle, U. (1998). Ethanol impairs migration of the prechordal plate in the zebrafish embryo. *Dev. Biol.* 201, 185–201. doi: 10.1006/dbio.1998.8995

Bruneel, B., and Witten, P. E. (2015). Power and challenges of using zebrafish as a model for skeletal tissue imaging.*Connect. Tissue Res.* 56, 161–173. doi: 10.3109/03008207.2015.1013193

Burd, L., Roberts, D., Olson, M., and Odendaal, H. (2007). Ethanol and the placenta: a review. *J. Matern. Fetal Neonatal. Med.* 20, 361–375.

Burton, D. F., Zhang, C., Boa-Amponsem, O., Mackinnon, S., and Cole, G. J. (2017). Long-term behavioral change as a result of acute ethanol exposure in zebrafish: evidence for a role for sonic hedgehog but not retinoic acid signaling. *Neurotoxicol. Teratol.* 61, 66–73. doi: 10.1016/j.ntt.2017.01.006

Bush, J. O., and Jiang, R. (2012). Palatogenesis: morphogenetic and molecular mechanisms of secondary palate development. *Development* 139, 231–243. doi: 10.1242/dev.067082

Carmichael, S. L., Ma, C., Rasmussen, S. A., Honein, M. A., Lammer, E. J., Shaw, G. M., et al. (2008). Craniosynostosis and maternal smoking. *Birth Defects Res. A. Clin. Mol. Teratol.* 82, 78–85.

Carvan, M. J. III, Loucks, E., Weber, D. N., and Williams, F. E. (2004). Ethanol effects on the developing zebrafish: neurobehavior and skeletal morphogenesis. *Neurotoxicol. Teratol.* 26, 757–768. doi: 10.1016/j.ntt.2004.06.016

Cedron, V. P., Weiner, A. M. J., Vera, M., and Sanchez, L. (2020). Acetaminophen affects the survivor, pigmentation and development of craniofacial structures in zebrafish (Danio rerio) embryos. *Biochem. Pharmacol.* 174:113816. doi: 10.1016/j.bcp.2020.113816

Chagin, A. S., Chrysis, D., Takigawa, M., Ritzen, E. M., and Savendahl, L. (2006). Locally produced estrogen promotes fetal rat metatarsal bone growth; an effect mediated through increased chondrocyte proliferation and decreased apoptosis. *J. Endocrinol.* 188, 193–203. doi: 10.1677/joe.1.06364

Charles, J. F., Sury, M., Tsang, K., Urso, K., Henke, K., Huang, Y., et al. (2017). Utility of quantitative micro-computed tomographic analysis in zebrafish to define gene function during skeletogenesis. *Bone* 101, 162–171. doi: 10.1016/j.bone.2017.05.001

Chawla, B., Swain, W., Williams, A. L., and Bohnsack, B. L. (2018). Retinoic acid maintains function of neural crest-derived ocular and craniofacial structures in adult zebrafish. *Invest. Ophthalmol. Vis. Sci.* 59, 1924–1935. doi: 10.1167/iovs.17-22845

Chiquet, B. T., Blanton, S. H., Burt, A., Ma, D., Stal, S., Mulliken, J. B., et al. (2008). Variation in WNT genes is associated with non-syndromic cleft lip with or without cleft palate. *Hum. Mol. Genet.* 17, 2212–2218. doi: 10.1093/hmg/ddn121

Clayton-Smith, J., Bromley, R., Dean, J., Journel, H., Odent, S., Wood, A., et al. (2019). Diagnosis and management of individuals with Fetal Valproate Spectrum Disorder; a consensus statement from the european reference network for congenital malformations and intellectual disability. *Orphanet. J. Rare Dis.* 14:180.

Cohen, S. P., LaChappelle, A. R., Walker, B. S., and Lassiter, C. S. (2014). Modulation of estrogen causes disruption of craniofacial chondrogenesis in Danio rerio. *Aquat. Toxicol.* 152, 113–120. doi: 10.1016/j.aquatox.2014.03.028

Cornille, M., Dambroise, E., Komla-Ebri, D., Kaci, N., Biosse-Duplan, M., Di Rocco, F., et al. (2019). Animal models of craniosynostosis. *Neurochirurgie* 65, 202–209. doi: 10.1016/j.neuchi.2019.09.010

Cubbage, C. C., and Mabee, P. M. (1996). Development of the cranium and paired fins in the zebrafish Danio rerio (Ostariophysi. *Cyprinidae). J. Morphol.* 229, 121–160. doi: 10.1002/(sici)1097-4687(199608)229:2<121::aid-jmor1>3.0.co;2-4

DeRoo, L. A., Wilcox, A. J., Drevon, C. A., and Lie, R. T. (2008). First-trimester maternal alcohol consumption and the risk of infant oral clefts in Norway: a population-based case-control study. *Am. J. Epidemiol.* 168, 638–646. doi: 10.1093/aje/kwn186

Dixon, M. J., Marazita, M. L., Beaty, T. H., and Murray, J. C. (2011). Cleft lip and palate: understanding genetic and environmental influences. *Nat. Rev. Genet.* 12, 167–178. doi: 10.1038/nrg2933

Dougherty, M., Kamel, G., Grimaldi, M., Gfrerer, L., Shubinets, V., Ethier, R., et al. (2013). Distinct requirements for wnt9a and irf6 in extension and integration mechanisms during zebrafish palate morphogenesis. *Development* 140, 76–81. doi: 10.1242/dev.080473

Dougherty, M., Kamel, G., Shubinets, V., Hickey, G., Grimaldi, M., and Liao, E. C. (2012). Embryonic fate map of first pharyngeal arch structures in the sox10: kaede zebrafish transgenic model. *J. Craniofac Surg.* 23, 1333–1337. doi: 10.1097/scs.0b013e318260f20b

Duncan, K. M., Mukherjee, K., Cornell, R. A., and Liao, E. C. (2017). Zebrafish models of orofacial clefts. *Dev. Dyn.* 246, 897–914. doi: 10.1002/dvdy.24566

Eames, B. F., DeLaurier, A., Ullmann, B., Huycke, T. R., Nichols, J. T., Dowd, J., et al. (2013). FishFace: interactive atlas of zebrafish craniofacial development at cellular resolution. *BMC Dev. Biol.* 13:23. doi: 10.1186/1471-213X-13-23

Eason, J., Williams, A. L., Chawla, B., Apsey, C., and Bohnsack, B. L. (2017). Differences in neural crest sensitivity to ethanol account for the infrequency of anterior segment defects in the eye compared with craniofacial anomalies in a zebrafish model of fetal alcohol syndrome. *Birth Defects Res.* 109, 1212–1227. doi: 10.1002/bdr2.1069

Ellies, D. L., Langille, R. M., Martin, C. C., Akimenko, M. A., and Ekker, M. (1997). Specific craniofacial cartilage dysmorphogenesis coincides with a loss of dlx gene expression in retinoic acid-treated zebrafish embryos. *Mech. Dev.* 61, 23–36. doi: 10.1016/s0925-4773(96)00616-8

Ellis, L. D., Soo, E. C., Achenbach, J. C., Morash, M. G., and Soanes, K. H. (2014). Use of the zebrafish larvae as a model to study cigarette smoke condensate toxicity. *PLoS One* 9:e115305. doi: 10.1371/journal.pone.0115305

Facciol, A., Tsang, B., and Gerlai, R. (2019). Alcohol exposure during embryonic development: an opportunity to conduct systematic developmental time course analyses in zebrafish. *Neurosci. Biobehav. Rev.* 98, 185–193. doi: 10.1016/j.neubiorev.2019.01.012

Ferdous, J., Mukherjee, R., Ahmed, K. T., and Ali, D. W. (2017). Retinoic acid prevents synaptic deficiencies induced by alcohol exposure during gastrulation in zebrafish embryos. *Neurotoxicology* 62, 100–110. doi: 10.1016/j.neuro.2017.05.011

Fernandes, Y., Rampersad, M., Jones, E. M., and Eberhart, J. K. (2019). Social deficits following embryonic ethanol exposure arise in post-larval zebrafish. *Addict. Biol.* 24, 898–907. doi: 10.1111/adb.12649

Fernandez, I., Santos, A., Cancela, M. L., Laize, V., and Gavaia, P. J. (2014). Warfarin, a potential pollutant in aquatic environment acting through Pxr signaling pathway and gamma-glutamyl carboxylation of vitamin K-dependent proteins. *Environ. Pollut.* 194, 86–95. doi: 10.1016/j.envpol.2014.07.015

Finer, L. B., and Zolna, M. R. (2016). Declines in unintended pregnancy in the United States, 2008-2011. *N. Engl. J. Med.* 374, 843–852. doi: 10.1056/nejmsa1506575

Fushimi, S., Wada, N., Nohno, T., Tomita, M., Saijoh, K., Sunami, S., et al. (2009). 17beta-Estradiol inhibits chondrogenesis in the skull development of zebrafish embryos. *Aquat. Toxicol.* 95, 292–298. doi: 10.1016/j.aquatox.2009.03.004

Gao, Y., Huang, E., Zhang, H., Wang, J., Wu, N., Chen, X., et al. (2013). Crosstalk between Wnt/beta-catenin and estrogen receptor signaling synergistically promotes osteogenic differentiation of mesenchymal progenitor cells. *PLoS One* 8:e82436. doi: 10.1371/journal.pone.0082436

Gasser, D. L., Yang, P., and Buetow, K. H. (1992). Palate teratogenicity and embryotoxicity of cyclosporin A in mice. *J. Craniofac Genet. Dev. Biol.* 12, 155–158.

Gardner, J. S., Guyard-Boileau, B., Alderman, B. W., Fernbach, S. K., Greene, C., and Mangione, E. J. (1998). Maternal exposure to prescription and non-prescription pharmaceuticals or drugs of abuse and risk of craniosynostosis. *Int. J. Epidemiol.* 27, 64–67. doi: 10.1093/ije/27.1.64

Gebuijs, I. G. E., Metz, J. R., Zethof, J., Carels, C. E. L., Wagener, F., and Von den Hoff, J. W. (2020). The anti-epileptic drug valproic acid causes malformations in the developing craniofacial skeleton of zebrafish larvae. *Mech. Dev.* 163:103632. doi: 10.1016/j.mod.2020.103632

Geier, M. C., Chlebowski, A. C., Truong, L., Massey Simonich, S. L., Anderson, K. A., and Tanguay, R. L. (2018). Comparative developmental toxicity of a comprehensive suite of polycyclic aromatic hydrocarbons. *Arch. Toxicol.* 92, 571–586. doi: 10.1007/s00204-017-2068-9

Gelineau-van Waes, J., Bennett, G. D., and Finnell, R. H. (1999). Phenytoin-induced alterations in craniofacial gene expression. *Teratology* 59, 23–34. doi: 10.1002/(sici)1096-9926(199901)59:1<23::aid-tera7>3.0.co;2-m

Granzow, J. W., Thaller, S. R., and Panthaki, Z. (2003). Cleft palate and toe malformations in a child with fetal methotrexate exposure. *J. Craniofac. Surg.* 14, 747–748. doi: 10.1097/00001665-200309000-00027

Gurvich, N., Berman, M. G., Wittner, B. S., Gentleman, R. C., Klein, P. S., and Green, J. B. (2005). Association of valproate-induced teratogenesis with histone deacetylase inhibition in vivo. *FASEB J.* 19, 1166–1168. doi: 10.1096/fj.04-3425fje

Hammond, C. L., and Moro, E. (2012). Using transgenic reporters to visualize bone and cartilage signaling during development in vivo. *Front. Endocrinol.* 3:91. doi: 10.3389/fendo.2012.00091

Hanumanthaiah, R., Thankavel, B., Day, K., Gregory, M., and Jagadeeswaran, P. (2001). Developmental expression of vitamin K-dependent gamma-carboxylase activity in zebrafish embryos: effect of warfarin. *Blood Cells Mol. Dis.* 27, 992–999. doi: 10.1006/bcmd.2001.0472

He, H., Wang, C., Tang, Q., Yang, F., and Xu, Y. (2018). Elucidation of possible molecular mechanisms underlying the estrogen-induced disruption of cartilage development in zebrafish larvae. *Toxicol. Lett.* 289, 22–27. doi: 10.1016/j.toxlet.2018.02.023

Herman, S. B., Guo, T., McGinn, D. M., Blonska, A., Shanske, A. L., Bassett, A. S., et al. (2012). Overt cleft palate phenotype and TBX1 genotype correlations in velo-cardio-facial/DiGeorge/22q11.2 *deletion syndrome patients. Am. J. Med. Genet. A* 158A, 2781–2787.

Heusinkveld, H. J., Schoonen, W. G., Hodemaekers, H. M., Nugraha, A., Sirks, J. J., Veenma, V., et al. (2020). Distinguishing mode of action of compounds inducing craniofacial malformations in zebrafish embryos to support dose-response modeling in combined exposures. *Reprod. Toxicol.* 96, 114–127. doi: 10.1016/j.reprotox.2020.06.002

Hillegass, J. M., Villano, C. M., Cooper, K. R., and White, L. A. (2008). Glucocorticoids alter craniofacial development and increase expression and activity of matrix metalloproteinases in developing zebrafish (Danio rerio). *Toxicol. Sci.* 102, 413–424. doi: 10.1093/toxsci/kfn010

Holden, L. L., Truong, L., Simonich, M. T., and Tanguay, R. L. (2020). Assessing the hazard of E-Cigarette flavor mixtures using zebrafish. *Food Chem. Toxicol.* 136:110945. doi: 10.1016/j.fct.2019.110945

Hou, J. W. (2004). Fetal warfarin syndrome.*Chang. Gung. Med. J.* 27, 691–695.

Howe, K., Clark, M. D., Torroja, C. F., Torrance, J., Berthelot, C., Muffato, M., et al. (2013). The zebrafish reference genome sequence and its relationship to the human genome. *Nature* 496, 498–503.

Hu, X., Gao, J. H., Liao, Y. J., Tang, S. J., and Lu, F. (2013). Dexamethasone alters epithelium proliferation and survival and suppresses Wnt/beta-catenin signaling in developing cleft palate. *Food Chem. Toxicol.* 56, 67–74. doi: 10.1016/j.fct.2013.02.003

Huang, W., Zheng, S., Xiao, J., Liu, C., Du, T., and Wu, K. (2020). Parental exposure to bisphenol A affects pharyngeal cartilage development and causes global transcriptomic changes in zebrafish (Danio rerio) offspring. *Chemosphere* 249:126537. doi: 10.1016/j.chemosphere.2020.126537

Hutson, J. R., Stade, B., Lehotay, D. C., Collier, C. P., and Kapur, B. M. (2012). Folic acid transport to the human fetus is decreased in pregnancies with chronic alcohol exposure. *PLoS One* 7:e38057. doi: 10.1371/journal.pone.0038057

Jentink, J., Loane, M. A., Dolk, H., Barisic, I., Garne, E., Morris, J. K., et al. (2010). Valproic acid monotherapy in pregnancy and major congenital malformations. *N. Engl. J. Med.* 362, 2185–2193. doi: 10.1056/nejmoa0907328

Jiang, Q., Lu, D., Wang, F., Zhang, Y., Cao, L., Gui, Y., et al. (2020). Folic acid supplement rescues ethanol-induced developmental defects in the zebrafish embryos. *Acta Biochim. Biophys. Sin.* 52, 536–545. doi: 10.1093/abbs/gmaa030

Johansen, A. M., Lie, R. T., Wilcox, A. J., Andersen, L. F., and Drevon, C. A. (2008). Maternal dietary intake of vitamin A and risk of orofacial clefts: a population-based case-control study in Norway. *Am. J. Epidemiol.* 167, 1164–1170. doi: 10.1093/aje/kwn035

Joore, J., van der Lans, G. B., Lanser, P. H., Vervaart, J. M., Zivkovic, D., Speksnijder, J. E., et al. (1994). Effects of retinoic acid on the expression of retinoic acid receptors during zebrafish embryogenesis. *Mech. Dev.* 46, 137–150. doi: 10.1016/0925-4773(94)90082-5

Kennedy, A. E., Kandalam, S., Olivares-Navarrete, R., and Dickinson, A. J. G. (2017). E-cigarette aerosol exposure can cause craniofacial defects in Xenopus laevis embryos and mammalian neural crest cells. *PLoS One* 12:e0185729. doi: 10.1371/journal.pone.0185729

Kibar, Z., Salem, S., Bosoi, C. M., Pauwels, E., De Marco, P., Merello, E., et al. (2011). Contribution of VANGL2 mutations to isolated neural tube defects. *Clin. Genet.* 80, 76–82. doi: 10.1111/j.1399-0004.2010.01515.x

Kimmel, C. B., DeLaurier, A., Ullmann, B., Dowd, J., and McFadden, M. (2010). Modes of developmental outgrowth and shaping of a craniofacial bone in zebrafish. *PLoS One* 5:e9475. doi: 10.1371/journal.pone.0009475

Kimmel, C. B., Miller, C. T., and Moens, C. B. (2001). Specification and morphogenesis of the zebrafish larval head skeleton. *Dev. Biol.* 233, 239–257. doi: 10.1006/dbio.2001.0201

Kramer, A. G., Vuthiganon, J., and Lassiter, C. S. (2016). Bis-GMA affects craniofacial development in zebrafish embryos (Danio rerio). *Environ. Toxicol. Pharmacol.* 43, 159–165. doi: 10.1016/j.etap.2016.02.018

Kuchler, E. C., Silva, L. A. D., Nelson-Filho, P., Saboia, T. M., Rentschler, A. M., Granjeiro, J. M., et al. (2018). Assessing the association between hypoxia during craniofacial development and oral clefts. *J. Appl. Oral. Sci.* 26:e20170234.

Laue, K., Pogoda, H. M., Daniel, P. B., van Haeringen, A., Alanay, Y., von Ameln, S., et al. (2011). Craniosynostosis and multiple skeletal anomalies in humans and zebrafish result from a defect in the localized degradation of retinoic acid. *Am. J. Hum. Genet.* 89, 595–606. doi: 10.1016/j.ajhg.2011.09.015

Lee, J., Choi, K., Park, J., Moon, H. B., Choi, G., Lee, J. J., et al. (2018). Bisphenol A distribution in serum, urine, placenta, breast milk, and umbilical cord serum in a birth panel of mother-neonate pairs. *Sci. Total Environ.* 626, 1494–1501. doi: 10.1016/j.scitotenv.2017.10.042

Lee, M. S., Bonner, J. R., Bernard, D. J., Sanchez, E. L., Sause, E. T., Prentice, R. R., et al. (2012). Disruption of the folate pathway in zebrafish causes developmental defects. *BMC Dev. Biol.* 12:12. doi: 10.1186/1471-213X-12-12

Lee, Y., Kim, Y. H., Yun, J. S., and Lee, C. J. (2013). Valproic acid decreases the proliferation of telencephalic cells in zebrafish larvae. *Neurotoxicol. Teratol.* 39, 91–99. doi: 10.1016/j.ntt.2013.07.004

Leslie, E. J., Taub, M. A., Liu, H., Steinberg, K. M., Koboldt, D. C., Zhang, Q. Y., et al. (2015). Identification of functional variants for cleft lip with or without cleft palate in or near PAX7. FGFR2, and NOG by Targeted Sequencing of GWAS Loci. *Am. J. Hum. Genet.* 96, 397–411. doi: 10.1016/j.ajhg.2015.01.004

Li, Y. X., Yang, H. T., Zdanowicz, M., Sicklick, J. K., Qi, Y., Camp, T. J., et al. (2007). Fetal alcohol exposure impairs Hedgehog cholesterol modification and signaling. *Lab. Invest.* 87, 231–240. doi: 10.1038/labinvest.3700516

Liszewski, W., Ritner, C., Aurigui, J., Wong, S. S., Hussain, N., Krueger, W., et al. (2012). Developmental effects of tobacco smoke exposure during human embryonic stem cell differentiation are mediated through the transforming growth factor-beta superfamily member, Nodal. *Differentiation* 83, 169–178. doi: 10.1016/j.diff.2011.12.005

Liu, S., Narumi, R., Ikeda, N., Morita, O., and Tasaki, J. (2020). Chemical-induced craniofacial anomalies caused by disruption of neural crest cell development in a zebrafish model. *Dev. Dyn.* 249, 794–815. doi: 10.1002/dvdy.179

Lofroth, M., Ghasemimehr, M., Falk, A., and Vult von Steyern, P. (2019). Bisphenol A in dental materials - existence, leakage and biological effects. *Heliyon* 5:e01711. doi: 10.1016/j.heliyon.2019.e01711

Loucks, E., and Carvan, M. J. I. I. I. (2004). Strain-dependent effects of developmental ethanol exposure in zebrafish. *Neurotoxicol. Teratol.* 26, 745–755. doi: 10.1016/j.ntt.2004.06.017

Lovely, C., Rampersad, M., Fernandes, Y., and Eberhart, J. (2017). Gene-environment interactions in development and disease. *Wiley Interdiscip. Rev. Dev. Biol.* 6:e247.

Lovely, C. B. (2020). Animal models of gene-alcohol interactions. *Birth Defects Res.* 112, 367–379. doi: 10.1002/bdr2.1623

Machado, R. G., and Eames, B. F. (2017). Using zebrafish to test the genetic basis of human craniofacial diseases. *J. Dent. Res.* 96, 1192–1199. doi: 10.1177/0022034517722776

Mammadova, A., Ackermans, M. M., Bloemen, M., Oostendorp, C., Zhou, H., Carels, C. E., et al. (2014). Effects of retinoic acid on proliferation and gene expression of cleft and non-cleft palatal keratinocytes. *Eur. J. Orthod.* 36, 727–734. doi: 10.1093/ejo/cjt104

Mansilla, M. A., Kimani, J., Mitchell, L. E., Christensen, K., Boomsma, D. I., Daack-Hirsch, S., et al. (2005). Discordant MZ twins with cleft lip and palate: a model for identifying genes in complex traits. *Twin Res. Hum. Genet.* 8, 39–46. doi: 10.1375/twin.8.1.39

Mao, X. Y., and Tang, S. J. (2010). Effects of phenytoin on Satb2 and Hoxa2 gene expressions in mouse embryonic craniofacial tissue. *Biochem. Cell Biol.* 88, 731–735. doi: 10.1139/o10-013

Marean, A., Graf, A., Zhang, Y., and Niswander, L. (2011). Folic acid supplementation can adversely affect murine neural tube closure and embryonic survival. *Hum. Mol. Genet.* 20, 3678–3683. doi: 10.1093/hmg/ddr289

Marrs, J. A., Clendenon, S. G., Ratcliffe, D. R., Fielding, S. M., Liu, Q., and Bosron, W. F. (2010). Zebrafish fetal alcohol syndrome model: effects of ethanol are rescued by retinoic acid supplement. *Alcohol* 44, 707–715. doi: 10.1016/j.alcohol.2009.03.004

Martin, S., McBride, M., McGarry, K., and Hill, C. (2020). Burden of cleft surgery-a 21-year follow-up of patients with cleft lip and palate. *Eur. J. Plastic Surg.* 43, 365–370. doi: 10.1007/s00238-020-01633-z

Massarsky, A., Abdel, A., Glazer, L., Levin, E. D., and Di Giulio, R. T. (2017). Exposure to 1,2-Propanediol Impacts Early Development of Zebrafish (Danio rerio) and Induces Hyperactivity. *Zebrafish* 14, 216–222. doi: 10.1089/zeb.2016.1400

Massarsky, A., Bone, A. J., Dong, W., Hinton, D. E., Prasad, G. L., and Di Giulio, R. T. (2016). AHR2 morpholino knockdown reduces the toxicity of total particulate matter to zebrafish embryos. *Toxicol. Appl. Pharmacol.* 309, 63–76. doi: 10.1016/j.taap.2016.08.024

Massarsky, A., Jayasundara, N., Bailey, J. M., Oliveri, A. N., Levin, E. D., Prasad, G. L., et al. (2015). Teratogenic, bioenergetic, and behavioral effects of exposure to total particulate matter on early development of zebrafish (Danio rerio) are not mimicked by nicotine. *Neurotoxicol. Teratol.* 51, 77–88. doi: 10.1016/j.ntt.2015.09.006

McCarthy, N., and Eberhart, J. K. (2014). Gene-ethanol interactions underlying fetal alcohol spectrum disorders. *Cell Mol. Life. Sci.* 71, 2699–2706. doi: 10.1007/s00018-014-1578-3

McCarthy, N., Wetherill, L., Lovely, C. B., Swartz, M. E., Foroud, T. M., and Eberhart, J. K. (2013). Pdgfra protects against ethanol-induced craniofacial defects in a zebrafish model of FASD. *Development* 140, 3254–3265. doi: 10.1242/dev.094938

Metzler, M. A., and Sandell, L. L. (2016). Enzymatic metabolism of vitamin A in developing vertebrate embryos. *Nutrients* 8:812. doi: 10.3390/nu8120812

Millacura, N., Pardo, R., Cifuentes, L., and Suazo, J. (2017). Effects of folic acid fortification on orofacial clefts prevalence: a meta-analysis. *Public Health Nutr.* 20, 2260–2268. doi: 10.1017/s1368980017000878

Miller, C. T., Schilling, T. F., Lee, K., Parker, J., and Kimmel, C. B. (2000). sucker encodes a zebrafish Endothelin-1 required for ventral pharyngeal arch development. *Development* 127, 3815–3828.

Moreman, J., Lee, O., Trznadel, M., David, A., Kudoh, T., and Tyler, C. R. (2017). Acute Toxicity, Teratogenic, and Estrogenic Effects of Bisphenol A and its alternative replacements bisphenol S, bisphenol F, and bisphenol AF in Zebrafish Embryo-Larvae. *Environ. Sci. Technol.* 51, 12796–12805. doi: 10.1021/acs.est.7b03283

Mork, L., and Crump, G. (2015). Zebrafish craniofacial development: a window into early patterning. *Curr. Top. Dev. Biol.* 115, 235–269. doi: 10.1016/bs.ctdb.2015.07.001

Muralidharan, P., Sarmah, S., and Marrs, J. A. (2015). Zebrafish retinal defects induced by ethanol exposure are rescued by retinoic acid and folic acid supplement. *Alcohol* 49, 149–163. doi: 10.1016/j.alcohol.2014.11.001

Ng, S. B., Buckingham, K. J., Lee, C., Bigham, A. W., Tabor, H. K., Dent, K. M., et al. (2010). Exome sequencing identifies the cause of a mendelian disorder. *Nat. Genet.* 42, 30–35. doi: 10.1038/ng.499

Palpant, N. J., Hofsteen, P., Pabon, L., Reinecke, H., and Murry, C. E. (2015). Cardiac development in zebrafish and human embryonic stem cells is inhibited by exposure to tobacco cigarettes and e-cigarettes. *PLoS One* 10:e0126259. doi: 10.1371/journal.pone.0126259

Pardo-Martin, C., Allalou, A., Medina, J., Eimon, P. M., Wahlby, C., and Fatih Yanik, M. (2013). High-throughput hyperdimensional vertebrate phenotyping. *Nat. Commun.* 4:1467.

Parker, B., and Connaughton, V. P. (2007). Effects of nicotine on growth and development in larval zebrafish. *Zebrafish* 4, 59–68. doi: 10.1089/zeb.2006.9994

Pashay Ahi, E., Walker, B. S., Lassiter, C. S., and Jonsson, Z. O. (2016). Investigation of the effects of estrogen on skeletal gene expression during zebrafish larval head development. *PeerJ* 4:e1878. doi: 10.7717/peerj.1878

Paterni, I., Granchi, C., and Minutolo, F. (2017). Risks and benefits related to alimentary exposure to xenoestrogens. *Crit. Rev. Food Sci. Nutr.* 57, 3384–3404. doi: 10.1080/10408398.2015.1126547

Phiel, C. J., Zhang, F., Huang, E. Y., Guenther, M. G., Lazar, M. A., and Klein, P. S. (2001). Histone deacetylase is a direct target of valproic acid, a potent anticonvulsant, mood stabilizer, and teratogen. *J. Biol. Chem.* 276, 36734–36741. doi: 10.1074/jbc.m101287200

Pinto, P., and Dougados, M. (2006). Leflunomide in clinical practice. *Acta Reumatol. Port* 31, 215–224.

Rattanasopha, S., Tongkobpetch, S., Srichomthong, C., Siriwan, P., Suphapeetiporn, K., and Shotelersuk, V. (2012). PDGFRa mutations in humans with isolated cleft palate. *Eur. J. Hum. Genet.* 20, 1058–1062. doi: 10.1038/ejhg.2012.55

Reynolds, K., Kumari, P., Sepulveda, L., Rincon, Gu, R., Ji, Y., et al. (2019). Wnt signaling in orofacial clefts: crosstalk, pathogenesis and models. *Dis. Model Mech.* 12:dmm037051. doi: 10.1242/dmm.037051

Rocha, M., Singh, N., Ahsan, K., Beiriger, A., and Prince, V. E. (2020). Neural crest development: insights from the zebrafish. *Dev. Dyn.* 249, 88–111. doi: 10.1002/dvdy.122

Rudel, R. A., Camann, D. E., Spengler, J. D., Korn, L. R., and Brody, J. G. (2003). Phthalates, alkylphenols, pesticides, polybrominated diphenyl ethers, and other endocrine-disrupting compounds in indoor air and dust. *Environ. Sci. Technol.* 37, 4543–4553. doi: 10.1021/es0264596

Sabbagh, H. J., Hassan, M. H., Innes, N. P., Elkodary, H. M., Little, J., and Mossey, P. A. (2015). Passive smoking in the etiology of non-syndromic orofacial clefts: a systematic review and meta-analysis. *PLoS One* 10:e0116963. doi: 10.1371/journal.pone.0116963

Saili, K. S., Tilton, S. C., Waters, K. M., and Tanguay, R. L. (2013). Global gene expression analysis reveals pathway differences between teratogenic and non-teratogenic exposure concentrations of bisphenol A and 17beta-estradiol in embryonic zebrafish. *Reprod. Toxicol.* 38, 89–101. doi: 10.1016/j.reprotox.2013.03.009

Sampson, P. D., Streissguth, A. P., Bookstein, F. L., Little, R. E., Clarren, S. K., Dehaene, P., et al. (1997). Incidence of fetal alcohol syndrome and prevalence of alcohol-related neurodevelopmental disorder. *Teratology* 56, 317–326. doi: 10.1002/(sici)1096-9926(199711)56:5<317::aid-tera5>3.0.co;2-u

Sarmah, S., Muralidharan, P., Curtis, C. L., McClintick, J. N., Buente, B. B., Holdgrafer, D. J., et al. (2013). Ethanol exposure disrupts extraembryonic microtubule cytoskeleton and embryonic blastomere cell adhesion, producing epiboly and gastrulation defects. *Biol. Open* 2, 1013–1021. doi: 10.1242/bio.20135546

Schilling, T. F., and Kimmel, C. B. (1997). Musculoskeletal patterning in the pharyngeal segments of the zebrafish embryo. *Development* 124, 2945–2960.

Schober, W., Szendrei, K., Matzen, W., Osiander-Fuchs, H., Heitmann, D., Schettgen, T., et al. (2014). Use of electronic cigarettes (e-cigarettes) impairs indoor air quality and increases FeNO levels of e-cigarette consumers. *Int. J. Hyg. Environ. Health* 217, 628–637. doi: 10.1016/j.ijheh.2013.11.003

Seda, M., Geerlings, M., Lim, P., Jeyabalan-Srikaran, J., Cichon, A. C., Scambler, P. J., et al. (2019). An FDA-approved drug screen for compounds influencing craniofacial skeletal development and craniosynostosis. *Mol. Syndromol.* 10, 98–114. doi: 10.1159/000491567

Soares, A. R., Pereira, P. M., Ferreira, V., Reverendo, M., Simoes, J., Bezerra, A. R., et al. (2012). Ethanol exposure induces upregulation of specific microRNAs in zebrafish embryos. *Toxicol. Sci.* 127, 18–28. doi: 10.1093/toxsci/kfs068

Spoorendonk, K. M., Peterson-Maduro, J., Renn, J., Trowe, T., Kranenbarg, S., Winkler, C., et al. (2008). Retinoic acid and Cyp26b1 are critical regulators of osteogenesis in the axial skeleton. *Development* 135, 3765–3774. doi: 10.1242/dev.024034

Staal, Y. C. M., Meijer, J., van der Kris, R. J. C., de Bruijn, A. C., Boersma, A. Y., Gremmer, E. R., et al. (2018). Head skeleton malformations in zebrafish (Danio rerio) to assess adverse effects of mixtures of compounds. *Arch. Toxicol.* 92, 3549–3564. doi: 10.1007/s00204-018-2320-y

Stuppia, L., Capogreco, M., Marzo, G., La Rovere, D., Antonucci, I., Gatta, V., et al. (2011). Genetics of syndromic and nonsyndromic cleft lip and palate. *J. Craniofac Surg.* 22, 1722–1726.

Sulik, K. K., Johnston, M. C., Ambrose, L. J., and Dorgan, D. (1979). Phenytoin (dilantin)-induced cleft lip and palate in A/J mice: a scanning and transmission electron microscopic study. *Anat. Rec.* 195, 243–255. doi: 10.1002/ar.1091950201

Sun, Y., Zhang, B., Luo, L., Shi, D. L., Wang, H., Cui, Z., et al. (2019). Systematic genome editing of the genes on zebrafish Chromosome 1 by CRISPR/Cas9. *Genome Res.* 30, 118-126.

Swartz, M. E., Lovely, C. B., McCarthy, N., Kuka, T., and Eberhart, J. K. (2020). Novel ethanol-sensitive mutants identified in an F3 forward genetic screen. *Alcohol. Clin. Exp. Res.* 44, 56–65. doi: 10.1111/acer.14240

Swartz, M. E., Sheehan-Rooney, K., Dixon, M. J., and Eberhart, J. K. (2011). Examination of a palatogenic gene program in zebrafish. *Dev. Dyn.* 240, 2204–2220. doi: 10.1002/dvdy.22713

Swartz, M. E., Wells, M. B., Griffin, M., McCarthy, N., Lovely, C. B., McGurk, P., et al. (2014). A screen of zebrafish mutants identifies ethanol-sensitive genetic loci. *Alcohol. Clin. Exp. Res.* 38, 694–703. doi: 10.1111/acer.12286

Tanko, L. B., Sondergaard, B. C., Oestergaard, S., Karsdal, M. A., and Christiansen, C. (2008). An update review of cellular mechanisms conferring the indirect and direct effects of estrogen on articular cartilage. *Climacteric* 11, 4–16. doi: 10.1080/13697130701857639

Tierney, P. A., Karpinski, C. D., Brown, J. E., Luo, W., and Pankow, J. F. (2016). Flavour chemicals in electronic cigarette fluids. *Tob Control* 25, e10–e15.

Van Otterloo, E., Williams, T., and Artinger, K. B. (2016). The old and new face of craniofacial research: how animal models inform human craniofacial genetic and clinical data. *Dev. Biol.* 415, 171–187. doi: 10.1016/j.ydbio.2016.01.017

van Rooij, I. A., Wegerif, M. J., Roelofs, H. M., Peters, W. H., Kuijpers-Jagtman, A. M., Zielhuis, G. A., et al. (2001). Smoking, genetic polymorphisms in biotransformation enzymes, and nonsyndromic oral clefting: a gene-environment interaction. *Epidemiology* 12, 502–507. doi: 10.1097/00001648-200109000-00007

Vandenberg, L. N., Chahoud, I., Heindel, J. J., Padmanabhan, V., Paumgartten, F. J., and Schoenfelder, G. (2010). Urinary, circulating, and tissue biomonitoring studies indicate widespread exposure to bisphenol A. *Environ. Health Perspect* 118, 1055–1070. doi: 10.1289/ehp.0901716

Wada, N., Javidan, Y., Nelson, S., Carney, T. J., Kelsh, R. N., and Schilling, T. F. (2005). Hedgehog signaling is required for cranial neural crest morphogenesis and chondrogenesis at the midline in the zebrafish skull. *Development* 132, 3977–3988. doi: 10.1242/dev.01943

Wagner, N. J., Camerota, M., and Propper, C. (2017). Prevalence and Perceptions of Electronic Cigarette Use during Pregnancy. *Matern. Child Health J.* 21, 1655–1661. doi: 10.1007/s10995-016-2257-9

Weigele, J., and Franz-Odendaal, T. A. (2016). Functional bone histology of zebrafish reveals two types of endochondral ossification, different types of osteoblast clusters and a new bone type. *J. Anat.* 229, 92–103. doi: 10.1111/joa.12480

Weigt, S., Huebler, N., Strecker, R., Braunbeck, T., and Broschard, T. H. (2011). Zebrafish (Danio rerio) embryos as a model for testing proteratogens. *Toxicology* 281, 25–36. doi: 10.1016/j.tox.2011.01.004

Weigt, S., Huebler, N., Strecker, R., Braunbeck, T., and Broschard, T. H. (2012). Developmental effects of coumarin and the anticoagulant coumarin derivative warfarin on zebrafish (Danio rerio) embryos. *Reprod. Toxicol.* 33, 133–141. doi: 10.1016/j.reprotox.2011.07.001

Williams, A. L., and Bohnsack, B. L. (2019). What's retinoic acid got to do with it? Retinoic acid regulation of the neural crest in craniofacial and ocular development. *Genesis* 57:e23308. doi: 10.1002/dvg.23308

Wilson, R. D., Genetics, C., Wilson, R. D., Audibert, F., Brock, J. A., Carroll, J., et al. (2015). Pre-conception folic acid and multivitamin supplementation for the primary and secondary prevention of neural tube defects and other folic acid-sensitive congenital anomalies. *J. Obstet. Gynaecol. Can.* 37, 534–552. doi: 10.1016/s1701-2163(15)30230-9

Winslow, M. M., Pan, M., Starbuck, M., Gallo, E. M., Deng, L., Karsenty, G., et al. (2006). Calcineurin/NFAT signaling in osteoblasts regulates bone mass. *Dev. Cell* 10, 771–782. doi: 10.1016/j.devcel.2006.04.006

Woo, G. H., Katayama, K., Bak, E. J., Ueno, M., Yamauchi, H., Uetsuka, K., et al. (2004). Effects of prenatal hydroxyurea-treatment on mouse offspring. *Exp. Toxicol. Pathol.* 56, 1–7. doi: 10.1016/j.etp.2004.04.011

Wu, T., Liang, K. Y., Hetmanski, J. B., Ruczinski, I., Fallin, M. D., Ingersoll, R. G., et al. (2010). Evidence of gene-environment interaction for the IRF6 gene and maternal multivitamin supplementation in controlling the risk of cleft lip with/without cleft palate. *Hum. Genet.* 128, 401–410. doi: 10.1007/s00439-010-0863-y

Xiong, K. M., Peterson, R. E., and Heideman, W. (2008). Aryl hydrocarbon receptor-mediated down-regulation of sox9b causes jaw malformation in zebrafish embryos. *Mol. Pharmacol.* 74, 1544–1553. doi: 10.1124/mol.108.050435

Xuan, Z., Zhongpeng, Y., Yanjun, G., Jiaqi, D., Yuchi, Z., Bing, S., et al. (2016). Maternal active smoking and risk of oral clefts: a meta-analysis. *Oral Surg. Oral Med. Oral Pathol. Oral Radiol.* 122, 680–690. doi: 10.1016/j.oooo.2016.08.007

Yan, Y. L., Jowett, T., and Postlethwait, J. H. (1998). Ectopic expression of hoxb2 after retinoic acid treatment or mRNA injection: disruption of hindbrain and craniofacial morphogenesis in zebrafish embryos. *Dev. Dyn.* 213, 370–385. doi: 10.1002/(sici)1097-0177(199812)213:4<370::aid-aja3>3.0.co;2-o

Zarella, C. S., Albino, F. P., Oh, A. K., Wood, B. C., Oluigbo, C. O., Myseros, J. S., et al. (2016). Craniosynostosis following fetal methotrexate exposure. *J. Craniofac. Surg.* 27, 450–452. doi: 10.1097/scs.0000000000002423

Zhang, C., Frazier, J. M., Chen, H., Liu, Y., Lee, J. A., and Cole, G. J. (2014). Molecular and morphological changes in zebrafish following transient ethanol exposure during defined developmental stages. *Neurotoxicol. Teratol.* 44, 70–80. doi: 10.1016/j.ntt.2014.06.001

Zhang, H., Yao, Y., Chen, Y., Yue, C., Chen, J., Tong, J., et al. (2016). Crosstalk between AhR and wnt/beta-catenin signal pathways in the cardiac developmental toxicity of PM2.5 *in zebrafish embryos. Toxicology* 35, 31–38. doi: 10.1016/j.tox.2016.05.014

Zhu, S. H., Sun, J. Y., Bonnevie, E., Cummins, S. E., Gamst, A., Yin, L., et al. (2014). Four hundred and sixty brands of e-cigarettes and counting: implications for product regulation. *Tob. Control* 23(Suppl. 3), iii3–iii9.

Zoupa, M., Zwart, E. P., Gremmer, E. R., Nugraha, A., Compeer, S., Slob, W., et al. (2020). Dose addition in chemical mixtures inducing craniofacial malformations in zebrafish (Danio rerio) embryos. *Food Chem. Toxicol.* 137:111117. doi: 10.1016/j.fct.2020.111117

5

Sialometric and Sialochemical Analysis in Individuals With Pulp Stones

Marilisa Carneiro Leão Gabardo[1], Prescila Mota de Oliveira Kublitski[1], Isabela Rodrigues Sette[1], Thaís Lauschner[1], Mariana Martins Juglair[1], Flares Baratto-Filho[1], João Armando Brancher[1] and Edgard Michel-Crosato[2]*

[1] *School of Health Sciences, Universidade Positivo, Curitiba, Brazil,*

[2] *Department of Dentistry, Universidade de São Paulo, São Paulo, Brazil*

Correspondence:
Marilisa Carneiro Leão Gabardo
marilisagabardo@gmail.com

The aim of this study was to analyze the saliva of patients with pulp stones, with sialometric and sialochemical tests. Eighty individuals, aged between18 and 65 years, of both sexes, were investigated. Patients were included in the pulp stone group when radiographic examination was suggestive of pulp stones in at least one permanent tooth, whereas those without this alteration were considered controls. Saliva was collected by stimulation, followed by salivary flowrate (SFR) and pH analysis tests. The organic components, such as urea (URE), glucose (GLU), total proteins (TPTs), alkaline phosphatase, creatinine (CRE), salivary amylase (SAM), and uric acid (URA), and the inorganic components, such as calcium, iron, and phosphorus, were evaluated by colorimetric techniques in an ultraviolet–visible (UV–vis) spectrophotometer. Differences among pulp stones and control groups were compared using Student's *t*-test, with a significance level of $p < 0.05$. In both groups prevailed the female. Statistically significant differences between groups were observed for pH ($p = 0.027$), SFR ($p = 0.002$), alkaline phosphatase ($p = 0.008$), and URA ($p = 0.005$). None of the inorganic components showed significant difference ($p > 0.05$). In the analyses stratified by sex, difference between groups was observed for pH ($p = 0.007$) and URA ($p = 0.003$) in women. In conclusion, sialometric and sialochemical alterations occurred in patients with pulp stones, with significantly higher levels of pH, SFR, alkaline phosphatase, and URA.

Keywords: dental pulp calcification, saliva, organic chemicals, inorganic chemicals, sialometry, sialochemistry

INTRODUCTION

Saliva is a complex biological fluid secreted continuously by salivary glands that performs numerous functions in the oral cavity, such as providing minerals to balance the process of dental demineralization and remineralization, and control of microbiota. This is possible because saliva contains numerous organic and inorganic components, which contribute to the equilibrium of the oral environment (Dawes et al., 2015). Saliva has also been described as a potential biological marker for systemic diseases (Zhang et al., 2012). The variation in salivary flowrate (SRF) and pH are related with systemic (Carramolino-Cuellar et al., 2018) and oral diseases (Foglio-Bonda et al., 2017). Diabetic patients present salivary glucose (GLU) alterations (Ladgotra et al., 2016), and higher levels of salivary urea (URE) and uric acid (URA) are commonly observed in patients with renal diseases

(Alpdemir et al., 2018). Such alterations have also been observed in the most prevalent oral diseases, for example, increased total protein (TPT) levels in the presence of dental caries (Pandey et al., 2015) and periodontal disease (Shaila et al., 2013). In the past decades, numerous studies have described, standardized, and validated analyses of salivary organic and inorganic components (Teixeira et al., 2012; Malathi et al., 2013; Shaila et al., 2013; Pandey et al., 2015; Buche et al., 2017; Khozeimeh et al., 2017; Saha et al., 2017; Alpdemir et al., 2018; De et al., 2018; Jeyasree et al., 2018; Riis et al., 2018; Alshahrani et al., 2019). Owing to the detection of serum constituents, saliva has also been used as a tool for diagnosis, monitoring, and management of patients with both oral and systemic diseases (Malamud, 2011). The chief advantage of saliva as a diagnostic/prognostic tool is the ease of collection, considering the non-invasive nature of the procedure when compared to blood test (Zhang et al., 2012; Dawes et al., 2015).

Pulp stones are characterized by calcifications in the pulp chamber commonly observed in the general population, both in young and elderly patients (Satheeshkumar et al., 2013), although the prevalence is higher in the latter (Horsley et al., 2009). Its reported rates range widely, depending on the method of diagnosis, reaching 36.53% (Jannati et al., 2019), 46.9% (Ravanshad et al., 2015), and 83.3% (Hsieh et al., 2018) of frequency. Although its origin has not been fully elucidated (Goga et al., 2008), its formation results from the natural aging process or as a response to injuries, such as traumatic occlusion and orthodontic movement (Ertas et al., 2017). Genetic causes (VanDenBerghe et al., 1999) and, currently, the identification of nanoparticles and nanobacteria are pointed out as etiological factors (Zeng et al., 2011), which have also been found in kidney stones (Chen et al., 2010).

The entire process of calcification formation is reduced to the adhesion of calcium crystals to the cells, which hinders the permeability of mitochondria and the transport through their pores, which determines oxidative stress, apoptosis, and expression of osteopontin (OPN), a glycoprotein phosphorylated secreted in the extracellular bone matrix (Senger et al., 1979). Macrophages phagocytize and digest a number of crystals, but some end up aggregating into a mass containing OPN and epithelial cell debris, giving rise to the calculus nuclei. This biomolecular mechanism, described by Kohri et al. (2012), is similar to atherosclerotic calcification. Thus, these tissue changes follow the same pattern, and pulp calcifications should not be an exception (Foster et al., 2018).

In the clinical context, the presence of pulp stones can pose a challenge in endodontic treatment because they partially or fully obliterate the pulp chamber thus closing entrances to the root canals, which aggravates or fully disables thorough cleaning and shaping of the root canal system (Qualtrough and Mannocci, 2011).

Interestingly, the incidence of pulp stones is higher in patients with diabetes and kidney disease (Nakajima et al., 2013), including urolithiasis (Movahhedian et al., 2018; Gabardo et al., 2019), and coronary artery disease (Alsweed et al., 2019), possibly due to the inflammatory process common to them (Gopal et al., 2016). The association between them and certain systemic conditions is also supported by the fact that the mechanism of mineralization of pulp stones is similar to calcifications in other organs in the body (Carson, 1998). However, the exact etiology of this process remains unclear (Milcent et al., 2019). Despite the lack of a direct relationship between the salivary composition and the pulp stones, these alterations may be an oral factor indicating the presence of systemic changes (Horsley et al., 2009; Satheeshkumar et al., 2013).

Therefore, the present study evaluated the sialometric and sialochemical profile of patients with pulp stones in order to identify possible changes in composition of their saliva. The null hypothesis is that alterations in inorganic and organic components are not present in the saliva of these individuals.

MATERIALS AND METHODS

The local ethics committee of Universidade Positivo for research on humans (Reg. No. 2.805.133) approved this case-control study. Individuals who signed the form of informed consent were included.

Initially, dental records of patients (18–65 years old) with radiographs (panoramic, periapical, or bitewing), who were under treatment at the Universidade Positivo Dental Clinic, were selected. Initially, a questionnaire with nine items, adapted from a study by Bhattarai et al. (2018), was applied as a screening tool to exclude individuals with cognitive impairment, viral diseases such as HIV and hepatitis, and recent history of oral surgery (<1 month). Individuals with oral infection; salivary gland problems; history of radiotherapy in the head and neck region; those under treatment with antibiotics, antihistamines, antipsychotics, antidepressants, or anti-inflammatory drugs; dry mouth; and pregnant women were also excluded.

For the pulp stones group, patients with at least one permanent tooth with a radiograph showing pulp stones were selected. In the control group, patients with no evident pulp stone on panoramic or full-mouth radiographs were included. The period of recruitment of subjects for saliva collection was from October 2018 to June 2019.

The power observed in the sample was calculated, considering the value of α = 5% and the rejection of the null hypothesis (existence of difference between the groups), which resulted in a value of 76%.

Pulp Stones Identification

Two trained and calibrated examiners (kappa = 0.88) preselected prospective individuals to be included in the pulp stones and control groups by analyzing radiographs from their dental records. A third examiner specialized in radiology (gold standard) reanalyzed the selected radiographs. In order to confirm the diagnosis, during the follow-up, bilateral bitewing radiographs were taken in patients with an initial finding of pulp stones. There was complete agreement between the previous and recent radiographic findings.

Saliva Collection and Sialometric Analysis

One sample of saliva of each participant (n = 80) was collected, and three trained examiners performed this phase. Patients were instructed to perform proper oral hygiene and refrain from consumption of alcoholic beverages in the 12 h prior to the collection (Gopal et al., 2016). Patients were asked to chew a 1- × 0.5-cm sterile rubber band for 5 min for stimulation of salivary flow (Priya, 2017). Bottles were weighed before collection, which were reweighed after completion of the procedure to measure the SFR. The difference in weights of the empty and full bottles, in grams, is equivalent to milliliters of saliva/minute (ml/min), as per the so-called gravimetric method. Following collection of saliva, pH was immediately measured using a pocket meter with a direct electrode (Q400BD, QUIMIS, Diadema, SP, Brazil), and the samples were stored at −20°C (Chiappin et al., 2007). All samples were collected at least 1 h after the last meal.

Sialochemical Analyses

Labtest Diagnóstica® (Lagoa Santa, MG, Brazil) colorimetric kits were used for sialochemical analyses of URE, GLU, TPT, alkaline phosphatase (Alpdemir et al., 2018), creatinine (CRE), salivary amylase (SAM; Gopal et al., 2016), URA, calcium (Ca), and iron (Biscaglia et al., 2016). The Quimifos kit (Ebram Produtos Laboratoriais Ltda., São Paulo, SP, Brazil) was used for phosphorus (P) measurement. **Table 1** shows the kits used with their respective wavelengths for reading and the unit of measurement of each compound.

Biochemical procedures were performed by a single operator on ultraviolet-visible (UV–vis) spectrophotometer (Model UV, 1601, UV Visible Spectrophotometer, Shimadzu, Kyoto, Japan) using quartz cuvettes. The device was calibrated prior to each test. All colorimetric analyses were performed according to the manufacturers' instructions.

Statistical Analyses

Initially, a descriptive analysis of the data was performed. After the normality (Shapiro–Wilk) and homogeneity of variance (Levene) tests were done, the data were submitted for Student's t-test to identify differences between the groups (pulp stones and control) and gender (male and female). Due to the sexual dimorphism observed in some salivary parameters, the analyses were also performed after stratification of the samples according to sex.

All analyses were performed using SPSS® (IBM® SPSS® Statistics v. 25.0, SPSS Inc., Chicago, IL, United States), with a significance level of 5%.

RESULTS

Among the 80 patients included in this study, 43 (53.8%) presented with pulp stones and 37 (46.3%) were included as controls.

In the pulp stones group, 30 (69.8%) individuals were female, while in the control group, the number was 33 (89.2%) (p = 0.054).

Regarding SFR and pH, in the total sample, the means and SD were 1.09 (0.60) and 7.81 (0.45), respectively. **Figure 1** shows the comparison of SFR and pH between the groups, wherein statistically significant differences were observed in both parameters, with higher mean values of both in the pulp stones (p = 0.002 and p = 0.027, respectively).

Table 2 shows the mean values of organic and inorganic components according to the groups. Statistically significant differences between groups were identified with higher mean values in the pulp stones group of ALP (p = 0.008) and URA (p = 0.005). None of the inorganic components showed significant difference ($p > 0.05$).

In the comparison between sexes in the same group, female individuals presented statistically significant lower levels of P in

TABLE 1 | Salivary components analyzed, colorimetric kit used with respective wavelength, and unit of measurement.

Salivary components	Colorimetric kit	Wavelength (nm)	Unit
	Organic		
URE	Urea CE (Labtest Diagnóstica S. A., Lagoa Santa, MG, Brazil)	600 (580–620)	mg/dl
GLU	Glucose Liquiform (Labtest Diagnóstica S. A., Lagoa Santa, MG, Brazil)	505 (490–520)	mg/dl
TPT	Total Protein Totais (Labtest Diagnóstica S. A., Lagoa Santa, MG, Brazil)	545 (530–55)	g/dl
ALP	Alkaline phosphatase (Labtest Diagnóstica S. A., Lagoa Santa, MG, Brazil)	590 (580–590)	U/L
CRE	Creatinine (Labtest Diagnóstica S. A., Lagoa Santa, MG, Brazil)	510 (500–540)	mg/dl
SAM	Salivary amylase (Labtest Diagnóstica S. A., Lagoa Santa, MG, Brazil)	660 (620–700)	U/dl
URA	Uric acid Liquiform (Labtest Diagnóstica S. A., Lagoa Santa, MG, Brazil)	520 (490–540)	mg/dl
	Inorganic		
Ca	Cálcio Liquiform (Labtest Diagnóstica S. A., Lagoa Santa, MG, Brazil)	570 (550–590)	mg/dl
Fe	Ferro sérico (Labtest Diagnóstica S. A., Lagoa Santa, MG, Brazil)	560 (540–580)	μg/dl
P	Quimifos (Ebram Produtos Laboratoriais Ltda., São Paulo, SP, Brazil)	340	mg/dl

URE, urea; GLU, glucose; TPT, total protein; ALP, alkaline phosphatase; CRE, creatinine; SAM, salivary amylase; URA, uric acid; Ca, calcium; Fe, iron; P, phosphorus.

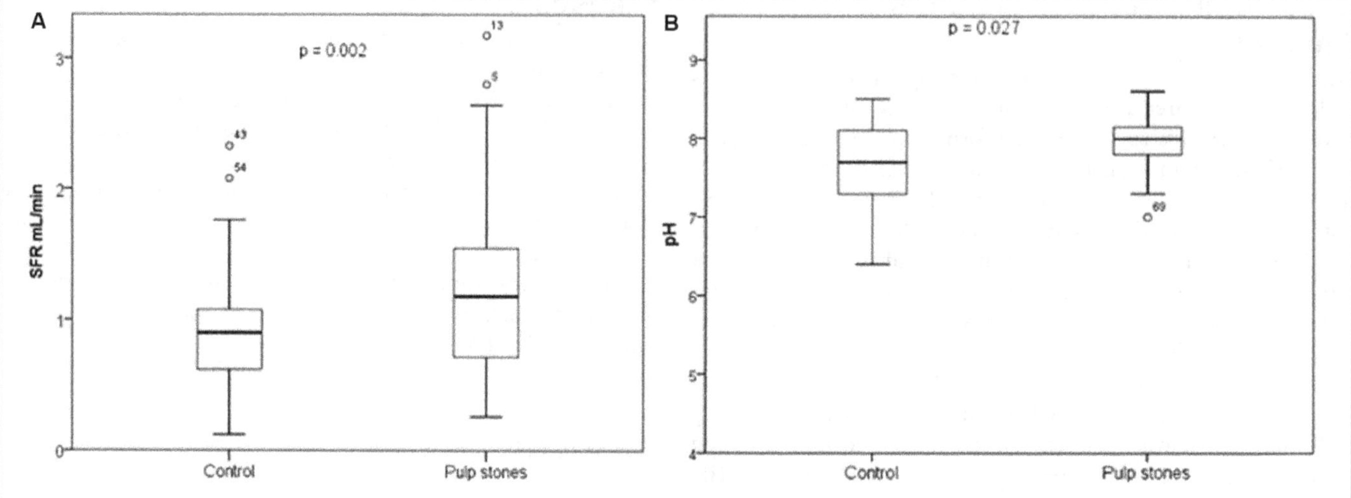

FIGURE 1 | Box plot representing **(A)** salivary flowrate (SFR) (ml/min) and **(B)** salivary pH, according to pulp stones and control groups. Student's *t*-test ($p < 0.05$).

the control group ($p = 0.011$). Similarly, in the pulp stones group, female individuals showed lower levels of URA ($p = 0.023$), SFR ($p = 0.038$), and ALP ($p = 0.034$).

In female, within the total sample, statistically significant differences were observed between the groups (pulp stones and control) for pH ($p = 0.007$) and for URA ($p = 0.003$) (**Table 3**).

DISCUSSION

In recent years, owing to rapid advancement in research, saliva has become well recognized as a pool of biological markers. However, to the best of our knowledge, this is the first study to evaluate biochemical parameters of saliva in individuals with pulp stones. The results presented in this study rejected the null hypothesis, indicating certain salivary changes, which include alterations in pH, SFR, ALP, and URA, in patients with pulp stones.

The choice for investigating pulp stones in this research was due to the high prevalence of this alteration observed in the general population (Horsley et al., 2009; Satheeshkumar et al., 2013; Jannati et al., 2019). With an origin not elucidated (Goga et al., 2008), some authors attributed its formation to aging, injuries, orthodontic movement (Ertas et al., 2017), and genetics (VanDenBerghe et al., 1999). What is known is that there are similarities in the calcification processes (Carson, 1998; Kohri et al., 2012; Foster et al., 2018), with an exacerbation of the inflammatory process (Gopal et al., 2016). Another highlight is that the incidence of pulp stones is higher in patients with diabetes and kidney disease (Nakajima et al., 2013), including urolithiasis (Movahhedian et al., 2018; Gabardo et al., 2019), and coronary artery disease (Alsweed et al., 2019). In addition, there are evidence in the literature that female individuals are more affected (Ravanshad et al., 2015; Jannati et al., 2019), but other authors have not confirmed this information (Hsieh et al., 2018; Babu et al., 2020).

From the clinical point of view, the pulp stones make endodontic treatment extremely difficult, as they cause obliterations that cannot allow an adequate chemical–surgical preparation (Qualtrough and Mannocci, 2011).

TABLE 2 | Absorbance of sialochemical tests for organic and inorganic components in total subjects in the pulp stones and control groups compared (n = 80).

Component	Pulp stones	Control	Total	*p*-value*
URE	12.98 (10.71)	10.67 (7.70)	11.91 (9.45)	0.278
GLU	3.08 (3.19)	3.32 (2.21)	3.19 (2.77)	0.702
TPT	0.74 (0.48)	0.75 (0.38)	0.74 (0.73)	0.947
ALP	16.41 (14.97)	9.19 (7.96)	13.07 (12.69)	**0.008**
CRE	0.10 (0.92)	0.11 (0.13)	0.11 (0.11)	0.820
SAM	595.59 (248.84)	528.86 (201.99)	564.73 (229.42)	0.196
URA	3.79 (2.64)	2.17 (2.37)	3.04 (2.63)	**0.005**
Ca	7.08 (5.92)	8.13 (13.66)	7.56 (10.19)	0.647
Fe	101.42 (46.08)	88.03 (67.23)	95.23 (56.86)	0.296
P	17.31 (5.87)	15.12 (7.39)	16.30 (6.67)	0.144

*Values presented as mean (± SD). URE, urea; GLU, glucose; TPT, total protein; ALP, alkaline phosphatase; CRE, creatinine; SAM, salivary amylase; UR, uric acid; Ca, calcium; Fe, iron; P, phosphorus. *Student's t-test. Bold values mean statistically significant (p < 0.05).*

TABLE 3 | Results of sialometric and sialochemical tests compared between groups, stratified by sex ($n = 80$).

Variable	Male		p-value*	Female		p-value*
	Pulp stones	Control		Pulp stones	Control	
SFR	1.55 (0.82)	1.20 (0.83)	0.465	1.08 (0.58)	0.90 (0.40)	0.157
pH	7.98 (0.21)	7.75 (0.48)	0.405	7.95 (0.33)	7.63 (0.55)	**0.007**
URE	15.61 (11.96)	14.61 (10.56)	0.883	11.85 (10.13)	10.19 (7.35)	0.458
GLU	3.16 (3.08)	2.19 (0.97)	0.555	3.05 (3.29)	3.46 (2.29)	0.567
TPT	0.57 (0.22)	0.80 (0.45)	0.171	0.82 (0.54)	0.74 (0.37)	0.520
ALP	23.68 (19.40)	6.07 (4.73)	0.099	13.26 (11.61)	9.57 (8.24)	0.156
CRE	0.08 (0.04)	0.07 (0.00)	0.600	0.11 (0.11)	0.11 (0.14)	0.981
SAM	627.06 (235.41)	683.48 (148.73)	0.661	581.96 (257.11)	510.12 (201.19)	0.219
URA	3.82 (2.83)	4.68 (1.97)	0.583	3.78 (2.59)	1.87 (2.26)	**0.003**
Ca	7.41 (6.93)	15.31 (11.32)	0.105	6.93 (5.54)	7.26 (13.81)	0.903
Fe	105.65 (34.11)	80.36 (48.77)	0.257	99.59 (50.81)	88.96 (69.67)	0.495
P	17.66 (5.69)	23.80 (3.03)	0.060	17.16 (6.04)	14.07 (7.07)	0.068

*Values presented as mean (de Almeida et al., 2008). SFR, salivary flowrate; URE, urea; GLU, glucose; TPT, total proteins; ALP, alkaline phosphatase; CRE, creatinine; SAM, salivary amylase; URA, uric acid; Ca, calcium; Fe, iron; P, phosphorus. *Student's t-test. Bold values mean statistically significant ($p < 0.05$).*

For clinical diagnosis of the systemic diseases, blood or urine samples are widely used, but recently, saliva emerges as a useful biofluid that provides rapid and accurate information for monitoring and management of patients with both oral and systemic diseases (Malamud, 2011; Rahim et al., 2015; Babu et al., 2020). In fact, it is not new that salivary compounds are a mixture of components derived from the salivary gland and blood, and both its volume and composition may vary depending on the environmental stimuli to which the individual is subjected (Malamud, 2011) or nutrition status. Thus, just as blood or urine GLU are affected by starvation or fullness, salivary components may be altered. In this sense, it is necessary to standardize a minimum time for collection after the meal. Invariably, this time varies between 1 h (Fregoneze et al., 2013), 2 h (Panchbhai et al., 2010), or more, after meal, so here, it was standardized that collection was carried out at least 1 h after food and dental hygiene.

It is known that pH and SFR changes can be observed in individuals with systemic (Carramolino-Cuellar et al., 2018) and oral disorders (Foglio-Bonda et al., 2017). SFR is an important parameter in the maintenance of oral health, and it is known that the value is directly proportional to the amount of salivary components (Teixeira et al., 2012). The normal range of SFR is 1–3 ml/min of stimulated saliva (de Almeida et al., 2008). In this study, SFR of individuals with pulp stones was higher than those in the control group. However, this result should be interpreted with caution once the SFR was not statistical different when stratified by sex in comparison between groups. However, in the comparison between sexes, in the pulp stones, men presented statistically significant higher SFR than women.

Regarding the pH levels, the main point to be investigated is that salivary pH was higher in individuals with pulp stones in the total analysis, and when the analysis was stratified by sex, female individuals with pulp stones also presented higher pH. Statistically significant difference was not observed in male individuals, but this could be due to the lower number of men in the present sample. It is assumed that the mechanism of formation of pulp stones is similar to that of calcifications occurring in other organs in the body (Carson, 1998). A study showed that kidney stones may form due to an increase in urinary pH, and high alkalinity of urine is a strong indicator of urolithiasis (Cong et al., 2014). Interestingly, a recent meta-analysis reported an association between pulp and kidney stones (Gabardo et al., 2019). It is possible that patients with pulp stones have higher pH levels in body fluids, thereby creating an environment conducive to formation of calcifications.

Although the mean difference of URE between pulp stones and control was not statistically significantly different, this organic component in the oral cavity is degraded by the ureases produced by the microbiota, resulting in the production of ammonia, contributing to the pH elevation (Sissons et al., 2007). In addition, studies have reported increase in levels of URE in patients with renal diseases (Alpdemir et al., 2018) and halitosis (Khozeimeh et al., 2017). Further studies should be conducted to investigate the association between salivary URE and pulp stones.

Increased concentration of GLU appears to be associated with an increase in SFR (Teixeira et al., 2012). The mean GLU value (3.19 mg/dl) of the samples in the present study was similar to that reported by Alshahrani et al. (2019) (3.39–4.28 mg/dl).

Total protein was not associated with pulp stones in the present study. Salivary TPT has many protective aspects, since they are adsorbed onto the surface of the enamel, forming a pellicle that regulates the process of demineralization and remineralization, in conjunction with other components, such as Ca (Humphrey and Williamson, 2001). Increased TPT levels have been reported in individuals undergoing orthodontic treatment (Teixeira et al., 2012), patients with dental caries (Pandey et al., 2015), and periodontal disease (Shaila et al., 2013). Similarly, higher ALP levels in saliva have been reported in patients with periodontitis (De et al., 2018; Jeyasree et al., 2018).

ALP is found in cells of the periodontium, such as fibroblasts, neutrophils, and osteoblasts, and is released during their migration to the site of infection (Safkan-Seppala and Ainamo, 1992). In addition, in edentulous, osteoporotic, or osteopenic individuals, the level of salivary ALP was significantly higher when compared to the control group, suggesting that this component may be an indicator of bone metabolism disorders (Saha et al., 2017). In the present study, salivary ALP was associated with pulp stones. It is possible that ALP is higher in the pulp fluids of teeth with pulp stones. It is well known that the equilibrium of tooth demineralization and remineralization is affected by ions such as Ca and P in saliva and, consequently, by ALP. One study has reported about development of caries with significant changes in P levels (Kaur et al., 2012). In the present study, a borderline association of P in both sexes it was observed (when stratified analysis was performed for the comparison between pulp stones and control). Higher levels of P were found in patients with renal diseases (Alpdemir et al., 2018) and diabetes (Ladgotra et al., 2016). Further studies should investigate salivary P levels in patients with pulp stones. Salivary Ca was not associated with pulp stones. Previously, higher salivary levels of Ca were observed in patients with renal disease (Alpdemir et al., 2018), diabetes (Ladgotra et al., 2016), and osteoporosis and osteopenia (Saha et al., 2017). Caries-free children may also demonstrate increased salivary Ca levels (Pandey et al., 2015).

Creatinine is a common parameter evaluated in patients with renal disease, and its analysis in saliva reflected the blood levels, thus can be used as a biomarker for the diagnosis of chronic kidney disease (Lasisi et al., 2016). In individuals with halitosis, decrease in CRE levels has been reported, contrary to the levels of URE and URA (Khozeimeh et al., 2017). The present result does not support that CRE could be a biomarker for pulp stones. On the other hand, URA was associated with kidney stones in this study. A previous analysis reported that the level of URA was associated with the development of arthritis and kidney stones, due to accumulation of URA crystals (Biscaglia et al., 2016). Riis et al. (2018) evaluated salivary URA levels in healthy individuals and did not observe differences among age groups, gender, and ethnicity.

It is possible that an association between URA and pulp stones was not observed in men in the present study due to the small sample size. Previous studies conducted on salivary URA demonstrated an association of the parameter with metabolic syndrome, cardiometabolic risk factors (Soukup et al., 2012), and body mass index (Martínez et al., 2017).

Salivary amylase is an enzyme that plays an important role in digestion of starch and protein. Teixeira et al. (2012) and Alshahrani et al. (2019) reported higher levels of SAM after the installation of fixed orthodontic appliances. Studies have also reported significant increase in SAM in diabetic patients, with levels reaching 2739.48 U/dl (Malathi et al., 2013) and 1671.42 U/dl (Ladgotra et al., 2016).

A previous study reported reduction in salivary Fe levels in individuals with dental caries (Buche et al., 2017). Another study concluded that patients undergoing procedures such as peritoneal dialysis and hemodialysis had a significant reduction in salivary Fe values (Alpdemir et al., 2018). In the present study, there was no statistically significant difference in salivary Fe levels between the groups.

It is important to highlight that the present study has some limitations. The study design (convenience sample) and the sample size, as well as the lack of previous history of orthodontic treatment and previous dental and occlusal trauma could present some important limitations. In addition, saliva compounds may be altered by many factors, and there is no guarantee that all patients respected the instructions before the saliva collection. Further long-term studies, with larger sample sizes are needed to confirm and understand the associations observed here.

To summarize, high prevalence of pulp stones has been reported globally (Jannati et al., 2019) and may be associated with other systemic conditions (Nakajima et al., 2013; Alsweed et al., 2019; Gabardo et al., 2019). Additionally, sialometric and sialochemical evaluations are relevant to research in this field, to understand the etiology of diseases and discover potential salivary biomarkers. Further studies should be conducted to evaluate more biomarkers associated with pulp stones as well as elucidate the association between pulp stones and systemic conditions.

CONCLUSION

Sialometric and sialochemical alterations occur in patients with pulp stones, with significantly higher levels of pH, SFR, ALP, and URA being reported in the present study.

ETHICS STATEMENT

The studies involving human participants were reviewed and approved by the Ethics Committee of Universidade Positivo for research on humans (Reg. No. 2.805.133). The patients/participants provided their written informed consent to participate in this study.

AUTHOR CONTRIBUTIONS

MG contributed to study conception and design, acquisition of data, analysis and interpretation of data, and drafting of the manuscript. PK contributed to acquisition of data and drafting of the manuscript. IS, TL, and MJ contributed to acquisition of data, analysis and interpretation of data. FB-F contributed to analysis and interpretation of data, and drafting of the manuscript. JB contributed to study conception and design, acquisition of data, and drafting of the manuscript. EM-C contributed to study conception and design, and critical revision. All authors contributed to manuscript revision, reading, and approving the submitted version.

REFERENCES

Alpdemir, M., Eryilmaz, M., Alpdemir, M. F., Topcu, G., Azak, A., and Yucel, D. (2018). Comparison of widely used biochemical analytes in the serum and saliva samples of dialysis patients. *J. Med. Biochem.* 37, 346–354. doi: 10.1515/jomb-2017-0056

Alshahrani, I., Hameed, M. S., Syed, S., Amanullah, M., Togoo, R. A., and Kaleem, S. (2019). Changes in essential salivary parameters in patients undergoing fixed orthodontic treatment: a longitudinal study. *Niger. J. Clin. Pract.* 22, 707–712. doi: 10.4103/njcp.njcp_606_18

Alsweed, A., Farah, R., Ps, S., and Farah, R. (2019). The prevalence and correlation of carotid artery calcifications and dental pulp stones in a saudi arabian population. *Diseases* 7:E50. doi: 10.3390/diseases7030050

Babu, N. A., Swarnalatha, C., Rao, A. P., Kumar, B. B., Tilak, B. P., Naidu, R. B., et al. (2020). Pulp stones as risk predictors for coronary artery disease. *Int. J. Prev. Med.* 11:7. doi: 10.4103/ijpvm.IJPVM_68_19

Bhattarai, K. R., Kim, H. R., and Chae, H. J. (2018). Compliance with saliva collection protocol in healthy volunteers: strategies for managing risk and errors. *Int. J. Med. Sci.* 15, 823–831. doi: 10.7150/ijms.25146

Biscaglia, S. C. C., Malagù, M., Pavasini, R., and Ferrari, R. (2016). Uric acid and coronary artery disease: an elusive link deserving further attention. *Int. J. Cardiol.* 15, 28–32. doi: 10.1016/j.ijcard.2015.08.086

Buche, B. O., Gusso, B., Torres, M. F., Dalledone, M., Bertoli, F. M. P., de Souza, J. F., et al. (2017). Association between decrease in salivary iron levels and caries experience in children. *Rev. Odonto Cienc.* 32, 94–98.

Carramolino-Cuellar, E., Lauritano, D., Silvestre, F. J., Carinci, F., Lucchese, A., and Silvestre-Rangil, J. (2018). Salivary flow and xerostomia in patients with type 2 diabetes. *J. Oral. Pathol. Med.* 47, 526–530. doi: 10.1111/jop.12712

Carson, D. A. (1998). An infectious origin of extraskeletal calcification. *Proc. Natl. Acad. Sci. U.S.A.* 95, 7846–7847. doi: 10.1073/pnas.95.14.7846

Chen, L., Huang, X. B., Xu, Q. Q., Li, J. X., Jia, X. J., and Wang, X. F. (2010). [Cultivation and morphology of nanobacteria in sera of patients with kidney calculi]. *Beijing Da Xue Xue Bao Yi Xue Ban.* 42, 443–446.

Chiappin, S., Antonelli, G., Gatti, R., and De Palo, E. F. (2007). Saliva specimen: a new laboratory tool for diagnostic and basic investigation. *Clin. Chim. Acta* 383, 30–40. doi: 10.1016/j.cca.2007.04.011

Cong, X., Gu, X., Sun, X., Ning, B., and Shen, L. (2014). Possible function of urinary pH and citrate on the ceftriaxone-induced nephrolithiasis. *Urology* 83, 63–67. doi: 10.1016/j.urology.2013.09.029

Dawes, C., Pedersen, A. M., Villa, A., Ekstrom, J., Proctor, G. B., Vissink, A., et al. (2015). The functions of human saliva: a review sponsored by the world workshop on oral medicine VI. *Arch. Oral. Biol.* 60, 863–874. doi: 10.1016/j.archoralbio.2015.03.004

De, A. P. R., Rahman, F., Adak, A., Sahoo, R., and Prakash, B. S. R. (2018). Estimation of salivary and serum alkaline phosphatase level as a diagnostic marker in type-2 diabetes mellitus with periodontal health and disease: a clinico-biochemical study. *J. Oral. Maxillofac Pathol.* 22:445. doi: 10.4103/jomfp.JOMFP_212_18

de Almeida, P. V., Gregio, A. M., Machado, M. A., de Lima, A. A., and Azevedo, L. R. (2008). Saliva composition and functions: a comprehensive review. *J. Contemp. Dent Pract.* 9, 72–80. doi: 10.5005/jcdp-9-3-72

Ertas, E. T., Veli, I., Akin, M., Ertas, H., and Atici, M. Y. (2017). Dental pulp stone formation during orthodontic treatment: a retrospective clinical follow-up study. *Niger. J. Clin. Pract.* 20, 37–42. doi: 10.4103/1119-3077.164357

Foglio-Bonda, P. L., Brilli, K., Pattarino, F., and Foglio-Bonda, A. (2017). Salivary flow rate and pH in patients with oral pathologies. *Eur. Rev. Med. Pharmacol. Sci.* 21, 369–374.

Foster, B. L., Ao, M., Salmon, C. R., Chavez, M. B., Kolli, T. N., Tran, A. B., et al. (2018). Osteopontin regulates dentin and alveolar bone development and mineralization. *Bone* 107, 196–207. doi: 10.1016/j.bone.2017.12.004

Fregoneze, A. P., de Oliveira Lira Ortega, A., Brancher, J. A., Vargas, E. T., de Paula Meneses, R., and Strazzeri Bonecker , M. J. (2013). Sialometric analysis in young patients with chronic renal insufficiency. spec care. *Dentist* 33, 118–122. doi: 10.1111/scd.12008

Gabardo, M. C. L., Wambier, L. M., Rocha, J. S., Kuchler, E. C., de Lara, R. M., Leonardi, D. P., et al. (2019). Association between pulp stones and kidney stones: a systematic review and meta-analysis. *J. Endod* 45, 1099.e2–1105.e2. doi: 10.1016/j.joen.2019.06.006

Goga, R., Chandler, N. P., and Oginni, A. O. (2008). Pulp stones: a review. *Int. Endod. J.* 41, 457–468. doi: 10.1111/j.1365-2591.2008.01374.x

Gopal, N., Rajagambeeram, R., Venkatkumar, S., Vijayan, M. V., Murugaiyan, S. B., Gopal, S. P., et al. (2016). Association of salivary osteopontin levels with glycaemic status and microalbuminuria - in patients with Type 2 diabetes mellitus. *J. Clin. Diagn. Res.* 10, BC06–BC8. doi: 10.7860/JCDR/2016/20156.8257

Horsley, S. H., Beckstrom, B., Clark, S. J., Scheetz, J. P., Khan, Z., and Farman, A. G. (2009). Prevalence of carotid and pulp calcifications: a correlation using digital panoramic radiographs. *Int. J. Comput. Assist. Radio.l Surg.* 4, 169–173. doi: 10.1007/s11548-008-0277-7

Hsieh, C. Y., Wu, Y. C., Su, C. C., Chung, M. P., Huang, R. Y., Ting, P. Y., et al. (2018). The prevalence and distribution of radiopaque, calcified pulp stones: a cone-beam computed tomography study in a northern taiwanese population. *J. Dent. Sci.* 13, 138–144. doi: 10.1016/j.jds.2017.06.005

Humphrey, S. P., and Williamson, R. T. (2001). A review of saliva: normal composition, flow, and function. *J. Prosthet. Dent.* 85, 162–169. doi: 10.1067/mpr.2001.113778

Jannati, R., Afshari, M., Moosazadeh, M., Allahgholipour, S. Z., Eidy, M., and Hajihoseini, M. (2019). Prevalence of pulp stones: a systematic review and meta-analysis. *J. Evid. Based Med.* 12, 133–139. doi: 10.1111/jebm.12331

Jeyasree, R. M., Theyagarajan, R., Sekhar, V., Navakumar, M., Mani, E., and Santhamurthy, C. (2018). Evaluation of serum and salivary alkaline phosphatase levels in chronic periodontitis patients before and after nonsurgical periodontal therapy. *J. Indian Soc. Periodontol.* 22, 487–491. doi: 10.4103/jisp.jisp_133_18

Kaur, A., Kwatra, K. S., and Kamboj, P. (2012). Evaluation of non-microbial salivary caries activity parameters and salivary biochemical indicators in predicting dental caries. *J. Indian Soc. Pedod. Prev. Dent.* 30, 212–217. doi: 10.4103/0970-4388.105013

Khozeimeh, F., Torabinia, N., Shahnaseri, S., Shafaee, H., and Mousavi, S. A. (2017). Determination of salivary urea and uric acid of patients with halitosis. *Dent. Res. J.* 14, 241–245.

Kohri, K., Yasui, T., Okada, A., Hirose, M., Hamamoto, S., Fujii, Y., et al. (2012). Biomolecular mechanism of urinary stone formation involving osteopontin. *Urol. Res.* 40, 623–637. doi: 10.1007/s00240-012-0514-y

Ladgotra, A., Verma, P., and Raj, S. S. (2016). Estimation of salivary and serum biomarkers in diabetic and non diabetic patients - A comparative study. *J. Clin. Diagn. Res.* 10, ZC56–ZC61. doi: 10.7860/JCDR/2016/19135.7995

Lasisi, T. J., Raji, Y. R., and Salako, B. L. (2016). Salivary creatinine and urea analysis in patients with chronic kidney disease: a case control study. *BMC Nephrol.* 17:10. doi: 10.1186/s12882-016-0222-x

Malamud, D. (2011). Saliva as a diagnostic fluid. *Dent. Clin. North Am.* 55, 159–178. doi: 10.1016/j.cden.2010.08.004

Malathi, L., Masthan, K. M., Balachander, N., Babu, N. A., and Rajesh, E. (2013). Estimation of salivary amylase in diabetic patients and saliva as a diagnostic tool in early diabetic patients. *J. Clin. Diagn Res.* 7, 2634–2636. doi: 10.7860/JCDR/2013/7574.3634

Martínez, A. D., Ruelas, L., and Granger, D. A. (2017). Association between BMI and salivary uric acid among mexican-origin infants, youth and adults: gender and developmental differences. *Dev. Psychobiol.* 59, 225–234. doi: 10.1002/dev.21492

Milcent, C. P. F., da Silva, T. G., Baika, L. M., Grassi, M. T., Carneiro, E., Franco, A., et al. (2019). Morphologic, structural, and chemical properties of pulp stones in extracted human teeth. *J. Endod.* 45, 1504–1512. doi: 10.1016/j.joen.2019.09.009

Movahhedian, N., Haghnegahdar, A., and Owji, F. (2018). How the prevalence of pulp stone in a population predicts the risk for kidney stone. *Iran. Endod. J.* 13, 246–250. doi: 10.22037/iej.v13i2.18181

Nakajima, Y., Inagaki, Y., Hiroshima, Y., Kido, J., and Nagata, T. (2013). Advanced glycation end-products enhance calcification in cultured rat dental pulp cells. *J. Endod.* 39, 873–878. doi: 10.1016/j.joen.2012.11.027

Panchbhai, A. S., Degwekar, S. S., and Bhowte, R. R. (2010). Estimation of salivary glucose, salivary amylase, salivary total protein and salivary flow rate in diabetics in India. *J. Oral. Sci.* 52, 359–368. doi: 10.2334/josnusd.52.359

Pandey, P., Reddy, N. V., Rao, V. A., Saxena, A., and Chaudhary, C. P. (2015). Estimation of salivary flow rate, pH, buffer capacity, calcium, total protein content and total antioxidant capacity in relation to dental caries severity, age and gender. *Contemp. Clin. Dent.* 6(Suppl. 1), S65–S71. doi: 10.4103/0976-237X.152943

Priya, Y. P. M. (2017). Methods of collection of saliva - a review. *Int. J. Oral Health Dent.* 3, 149–153.

Qualtrough, A. J., and Mannocci, F. (2011). Endodontics and the older patient. *Dent. Update* 38, 559–562.

Rahim, M. A., Rahim, Z. H., Ahmad, W. A., and Hashim, O. H. (2015). Can saliva proteins be used to predict the onset of acute myocardial infarction among high-risk patients? *Int. J. Med .Sci.* 12, 329–335. doi: 10.7150/ijms.11280

Ravanshad, S., Khayat, S., and Freidonpour, N. (2015). The prevalence of pulp stones in adult patients of shiraz dental school, a radiographic assessment. *J. Dent.* 16, 356–361.

Riis, J. L., Bryce, C. I., Matin, M. J., Stebbins, J. L., Kornienko, O., Huisstede, L. V., et al. (2018). The validity, stability, and utility of measuring uric acid in saliva. *Biomark Med.* 12, 583–596. doi: 10.2217/bmm-2017-0336

Safkan-Seppala, B., and Ainamo, J. (1992). Periodontal conditions in insulin-dependent diabetes mellitus. *J. Clin. Periodontol.* 19, 24–29. doi: 10.1111/j.1600-051x.1992.tb01144.x

Saha, M. K., Agrawal, P., Saha, S. G., Vishwanathan, V., Pathak, V., Saiprasad, S. V., et al. (2017). Evaluation of correlation between salivary calcium, alkaline phosphatase and osteoporosis- a prospective, comparative and observational study. *J. Clin. Diagn. Res.* 11, ZC63–ZC66. doi: 10.7860/JCDR/2017/24960.9583

Satheeshkumar, P. S., Mohan, M. P., Saji, S., Sadanandan, S., and George, G. (2013). Idiopathic dental pulp calcifications in a tertiary care setting in South India. *J. Conserv. Dent.* 16, 50–55. doi: 10.4103/0972-0707.105299

Senger, D. R., Wirth, D. F., and Hynes, R. O. (1979). Transformed mammalian cells secrete specific proteins and phosphoproteins. *Cell* 16, 885–893. doi: 10.1016/0092-8674(79)90103-x

Shaila, M., Pai, G. P., and Shetty, P. (2013). Salivary protein concentration, flow rate, buffer capacity and pH estimation: a comparative study among young and elderly subjects, both normal and with gingivitis and periodontitis. *J. Indian Soc. Periodontol.* 17, 42–46. doi: 10.4103/0972-124X.107473

Sissons, C. H., Anderson, S. A., Wong, L., Coleman, M. J., and White, D. C. (2007). Microbiota of plaque microcosm biofilms: effect of three times daily sucrose pulses in different simulated oral environments. *Caries Res.* 41, 413–422. doi: 10.1159/000104801

Soukup, M., Biesiada, I., Henderson, A., Idowu, B., Rodeback, D., Ridpath, L., et al. (2012). Salivary uric acid as a noninvasive biomarker of metabolic syndrome. *Diabetol. Metab. Syndr.* 4:14. doi: 10.1186/1758-5996-4-14

Teixeira, H. S. K. S., Ribeiro, J. S., Pereira, B. R., Brancher, J. A., and Camargo, E. S. (2012). Calcium, amylase, glucose, total protein concentrations, flow rate, pH and buffering capacity of saliva in patients undergoing orthodontic treatment with fixed appliances. *Dental. Press J. Orthod.* 17, 157–161.

VanDenBerghe, J. M., Panther, B., and Gound, T. G. (1999). Pulp stones throughout the dentition of monozygotic twins: a case report. *Oral. Surg. Oral. Med. Oral. Pathol. Oral. Radiol,. Endod.* 87, 749–751. doi: 10.1016/s1079-2104(99)70174-5

Zeng, J., Yang, F., Zhang, W., Gong, Q., Du, Y., and Ling, J. (2011). Association between dental pulp stones and calcifying nanoparticles. *Int. J. Nanomedicine.* 6, 109–118. doi: 10.2147/IJN.S13267

Zhang, A., Sun, H., and Wang, X. (2012). Saliva metabolomics opens door to biomarker discovery, disease diagnosis, and treatment. *Appl. Biochem. Biotechnol.* 168, 1718–1727. doi: 10.1007/s12010-012-9891-5

6

Pattern of Morphological Variability in Unrepaired Unilateral Clefts With and Without Cleft Palate May Suggest Intrinsic Growth Deficiency

Benny S. Latief[1], Mette A. R. Kuijpers[2], Adam Stebel[3,4], Anne Marie Kuijpers-Jagtman[5,6,7] and Piotr S. Fudalej[7,8,9]*

[1] Department of Oral and Maxillofacial Surgery, Faculty of Dentistry, Universitas Indonesia, Jakarta, Indonesia, [2] Department of Dentistry – Orthodontics and Craniofacial Biology, Radboud University Medical Center, Radboud Institute for Health Sciences, Nijmegen, Netherlands, [3] Department of Maxillofacial Surgery, F. D. Roosevelt University Hospital, Banská Bystrica, Slovakia, [4] Department of Stomatology and Maxillofacial Surgery, Faculty of Medicine, Comenius University, Bratislava, Slovakia, [5] Faculty of Dentistry, Universitas Indonesia, Jakarta, Indonesia, [6] Department of Orthodontics, University Medical Center Groningen, Groningen, Netherlands, [7] Department of Orthodontics and Dentofacial Orthopedics, University of Bern, Bern, Switzerland, [8] Department of Orthodontics, Jagiellonian University, Kraków, Poland, [9] Department of Orthodontics, Institute of Dentistry and Oral Sciences, Palacký University Olomouc, Olomouc, Czechia

***Correspondence:**
Piotr S. Fudalej
piotr.fudalej@uj.edu.pl

In individuals with cleft lip and palate (CLP) an iatrogenic effect of operations on subsequent maxillary growth is well-known. Much less is known about the association between occurrence of CLP and intrinsic growth deficiency of the maxillofacial complex. The aim of this study was to compare morphological variability in subjects with unilateral cleft lip and alveolus/palate and unaffected controls using geometric morphometric methods. The research hypothesis was that if subjects with *unrepaired* unilateral CLP have intrinsic growth deficiency, the pattern of their craniofacial growth variation may differ from that in unaffected individuals. Lateral cephalograms were available of three groups of the same ethnic background (Proto-Malayid): (a) non-syndromic *unrepaired* unilateral complete cleft lip, alveolus, and palate (UCLP), $N = 66$, mean age 24.5 years (b) non-syndromic *unrepaired* unilateral complete cleft lip and alveolus (UCLA), $N = 177$, mean age 23.7 years, and (c) NORM ($N = 50$), mean age 21.2 years without a cleft. Using geometric morphometrics shape variability in groups and shape differences between groups was analyzed. Principal component analysis (PCA) was used to examine shape variability, while differences between groups and sexes were evaluated with canonical variate analysis. Sexual dimorphism was evaluated with discriminant function analysis (DA). Results showed that in comparison to NORM subjects, shape variability in UCLA and UCLP is more pronounced in the antero-posterior than in vertical direction. Pairwise comparisons of the mean shape configurations (NORM vs. UCLA, NORM vs. UCLP, and UCLA vs. UCLP) revealed significant differences between cleft and non-cleft subjects. The first canonical variate (CV1, 68.2% of variance) demonstrated that differences were associated with maxillary shape and/or position and incisor inclination, while in females, the CV1 (69.2% of variance) showed a combination of differences of "maxillary shape and/or position and incisor inclination" and inclination of the cranial base. Shape variability demonstrated considerable differences in subjects with UCLA,

UCLP, and NORM. Moreover, in subjects with a cleft, within-sample variability was more pronounced in the antero-posterior direction, while in non-cleft subjects, within-sample variability was more pronounced in the vertical direction. These findings may suggest that subjects with unilateral clefts have intrinsic growth impairment affecting subsequent facial development.

Keywords: unilateral cleft lip and palate, unilateral cleft lip, unrepaired clefts, geometric morphometrics, maxillary growth, facial morphology intrinsic growth deficiency in clefts

INTRODUCTION

Cleft lip with or without cleft palate shows a large phenotypic variation ranging from complete open clefts of the lip, alveolus and palate to microforms and subclinical phenotypes like submucous cleft lip or palate. All of them have their own specific phenotype and the related problems are different for each type of cleft. Surgical rehabilitation of patients with cleft lip and palate aims at restoration of the anatomy, function, and aesthetics of the face, but is associated with growth disturbance of the midface. Identification of factor(s) leading to maxillofacial growth disturbance in individuals with cleft lip and palate (CLP) is critical for improvement of treatment results. To date, numerous animal experiments have shown that scar tissue that develops after the palatal surface has been denuded to close the cleft and the palate, is a strong inhibitor of maxillary growth and the adverse growth effect persists into adulthood (Li et al., 2015).

Much less is known about the association between occurrence of CLP and intrinsic growth deficiency of the maxillofacial complex. The theoretical ground for it is that the processes causing lack of fusion of maxillary/nasal prominences during embryonic life could also lead to impaired growth. One way to assess this would be to compare craniofacial morphology in subjects with unoperated CLP with their non-cleft counterparts. However, for obvious reasons it is difficult to collect a large sample of untreated CLP individuals. Several investigations on untreated clefts produced conflicting results and demonstrated that the maxilla could be smaller (Capelozza et al., 1993; Liao and Mars, 2005), comparable (Shetye and Evans, 2006; Diah et al., 2007), or larger (Ortiz-Monasterio et al., 1974) than in non-cleft controls. Data for unoperated bilateral clefts is even more scarce and comprise mostly case reports (Will, 2000). These inconsistent findings may be due to the error of the method, different ages of evaluation, or the use of samples with mixed cleft types.

An alternative approach is a comparison of variability of craniofacial morphology in subjects with unoperated CLP with non-cleft individuals using geometric morphometry, a statistical method to analyze shape (Halazonetis, 2004; Zelditch et al., 2012). This method has been used in a few studies comparing two- or three-dimensionally craniofacial morphology of patients operated for a cleft, but comparisons between individuals with unoperated clefts and non-cleft controls are scarce (Toro-Ibacache et al., 2014; Liberton et al., 2020). Our recent study (Latif et al., 2020) demonstrated differences in facial variation between subjects with unrepaired bilateral clefts and non-cleft controls. Variability was mainly present in the vertical direction in non-cleft subjects, while in bilateral CLP subjects the anteroposterior component of variation was marked. We suggested that this difference might point to intrinsic growth impairment in bilateral CLP.

The aim of this study was to compare facial morphological variability in subjects with unilateral cleft lip and alveolus/palate and unaffected controls using geometric morphometric methods. The research hypothesis (H_R) tested in this study was that the patterns of craniofacial shape variations in subjects with unilateral cleft lip and alveolus/palate and unaffected controls is different.

SUBJECTS AND METHODS

Sample

The study sample consisted of three groups from the same ethnic background (Proto-Malayid): (**a**) group comprising 66 subjects (37 males, 29 females, mean age 24.5 years, SD 10.5, range 14–61 years) with a non-syndromic *unrepaired* unilateral complete cleft lip, alveolus, and palate (UCLP group), (**b**) group comprising 177 subjects (104 males, 73 females, mean age 23.7 years, SD 10.9, range 14–72 years) with a non-syndromic *unrepaired* unilateral complete cleft lip and alveolus (UCLA group), and (**c**) group comprising 50 subjects (25 males, 25 females, mean age 21.2 years, SD 3.2, range 15–31 years)—NORM group.

The cleft sample was collected between 1986 and 1997 during nine charity missions in the province of East Nusa Tenggara, Indonesia, as part of a larger study as described earlier (Latief et al., 2010) in cooperation between the University of Brawijaya, Faculty of Medicine (Malang, Indonesia), Universitas Indonesia, Faculty of Dentistry (Jakarta, Indonesia), University Medical Centre Leiden, Department of Oral and Maxillofacial Surgery (Leiden, Netherlands) and the Radboud University Medical Centre (Nijmegen, Netherlands). The inclusion criteria were Proto-Malayid origin, complete unrepaired non-syndromic UCLA or UCLP, non-syndromic cleft as ascertained from medical records and clinical examination; the exclusion criteria were additional submucosal cleft and/or Simonart's band, earlier surgical repair or orthodontic treatment, lack of adequate contacts between opposing molars, age younger than 14 years.

The NORM group was collected in 1997 and consisted of 50 healthy volunteers from the city of Kupang (capital of the province East Nusa Tenggara). The inclusion criteria were Proto-Malayid origin, no cleft or other craniofacial anomaly, no clefts in the family history, normal occlusal relationship (Angle Class I); The exclusion criteria were earlier orthodontic or surgical treatment in the maxillofacial region, and age younger than 14 years. All study participants (clefts and controls) signed the informed consent.

The Bioethics Committee of the University of Indonesia approved this investigation in 2015 (Ref #: *1/EthEx/FKGUI/II/2015*).

Methods

Lateral cephalograms taken prior to surgical closure of the cleft were available for further analysis. The radiographs were taken in a mobile custom-built radiographic setup including a cephalostat with a focus-film distance of 1.70 m. The film cassette was 24 × 30 cm with a high-speed intensifying screen to shorten the exposure time. Considering field conditions during imaging of cleft and non-cleft subjects, it is likely that the radiographic magnification factor could not have been kept constant. Therefore, only facial shape (i.e., without information about the size) was evaluated in this study. The cephalograms were scanned at 300 dpi resolution.

Facial morphology was evaluated on lateral radiographs of the head (cephalograms). Because the contour of the soft tissues was blurred and difficult to identify, the assessment of the facial morphology was limited to bony structures. The geometry of the cranial base, the maxillary complex, the mandible, and the anterior dentition was captured using 18 anatomical landmarks (**Figure 1**). We used the same landmarks as in the study by Latif et al. (2020), which seemed sufficient to represent key anatomical structures of the craniofacial skeleton.

The landmarks were digitized by one investigator (PF) on the scan of each radiograph with the tpsDig2 program, version 2.18[1]. Two-dimensional landmark coordinates were extracted and exported in TPS format to be used for the geometric morphometric analyses with the MorphoJ software package, version 1.06d (Klingenberg, 2011). The sample was checked for outliers—none was detected.

To assess the intra-observer reliability 28 images were randomly selected and re-digitized by the same investigator (PF) after a minimum of 1 month. Random error was expressed as the Procrustes distance between the redigitizations in shape space in comparison with the total shape variance.

Statistical Analysis

Two areas were analyzed in this investigation: shape variability in the groups and shape differences between the groups. First, principal component analysis (PCA) was used to examine shape variability. The effect of group, age, and sex on the shape was evaluated with multivariate regression analysis, where Procrustes shape coordinates were dependent variables and the group, age, and sex were covariates. Differences between the UCLP, UCLA, and NORM groups, i.e., the Procrustes distances between group means, for males and females were assessed using canonical variate analysis (CVA), which is a method used to find the shape features that best distinguish among multiple groups of subjects (Zelditch et al., 2012). Sexual dimorphism in the UCLA, UCLP, and NORM groups was evaluated with discriminant function analysis (DA; equivalent to CVA but used for comparisons between two groups only). Analogous as in CVA, also in DA the Procrustes distances between males and females were established.

All analyses and statistical tests were performed in MorphoJ and PAST v.3 software (Øyvind Hammer, University of Oslo, Norway). Permutation tests (100,000 permutation runs) with a significance level of 0.05 were used to establish intergroup differences in facial shapes. The visualization of facial shape changes was carried out in MorphoJ and Viewbox 4.1 (dHAL Software, Kifissia, Greece).

[1]http://life.bio.sunysb.edu/morph/

RESULTS

Method Error

The measurement error was relatively small in the redigitized subsample—it was equal to 7.29% of the total variation.

Within-Sample Shape Variability

The plot depicting overall shape variability in the sample (**Figure 2**) implies shape differences between groups. The pattern of scatter of individual shapes with a concentration of NORM shapes in the upper right region of the plot (i.e., PC1 and PC2 are > 0) and few NORM shapes in the lower left region of the plot (i.e., PC1 and PC2 are < 0) suggests that non-cleft subjects differ from subjects with a cleft. The principal components 1 through 5, each accounting for at least 5% of variance, explained in total 60.3% of variance among individuals (**Table 1** and **Supplementary Table 1** presents variance explained by all principal components). The first major axis of shape variation (PC1, 21.3% of variance) demonstrates shape patterns in the vertical direction, while PC2 (14.1% of variance) depicts mainly anteroposterior shape patterns, particularly of the size and/or position of the mandible relative to the cranial base and maxillary complex. **Figure 3** shows shape variability separately in UCLP, UCLA, and NORM groups. In comparison to non-cleft subjects, shape variability in individuals with unilateral clefts is more pronounced in the antero-posterior than in vertical direction. **Supplementary Table 2** demonstrates variability for each landmark in x and y directions.

Age-Shape Correlation

Regression analysis (**Table 2**) with group, sex, and age as covariates and PC1–PC5 as dependent variables showed a limited effect of the age on the facial shape variability—the age "weighted" considerably less than group and sex. This indicates that a subject's age was not a predictor of the facial shape, either in males or in females, or with or without a cleft.

Sexual Dimorphism

Sexual dimorphism was detected in UCLA and NORM groups but not in UCLP group (**Table 3**). The Procrustes distance between mean shapes for males and females was largest for non-cleft subjects (NORM) and smallest for subjects of the UCLP group. The non-cleft males had a shorter anterior facial height and flatter mandibular plane than females (**Figure 4**), while

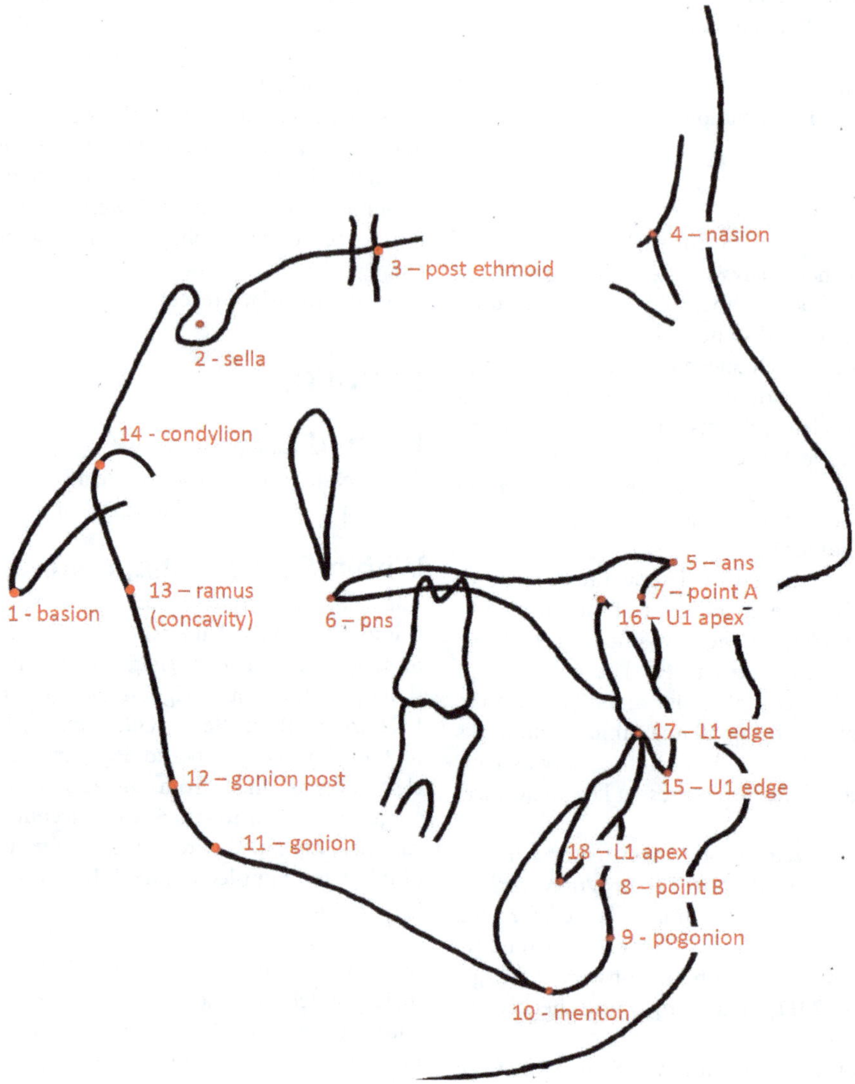

FIGURE 1 | Drawing of a cephalogram illustrating the anatomical landmarks used in this study.

the males and females with UCLA had subtle differences in vertical proportions.

Differences Between UCLP, UCLA, and NORM Groups

The inter-group differences between the mean shape configurations in each group were analyzed with CVA (**Table 4**). Pairwise comparisons (NORM vs. UCLA, NORM vs. UCLP, and UCLA vs. UCLP) in males and females revealed statistically significant differences between subjects with and without a cleft. In males, the first canonical variate (CV1, 68.2% of variance) demonstrated that differences were associated with maxillary shape and/or position and incisor inclination, while in females, the CV1 (69.2% of variance) showed a combination of differences of "maxillary shape and/or position and incisor inclination" and inclination of the cranial base (**Figure 5**).

DISCUSSION

In the current study we used geometric morphometrics (GM) to evaluate craniofacial shape. This novel method has been commonly used in anatomy and anthropology. We are aware that the vast majority of studies evaluating craniofacial shape in cleft and non-cleft population has used conventional cephalometrics as a shape descriptor. However, cephalometric analysis has inherent problems regarding its applicability as shape measure; it provides only a partial and localized description of shape and is confounded by our biases regarding the reference structures. As a result (a) the measurements are often conflicting, (b) many measurements are needed for a comprehensive shape description, (c) it is not trivial to compare the craniofacial pattern between different individuals, and (d) classification of shape is based on a limited subset of all possible measurements and might therefore be biased by that particular selection.

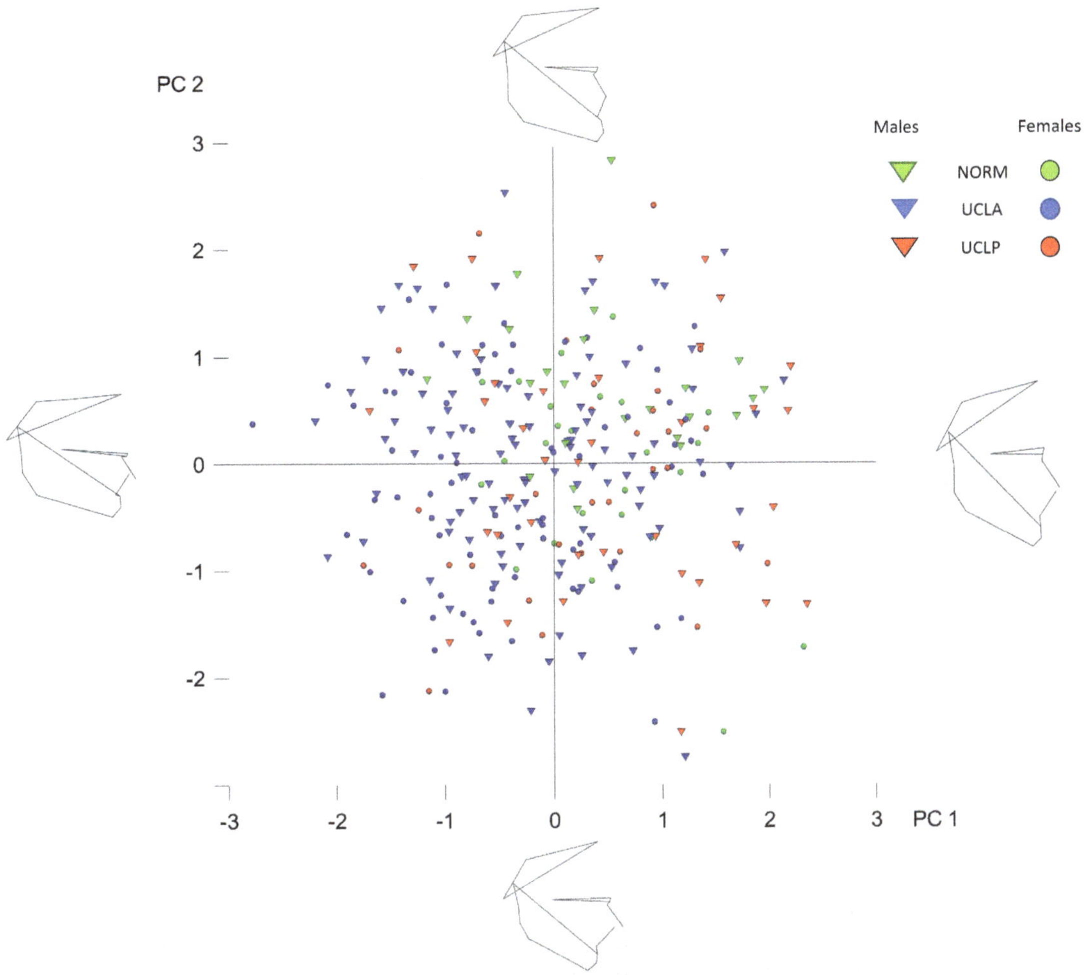

FIGURE 2 | Principal component analysis of shape variables in the whole sample (subjects with and without cleft pooled together). The figure presents the variation in the whole sample along PC axes 1 and 2 (PC1 and PC2). Each "point" represents a single subject. The numbers (1, 2, 3, -1, -2, -3) on the axes denote standard deviation (SD).

In comparison to conventional cephalometrics, GM allows for (a) comprehensive description of the overall craniofacial shape with measurements, which are not conflicting because they are unrelated statistically; (b) easy assessment of the degree of variation from the mean; (c) it is relative insensitive to errors in landmark identification (Halazonetis, 2004). These advantages make GM an interesting alternative in studies of the craniofacial shape (Wellens et al., 2013; Urbanova et al., 2016; Jaklová et al., 2020; Segna et al., 2020). Unfortunately, the "non-intuitive" mathematical methods of GM can present a challenge in interpretation of results.

Studies exploring the craniofacial shape in humans without congenital malformations (Rosas et al., 2008; Wellens and Kuijpers-Jagtman, 2016; Katsadouris and Halazonetis, 2017; Paoloni et al., 2017) demonstrated that the largest variability of the shape concerned the vertical direction (i.e., *dolichocephalic* vs. *brachycephalic* shape) irrespective of the ethnic background or population origin. Although contemporary populations from Europe are more *dolichocephalic* than those coming from Asia (African populations are relatively most *brachycephalic)*, vertical variability (i.e., different degree of *dolichocephalic/brachycephalic* facial pattern) prevails over variability in antero-posterior direction (Rosas et al., 2008). Thus, our research hypothesis was that if subjects with unilateral cleft lip and palate do have intrinsic growth deficiency, the pattern of their craniofacial

TABLE 1 | Proportion of variance in a sample comprising subjects with clefts (UCLP and UCLA) (N = 243) and without clefts (N = 50) described by principal components (PCs), explaining at least 5% of variance each, in shape space.

Principal component (PC)	% Variance	Cumulative %
PC1	21.3%	21.3%
PC2	14.1%	35.4%
PC3	11.8%	47.2%
PC4	8.1%	55.3%
PC5	5%	60.3%
Remaining PCs	*39.7%*	*100%*

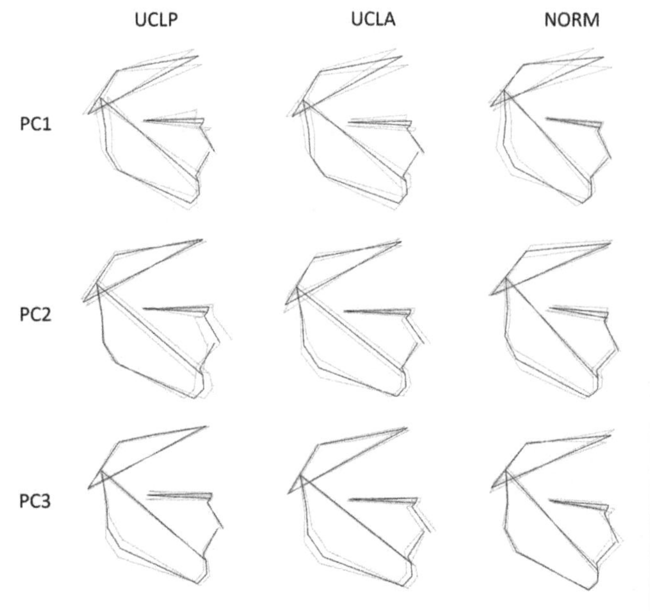

FIGURE 3 | Variation in subjects with unilateral cleft lip and palate (UCLP), unilateral cleft lip and alveolus (UCLA), and in unaffected subjects (NORM) along the first three principal components (PC1–PC3). The black shape is the mean shape, the red shapes correspond with the shape at -3 SD and +3 SD for each axis (PC1–PC3) and each group (UCLP, UCLA, NORM).

growth variation may differ from the pattern of variation in unaffected individuals.

In our previous study on individuals with bilateral orofacial clefts, we found evidence that subjects with unrepaired *bilateral* CLA and *bilateral* CLP did demonstrate a disparate pattern of craniofacial variation. Unaffected subjects and individuals with a bilateral cleft differed mostly in respect to the position of the (pre)maxilla, which was more protruded in the BCLA and BCLP groups than in controls (Latif et al., 2020). The aim of the current study was to test whether the difference in craniofacial shape variation between subjects with unrepaired unilateral orofacial clefts and their non-affected counterparts is comparable to the disparity between subjects with bilateral orofacial clefts and unaffected ones.

In the present study we found that subjects with a unilateral cleft had a considerably different pattern of craniofacial variation. In UCLA and UCLP groups PC1 through PC3 (cumulative variance: 47.2%) depicted a variation in both vertical and anteroposterior direction. Both directions of variation are easily discernible in **Figure 3**, with a possible exception of PC3 in the UCLP group, where anteroposterior variation of the maxilla was limited. In the NORM group, in contrast, variation in anteroposterior direction along the axes for PC1 and PC2 was limited, particularly for the maxilla (**Figure 3**). Furthermore, comparison of patterns of variation between subjects with different cleft types (UCLA and UCLP groups) demonstrates a lack of significant differences between the groups. PC1 shows an almost identical pattern of variation in the UCLA and UCLP groups, while PC2 indicates more anteroposterior variation in UCLP than in the UCLA group. The similarity of patterns of variation for subjects with a different type of the cleft on one side and the difference in patterns of variation between subjects with and without a cleft on the other side are visualized by clear separation of groups with and without a cleft along Canonical Variate 1 axis (**Figure 5**). Therefore, our findings imply that the orofacial cleft may be associated with intrinsic deficiency of growth of the structures affected by the cleft.

In exploratory studies such as the present one it is impossible to identify mechanisms responsible for growth deficiency in the cleft anomaly. Instead they serve as a tool to corroborate that such growth deficiency is possible. It is particularly important in subjects with unilateral cleft lip and alveolus/palate because there is an ongoing controversy encompassing the problem of

TABLE 2 | Multivariate regression analysis with group, sex, and age as covariates (independent variables) and principal components 1–5 (PC1–PC5) as dependent variables.

		Coeff.	Std. Err.	p	R^2
pc1	Sex	−6.51	4.07	0.110	0.009
	Age	−0.08	0.20	0.706	0.000
	Group	0.30	3.24	0.925	0.000
pc2	Sex	−7.94	3.20	0.014	0.023
	Age	0.50	0.16	0.002	0.031
	Group	−5.64	2.55	0.028	0.011
pc3	Sex	−9.93	2.91	0.001	0.043
	Age	0.52	0.15	0.000	0.046
	Group	−1.80	2.32	0.439	0.000
pc4	Sex	−6.25	2.46	0.012	0.023
	Age	0.01	0.12	0.910	0.001
	Group	4.35	1.96	0.027	0.018
pc5	Sex	−4.16	1.79	0.021	0.014
	Age	−0.38	0.09	0.000	0.034
	Group	9.31	1.43	0.000	0.111

Wilks λ = 0.6596; F: 8.508; df1: 15; df2: 784.4; p-value (the whole model) < 0.001.
Tests on independent variables:
(1) Sex: Wilks λ = 0.894; p < 0.001.
(2) Age: Wilks λ = 0.862; p < 0.001.
(3) Group: Wilks λ = 0.832; p < 0.001.
Tests on dependent variables:
(1) pc1: R^2 = 0.009, p = 0.451.
(2) pc2: R^2 = 0.066, p < 0.001.
(3) pc3: R^2 = 0.084, p < 0.001.
(4) pc4: R^2 = 0.04, p = 0.008.
(5) pc5: R^2 = 0.1749, p < 0.001.

TABLE 3 | Sexual dimorphism in groups assessed with discriminant function analysis (DA).

	Groups		
	UCLP	UCLA	NORM
Procrustes distance	0.01405	0.02072	0.04035
95%CI	0.01212–0.02713	0.00706–0.01587	0.01217–0.02759
p-value	0.896	<0.001	<0.001

P-values for permutation tests (100,000 permutation runs).

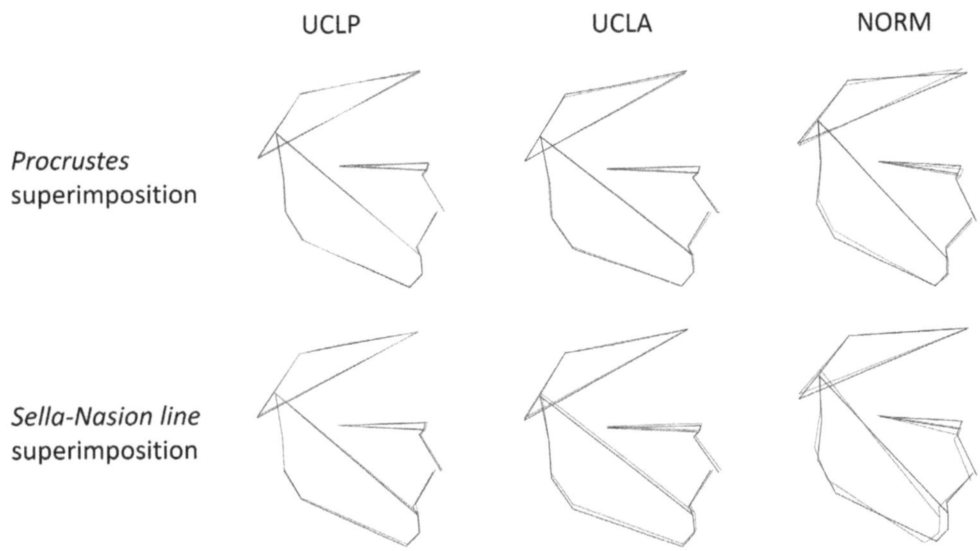

FIGURE 4 | Visualization of sexual dimorphism in subjects with unilateral cleft lip and palate (UCLP), unilateral cleft lip and alveolus (UCLA), and in unaffected subjects (NORM) based on discriminant function analysis. Black color—males, blue—females.

the impact of intrinsic growth deficiency vs. surgical iatrogenesis on subsequent craniofacial development. As discussed in our previous paper (Latif et al., 2020) "In theory, if facial growth deficiency is exclusively the result of treatment of the cleft deformity, one could expect that the pattern of variations of the shape of the face in untreated clefts is comparable with the pattern of variations in subjects without an orofacial cleft. If the opposite is true, the pattern of facial shape variations in untreated and treated clefts should be different." Publications to date demonstrated somewhat contradictory results—Lambrecht et al. (2000) reviewed studies assessing craniofacial morphology in unrepaired unilateral cleft lip and palate in comparison with non-cleft individuals and found that the maxillary complex in the cleft anomaly can be retruded (one study found retrusion), normal (three studies), or protruded (six studies). Later publications (Shetye and Evans, 2006; Chen et al., 2012) implied that in unrepaired unilateral cleft lip and palate although the length of the maxilla appears to be somewhat shorter in many patients, sagittal growth does not seem to be significantly disturbed. Our findings seem to disagree with the results of these studies assessing craniofacial morphology as

TABLE 4 | Pairwise differences between groups in facial shape configurations assessed with canonical variate analysis (CVA).

		UCLA	UCLP
Both sexes	NORM	0.0353 ($p < 0.001$)	0.0311 ($p < 0.001$)
	UCLA		0.0286 ($p < 0.001$)
Males	NORM	0.0373 ($p < 0.001$)	0.0386 ($p < 0.001$)
	UCLA		0.0319 ($p < 0.001$)
Females	NORM	0.041 ($p < 0.001$)	0.0371 ($p < 0.001$)
	UCLA		0.0313 ($p < 0.001$)

P-values from permutation tests (100,000 permutation runs) in brackets.

we found evidence for an intrinsic growth deficiency within the craniofacial complex, while most clinical studies revealed little maxillofacial growth disturbance in adults with unrepaired cleft lip and palate. There may be several explanations for this discrepancy.

First, the investigations mentioned above had rather small sample sizes which increases uncertainty for *generalizability* of findings. Second, the spatial position of the maxilla is typically assessed by measuring the angle between the point A and cranial base (or Frankfurt horizontal plane). The larger the angle, the more protruded the maxilla. However, in unrepaired cleft lip and palate when there is discontinuity of the orbicularis muscle and a wide cleft, the anterior part of the larger segment (on which point A is located) can be rotated forward. The repair of the cleft can result in maxillary remodeling and posterior dislocation of point A. In other words, location of point A in the unrepaired cleft and non-cleft maxilla is not completely homologous. Finally, conventional cephalometric analysis as used in earlier studies has significant limitations such as the use of many inter-related landmarks and angles to characterize morphology of the anatomical structure (Moyers and Bookstein, 1979; Bookstein, 2016). In effect the change of a given angle (e.g., sella-nasion-point A) cannot be precisely ascribed to the change of a structure (e.g., position of point A on the surface of maxilla) because the change of reference line (e.g., sella-nasion, dependent on position of both sella and nasion landmarks) might well be responsible for it (Halazonetis, 2004). Therefore the use of geometric morphometrics to analyze shape is a better choice.

The pattern of shape variation in subjects with unrepaired **unilateral** clefts is **similar** to that found in **bilateral** clefts (Latif et al., 2020). The variation along the PC1 axis in UCLA, UCLP, and pooled bilateral cleft lip and alveolus (BCLA)—bilateral cleft lip, alveolus, and palate (BCLP) groups is a combination of variation in vertical and anteroposterior direction. Both

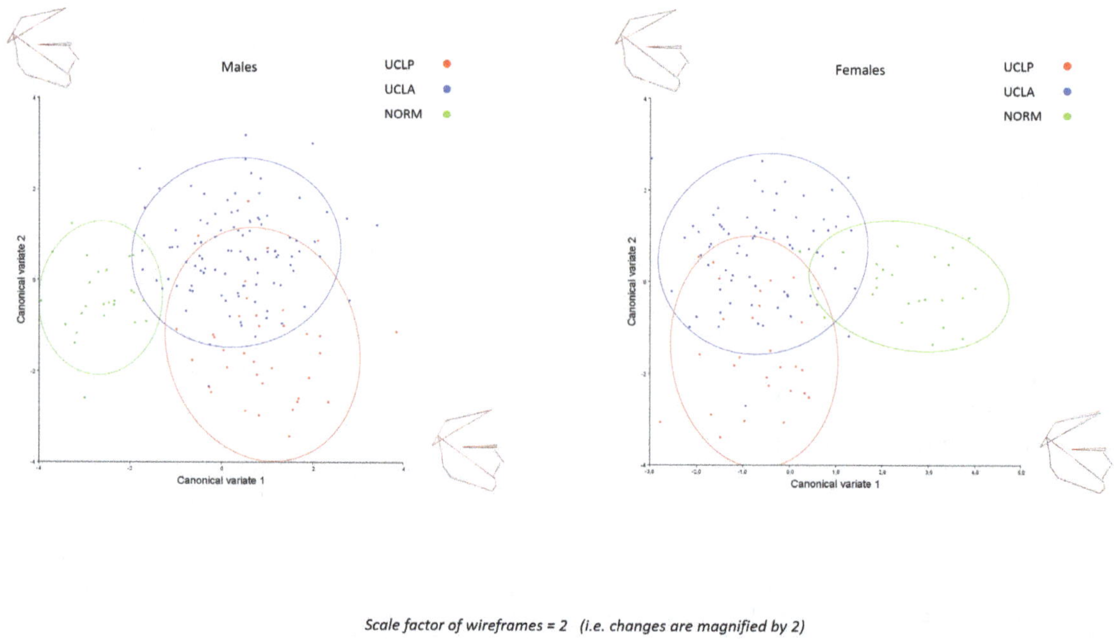

FIGURE 5 | Canonical variate analysis of males and females with unilateral cleft lip and palate (UCLP), with unilateral cleft lip and alveolus (UCLA), and in unaffected individuals (NORM).

components (directions) are easily recognizable on the plots. A subtle difference is that the anteroposterior component in the BCLA-BCLP group is more pronounced than in UCLA and UCLP groups. This may reflect a more variable position of the pre-maxilla in subjects with bilateral clefts but could also be due to a significantly smaller sample size in the BCLA-BCLP group. The variation along the PC2 axis is also a combination of variation in the vertical and anteroposterior direction. However, in the BCLA-BCLP group the vertical component is stronger than along PC1 axis; in UCLA and UCLP groups the vertical component is weaker than the anteroposterior component, especially in subjects with UCLP. A comparison with the control group (in both studies the same group of non-cleft subjects was used) demonstrates that cleft vs. non-cleft differences are considerably larger than discrepancies between groups with different cleft types. To understand the effect of treatment and intrinsic growth deficiency it would be interesting to be able to compare a treated group with the same ethnicity and a control group.

The strengths of this investigation are a large sample size, the use of controls derived from the same ethnic group, and the use of geometric morphometrics for characterization of craniofacial variability. Nevertheless, this study has several limitations mentioned previously (Latif et al., 2020). In summary, some subjects were relatively young (i.e., 14–18 years of age) when the cephalogram was collected. The age of subjects should be viewed in the context of achievement of relative stability of craniofacial structures. Indonesian populations, as other from equatorial regions, start and finish their maturation phase earlier.

Nevertheless, the literature on unoperated cleft uses the age of 13 years to pinpoint the start of the adulthood stage (Latief et al., 2010). Certainly, the aging affects facial soft tissues; however, its effect on the skeleton is limited, when assessed with geometric morphometrics, provided a subject has adequate occlusal contacts between opposing teeth (otherwise a loss of opposing teeth can result in loss of occlusal support and decrease of facial height). In our study we excluded subjects who had missing occlusal contacts between opposing teeth. We used 2D cephalograms, although 3D imaging is currently the method of choice, but this is not a feasible option in a low-income country and an isolated population. The soft tissue profile was difficult to identify so we were restricted to analysis of the hard tissues only. In future research the presently available handheld 3D cameras may facilitate soft tissue analysis of patients and controls in remote areas. Finally, the lack of information on magnification of facial structures on cephalograms prevented us from analyzing the size and allometry in subjects with and without a cleft.

CONCLUSION

Shape variability demonstrates considerable differences in subjects with unrepaired complete unilateral cleft lip and alveolus (UCLA) and complete unilateral cleft lip, alveolus and palate (UCLP) and non-cleft subjects (NORM). Moreover, in subjects with a cleft, within-sample variability was more pronounced in the antero-posterior direction, while in non-cleft subjects, within-sample variability was more pronounced in the vertical direction. These findings may suggest that subjects with unilateral clefts have intrinsic growth impairment affecting subsequent facial development.

ETHICS STATEMENT

The studies involving human participants were reviewed and approved by the Bioethics Committee of the University of Indonesia (Ref#: 1/EthEx/FKGUI/II/2015). Written informed consent for participation was not required for this study in accordance with the national legislation and the institutional requirements.

AUTHOR CONTRIBUTIONS

PF, MK, and AK-J conceived and designed the study. BL and AK-J collected the data. PF digitized the radiographs. PF and MK performed analyses. BL, MK, AS, AK-J, and PF contributed to the data interpretation. BL, AS, and PF wrote the draft manuscript. All authors critically revised, finalized, and approved the manuscript.

REFERENCES

Bookstein, F. L. (2016). Reconsidering the inappropriateness of conventional cephalometrics. *Am. J. Orthod. Dentofacial. Orthop.* 149, 784–797. doi: 10.1016/j.ajodo.2015.12.011

Capelozza, L. Jr., Taniguchi, S. M., and da Silva, O. G. Jr. (1993). Craniofacial morphology of adult unoperated complete unilateral cleft lip and palate patients. *Cleft. Palate Craniofac. J.* 30, 376–381. doi: 10.1597/1545-1569_1993_030_0376_cmoauc_2.3.co_2

Chen, Z. Q., Wu, J., and Chen, R. J. (2012). Sagittal maxillary growth pattern in unilateral cleft lip and palate patients with unrepaired cleft palate. *J. Craniofac. Surg.* 23, 491–493. doi: 10.1097/SCS.0b013e3182413f88

Diah, E., Lo, L. J., Huang, C. S., Sudjatmiko, G., Susanto, I., and Chen, Y. R. (2007). Maxillary growth of adult patients with unoperated cleft: answers to the debates. *J. Plast. Reconstr. Aesthet. Surg.* 60, 407–413. doi: 10.1016/j.bjps.2006.10.004

Halazonetis, D. J. (2004). Morphometrics for cephalometric diagnosis. *Am. J. Orthod. Dentofacial. Orthop.* 125, 571–581. doi: 10.1016/j.ajodo.2003.05.013

Jaklová, L., Borský, J., Jurovčík, M., Hoffmannová, E., Černý, M., Dupej, J., et al. (2020). Three-dimensional development of the palate in bilateral orofacial cleft newborns 1 year after early neonatal cheiloplasty: classic and geometric morphometric evaluation. *J. Craniomaxillofac. Surg.* 48, 383–390. doi: 10.1016/j.jcms.2020.02.019

Katsadouris, A., and Halazonetis, D. J. (2017). Geometric morphometric analysis of craniofacial growth between the ages of 12 and 14 in normal humans. *Eur. J. Orthod.* 39, 386–394. doi: 10.1093/ejo/cjw070

Klingenberg, C. P. (2011). MorphoJ: an integrated software package for geometric morphometrics. *Mol. Ecol. Resour.* 11, 353–357. doi: 10.1111/j.1755-0998.2010.02924.x

Lambrecht, J. T., Kreusch, T., and Schulz, L. (2000). Position, shape, and dimension of the maxilla in unoperated cleft lip and palate patients: review of the literature. *Clin. Anat.* 13, 121–133. doi: 10.1002/(sici)1098-2353(2000)13:2<121::aid-ca6>3.0.co;2-k

Latief, B. S., Lekkas, C., and Kuijpers, M. A. (2010). Maxillary arch width in unoperated adult bilateral cleft lip and alveolus and complete bilateral cleft lip and palate. *Orthod. Craniofac. Res.* 13, 82–88. doi: 10.1111/j.1601-6343.2009.01479.x

Latif, A., Kuijpers, M. A. R., Rachwalski, M., Latief, B. S., Kuijpers-Jagtman, A. M., and Fudalej, P. S. (2020). Morphological variability in unrepaired bilateral clefts with and without cleft palate evaluated with geometric morphometrics. *J. Anat.* 236, 425–433. doi: 10.1111/joa.13118

Li, J., Johnson, C. A., Smith, A. A., Salmon, B., Shi, B., Brunski, J., et al. (2015). Disrupting the intrinsic growth potential of a suture contributes to midfacial hypoplasia. *Bone* 81, 186–195. doi: 10.1016/j.bone.2014.04.020

Liao, Y. F., and Mars, M. (2005). Long-term effects of clefts on craniofacial morphology in patients with unilateral cleft lip and palate. *Cleft. Palate Craniofac. J.* 42, 601–609. doi: 10.1597/04-163r.1

Liberton, D. K., Verma, P., Almpani, K., Fung, P. W., Mishra, R., Oberoi, S., et al. (2020). Craniofacial analysis may indicate co-occurrence of skeletal malocclusions and associated risks in development of cleft lip and palate. *J. Dev. Biol.* 8:2. doi: 10.3390/jdb8010002

Moyers, R. E., and Bookstein, F. L. (1979). The inappropriateness of conventional cephalometrics. *Am. J. Orthod.* 75, 599–617. doi: 10.1016/0002-9416(79)90093-9

Ortiz-Monasterio, F., Olmedo, A., Trigos, I., Yudovich, M., Velazquez, M., and Fuente-del-Campo, A. (1974). Final results from the delayed treatment of patients with clefts of the lip and palate. *Scand. J. Plast. Reconstr. Surg.* 8, 109–115. doi: 10.3109/02844317409084379

Paoloni, V., Lione, R., Farisco, F., Halazonetis, D. J., Franchi, L., and Cozza, P. (2017). Morphometric covariation between palatal shape and skeletal pattern in Class II growing subjects. *Eur. J. Orthod.* 39, 371–376. doi: 10.1093/ejo/cjx014

Rosas, A., Bastir, M., Alarcón, J. A., and Kuroe, K. (2008). Thin-plate spline analysis of the cranial base in African, Asian and European populations and its relationship with different malocclusions. *Arch. Oral Biol.* 53, 826–834. doi: 10.1016/j.archoralbio.2008.02.005

Segna, E., Khonsari, R. H., Meazzini, M. C., Battista, V., Picard, A., and Autelitano, L. (2020). Maxillary shape at the end of puberty in operated unilateral cleft lip and palate: a geometric morphometric assessment using computer tomography. *J. Stomatol. Oral Maxillofac. Surg.* 121, 9–13. doi: 10.1016/j.jormas.2019.06.004

Shetye, P. R., and Evans, C. A. (2006). Midfacial morphology in adult unoperated complete unilateral cleft lip and palate patients. *Angle Orthod.* 76, 810–816.

Toro-Ibacache, V., Cortés Araya, J., Díaz Muñoz, A., and Manríquez, S. G. (2014). Morphologic variability of nonsyndromic operated patients affected by cleft lip and palate: a geometric morphometric study. *Am. J. Orthod. Dentofacial. Orthop.* 146, 346–354. doi: 10.1016/j.ajodo.2014.06.002

Urbanova, W., Klimova, I., Brudnicki, A., Polackova, P., Kroupova, D., Dubovska, I., et al. (2016). The Slav-cleft: a three-center study of the outcome of treatment of cleft lip and palate. Part 1: craniofacial morphology. *J. Craniomaxillofac. Surg.* 44, 1767–1776. doi: 10.1016/j.jcms.2016.06.010

Wellens, H. L., and Kuijpers-Jagtman, A. M. (2016). Connecting the new with the old: modifying the combined application of *Procrustes* superimposition and principal component analysis, to allow for comparison with traditional lateral cephalometric variables. *Eur. J. Orthod.* 38, 569–576. doi: 10.1093/ejo/cjv096

Wellens, H. L., Kuijpers-Jagtman, A. M., and Halazonetis, D. J. (2013). Geometric morphometric analysis of craniofacial variation, ontogeny and modularity in a cross-sectional sample of modern humans. *J. Anat.* 222, 397–409. doi: 10.1111/joa.12027

Will, L. A. (2000). Growth and development in patients with untreated clefts. *Cleft. Palate Craniofac. J.* 37, 523–526. doi: 10.1597/1545-1569(2000)037<0523:gadipw>2.0.co;2

Zelditch, M. L., Swiderski, D. L., and Sheets, H. D. (2012). *Geometric Morphometrics for Biologists. A Primer.* San Diego, CA: Elsevier Academic Press.

7

Anatomy and Development of the Mammalian External Auditory Canal: Implications for Understanding Canal Disease and Deformity

Mona Mozaffari[1], Robert Nash[2] and Abigail S. Tucker[1]*

[1] Centre for Craniofacial and Regenerative Biology, King's College London, Guy's Hospital, London, United Kingdom,

[2] Department of Paediatric Otolaryngology, Cochlear Implants, Great Ormond Street Hospital for Children NHS Trust, London, United Kingdom

***Correspondence:**
Mona Mozaffari
monireh.mozaffari@kcl.ac.uk

The mammalian ear is made up of three parts (the outer, middle, and inner ear), which work together to transmit sound waves into neuronal signals perceived by our auditory cortex as sound. This review focuses on the often-neglected outer ear, specifically the external auditory meatus (EAM), or ear canal. Within our complex hearing pathway, the ear canal is responsible for funneling sound waves toward the tympanic membrane (ear drum) and into the middle ear, and as such is a physical link between the tympanic membrane and the outside world. Unique anatomical adaptations, such as its migrating epithelium and cerumen glands, equip the ear canal for its function as both a conduit and a cul-de-sac. Defects in development, or later blockages in the canal, lead to congenital or acquired conductive hearing loss. Recent studies have built on decades-old knowledge of ear canal development and suggest a novel multi-stage, complex and integrated system of development, helping to explain the mechanisms underlying congenital canal atresia and stenosis. Here we review our current understanding of ear canal development; how this biological lumen is made; what determines its location; and how its structure is maintained throughout life. Together this knowledge allows clinical questions to be approached from a developmental biology perspective.

Keywords: hearing, deafness, external ear, ear canal, ear deformities, congenital

INTRODUCTION

Hearing places us within our external environment, allowing us to experience a multi-dimensional world, to listen and to communicate. Sound is essentially a series of pressure waves in our airborne environment. That we can "hear" these waveforms involves a complex array of neurophysiological mechanisms which begin at the outer ear and end at the auditory cortex. The mammalian ear is a crucial and fascinating sensory organ formed from the integration of three parts (**Figure 1**). The pinna or auricle directs sound waves into the external auditory Meatus (EAM), which then funnels sound waves toward the ear drum or tympanic membrane (TM), causing it to displace and move the ossicular chain of bones in the air-filled middle ear. The middle ear ossicles connect the TM to the much smaller oval window of the inner ear. This intricate leverage mechanism corrects the impedance mismatch between gas and liquid allowing airborne sound waves to move hair cells in the fluid-filled cochlea, generating neural signals that are transmitted to the auditory cortex *via* the cochlear nerve.

Hearing loss is most commonly caused due to pathology in the inner ear, referred to as sensorineural hearing loss, which consequently receives the lion's share of scientific research (Cunningham and Tucci, 2017). However, there are limited options for treating sensorineural hearing loss with many potential treatments in the experimental phase (Devare et al., 2018). Currently, the clinician's arsenal is best equipped to treat middle ear disease, which consequently receives the lion's share of clinical attention (Cunningham and Tucci, 2017). This leaves the outer ear, which is also indispensable for hearing, but is comparatively overlooked. Pathologies of the ear canal can cause hearing loss, recurrent infection, and complications including cranial nerve palsy and intracranial sepsis (Ostrowski and Wiet, 1996). Management of hearing loss in this part of the ear may be particularly challenging, as the interaction between the anatomy and physiology of the canal, and the pathologies that affect it, may complicate the two most commonly used techniques of hearing rehabilitation – hearing aids and hearing restoration surgery.

In this review we focus in on the ear canal or EAM. We discuss the anatomy of the canal and the epithelial dynamics involved in canal homeostasis. We then turn to the congenital and acquired defects of the canal, and how they are currently treated, before investigating canal development. As anatomical and molecular details are added to our understanding of ear development, compelling questions are beginning to emerge. What factors determine the development of the ear canal's specialized epithelium? And how does the canal integrate with the middle ear to form a functioning structure?

EAR CANAL ANATOMY AND FUNCTION

With certain exceptions, the EAM is similar across all mammals; a deep-set structure on either side of the skull ending in an ear drum cul-de-sac medially and opening to a pinna laterally (**Figure 1**). In adult humans, the EAM is typically 25 mm in length and 8 mm in diameter (Areias et al., 2016). Rather than a horizontal tube its shape is that of a soft sigmoid, tilted to face downward and inward as it projects medially (van Spronsen et al., 2014). This curved path varies between individuals (van Spronsen et al., 2014). Finite element modeling of the ear has highlighted the importance of a patent EAM in hearing higher frequency sound (which is crucial for speech recognition) (Areias et al., 2016). Lower frequencies with wavelengths larger than the canal itself are not affected by variations in canal diameter, however, as sound waves concertina at higher frequency, variations in canal dimension have a discernible effect on sound transmission. In particular, the segment of canal closest to the TM plays an important part in high frequency sound transmission (Areias et al., 2016). Variation in this pretympanic area, namely a deeper pretympanic recess, therefore can influence acquisition of high frequency sound, and has also been linked to increased susceptibility to chronic otitis externa (van Spronsen et al., 2014). Such biomechanical modeling at a patient-level would provide valuable information in understanding stenotic canal disease and measuring treatment outcomes.

In contrast to the deep canal observed in most mammals, in sauropsids (reptiles and birds) and amphibia, the ear canal is typically shallow or non-existent (**Figures 2A,B**). Indeed, we can consider a deep canal to be a specific mammalian trait. It has been proposed that a cavitated middle ear and tympanic membrane evolved multiple times in land vertebrates (tetrapods), therefore the deep mammalian ear is not homologous to the shallow ear canal of other land vertebrates (Tucker, 2017). A deep canal is observed in both therian mammals (placentals and marsupials) and monotremes (egg laying platypus and echidna), however, monotremes do not have pinna, suggesting that this was a later therian adaptation as monotremes diverged from other mammals relatively early in evolutionary time (**Figures 2C,F**; Manger et al., 1998). The deep canal means that the mammalian tympanic membrane is protected within the head and therefore potentially at less risk of damage. Despite this, damage to the mammalian tympanic membrane is fairly common, with perforations being caused by loud noises, bangs to the head and from middle ear infections (Mozaffari et al., 2020). A deep canal also provides a means for funneling and thereby focusing sound waves, as discussed above.

Depending on the position of the middle ear with respect to the exit position of the canal, the relative length of the canal can vary across mammals. For example, in the platypus the ear canal exits high on the head, next to the eye, so that both the eye and ear are not submerged while the animal is swimming (Manger et al., 1998). This results in the development of a very long canal (**Figure 2C**). How the developing ear canal reaches the middle ear, finding its way to varying exit sites in different species, remains a largely unanswered question.

A deep-set lumen requires structural support. In humans, the inner two-thirds of the EAM is bony (typically 16 mm in length in the human adult) and the outer third is cartilaginous (around 8 mm in length), encasing the canal with a semi-rigid wall (Standrig et al., 2016). How the mammalian ear canal evolved remains an intriguing question. Did pinna cartilage elongate inward to meet the bony canal or did the cartilaginous canal evolve separately from the pinna? The latter appears more likely as monotremes have no pinna but still have a cartilaginous support that forms around the developing EAM (**Figures 2D,E**; Anthwal et al., 2020). Cartilage support for the EAM, therefore, likely predates pinna evolution.

The newborn human ear canal is soft and rudimentary along its length (Abdel-Aziz, 2013). The osseous canal is not evident during embryonic development so appears to develop postnatally (Ikari et al., 2013). The specifics of its development, however, remain vague. It is not yet known whether the tympanic ring, which is a membranous bone, extends posterolaterally to take part in creation of the osseous canal, or whether the osseous canal forms by endochondral ossification of an initially fibrocartilaginous scaffold. Both scenarios are described in textbooks and articles, however, there are as yet no published studies demonstrating the process (Abdel-Aziz, 2013; Standrig et al., 2016). The cartilaginous canal appears prior to and apparently independent of the osseous canal (Ikari et al., 2013).

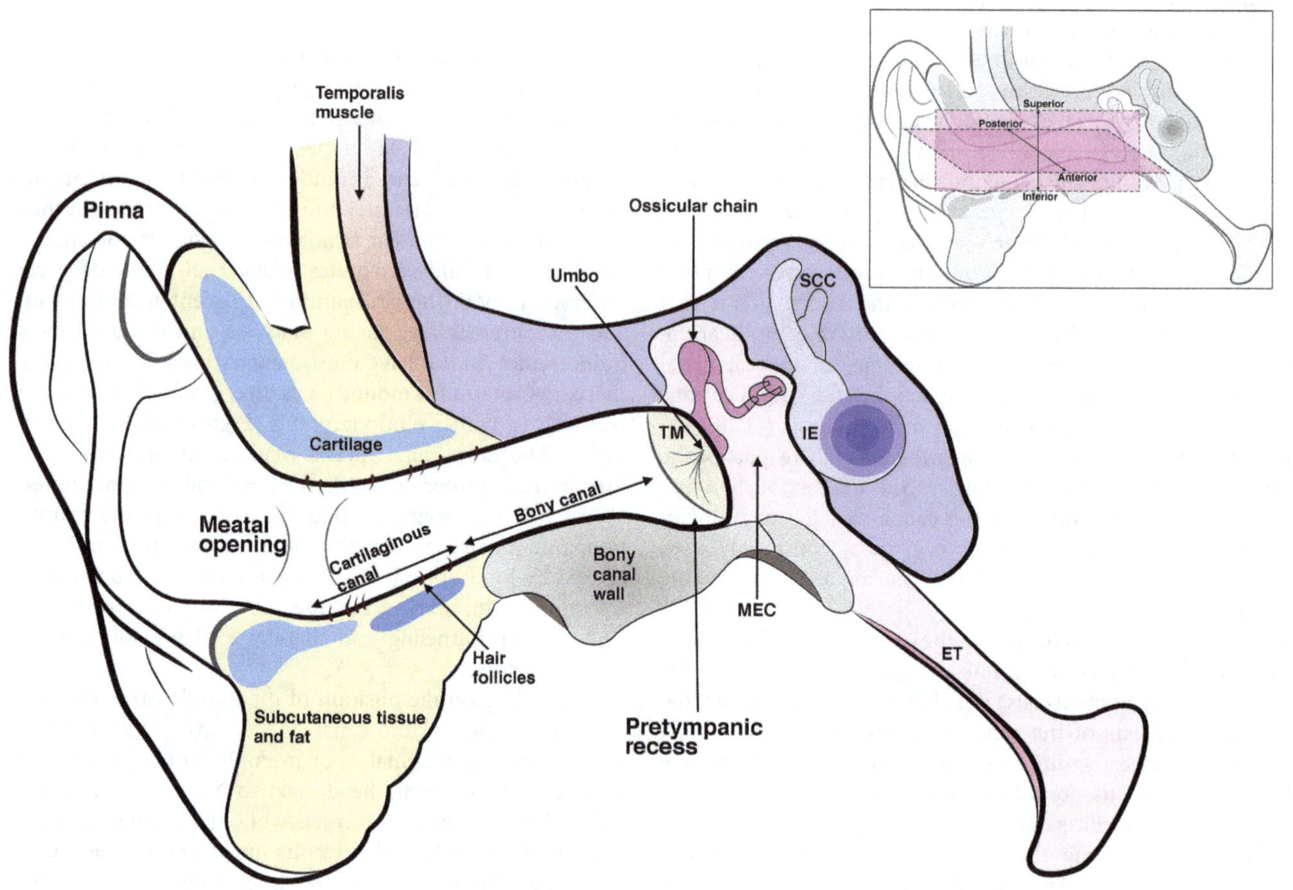

FIGURE 1 | Schematic diagram of the three-part ear; the external ear, which includes the pinna and ear canal; the middle ear which includes the tympanic membrane (TM), middle ear cavity (MEC), and the ossicles. The malleus inserts into the TM at the umbo. The middle ear connects to the nasopharynx *via* the eustachian tube (ET). The inner ear (IE) includes the cochlea and semi-circular canals. The ear canal is enclosed in its inner two-thirds by a bony wall and its outer third by a cartilaginous wall, which is lined by hair-bearing skin. The ear canal lumen varies in shape but typically has a pretympanic recess and meatal opening. Inset shows anterior, posterior, superior, and inferior axes as referred to in the text.

From around 15 gestational weeks, a chain of bar like cartilages form inferiorly between the tragus and helix. The anterior cartilage of the tragus and the posterior cartilage of the helix develop early and are consistent in shape; ring and plate-like, respectively (Ikari et al., 2013). Rather than fibrocartilage, glial fibrillary acid protein (GFAP) positive elastic cartilage makes up the outer cartilaginous canal (Ikari et al., 2013). The cartilages transform morphology *via* intermediate circular and triangle shapes to become H-shaped cartilage wrapping their arms upward around the developing EAM epithelium (Ikari et al., 2013). Interestingly, these bars of cartilage appear to develop along a fascial condensation linking Reichert's cartilage and the tragus (Ikari et al., 2013). No evidence of a corresponding fascial plane extending out from Meckel's cartilage has been described that would potentially precede a superior wall (**Figure 1** insert). Unlike the anterior canal, the posterosuperior canal is usually deficient of cartilage in the adult (Standrig et al., 2016). There is significant individual variation in canal shape, which is perhaps not surprising given the complex of irregular shaped cartilages that interlink to form the cartilaginous ear canal (Bartel-Friedrich and Wulke, 2007). Clinically, this variability appears to be of little consequence. Inevitable gaps between the jigsaw of connecting cartilages does, however, provide a likely explanation for the etiology of congenital auricular pseudocysts that can occur in multiples between the perichondrium and the skin of the external ear, requiring drainage and pinna reconstruction (Secor et al., 1999).

The lining of the ear canal is continuous with skin covering the pinna laterally and the outer layer of the tympanic membrane medially (Mallo, 2000). Being an anatomical cul-de-sac ending at the TM, the ear canal is lined with specialized skin capable of migrating, such that it can self-clean with the epidermal layer sloughing off and moving outward – as opposed to upward in skin elsewhere (Alberti, 1964; Fuchs and Horsley, 2008). A failure of this self-cleaning mechanism leads to the build-up of sloughed off keratinocytes in the canal, causing hearing impairment from blockage and localized tissue damage from chronic inflammation (Naiberg et al., 1984). Indeed, failure to remove ear canal skin is also observed in keratosis obturans and ear canal cholesteatoma, which are uncommon but well

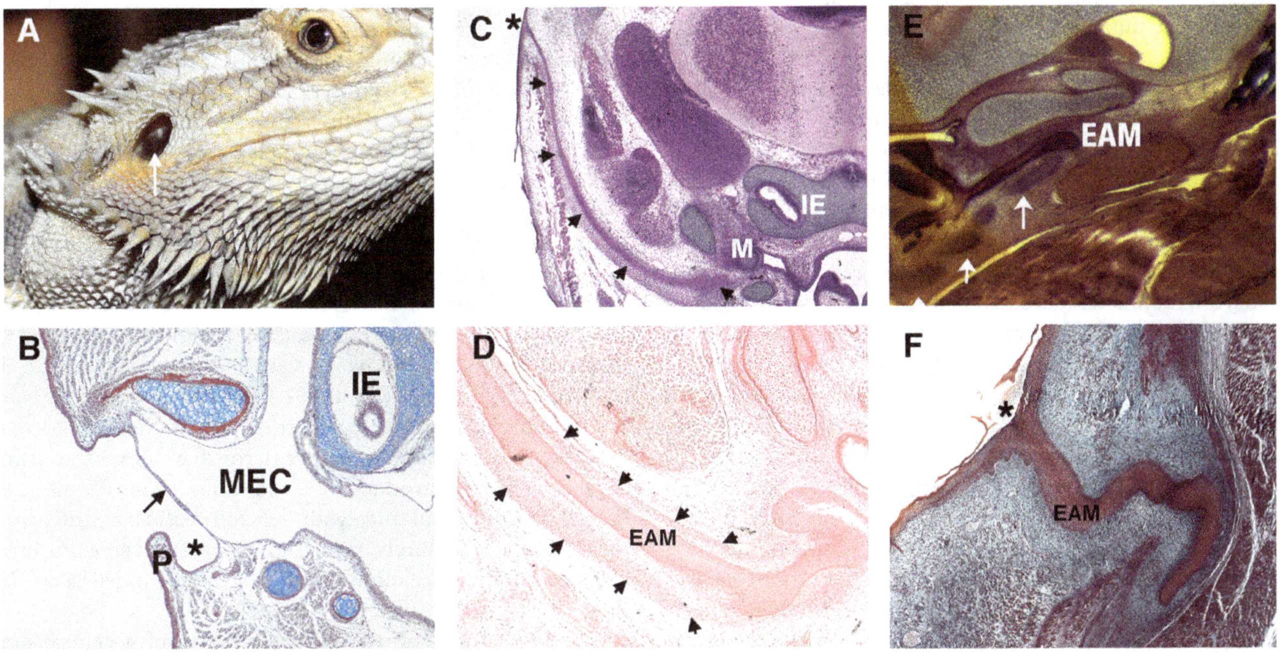

FIGURE 2 | Variations in the non-mammalian ear canal. **(A)** Bearded dragon (*Pogona vitticeps*) with superficial tympanic membrane outlined by arrow. **(B–F)** Histology sections. **(B)** Sagittal trichrome section of gecko ear showing a shallow ear canal (star) and superficial tympanic membrane (arrow). **(C,D)** Developing platypus (*Ornithorhynchus anatinus*) EAM **(C)** Frontal section of platypus ear at 2 days post hatching (2 p.h.). The developing ear canal (arrows) is long extending from extending form the top of the head to the malleus. There is no pinna at the canal opening (marked by *). **(D)** Frontal section of developing ear canal in 10 p.h. day platypus. The EAM develops in a sheath of condensed mesenchyme (arrows). **(E,F)** Developing echidna (*Tachyglossus aculeatus*) EAM **(E)** Horizontal section through the EAM of 55–65 p.h. (arrows) days echidna demonstrating cartilage support (arrows) around the developing EAM. **(F)** Horizontal trichrome section through EAM of an echidna at 18 p.h. days showing a tortuous path to the opening (star). P, Pinna; MEC, middle ear cavity; IE, inner ear; EAM, external auditory meatus.

recognized diseases of the external ear discussed further below (Naiberg et al., 1984; Persaud et al., 2004).

Experiments tracing the movement of ink-tattooed ear canal skin cells in mammals (including humans) show these labeled cells moving laterally, out of the canal over time (Alberti, 1964; Michaels and Soucek, 1991). This movement occurs roughly at the rate of fingernail growth with anterior canal skin demonstrating the fastest migration (Alberti, 1964). Does this migratory pattern have an epicenter at the tympanic membrane? Dated dye experiments suggest a radial pattern of epidermal cell migration spoking away from the umbo, at the center of the TM (Michaels and Soucek, 1990). More recent experiments using BrdU to chase and label proliferating cells suggest a more involved and dynamic source of stem and progenitor cells that migrate in different directions in different parts of the TM (Knutsson et al., 2011; Chari et al., 2018). Frumm et al. add further detail to the migratory nature of the keratinocytes in the tympanic membrane's outer layer. Using a combination of lineage tracing, live imaging and single cell sequencing, they demonstrate that the TM epidermis has distinct stem cell and committed progenitor regions, located close to supporting mesenchyme (the manubrium and annulus respectively). The progeny of these cells migrate out across the TM, maintaining a thin vibratory surface (Frumm et al., 2020).

There are distinctions in the morphology of the skin that covers the bony canal versus the skin that covers the cartilaginous canal in humans. The former is thin and flush against the canal wall bone, whilst the latter is thickened with a spongey subcutaneous layer possessing modified sebaceous glands called cerumen glands. The bony canal skin, does not possess ceruminous glands or hair follicles (Standrig et al., 2016). Our observations of human cranial skin verses ear canal skin development suggest the latter develops precociously in relation to skin (Fons et al., 2020). This has interesting implications for experimental comparisons drawn between ear canal skin and skin elsewhere, as well as clinical implications, where skin from the limbs is used to reconstruct the canal lumen. If a different developmental timeline leads to different skin biology, transplanting skin into a reconstructed ear canal may not be the ideal graft tissue.

The cerumen glands are responsible for the production of ear wax. Serous secretions and sebum from the cerumen glands mix with sloughed keratinized squames. A natural lubricant, ear wax aids the self-cleaning function of the ear canal, and is thought to have antimicrobial properties (Shokry and Filho, 2017). Interestingly, a little like tongue rolling ability, ear wax type is a dimorphic trait. Whether your wax is wet or dry is determined by one single-nucleotide polymorphism (SNP) of a single gene (ABCC11) (Toyoda et al., 2009). Patients with dry wax, which lacks oily components, are at higher risk of suffering from cerumen impaction. Impacted ear wax is the single most common ear canal ailment to affect patients and may require regular removal, especially in those using hearing aids (Schwartz et al., 2017). The human ABCC11 gene has no orthologous gene in mammals, except for primates. In mice, cerumen production is from a single large gland, the glandula ceruminosa, which opens into a single duct near the TM (Gruneberg, 1971). Layout of glands and secretion type is likely to be species specific and relate to size and position of the canal. In mice, this gland is present from E15 (Gruneberg, 1971). Human ceruminous glands are noted at around 19 gestational weeks in published literature (Perry and Shelley, 1955). It is likely that ceruminous glands evolved from modified sebaceous glands, as like sebaceous glands these are holocrine glands, were the cells burst to release their content (Niemann and Horsley, 2012). Sebaceous glands fail to develop normally in patients with hypohidrotic ectodermal dysplasia (XLHED), suggesting involvement of the ectodysplasin (EDA) receptor signaling pathway in the development of sebaceous glands (del-Pozo et al., 2019). Similarly, Eda mutant mice have defects in sebaceous glands, with addition of Eda stimulants able to rescue the defect (Kowalczyk-Quintas and Schneider, 2014). Meibomian glands, another example of a modified sebaceous gland, also fail to develop in rodent models carrying hypomorphic mutations in the Edar signaling pathway consistent with an XLHED phenotype, with increased Edar signaling leading to larger meibomian glands (Chang et al., 2009). Recently Edar has been shown to be expressed in developing rat cerumen glands, highlighting a conserved role for this pathway in these holocrine glands (del-Pozo et al., 2019). In addition to the Eda pathway, Wnt and hedgehog signaling have been shown to play a role in skin sebaceous gland development and therefore may have a role also in cerumen gland development (Allen et al., 2003; Niemann et al., 2003). Further study into the developmental mechanisms of these unique glands would certainly be revealing.

DEVELOPMENT OF THE EAR CANAL AND HOW IT REACHES ITS TARGET

The ear canal develops in two parts, the outer part or primary canal, and the inner part or meatal plug (Fons et al., 2020; **Figure 3**). At around Carnegie stage 17 (6 weeks post conception and equivalent to E12.0 in mice), the primary canal begins to form either by the first cleft deepening or as a new invagination within the 1st arch. Supporting the latter scenario is a recent study unexpectedly suggesting the murine ear canal forms entirely within the first arch (Minoux et al., 2013). This is unexpected because it had previously been assumed that the ear canal forms within the first cleft (Grevellec and Tucker, 2010). The meatal plug then forms as a plug of cells adjacent to this cleft. (Michaels and Soucek, 1991). This plug of cells will continue to extend inward into the surrounding mesenchyme becoming a finger-like projection pointing to the developing middle ear cavity (MEC) (**Figure 3B**; Nishimura and Kumoi, 2017). Temporal and situational differences in cell proliferation appear to influence the extension and directional growth of the meatal plug as it begins to develop (Fons et al., 2020). Both human and mouse display a distinctive duality in EAM development: the outer, primary canal (which will become the cartilaginous canal) develops differently to the inner, meatal plug (which will become the osseous canal) (Fons et al., 2020). Initially open, the primary canal closes for some time before opening again along with the meatal plug, to form one long lumen (Fons et al., 2020) (**Figures 3C,E**). This closure has been linked to the removal of periderm (Fons et al., 2020). In mouse embryos, a superficial layer of periderm, denoted by keratin 8 staining, acts as a non-stick Teflon layer to keep the primary canal open in early development (Fons et al., 2020).

Programmed cell death, or apoptosis, is a ubiquitous event in development. Its role in ear canal development has been previously alluded to in experiments noting the emergence of TUNEL-positive cells at E15.5 in mice with the surprising lack of them around the time of canal opening, up to 12 days postnatally (Nishizaki et al., 1998). Inhibiting apoptosis in culture and staining K8 positive peridermal cells demonstrated that it is the apoptotic death of the periderm that allows the primary canal to close at around E15.5 in mice (Fons et al., 2020). Indeed, in *Grhl3* null mice with deficient periderm, the primary canal closed prematurely, providing a hopeful avenue for further research into the etiopathology of congenital aural atresia (CAA) (Fons et al., 2020).

The canal finally opens by the creation of a central lumen (**Figure 3E**). This occurs at around 16 weeks in human fetal samples, and is preceded by a precocious program of differentiation, ahead of developing skin elsewhere, and involves the apoptotic cell death of the cornified loricrin-positive layer of squamous epithelium (**Figure 3D**). The complex and multistage development of the ear canal may account for the variability, both in form and occurrence, of CAA.

As with much of craniofacial development, the EAC is in essence an epithelial structure taking shape in relation to, and influenced by, its surrounding structures. How does the developing ear canal find its path to the middle ear cavity? Current knowledge tells us some detail about these relative relations and signaling pathways, putting the tympanic ring in a lead role. When tympanic ring formation is disrupted using retinoic acid, the EAC also fails to form (Mallo and Gridley, 1996). And when the tympanic ring is duplicated in *Hoxa2* null mutant mice, a duplication of the EAC is also noted, as the second arch transforms to a first arch fate (Rijli et al., 1993). In keeping with this phenotype, overexpression of *Hoxa2* in the first arch neural crest leads to a duplication of the pinna and loss of the EAM (Minoux et al., 2013). Additionally, *Prx1*, *Gas1*, *Tshirt (Tsh)*, and *Goosecoid (Gsc)* have all been shown to cause EAC defects in the presence of hypoplastic or absent tympanic rings (Rivera-Perez et al., 1995; Mallo, 2001; Seppala et al., 2007; Feenstra et al., 2011). Whilst EAC defects are observed in mouse mutants of *Prx1* and *Gas1*, *TSH*, and *GSC* have been corroborated in human genome wide sequencing studies also (Feenstra et al., 2007). Interestingly, mutations in *Gsc* and *Prx1* also cause hypomorphism of the malleal manubrium - an essential link in sound transduction from outside world to cochlea. Experiments in knock out mice as well as associative data corroborating human CT scans and intra-operative findings, indicate an essential role for the EAC in the induction and proper positioning of the manubrium within the eardrum (Mallo, 2000; Ishimoto et al., 2004). Not unlike an anatomical love triangle,

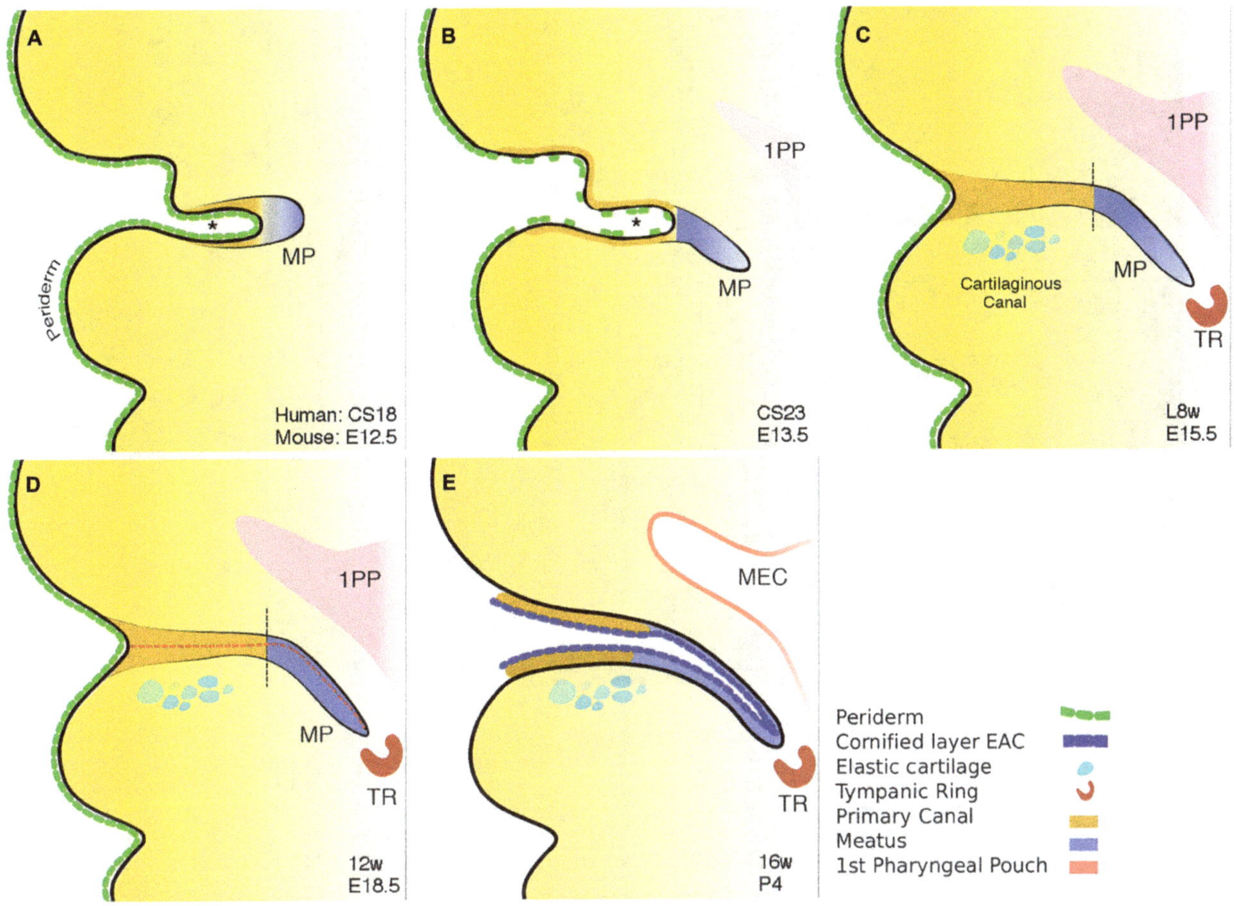

FIGURE 3 | Schematic of mammalian ear canal development. **(A)** Invagination of the primary canal (marked by *) with a meatal plug at its tip. **(B)** Extension of the meatus toward the forming middle ear, driven by a potential signal from the tympanic ring. At the same time selective loss of periderm is observed in the primary canal caused by apoptosis. **(C)** Closure of the primary canal (following loss of periderm layer) and further extension of the meatal plug to reach the tympanic ring. **(D)** Loricrin expression (red dashed line) marks the site of opening of the canal. **(E)** Following keratinocyte differentiation, the whole external ear canal opens, with the upper/rostral wall of the meatal plate forming the outer surface of the tympanic membrane. Vertical black dashed lines in **C** and **D** between brown and blue regions represent the two distinct parts of the ear canal. Schematic taken from Fons et al. (2020).

these findings indicate that formation of the EAM depends on formation of the tympanic ring. In turn formation of the manubrium depends on formation of the EAM.

CONGENITAL DISEASE OF THE EXTERNAL AUDITORY MEATUS

Congenital aural atresia is a spectrum of defects affecting the EAM at birth. The EAM may fail to form partially, completely or be narrowed. Occurring in around 1 in 10,000 to 20,000 live births, CAA affects males more than females and is typically unilateral, involving the right side more commonly than the left (Abdel-Aziz, 2013). Over the years, a number of systems for classifying CAA have been proposed (Altmann, 1955; Schuknecht, 1989; Jahrsdoerfer et al., 1992). More typically, clinicians group CAA patients into complete atresia (complete obliteration of the canal usually in combination with a bony atretic plate), stenosis (in which there is a continuous lumen to an at least partial tympanic membrane) or partial atresia (variable presence of a canal lumen lateral to an atretic plate) (**Figure 4**; Tian-Yu and Bulstrode, 2019). Complete atresia and stenosis are much more common than partial atresia, which is rare (Nicholas and Kesser, 2013). Severity of canal atresia has been linked with an early arrest in EAM development, although this does not account for the striking difference in the incidence of complete verses partial atresia (Abdel-Aziz, 2013; Nicholas and Kesser, 2013). Recent studies described above, examining EAM development at a range of timepoints and using molecular cues suggest a more involved etiology at play, which may, for example, begin to explain the surprising rarity of partial in comparison to complete atresia (Fons et al., 2020).

GENETIC BASIS OF CAA

Congenital atresia is often associated with pinna and middle ear defects (Kountakis et al., 1995). Less frequently inner

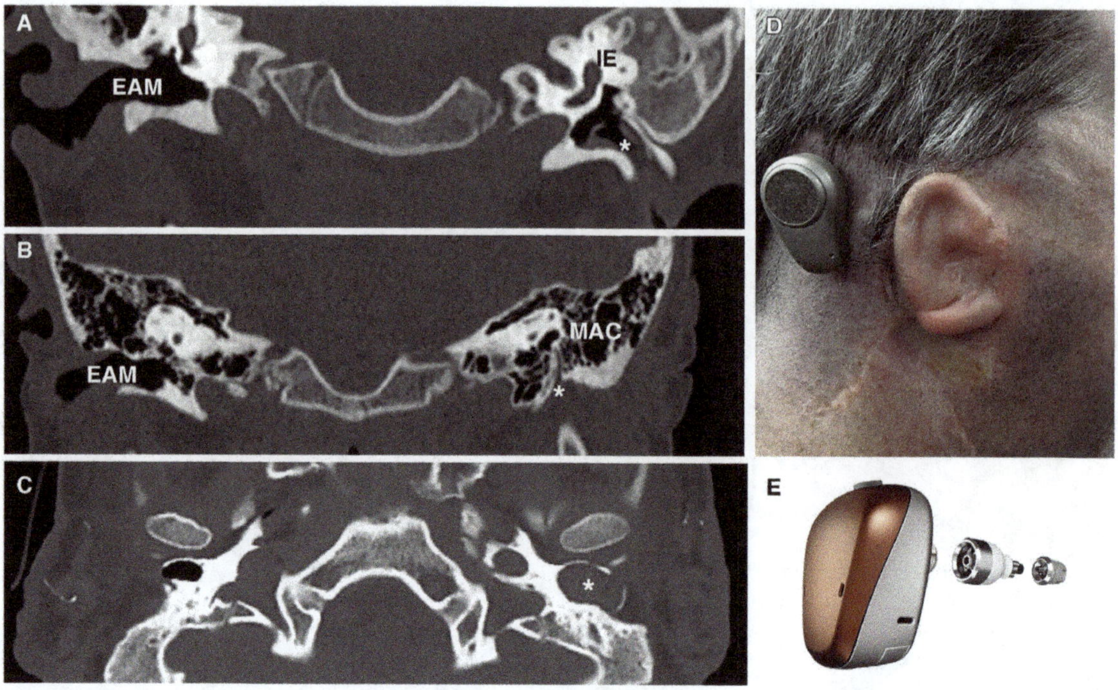

FIGURE 4 | Patient photograph and scans of congenital aural atresia. **(A)** Congenital aural stenosis. Coronal CT scan shows a normal, patent right ear canal and a stenotic left ear canal marked by *. **(B)** Complete congenital aural atresia. Coronal CT scan shows a normal ear canal on the right and an atretic plate on the left with no ear canal. **(C)** Congenital aural stenosis and cholesteatoma. Axial CT scan of a patient with congenital aural stenosis and left-sided cholesteatoma. The bony ear canal has been widened and remodeled by the collecting keratin (marked by *). **(D)** Photograph of a patient with Treacher-Collins syndrome and complete aural atresia of the left ear canal. The patient has been fitted with an osseointegrated hearing device visible behind the pinna. **(E)** Example of an osseointegrated device. Computer-generated image of a BAHA Connect (Image courtesy of Cochlear Bone Anchored Solutions AB, ©2020). EAM, external auditory meatus; IE, inner ear; MAC, mastoid air cells.

ear deformities and deformities of the stapes footplate are also present (Vrabec and Lin, 2010). Associations with other craniofacial abnormalities such as facial asymmetry and cleft lip/palate are also common (Abdel-Aziz, 2013). In some patients, these craniofacial defects are part of syndromic conditions such as Treacher-Collins, de Grouchy (chromosome 18q deletion), and Branchio-Oto-Renal syndrome (**Figure 4D**; Abdel-Aziz, 2013). Genetic analysis of syndromic patients can provide valuable genetic background to the etiology of both monogenic and syndromic CAA. For example, Genotype-phenotype mapping of chromosome 18q deletions (responsible for de Grouchy syndrome) has consistently shown the critical region for CAA in these patients to be 18q22.3 (Feenstra et al., 2007). Further delineating critical regions have highlighted candidate genes to investigate, with a loss of function mutation in the gene *TSHZ1*, known to be essential for murine middle ear development, being responsible for CAA both in isolated cases and in 18q deletion syndrome (Feenstra et al., 2011). A similar approach in a cohort of patients with the syndrome SAMS (short stature, auditory atresia, mandibular hypoplasia, and skeletal abnormalities) has identified mutations in the *Goosecoid (GSC)* gene as a causative factor (Parry et al., 2013). *GSC* is an important regulator of neural crest/mesoderm cell fate and has been shown to modulate tympanic ring development (Rivera-Perez et al., 1995). A canal defect in these patients may therefore be secondary to a tympanic ring defect, assigning a key signaling role to the tympanic ring (Mallo and Gridley, 1996).

Mutations in *HOXA2* have been characterized in a number of families with microtia (Alasti et al., 2008). Only one of these families, however, were noted to have additional EAM defects, with shortened and stenotic canals (Alasti et al., 2008). Mouse studies analyzing hypomorphic *Hoxa2* mutants with 45% the normal level of *Hoxa2,* and conditional mice, where loss was activated relatively late at E12.5, did not show any defects other than stapes and pinna deformity, respectively (Mallo and Gridley, 1996; Minoux et al., 2013). This is consistent with observations that *Hoxa2* requirement in craniofacial development is temporal (Santagati et al., 2005). It may be that low *Hoxa2* levels only effect EAM development in the early embryonic period by affecting arch fate, converting second arch to a first arch fate. That Alasti et al. report stenotic and shorted canals rather than completely atretic canals is interesting because it contradicts previous thinking that earlier mutations in EAM development lead to more severe anatomical defects (Abdel-Aziz, 2013; Nicholas and Kesser, 2013). It is likely that a more complex molecular basis is at play.

Genes discussed thus far play an indirect role in ear canal development, presumably due to their effect on the tympanic ring. *Foxi3*, in contrast, is likely involved in the development of the ear canal epithelium itself, making it a particularly interesting gene in the study of outer ear embryology (Tassano et al., 2015). Famously identified in hairless dogs, the *Foxi* family of genes are expressed in the ectoderm and play important roles in early arch patterning and thus early craniofacial development (Mukherjee et al., 2018). To date, mutations in *Foxi3* have been implicated in ear canal defects in mice, dog, and human, suggesting it plays a role in cases of canal atresia (Tassano et al., 2015). What is currently known about the role of *Foxi3* in EAC development is limited and associational. Unfortunately, *Foxi3* homozygous null mutants do not survive postnatally, and heterozygous mutants do not show a phenotype. A conditional mouse model would provide an intriguing avenue for further research, in particular into the mechanisms underlying the initiation of a meatal plug in early EAM development.

Given that CAA is a phenotype observed in multiple syndromes, it is not surprising that multiple genes have been associated with its etiopathology. The exciting next step will be to harness this information, using conditional knock outs or culture setups, to answer questions such as, what are the signaling pathways allowing the tympanic ring, ear canal, and manubrium to communicate?

TREATMENT OF CONGENITAL EAR CANAL DISEASE

Dividing canal atresia into complete, partial and stenotic is important to the clinician as it maps patients to key treatment considerations: hearing outcome, likelihood of cholesteatoma (erosive keratin-filled cysts that form when EAM skin cannot migrate out as normal) and the feasibility of achieving a self-cleaning ear should atresiaplasty be considered (Edfeldt and Strömbäck, 2015).

Esthetics aside, hearing loss is the main problem in complete atresia, as the absence of a lumen precludes the possibility of cholesteatoma forming. Despite significant advances in surgical technique and patient selection, atresiaplasty remains a difficult operation with typically poor outcomes and risk to the facial nerve, which is characteristically laterally placed, and therefore unexpectedly closer to the surgeon's drill (Edfeldt and Strömbäck, 2015). Surgical atresiaplasty predates the use of bone anchored hearing aids (BAHAs), and it is still performed in healthcare settings with limited access to audiological services (Yellon, 2011). Complications include restenosis, recurrent keratinous debris build up, poor hearing outcomes (in one study as many as 93% of patients still required a hearing aid post-op) and facial palsy resulting from altered and variable anatomy of the facial nerve in CAA (Bauer et al., 1994). Once the neo-lumen is created, it is covered with skin grafts taken from elsewhere or pedicled from postauricular skin. Restenosis is prevented by performing a wide canalplasty, although this may have cosmetic implications. As there is no native canal skin to use, the neo-lumen has no capacity to clear desquamated debris, requiring regular aural microsuction (Li et al., 2016). Hearing outcomes are typically poor despite the opening of the canal and patients may still need a hearing augmentation device as well. Meatoplasty, where the stenotic canal is widened, is more frequently considered in cases of congenital aural stenosis. These patients carry a much greater risk of cholesteatoma to the presence of a narrow canal, which may inhibit epithelial migration (Cole and Jahrsdoerfer, 1990). Furthermore, native canal skin is often available for canal reconstruction reducing chances of post-operative complications, making surgery a more straightforward decision (Cole and Jahrsdoerfer, 1990).

Given the difficulties relating to surgical correction of ear canal atresia, bone conduction devices and auditory implants are often considered instead of atresiaplasty (Nadaraja et al., 2013). Bone conduction devices bypass the outer and middle ear by transmitting sound vibrations to the cochlea *via* the skull. Their connection to the skull may be temporary, using methods such as a headband or adhesive; or it may involve the placement of an auditory implant (**Figure 4E**). Auditory implants can be classified into percutaneous devices, active and passive transcutaneous devices, and middle ear implants. Patient factors, middle ear anatomy and clinician preference determines which devices can be offered (Kohan and Ghossaini, 2019). The option of implantable hearing aids is attractive, however, they require near to normal middle ear anatomy and thus are not suitable for many CAA patients.

In reality, in Europe and the United States, the majority of patients receive bone anchored hearing aids (Yellon, 2011). Whilst these provide good hearing rehab, they are visible, can cause skin irritation and infection and of course do not create a continuous hearing response (they are taken on and off), which is particularly important for spontaneous learning in young patients (Yellon, 2011). Therefore, a surgical approach which reconstructs the ear canal with few complications and without the need for further device-assisted hearing, is attractive. Recent research investigating epithelial dynamics in the developing ear canal may provide new avenues to explore the biological basis of atresiaplasty complications (Fons et al., 2020). For example, surgeons note the greater frequency of restenosis in the lateral reconstructed canal, which is cartilage-lined (Moon et al., 2012). As the bony and cartilaginous parts of the canal develop in different ways (primary canal verses an extending meatal plate), the development may explain these differences in response after surgery. It would therefore be interesting to study whether there is an inbuilt signaling difference in the outer and inner parts of the EAM that influences their response to injury. A better understanding of EAM development would also further clarify the variable anatomy in CAA, e.g., the route of the facial nerve, easing technical challenges faced by surgeons.

ACQUIRED DISEASE OF THE EXTERNAL AUDITORY MEATUS

Acquired disease of the EAM includes of course the breadth of traumatic, infective and rarely neoplastic disease and its comprehensive review is beyond the scope of this review. These can all lead to a post-inflammatory canal atresia, sometimes referred to as stenosing otitis externa (Lavy and Fagan, 2000). Current treatment involves regular aural hygiene or meatoplasty to expand the canal opening. There is experimental evidence in Guinea pigs for the use of Mitomycin C (an inhibitor of fibroblastic activity) in preventing post-inflammatory canal stenosis (Yoon et al., 2010). Human studies, however, have had contradictory results and further controlled trials are needed to evaluate its potential role in preventing restenosis (Banthia and Selesnick, 2003; Battelino et al., 2005). Here, we focus on ear canal diseases that may be further understood through the lens of developmental biology.

Specific to the specialized biology of ear canal skin and its ability to migrate are two distinct diseases: keratosis obturans (KO) and ear canal cholesteatoma. KO is a rare disease in which squamous debris builds up in the ear canal, often leading to an expansion of canal diameter before presenting with acute pain. Current treatment is regular microsuction to maintain a patent ear canal (Persaud et al., 2004). As with healthy patients, the TM of individuals diagnosed with KO can be labeled with dye to observe the migration of the epidermal layer. One such study suggests that either delayed or disrupted epidermal migration may be the cause of KO (Corbridge et al., 1996). External ear canal cholesteatoma (EECC) is also rare and was for a long time grouped together with keratosis obturans as the same disease (Persaud et al., 2018). Whilst ear canal skin in KO is intact with layers of squames building up above it, in EECC there are focal ulcerations in canal skin and the organization of keratinous squames is random. Importantly there is bony necrosis with focal areas of deep sequestered bone (Persaud et al., 2018). As such, drawing a diagnostic distinction is important, as whilst KO can be managed conservatively, EECC typically requires surgical removal of all the cholesteatoma and reconstruction of the ear canal (Persaud et al., 2018). The etiopathology of EECC remains uncertain with disordered epithelial migration and/or cerumen gland dysfunction thought to play a role (Jackler et al., 2015). Localized differences in epithelial cell migration in the tympanic membrane have recently been proposed to underly propensity to middle ear cholesteatoma formation and may provide clues to the etiology of canal cholesteatoma also (Frumm et al., 2020). The underlying pathology of another category of cholesteatoma, congenital cholesteatoma of the middle ear, also remains controversial. Whilst current consensus rests with an epidermoid formation origin within the middle ear, another proposed theory suggests that an errant developing EAC extending beyond the tympanic ring and into the mastoid cavity may be at fault (Aimi, 1983). What determines epithelial behavior in the ear canal, driving it to focal erosion in EECC rather than circumferential upward layering into the lumen as in KO? Further understanding the epithelial dynamics that bestow EAM skin its migratory potential and its regenerative capacity will certainly begin to answer this question.

FUTURE QUESTIONS

Of the three-part mammalian ear, the external auditory canal receives arguably the least attention. Although this has not always been the case. Until the mid-twentieth century and the advent of hearing aids, an exaggerated external ear in the form of an ear trumpet was the most commonly used hearing device, emphasizing the valuable role of the external ear in hearing. Congenital disease of the EAM is thankfully rare but crucially important. Infancy is an irretrievable period in which to develop speech and language, which can determine the rest of a child's life. Clarity and spontaneity of hearing, as well as decibels gained, at this age is critical. Thus, current treatment options, BAHAs or complication-prone canalplasties, leave room for improvement. Better understanding the mechanisms underlying EAM development will provide valuable knowledge toward improving treatment options both for congenital canal atresia and also treatment of acquired canal disease that involves epithelial dysfunction, such as keratosis obturans or canal cholesteatoma.

Recent research has pushed forward valuable but dated, largely histology-based, knowledge of EAC development and created new questions. How exactly does the ear canal open along its length, creating innermost a single-cell layer thin tympanic membrane, a thinly lined osseous canal and a spongier outer cartilaginous canal? What determines the different behavior of epithelium along the canal postnatally? During development, how do the different part of the complex mammalian ear communicate and eventually integrate? Answering these questions will pave the way to answering the clinical quandaries that affect patients' lives. How to create a self-cleaning ear? How to recreate the external ear epithelium? Which pathways can be modified in the face of congenital ear disease? Looking to developmental biology for the answers will be key.

AUTHOR CONTRIBUTIONS

MM was responsible for conception and writing of the manuscript. AT contributed to the manuscript conception and reviewed the manuscript throughout the writing process. RN provided clinical images and reviewed clinical sections of the manuscript. All authors read and contributed to the manuscript and discussion.

ACKNOWLEDGMENTS

Monotreme images were provided by the zoological museum in Cambridge University and the Hill Collection at the Berlin Museum fur Naturkunde. Thanks to Neal Anthwal for discussions on the monotreme ear. Thanks to Francis Smith for insightful conversations on syndromic ear canal deformity.

REFERENCES

Abdel-Aziz, M. (2013). Congenital aural atresia. *J. Craniofac. Surg.* 24, e418–e422.

Aimi, K. (1983). Role of the tympanic ring in the pathogenesis of congenital cholesteatoma. *Laryngoscope* 93, 1140–1146.

Alasti, F., Sadeghi, A., Sanati, M. H., Farhadi, M., Stollar, E., Somers, T., et al. (2008). A mutation in HOXA2 is responsible for autosomal-recessive microtia in an iranian family. *Am. J. Hum. Genet.* 82, 982–991. doi: 10.1016/j.ajhg.2008.02.015

Alberti, P. W. (1964). Epithelial migration on the tympanic membrane. *J. Laryngol. Otol.* 78, 808–830.

Allen, M., Grachtchouk, M., Sheng, H., Grachtchouk, V., Wang, A., Wei, L., et al. (2003). Hedgehog signaling regulates sebaceous gland development. *Am. J. Pathol.* 163, 2173–2178. doi: 10.1016/s0002-9440(10)63574-2

Altmann, F. (1955). LXXVII congenital atresia of the ear in man and animals. *Ann. Otol. Rhinol. Laryngol.* 64, 824–858. doi: 10.1177/000348945506400313

Anthwal, N., Fenelon, J., Johnston, S. D., Renfree, M. B., and Tucker, A. S. (2020). Transient role of the middle ear as a lower jaw support across mammals. *eLife* 9, 1–36.

Areias, B., Santos, C., Natal Jorge, R. M., Gentil, F., and Parente, M. P. L. (2016). Finite element modelling of sound transmission from outer to inner ear. *Proc. Inst. Mech. Eng. Part H J. Eng. Med.* 230, 999–1007. doi: 10.1177/0954411916666109

Banthia, V., and Selesnick, S. H. (2003). Mitomycin-C in the postsurgical ear canal. *Otolaryngol. Head Neck Surg.* 128, 882–886. doi: 10.1016/s0194-5998(03)00468-6

Bartel-Friedrich, S., and Wulke, C. (2007). Classification and diagnosis of ear malformations. *GMS Curr. Top. Otorhinolaryngol. Head Neck Surg.* 6, 1865–1011.

Battelino, S., Hocevar-Boltezar, I., and Zargi, M. (2005). Intraoperative use of mitomycin C in fibrous atresia of the external auditory canal. *Era Nose Throat. J.* 84, 776–779. doi: 10.1177/014556130508401213

Bauer, G. P., Wiet, R. J., and Zappia, J. J. (1994). Congenital aural atresia. *Laryngoscope* 104, 1219–1224.

Chang, S. H., Jobling, S., Brennan, K., and Headon, D. J. (2009). Enhanced edar signalling has pleiotropic effects on craniofacial and cutaneous glands. *PLoS One* 4:e7591. doi: 10.1371/journal.pone.0007591

Chari, D. A., Frumm, S. M., Akil, O., and Tward, A. D. (2018). Cellular dynamics in early healing of mouse tympanic membranes. *Otol. Neurotol.* 40, e160–e166.

Cole, R. R., and Jahrsdoerfer, R. A. (1990). The risk of cholesteatoma in congenital aural stenosis. *Laryngoscope* 100, 576–578.

Corbridge, R. J., Michaels, L., and Wright, T. (1996). Epithelial migration in keratosis obturans. *Am. J. Otolaryngol. Head Neck Med. Surg.* 17, 411–414. doi: 10.1016/s0196-0709(96)90076-9

Cunningham, L. L., and Tucci, D. L. (2017). Hearing loss in adults. *N. Engl. J. Med.* 377, 2465–2473.

del-Pozo, J., MacIntyre, N., Azar, A., Headon, D., Schneider, P., and Cheeseman, M. (2019). Role of ectodysplasin signalling in middle ear and nasal pathology in rat and mouse models of hypohidrotic ectodermal dysplasia. *DMM Dis. Model. Mech.* 12:dmm037804. doi: 10.1242/dmm.037804

Devare, J., Gubbels, S., and Raphael, Y. (2018). Outlook and future of inner ear therapy. *Hear Res.* 368, 127–135. doi: 10.1016/j.heares.2018.05.009

Edfeldt, L., and Strömbäck, K. (2015). Surgical treatment of congenital aural atresia-is it still justified? *Acta Otolaryngol.* 135, 226–232. doi: 10.3109/00016489.2014.979437

Feenstra, I., Vissers, L., Orsel, M., van Kessel, A. G., Brunner, H. G., Veltman, J. A., et al. (2007). Genotype-Phenotype mapping of chromosome 18q Deletions by high resolution array CGH. *Am. J. Med. Genet. Part A* 143, 1858–1867. doi: 10.1002/ajmg.a.31850

Feenstra, I., Vissers, L. E. L. M., Pennings, R. J. E., Nillessen, W., Pfundt, R., Kunst, H. P., et al. (2011). Disruption of teashirt zinc finger homeobox 1 is associated with congenital aural atresia in humans. *Am. J. Hum. Genet.* 89, 813–819. doi: 10.1016/j.ajhg.2011.11.008

Fons, J. M., Mozaffari, M., Malik, D., Marshall, A. R., Connor, S., Greene, N. D. E., et al. (2020). Epithelial dynamics shed light on mechanisms underlying ear canal defects. *Development* 147:dev194654. doi: 10.1242/dev.194654

Frumm, S. M., Yu, S. K., Chang, J., Byrnes, L. E., Sneddon, J. B., Tward, A. D., et al. (2020). Article a hierarchy of proliferative and migratory keratinocytes maintains the tympanic membrane. *Cell Stem Cell* 28, 1–16. doi: 10.1016/j.stem.2020.10.006

Fuchs, E., and Horsley, V. (2008). More than one way to skin. *Genes Dev.* 22, 976–985. doi: 10.1101/gad.1645908

Grevellec, A., and Tucker, A. S. (2010). The pharyngeal pouches and clefts: development, evolution, structure and derivatives. *Semin. Cell Dev. Biol.* 21, 325–332. doi: 10.1016/j.semcdb.2010.01.022

Gruneberg, H. (1971). The glandular aspects of the tabby syndrome in the mouse. *J. Embryol. Exp. Morph.* 25, 1–19.

Ikari, Y., Katori, Y., Ohtsuka, A., Francisco Rodríguez-Vázquez, J., Abe, H., Kawase, T., et al. (2013). Fetal development and variations in the cartilages surrounding the human external acoustic meatus. *Ann. Anat.* 195, 128–136. doi: 10.1016/j.aanat.2012.07.009

Ishimoto, S. I., Ito, K., Kondo, K., Yamasoba, T., and Kaga, K. (2004). The role of the external auditory canal in the development of the malleal manubrium in humans. *Arch. Otolaryngol. Head Neck Surg.* 130, 913–916. doi: 10.1001/archotol.130.8.913

Jackler, R. K., Santa Maria, P. L., Varsak, Y. K., Nguyen, A., and Blevins, N. H. (2015). A new theory on the pathogenesis of acquired cholesteatoma: mucosal traction. *Laryngoscope* 125, S1–S14.

Jahrsdoerfer, R. A., Yeakley, J. W., Aguilar, E. A., Cole, R. R., and Gray, L. C. (1992). Grading system for the selection of patients with congenital aural atresia. *Otol. Neurotol.* 13, 6–12.

Knutsson, J., von Unge, M., and Rask-Andersen, H. (2011). Localization of progenitor/stem cells in the human tympanic membrane. *Audiol. Neurotol.* 16, 263–269. doi: 10.1159/000320612

Kohan, D., and Ghossaini, S. N. (2019). Osseointegrated auditory devices—transcutaneous: sophono and baha attract. *Otolaryngol. Clin. N. Am.* 52, 253–263. doi: 10.1016/j.otc.2018.11.013

Kountakis, S., Helidonis, E., and Jahrsdoerfer, R. A. (1995). Microtia grade as an indicator of middle ear development in aural atresia. *JAMA Otolaryngol. Head Neck Surg.* 121, 885–886. doi: 10.1001/archotol.1995.01890080053010

Kowalczyk-Quintas, C., and Schneider, P. (2014). Ectodysplasin A (EDA) - EDA receptor signalling and its pharmacological modulation. *Cytokine Growth Fact. Rev.* 25, 195–203. doi: 10.1016/j.cytogfr.2014.01.004

Lavy, J., and Fagan, P. (2000). Chronic stenosing external otitis/postinflammatory acquired atresia: a review. *Clin. Otolaryngol. Allied Sci.* 25, 435–439. doi: 10.1046/j.1365-2273.2000.00388.x

Li, C.-L., Chen, Y., Chen, Y.-Z., Fu, Y.-Y., and Zhang, T.-Y. (2016). Congenital aural stenosis: clinical features and long-term outcomes. *Nat. Sci. Rep.* 6:27063.

Mallo, M. (2000). Assembling a functional tympanic membrane: signals from the external acoustic meatus coordinate development of the malleal manubrium. *Development* 127, 4127–4136.

Mallo, M., and Gridley, T. (1996). Development of the mammalian ear: coordinate regulation of formation of the tympanic ring and the external acoustic meatus. *Development* 122, 173–179.

Mallo, M. S. (2001). Formation of the middle ear: recent progress on the developmental and molecular mechanisms. *Dev. Biol.* 231, 410–419. doi: 10.1006/dbio.2001.0154

Manger, P. R., Hall, L. S., and Pettigrew, J. D. (1998). The development of the external features of the platypus (*Ornithorhynchus anatinus*). *Philos. Trans. R. Soc. B Biol. Sci.* 353, 1115–1125.

Michaels, L., and Soucek, S. (1990). Auditory epithelial migration on the human tympanic membrane: II. The existence of two discrete migratory pathways and their embryologic correlates. *Am. J. Anat.* 189, 189–200. doi: 10.1002/aja.1001890302

Michaels, L., and Soucek, S. (1991). Auditory epithelial migration. III. development of the stratified squamous epithelium of the tympanic membrane and external canal in the mouse. *Am. J. Anat.* 191, 280–292. doi: 10.1002/aja.1001910307

Minoux, M., Kratochwil, C. F., Ducret, S., Amin, S., Kitazawa, T., Kurihara, H., et al. (2013). Mouse Hoxa2 mutations provide a model for microtia and auricle duplication. *Development* 140, 4386–4397. doi: 10.1242/dev.098046

Moon, I. J., Cho, Y. S., Park, J., Chung, W. H., Hong, S. H., and Chang, S. O. (2012). Long-term stent use can prevent postoperative canal stenosis in patients with congenital aural atresia. *Otolaryngol. Head Neck Surg.* 146, 614–620. doi: 10.1177/0194599811426257

Mozaffari, M., Jiang, D., and Tucker, A. S. (2020). Developmental aspects of the tympanic membrane: shedding light on function and disease. *Genesis* 58, 1–10. doi: 10.1016/j.devcel.2010.12.010

Mukherjee, A., Hollern, D. P., Williams, O. G., Rayburn, T. S., Byrd, W. A., Yates, C., et al. (2018). A review of FOXI3 regulation of development and possible roles in cancer progression and metastasis. *Front. Cell. Dev. Biol.* 6:69. doi: 10.3389/fcell.2018.00069

Nadaraja, G. S., Gurgel, R. K., Kim, J., and Chang, K. W. (2013). Hearing outcomes of atresia surgery versus osseointegrated bone conduction device in patients with congenital aural atresia?: a systematic review. *Otol. Neurotol.* 34, 1394–1399. doi: 10.1097/mao.0b013e3182a36065

Naiberg, J., Berger, G., and Hawke, M. (1984). The pathologic features of keratosis obturans and cholesteatoma of the external auditory canal. *Arch. Otolaryngol.* 110, 690–693.

Nicholas, B. D., and Kesser, B. W. (2013). Unilateral aural atresia: current management issues and results. *Curr. Otorhinolaryngol. Rep.* 1, 92–98. doi: 10.1007/s40136-013-0014-9

Niemann, C., and Horsley, V. (2012). Development and homeostasis of the sebaceous gland. *Semin. Cell. Dev. Biol.* 23, 928–936. doi: 10.1016/j.semcdb.2012.08.010

Niemann, C., Unden, A. B., Lyle, S., Zouboulis, C. C., Toftgård, R., and Watt, F. M. (2003). Indian hedgehog and β-catenin signaling: role in the sebaceous lineage of normal and neoplastic mammalian epidermis. *Proc. Natl. Acad. Sci. U.S.A.* 100(Suppl. 1), 11873–11880. doi: 10.1073/pnas.1834202100

Nishimura, Y., and Kumoi, T. (2017). The embryologic development of the human external auditory meatus. *Acta Otolaryngol.* 112, 496–503. doi: 10.3109/00016489209137431

Nishizaki, K., Anniko, M., Orita, Y., Masuda, Y., Yoshino, T., Kanda, S., et al. (1998). Programmed cell death in the development of the mouse external auditory canal. *Anat. Rec.* 252, 378–382. doi: 10.1002/(sici)1097-0185(199811)252:3<378::aid-ar5>3.0.co;2-#

Ostrowski, V. B., and Wiet, R. J. (1996). Pathologic conditions of the external ear and auditory canal. *Medquest Commun. LLC* 100, 223–237. doi: 10.3810/pgm.1996.09.79

Parry, D. A., Logan, C. V., Stegmann, A. P. A., Abdelhamed, Z. A., Calder, A., Khan, S., et al. (2013). SAMS, a syndrome of short stature, auditory-canal atresia, mandibular hypoplasia, and skeletal abnormalities is a unique neurocristopathy caused by mutations in Goosecoid. *Am. J. Hum. Genet.* 93, 1135–1142. doi: 10.1016/j.ajhg.2013.10.027

Perry, E. T., and Shelley, W. B. (1955). The histology of the human ear canal with special refernece to the ceruminous gland. *J. Invest. Dermatol.* 25, 439–451. doi: 10.1038/jid.1955.149

Persaud, R., Hajioff, D., Trinidade, A., Khemani, S., Bhattacharyya, M. N., Papadimitriou, N., et al. (2018). Evidence-based review of aetiopathogenic theories of congenital and acquired cholesteatoma. *J. Laryngol. Otol.* 121, 1013–1019. doi: 10.1017/s0022215107000503

Persaud, R. A. P., Hajioff, D., Thevasagayam, M. S., Wareing, M. J., and Wright, A. (2004). Keratosis obturans and external ear canal cholesteatoma: how and why we should distinguish between these conditions. *Clin. Otolaryngol. Allied Sci.* 29, 577–581. doi: 10.1111/j.1365-2273.2004.00898.x

Rijli, F. M., Mark, M., Lakkaraju, S., Dierich, A., Dollé, P., and Chambon, P. (1993). A homeotic transformation is generated in the rostral branchial region of the head by disruption of Hoxa-2, which acts as a selector gene. *Cell* 75, 1333–1349. doi: 10.1016/0092-8674(93)90620-6

Rivera-Perez, J. A., Mallo, M., Gendron-Maguire, M., Gridley, T., and Behringer, R. R. (1995). Goosecoid is not an essential component of the mouse gastrula organizer but is required for craniofacial and rib development. *Development* 121, 3005–3012.

Santagati, F., Minoux, M., Ren, S. Y., and Rijli, F. M. (2005). Temporal requirement of Hoxa2 in cranial neural crest skeletal morphogenesis. *Development* 132, 4927–4936. doi: 10.1242/dev.02078

Schuknecht, H. F. (1989). Congenital aural atresia. *Laryngoscope* 99, 908–917.

Schwartz, S. R., Magit, A. E., Rosenfeld, R. M., Ballachanda, B. B., Hackell, J. M., Krouse, H. J., et al. (2017). Clinical practice guideline (update): earwax (cerumen impaction). *Otolaryngol. Head Neck Surg.* 156, 1–29.

Secor, C. P., Farrell, H. A., and Haydon, R. C. (1999). Auricular endochondral pseudocysts: diagnosis and management. *Plast. Reconstr. Surg.* 103, 1451–1457. doi: 10.1097/00006534-199904050-00014

Seppala, M., Depew, M. J., Martinelli, D. C., Fan, C.-M., Sharpe, P. T., and Cobourne, M. T. (2007). Gas1 is a modifier for holoprosencephaly and genetically interacts with sonic hedgehog. *J. Clin. Invest.* 117, 1575–1584. doi: 10.1172/jci32032

Shokry, E., and Filho, N. R. A. (2017). Insights into cerumen and application in diagnostics: past, present and future prospective. *Biochem. Medica* 27:030503.

Standrig, S., Anand, N., Birch, R., Collins, P., Crossman, A. R., and Gleeson, M. (2016). *Gray's Anatomy 40th Edition*, 41st Edn. Amsterdam: Elsevier, 639–661.

Tassano, E., Jagannathan, V., Drögemüller, C., Leoni, M., Hytönen, M. K., Severino, M., et al. (2015). Congenital aural atresia associated with agenesis of internal carotid artery in a girl with a FOXI3 deletion. *Am. J. Med. Genet. Part A* 167, 537–544. doi: 10.1002/ajmg.a.36895

Tian-Yu, Z., and Bulstrode, N. (2019). International consensus recommendations on microtia, aural atresia and functional ear reconstruction. *J. Int. Adv. Otol.* 15, 204–208.

Toyoda, Y., Sakurai, A., Mitani, Y., Nakashima, M., Yoshiura, K., Nakagawa, H., et al. (2009). Earwax, osmidrosis, and breast cancer: why does one SNP (538G>A) in the human ABC transporter ABCC11 gene determine earwax type? *FASEB J.* 23, 2001–2013. doi: 10.1096/fj.09-129098

Tucker, A. S. (2017). Major evolutionary transitions and innovations: the tympanic middle ear. *Philos. Trans. R. Soc. B Biol. Sci.* 372, 1–11.

van Spronsen, E., Geerse, S., Mirck, P. G. B., van der Baan, S., Fokkens, W. J., and Ebbens, F. A. (2014). The shape of the osseous external auditory canal and its relationship to chronic external otitis. *Otol. Neurotol.* 35, 1790–1796. doi: 10.1097/mao.0000000000000430

Vrabec, J. T., and Lin, J. W. (2010). Inner ear anomalies in congenital aural atresia. *Otol. Neurotol.* 31, 1421–1426. doi: 10.1097/mao.0b013e3181f7ab62

Yellon, R. F. (2011). Atresiaplasty versus BAHA for congenital aural atresia. *Laryngoscope* 121, 2–3. doi: 10.1002/lary.21408

Yoon, Y. H., Park, J. Y., and Park, Y. H. (2010). The preventive effect of mitomycin-C on the external auditory canal fibrosis in an experimentally induced animal model. *Am. J. Otolaryngol. Head Neck Med. Surg.* 31, 9–13. doi: 10.1016/j.amjoto.2008.08.013

8

Caspase-12 is Present During Craniofacial Development and Participates in Regulation of Osteogenic Markers

Barbora Vesela[1]*, Adela Kratochvilova[1], Eva Svandova[1], Petr Benes[2], Kamila Rihova[2], Anne Poliard[3] and Eva Matalova[1,4]

[1] Laboratory of Odontogenesis and Osteogenesis, Institute of Animal Physiology and Genetics, Academy of Sciences, Brno, Czechia, [2] Department of Experimental Biology, Faculty of Science, Masaryk University, Brno, Czechia, [3] Laboratory of Orofacial Pathologies, Imaging and Biotherapies, UFR Odontology Montrouge, Paris University, Paris, France, [4] Department of Physiology, Faculty of Veterinary Medicine, University of Veterinary and Pharmaceutical Sciences, Brno, Czechia

***Correspondence:**
Barbora Vesela
veselab.lab@gmail.com

Caspases are evolutionary conserved proteases traditionally known as participating in apoptosis and inflammation but recently discovered also in association with other processes such as proliferation or differentiation. This investigation focuses on caspase-12, ranked among inflammatory caspases but displaying other, not yet defined functions. A screening analysis pointed to statistically significant ($P < 0.001$) increase in expression of caspase-12 in a decisive period of mandibular bone formation when the original mesenchymal condensation turns into vascularized bone tissue. Immunofluorescence analysis confirmed the presence of caspase-12 protein in osteoblasts. Therefore, the osteoblastic cell line MC3T3-E1 was challenged to investigate any impact of caspase-12 on the osteogenic pathways. Pharmacological inhibition of caspase-12 in MC3T3-E1 cells caused a statistically significant decrease in expression of some major osteogenic genes, including those for alkaline phosphatase, osteocalcin and Phex. This downregulation was further confirmed by an alkaline phosphatase activity assay and by a siRNA inhibition approach. Altogether, this study demonstrates caspase-12 expression and points to its unknown physiological engagement in bone cells during the course of craniofacial development.

Keywords: caspase-12, bone, osteoblast, differentiation, alkaline phosphatase

INTRODUCTION

Caspases are evolutionary conserved proteases traditionally associated with apoptosis and inflammation (Van Opdenbosch and Lamkanfi, 2019). Recently, particular attention has been paid to their novel roles in other processes, such as differentiation, proliferation or autophagy (Shalini et al., 2015; Nakajima and Kuranaga, 2017; Tsapras and Nezis, 2017). The most common investigated caspases include apical proapoptotic caspase-8 and caspase-9, pro-inflammatory caspase-1, and the executive caspases-3 and -7, while others are rather neglected.

Caspase-12 is usually ranked as an inflammatory caspase (Bolívar et al., 2019), however, its exact effect remains unknown. Early studies have suggested the participation of caspase-12 in endoplasmic reticulum stress-induced apoptosis (Nakagawa et al., 2000; Shiraishi et al., 2006).

Later, characterization of *Casp12*$^{-/-}$ deficient mice described a suppressive effect of caspase-12 on caspase-1, resulting in an enhanced vulnerability to sepsis (Saleh et al., 2006). Recently, these apoptotic or septic-related roles were not confirmed and its functions remain enigmatic (Salvamoser et al., 2019). Caspase-12 expression was previously described in several tissues (Nakagawa and Yuan, 2000; Kalai et al., 2003; Veselá and Matalová, 2015) in relation to development.

The mandibular bone develops from a mesenchymal condensation where osteoblasts differentiate directly from mesenchymal progenitor cells through an intramembranous process, as most craniofacial bones. In the mouse, a vascularized bone containing all three basic cell types (osteoblasts, osteocytes, osteoclasts) begins to form only 2 days after condensation is achieved. This short but critical period is accompanied by dynamic changes in expression of several specific genes as demonstrated recently for osteogenesis and vascularization synchrony (Veselá et al., 2019). Pilot data (presented here) pointed to a significant increase in caspase-12 expression within this period of mandibular bone development.

The purpose of this investigation was to develop this initial finding and to study caspase-12 in the context of mandibular development. The spatio-temporal analysis was performed to investigate caspase-12 expression pattern in forming mandible with a special focus on bone. Since caspase-12 was strongly present in osteoblasts and since a strong impact on osteoblastic differentiation was demonstrated after general inhibition of the caspases (Mogi and Togari, 2003; Kratochvílová et al., 2020), our aim was to determine whether caspase-12 participates in modulation of the osteogenic pathways.

MATERIALS AND METHODS

Samples

Mice (strain CD1) were purchased from the Laboratory Animal Breeding and Experimental Facility, Masaryk University Brno and kept in the facilities of the Institute of Animal Physiology and Genetics, Czech Academy of Sciences, Czech Republic. Mouse heads were taken as fresh *post-mortem* samples. Embryonic (E) and postnatal (P) stages E13, E15, E18, P1, and P12 were examined. For PCR Array, fresh mandibles at stages E13 and E15 were dissected and cut into 250 μm slices using a McIlwain tissue chopper as described previously (Minaříková et al., 2015). Seven mandibles were used as one biological sample. Tissue slices with region of interest (mandibular bone surrounding the first mouse molar) were selected and the mandibular bone was separated under a stereoscope. The samples were lysed by RLT buffer (Qiagen) for RNA isolation. For immunofluorescence, samples were fixed in 4% paraformaldehyde, dehydrated (ethanol series), treated with xylene, and embedded in paraffin.

Cell Cultures

A cell line of osteoblastic precursors, MC3T3-E1, was purchased from the European Collection of Cell Culture (ECACC 99072810) and differentiated for 21 days as described previously (Kratochvílová et al., 2020). Growth medium was composed of MEM Alpha (Gibco, United States), 10% fetal bovine serum (FBS), penicillin/streptomycin (1,000 U/ml, 100 μg/ml). Osteogenic differentiation was performed in the same medium containing β-glycerolphosphate (10 mM) and ascorbic acid (50 μg/ml). Medium was changed every second day. During differentiation process, cells were passaged on average once a week to avoid the deposition of thick layer of extracellular matrix which prevents efficiency of cell treatments. Cells differentiated in this way created and deposited cell matrix, expressed osteogenic markers at high levels and were prepared for caspase-12 downregulation. MC3T3-E1 cells were examined before differentiation and then every 7 days to measure levels of caspase-12 expression. After 3 weeks of differentiation, cells were seeded at a density of 5,000 cell/cm^2. Caspase-12 Inhibitor Z-ATAD-FMK (FMK013, R&D Systems) was used for inhibition of caspase-12 proteolytic activity in cell culture. It was dissolved in DMSO, and applied at a final concentration of 100 μM as recommended by the manufacturer. The control group was treated with the same concentration of DMSO as used for the experimental samples to exclude any side effect of this solvent. Cells were harvested after 6 days of inhibition (protocols previously published e.g., in Kratochvílová et al., 2020) and prepared for RNA isolation, western blot, histological staining, and immunofluorescence.

RNA Isolation, PCR Arrays, Real-Time PCR

RNA was isolated by RNeasy Mini Kit (Qiagen), then mRNA was transcribed into cDNA using SuperScript VILO (Invitrogen). The Apoptosis PCR Array (PAMM-012Z, Qiagen) was used for analysis of gene expression in developing mandibular bone while the Osteogenesis PCR Array (Qiagen, PAMM-024Z) was used for analysis of osteogenic markers in MC3T3-E1 inhibited by caspase-12 inhibitor. The panel of housekeeping genes included: Actb, B2m, Gapdh, Gusb, and Hsp90ab1. The PCR Array format also included positive and negative controls. $N = 3$ in each group.

Real-time PCR was performed in 10 μl of a final reaction mixture containing the one-step GB Ideal PCR Master Mix (Generi Biotech). Alkaline phosphatase (Mouse *Alpl*, Mm00475834_m1), Osteocalcin (Mouse *Bglap*, Mm03413826_mH), Phex (Mouse *Phex*, Mm00448119_m1) and Dentin matrix protein 1 (Mouse *Dmp1*, Mm01208363_m1) expression was detected by using a TaqMan Gene Expression Assay (Thermo Fisher Scientific) with normalization based on actin levels (Mouse Actb, Mm02619580_g1).

Immunofluorescence

Frontal sections (5 μm) of mouse heads were used for immunofluorescent detection. Histological sections were deparaffinized in xylene and rehydrated in a gradient series of ethanol, finishing in water. Sections were pre-treated in citrate buffer (98°C/10 min) for antigen retrieval and then incubated with primary Anti-Caspase-12 antibody (2202, Cell Signaling, Danvers, MA) overnight. For immunofluorescence, cells grown on glass were fixed, pre-treated with 0.1% triton and incubated with the primary antibodies for caspase-12 (see above) or osteocalcin (ab93876, Abcam). Primary antibodies were followed by incubation with secondary anti-rabbit antibody Alexa Fluor 488 (Thermo Fisher Scientific, United States) (1:200) for 40 min at RT. Nuclei were detected by ProLong Gold Antifade reagent with DAPI (Thermo Fisher Scientific, United States). For immunohistochemistry, mandibular slices were treated as described above. Incubation with primary antibodies: osteocalcin, caspase-12 and Runx2 (sc10758, Santa Cruz Biotechnology) was followed by treatment with the peroxidase-conjugated streptavidin-biotin system (Vectastain) and the chromogen substrate diaminobenzidine (DAB, K3466; Dako). Slides were counterstained with hematoxylin. Negative and positive controls for Caspase-12 primary antibody are included in **Supplementary Figure 1**.

Western Blot

MC3T3-E1 cells were harvested and lysed by boiling in sodium dodecyl sulfate (SDS)-loading buffer containing 0.1 M Tris (pH 6.8), 16% v/v glycerol, 3.2% w/v SDS, 10% v/v β-mercaptoethanol and 0.005% w/v bromophenol blue. Cell lysates were subjected to sodium dodecyl sulfate polyacrylamide gel electrophoresis (SDS-PAGE) and electroblotted to polyvinylidene fluoride (PVDF) membrane (Millipore). The blot was probed with anti-Caspase-12 Antibody (2202, Cell Signaling) and developed with anti-rabbit IgG secondary antibody conjugated with horseradish peroxidase (A4914, Sigma-Aldrich, St. Louis, MI) by standard procedure using Clarity Max Western ECL Substrate (Biorad).

siRNA Gene Silencing

Differentiated MC3T3-E1 cells were seeded at density 7,000 cells/cm^2. Next day cells were transfected with 20 nM Silencer Select pre-designed siRNA *Casp12* (ID: s63375, Catalog No. 4390771, Ambion) using Lipofectamine RNAiMAX Reagent (13778, Life Technologies) according to the producer's instructions. Silencer Select Negative Control No. 1 siRNA (Catalog No. 4390843, Ambion) was used as a control. Cells were treated for 3 days; the medium with siRNA-Lipofectamine complexes was changed after 48 h of cultivation. $N = 4$ in each group.

Staining for Alkaline Phosphatase Activity

Fixed cells were stained with 300 μl of Fast blue mixture containing 4 mg of naphthol AS-TR phosphate disodium salt (Sigma, N6125) in 150 μl of N,N-dimethylformamide (Fluka, 40248) and 12 mg of Fast blue BB Salt hemi(zinc chloride) salt (Sigma, F3378) in 15 ml of 0.1 M Tris-HCl buffer (pH 9.6) for 10 min in the dark. $N = 3$ in each group.

Statistical Analysis

PCR Arrays data were statistically evaluated by Qiagen Gene Globe as recommended by the manufacturer (available on-line). Statistical significance was determined as $P < 0.05$, the threshold of fold regulation as ±2. Three biological replicates were evaluated in each group. Real-time PCR expression levels were calculated using the ΔΔCT method and results were analyzed using two-tailed *t*-test.

RESULTS

Caspase-12 Is Among Apoptosis-Related Genes Expressed During Mandibular Bone Development

To evaluate apoptosis-related gene expression during mouse mandibular bone development, apoptotic PCR Array was used. Among the 84 tested genes, 7 were significantly increased and 11 decreased more than 2-fold between prenatal stages E13 and E15 (**Figure 1**). The most prominent change in gene expression was detected for caspase-12 (11.4-fold upregulation, $P < 0.001$). Other significantly upregulated genes included caspase-1 (2.26, $P = 0.0047$) caspase-14 (3.83, $P = 0.0484$) Il10 (2.37, $P = 0.0216$), Tnfrsf11b (gene for osteoprotegerin; 2.03, $P = 0.0062$), Tnfsf10 (gene for Trail; 5.45, $P < 0.001$), and Trp73 (3.81, $P = 0.0486$) while Abl1 (−2.14, $P = 0.003$), Bcl2 (−3.4, $P = 0.0034$), Bcl2l10 (−3.46, $P = 0.0403$), Bid (−2.09, $P = 0.0014$), Birc5 (−2.03, $P < 0.001$), Cideb (−2.83, $P = 0.0127$) Dapkl (−2.06, $P = 0.003$), Dffb (−2.5, $P = 0.0174$), Igflr (−2.55, $P = 0.0033$), Tnfrsf10b (gene for DR5; −2.12, $P = 0.0026$), and Traf3 (−2.02, $P = 0.0026$) were significantly downregulated.

Caspase-12 Protein Is Present in Developing Mandibular Bone and Adjacent Structures

To ascertain the increase in *Casp12* mRNA expression between stages E13 and E15, at the protein level and precise caspase-12 localization, immunofluorescent analyses were performed on the developing mandibular bone at the area surrounding the first molar. At E13, when the mandibular bone starts to develop, caspase-12 protein was observed in the condensed mesenchymal cells (**Figure 2A**). Moreover, caspase-12 was also detected in adjacent mandibular structures involving the Meckel's cartilage (**Figure 2B**), oral epithelium (**Figure 2C**) and tooth epithelium (**Figure 2D**). At E15, the mandibular bone contained all three types of bone cells, osteoclast, osteoblasts and osteocytes, and formed calcified extracellular matrix. At this stage, caspase-12 was still expressed in the developing bone, especially by osteoblasts (**Figure 2E**). Expression of caspase-12 in Meckel's cartilage was maintained but more pronounced than at E13 (**Figure 2F**). Oral and tooth epithelium were still positive, moreover some weak signal of caspase-12 was observed in dental pulp (**Figures 2G,H**). Next, prenatal stage E18 and postnatal stages P1 and P12 were examined to further delineate caspase-12 expression during the mineralized tissue development. At all these stages, caspase-12 was also detected in the mandibular bone, predominantly in osteoblasts (**Figures 3A,C,E**). In the tooth, caspase-12 was observed in differentiating ameloblasts and odontoblasts with the most evident signal around birth (**Figures 3B,D,F**).

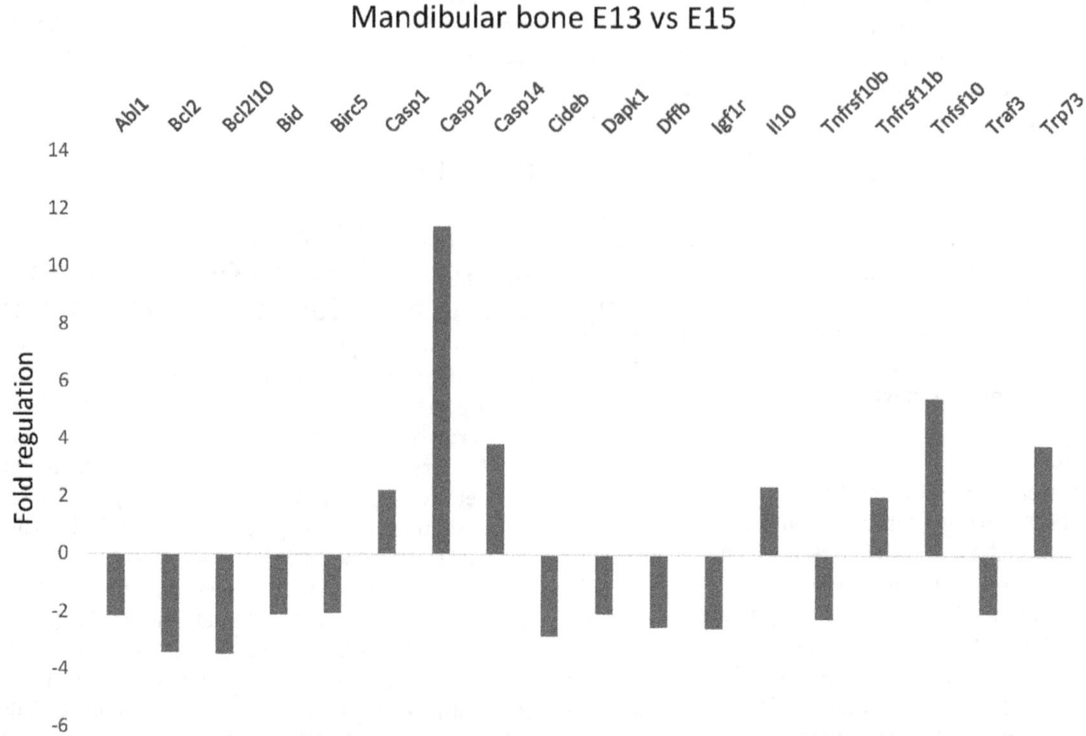

FIGURE 1 | Apoptosis-related gene expression in the developing mandible. Changes in expression of apoptosis-related genes in developing mandibular bone in the mouse. Analysis shows fold regulations (–2/+2 is used as the threshold) of gene expression between the prenatal/embryonic (E) days 13 and 15 detected by PCR Array. Statistically significant ($P < 0.05$) changes are displayed.

Caspase-12 Is Abundantly Present in Osteoblasts

To confirm the presence of the caspase-12 protein in osteoblasts *in vivo*, serial sections of mandibular bone at stage E15 were used. Expression of caspase-12 (**Figure 4A**) overlapped with localization of the osteoblastic markers osteocalcin (**Figure 4B**) and Runx2 (**Figure 4C**). To get closer insight into caspase-12 function in osteoblasts, expression of caspase-12 was evaluated in MC3T3-E1, an osteoblast cell line derived from calvaria. *Casp12* mRNA was expressed at a similar level, both in undifferentiated and MC3T3-E1 cells induced to differentiate toward an osteoblast phenotype (**Figure 4D**). *Casp12* mRNA expression remained stable during all the course of the differentiation process (data not shown). Western blot analysis revealed the presence of both the full length (55 kDa) and cleaved (42 kDa) forms of the caspase-12 protein in MC3T3-E1 cells (**Figure 4E**). The amount of non-cleaved full length form increased after treatment with caspase-12 inhibitor. Furthermore, caspase-12 protein presence in MC3T3-E1 cells was confirmed by immunofluorescence analysis (**Figure 4F**).

Osteoblastic Markers Are Downregulated After Caspase-12 Inhibition

As caspase-12 is produced by osteoblastic cells, its possible role was explored through inhibition studies. Differentiated MC3T3-E1 were treated for 6 days with the caspase-12 Inhibitor Z-ATAD-FMK and an Osteogenic PCR Array was performed. Analysis revealed a statistically significant downregulation in expression of 3 important osteogenic genes (**Figure 5A1**): *Alpl* (alkaline phosphatase) was decreased more than 3-times, *Bglap* (osteocalcin) decreased more than 2.5-times and expression of *Phex* (Phosphate-regulating neutral endopeptidase, X-linked) decreased more than 2-times. Downregulation of these genes was further confirmed by real-time PCR. *Alpl* expression (**Figure 5B**) decreased to 37% compared to control ($P < 0.001$), *Bglap* expression (**Figure 5C**) decreased to 39% ($P = 0.0047$) and *Phex* expression (**Figure 5D**) decreased to 54% ($P = 0.0196$) of the normal value. Only one upregulated gene (*Col2a1*, 3.32-times increased, $P < 0.001$) was detected after caspase-12 inhibition (A_2). The whole osteogenic panel showing gene expression in individual samples is presented in a heatmap (**Supplementary Figure 2**) At the protein level, a weaker staining for alkaline phosphatase activity and osteocalcin immunofluorescence were observed in caspase-12 inhibited samples as compared to the controls (respectively, **Figures 5E–H**).

Osteoblastic Markers Are Downregulated After *Casp12* Gene Silencing

To further confirm the involvement of caspase-12 in the regulation of gene expression of the above mentioned genes,

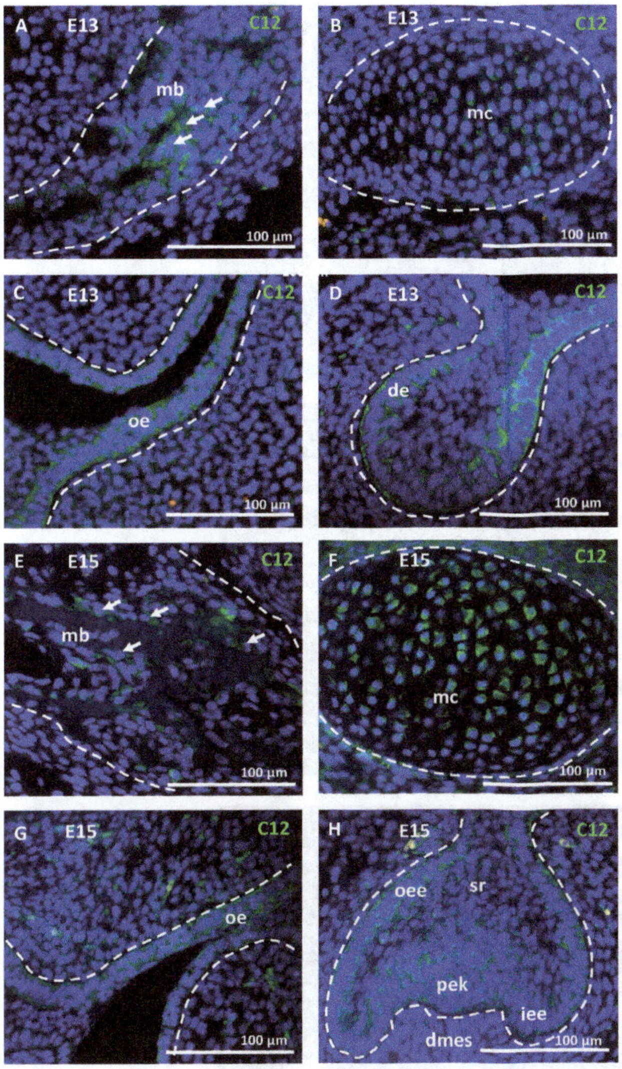

FIGURE 2 | Caspase-12 protein in prenatal development. Immunofluorescence analysis of caspase-12 (green) in developing mandibular bone and adjacent structures of the lower jaw. Caspase-12 at the stage E13 was localized in the mandibular bone **(A)**, Meckel's cartilage **(B)**, oral epithelium **(C)**, and first lower molar **(D)**. Caspase-12 positivity at the stage E15 was localized in the mandibular bone **(E)**, Meckel's cartilage **(F)**, oral epithelium **(G)**, and developing first lower molar **(H)**. Scale bar: 100 μm, counterstained by DAPI (blue). Arrows point to osteoblasts. mb, mandibular bone; mc, Meckel's cartilage; oe, oral epithelium; de, dental epithelium; oee, outer enamel epithelium; dmes, dental mesenchyme; iee, inner enamel epithelium; sr, stellate reticulum; pek, primary enamel knot.

a *Casp12* gene silencing approach was performed. Silencing was efficient since 3 days after transfection of differentiated MC3T3-E1 cells with a specific siRNA, *Casp12* gene expression (**Figure 6A**) decreased to 14% compared to control ($P < 0.001$). This efficient silencing was confirmed at the protein level (**Figures 6B,C**). Similarly, as observed with the caspase-12 inhibitor, expression of *Alpl* (**Figure 6D**), *Bglap* (**Figure 6E**), and *Phex* (**Figure 6F**) were significantly downregulated. *Alpl* decreased to 37% ($P = 0.0011$), *Bglap* to 48% ($P < 0.001$), and *Phex* to 23% ($P < 0.001$). In addition, a temporal silencing effect of *Casp12* siRNA, on *Bglap* gene expression was shown (**Supplementary Figure 3**). To further support the hypothesis on a novel role of caspase-12 in mineralization, expression of *Dmp1*, a critical marker for bone and dentin mineralization, not included in the osteogenic array, was analyzed. Expression of *Dmp1* dropped to 1% ($P < 0.001$) after *Casp12* gene silencing (**Figure 6G**).

DISCUSSION

Caspase-12 is a cysteine protease with yet unclear roles supported by often conflicting results. So far, caspase-12 protein was detected in some organs including heart, lungs, nose and hair follicles (Kalai et al., 2003; Veselá and Matalová, 2015). Several caspases were previously reported also in craniofacial bones (Svandova et al., 2018) but caspase-12 was investigated in this context for the first time. The initial examination related to mandibular bone and based on mRNA expression was focused on the period when the bone initially forms from the original mesenchymal condensation. This is essential also for further tooth-bone interactions heading for a dynamic anchorage of the tooth within the jaw in the context of functional dentition. Therefore, the spatio-temporal caspase-12 analysis was focused on the bone but also on the adjacent tooth developing in synchrony.

Since the strongest expression of caspase-12 in bone was identified within osteoblasts, further analysis was focused on this cell population. Caspase-12 was expressed in osteocalcin and Runx2-positive cells *in vivo* and both forms, full length procaspase-12 and cleaved active caspase-12, were identified in MC3T3-E1 cells. This osteoblastic cell line has a calvarial origin and is a valuable *in vitro* model for craniofacial bone research (Sudo et al., 1983). So far, caspase-12 expression in osteoblasts was considered mostly in the context of cell death and pathological conditions. For example, increased activation of caspase-12 was associated with endoplasmic reticulum stress and osteoblast apoptosis caused by fluorosis (Liu et al., 2015). In the present investigation, caspase-12 was observed in osteoblastic cells without a link to apoptosis, therefore other roles of this protease should be considered in the forming bone.

To tackle the question of these possible novel roles of caspase-12 in osteoblasts, functional experiments at the mRNA as well as protein levels were performed using the MC3T3-E1 cells. Notably, pharmacological inhibition of caspase-12 protein caused a significant downregulation of expression of the essential osteoblastic genes *Alpl*, *Bglap* and *Phex*. A similar decrease was previously observed following a general caspase inhibition in MC3T3-E1 cells (Kratochvílová et al., 2020). Therefore, caspase-12 is likely to be at least one of the major contributors to this modulatory effect within the osteogenic pathways. To further support our findings and exclude any non-specificity of the Z-ATAD-FMK inhibitor (Roy et al., 2008), *Casp12* gene silencing, using a specific siRNA, was performed and the significant decrease in all three genes was confirmed.

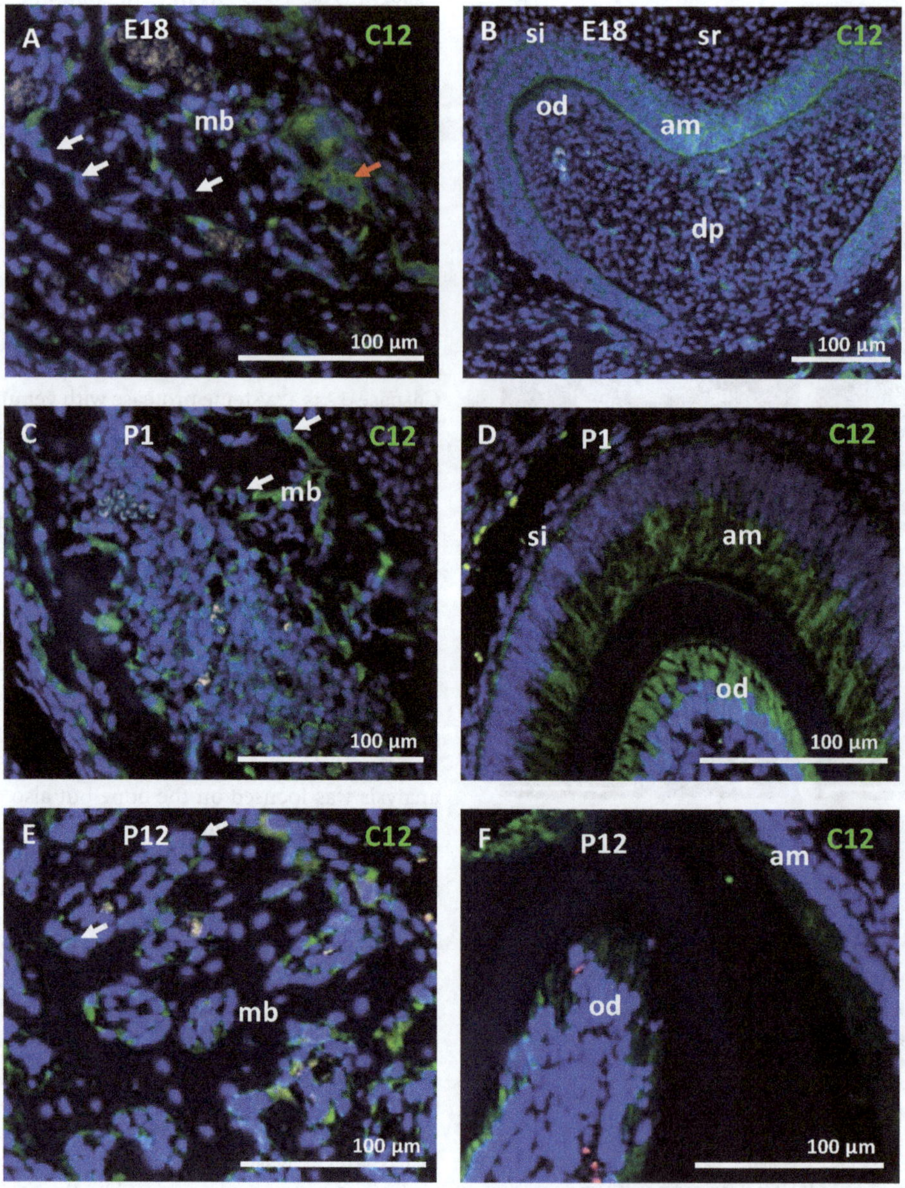

FIGURE 3 | Caspase-12 protein in perinatal and postnatal development. Immunofluorescence analysis of caspase-12 (green) in mandibular bone and the first lower molar at perinatal stages (E18 and P1) and postnatal stage P12. Caspase-12 was localized in the mandibular bone, predominantly in osteoblasts **(A,C,E)** at all of these stages. In the developing tooth, caspase-12 was positive mainly in ameloblasts and odontoblasts **(B,D,F)**. Scale bar: 100 µm, counterstained by DAPI (blue). White arrows point to osteoblasts, a red arrow points to osteoclasts. mb, mandibular bone; si, stratum intermedium; sr, stellate reticulum; dp, dental pulp; am, ameloblasts; od, odontoblasts.

Despite running attempts to understand the mechanism of the caspase-12 effect in development and homeostasis, little information is yet available (Salvamoser et al., 2019). One of the proposed mechanisms of caspase-12 functions was the recruitment of caspase-1 from its activation complexes and thus negative regulation of the inflammasome, but this function was not confirmed (Saleh et al., 2006; Vande Walle et al., 2016). Notably, in our original PCR Array based panel of pro-apoptotic molecules, caspase-1 expression was elevated along with caspase-12 which suggests an involvement of both caspases. Up to now, interactions between caspase-1 and caspase-12 at the protein level were essentially observed in inflammatory processes (Roy et al., 2008).

One of the caspases known to activate caspase-12 is caspase-7 (Rao et al., 2001). It is also expressed during craniofacial development, particularly in the mandibular bone where its lack causes a significant decrease in adult bone volume (Svandova et al., 2014). So far, caspase-7 and caspase-12 interplay was shown as an important step during neuronal death (De La Cadena et al., 2014). Their co-localization within mandibular osteoblasts

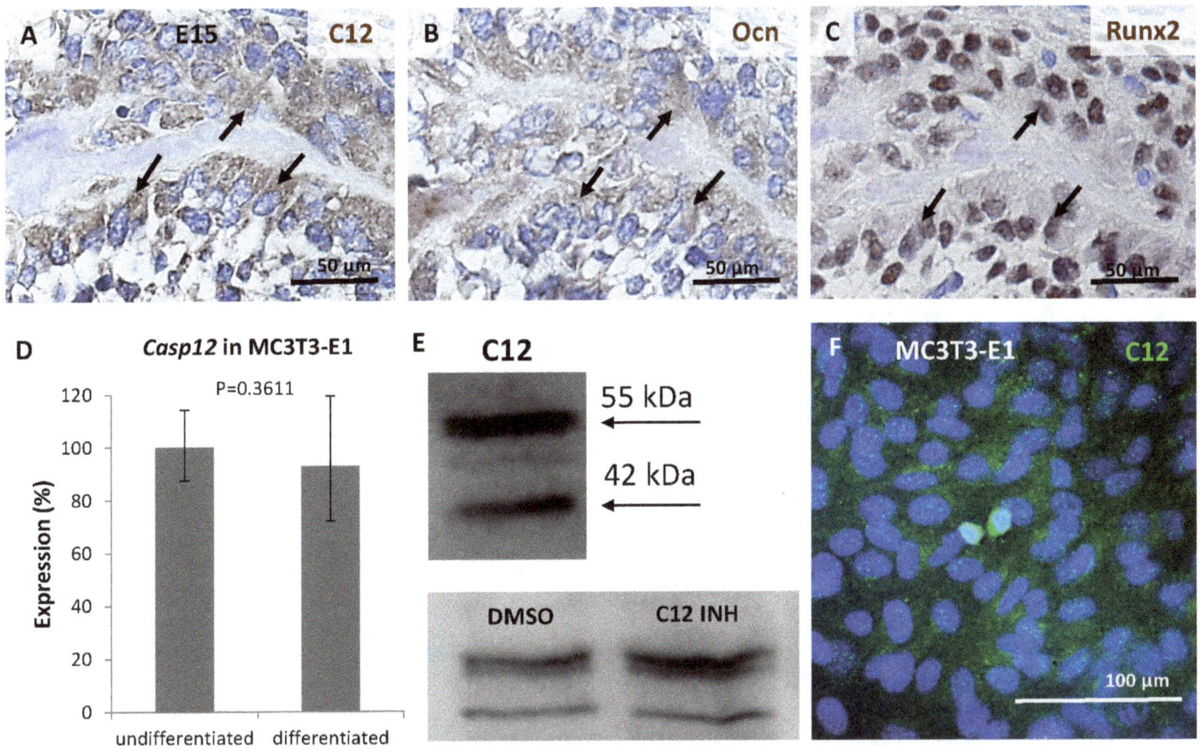

FIGURE 4 | Expression of caspase-12 in osteoblasts. Comparison of serial sections of the mouse mandibular bone at the prenatal/embryonic **(E)** day 15 showing co-localization of caspase-12 **(A)** with osteoblastic markers osteocalcin **(B)** and Runx2 **(C)** within the bone. Positive cells are brown, counterstained by hematoxylin (blue). Arrows point to cells in the same region. Scale bar: 50 µm. Expression of caspase-12 in undifferentiated and differentiated MC3T3-E1 cells **(D)** showing stable expression of *Casp12* after 21 days of differentiation. Western blot analysis **(E)** and immunofluorescence **(F)** confirmed the presence of caspase-12 protein in MC3T3-E1. E: 55 kDa-full length caspase-12, 42 kDa-cleaved caspase-12, DMSO: caspase-12 forms after DMSO treatment, C12 INH: caspase-12 forms after specific inhibitor treatment. F: Caspase-12 in green, DAPI in blue. Scale bar: 100 µm.

raises the possibility that caspase 7 could also participate in the non-apoptotic functions of caspase-12 within the bone.

Due to yet undefined roles and mechanisms related to caspase-12, the position of this caspase within the caspase networks is not yet understood. Based on our findings demonstrating a reduction of alkaline phosphatase activity upon caspase-12 inhibition/silencing and on earlier published data reporting a similar effect after inhibition of caspase-2, −3, and −8 (Mogi and Togari, 2003), caspase-12 could therefore be involved in the same caspase cascade.

Adding to the complexity, inter-species differences in caspase-12 functions are expected based on structural findings and activation processing of this caspase (Roy et al., 2008). Indeed, in humans, most people express a truncated form of caspase-12 lacking the catalytic domain and only about 20% of African descent people express the full length protease known to be a risk factor for developing sepsis (Saleh et al., 2004). In contrast in mice, the full length form is always expressed and can thus undergo proteolytic cleavage (Kalai et al., 2003). Until now, caspase-12 substrates have not been fully defined (Van Opdenbosch and Lamkanfi, 2019). One suggested option is caspase-12 autoprocessing (Roy et al., 2008), which is supported by increased amount of full length protein after caspase-12 inhibition observed also in our study.

Despite the complicated understanding of caspase-12 action mechanisms, the present investigation showed a clear-cut effect of its modulation on expression of important osteogenic genes necessary for proper osteogenic regulation. Caspase-12 deficient bone phenotype has not yet been analyzed but alkaline phosphatase deficiency in mice causes hypophosphatasia and impaired mineralization of bone and cartilage (Fedde et al., 1999), osteocalcin-deficient mice develop higher bone mass phenotype with bone defects (Ducy et al., 1996) and *Phex* mutation is associated with X-linked dominant hypophosphatemic rickets involving impaired bone mineralization (Francis et al., 1997). Therefore, all three caspase-12 regulated markers, alkaline phosphatase, osteocalcin and Phex are molecules associated with the regulation of bone mineralization. In accordance with these data, expression of *Dmp1*, another important factor in bone mineralization (Lorenz-Depiereux et al., 2006), was affected by *Casp12* gene silencing. This finding points to novel functions of caspase-12 in osteoblast differentiation. This conclusion would be in agreement with the latest data coming from analysis of caspase-1/-11/-12 triple mutant mice which did not reveal any critical functions of caspase-12 in apoptosis or inflammatory response (Salvamoser et al., 2019) and other functions thus become highly probable. The present investigation is therefore the first indication of such a novel function in craniofacial bone

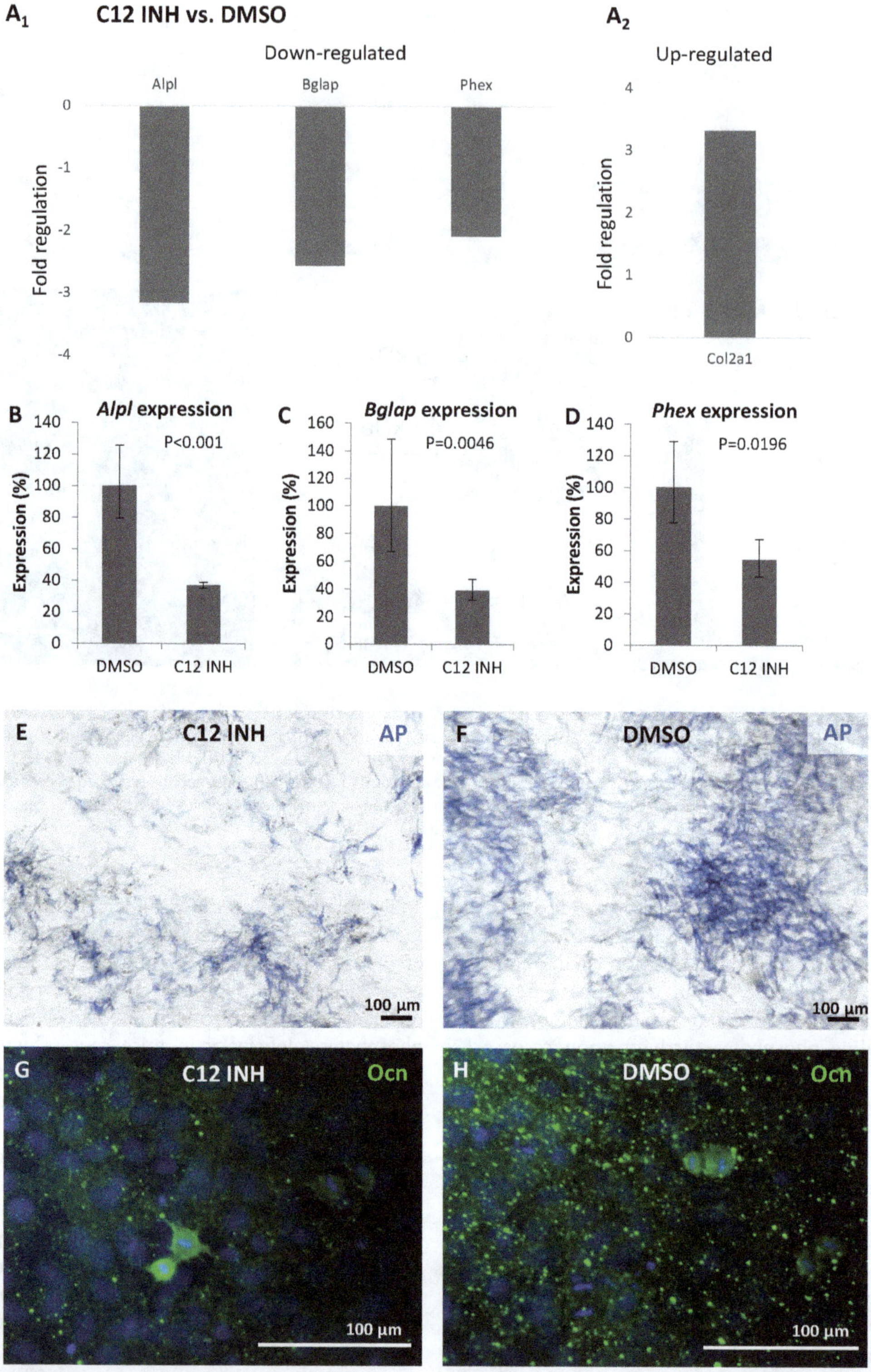

FIGURE 5 | Inhibition of caspase-12 in MC3T3-E1 cells. Changes in gene expression of osteogenesis-related genes **($A_{1,2}$)** in differentiated MC3T3-E1 cells after inhibition of caspase-12 by the specific inhibitor Z-ATAD-FMK, and DMSO-treated cells used as a control. Analysis shows fold regulations (–2/+2 is used as the threshold) of gene expression, statistically significant ($P < 0.05$) changes are displayed. Real-time PCR confirmed statistically significant decrease of *Alpl* **(B)**, *Bglap* **(C)**, and *Phex* **(D)** in inhibited MC3T3-E1. Results are presented as means ± standard deviations and were analyzed using two-tailed *t*-test. Staining for activation of alkaline phosphatase (blue) in MC3T3-E1 cells after caspase-12 inhibition **(E)** compared to control **(F)**. Immunofluorescence staining of osteocalcin expression (green) in differentiated MC3T3-E1 after inhibition of caspase-12 **(G)** compared to control **(H)**. Scale bar: 100 μm, counterstained by DAPI (blue).

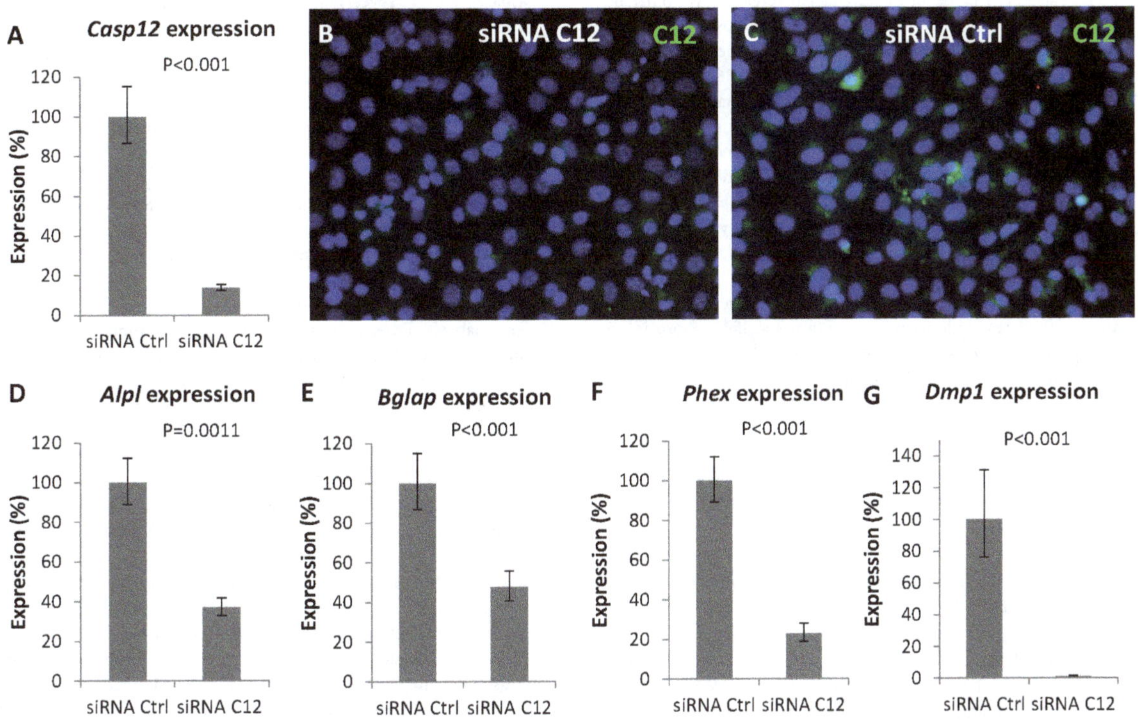

FIGURE 6 | Gene silencing of *Casp12* in MC3T3-E1. Gene silencing of *Casp12* in MC3T3-E1 cells using specific siRNA showed statistically significant reduction of *Casp12* expression **(A)**. Real-time PCR confirmed statistically significant decrease in expression of *Alpl* **(D)**, *Bglap* **(E)**, *Phex* **(F)**, and *Dmp1* **(G)** after *Casp12* silencing. Results are presented as means ± standard deviations and were analyzed using two-tailed *t*-test. Immunofluorescence detection of caspase-12 (green) protein in MC3T3-E1 after Casp12 gene silencing **(B)** compared to control **(C)**, DAPI in blue.

formation. Further studies should help to unravel the complex interactions between caspase-12 and its partners and understand its apoptosis-independent functions.

ETHICS STATEMENT

Ethical review and approval was not required for the animal study because the research did not include experiments in living animals, all the samples were obtained post-mortem. According to the recent law in the Czechia (359/2012 Sb.), post-mortem collection of animal samples is not considered as an experiment (paragraph 3, letter t) and thus does not require approval by any specific committee.

AUTHOR CONTRIBUTIONS

EM designed the study. BV planned the experiments. BV, AK, ES, and KR performed the experiments. PB and AP analyzed the data. BV, EM, and AP wrote the manuscript. All authors contributed to the article and approved the submitted version.

ACKNOWLEDGMENTS

We thank to Wim Declercq for helpful comments to the manuscript.

REFERENCES

Bolívar, B. E., Vogel, T. P., and Bouchier-Hayes, L. (2019). Inflammatory caspase regulation: maintaining balance between inflammation and cell death in health and disease. *FEBS J.* 286, 2628–2644. doi: 10.1111/febs.14926

De La Cadena, S. G., Hernández-Fonseca, K., Camacho-Arroyo, I., and Massieu, L. (2014). Glucose deprivation induces reticulum stress by the PERK pathway and caspase-7- and calpain-mediated caspase-12 activation. *Apoptosis* 19, 414–427. doi: 10.1007/s10495-013-0930-7

Ducy, P., Desbois, C., Boyce, B., Pinero, G., Story, B., Dunstan, C., et al. (1996). Increased bone formation in osteocalcin-deficient mice. *Nature* 382, 448–452. doi: 10.1038/382448a0

Fedde, K. N., Blair, L., Silverstein, J., Coburn, S. P., Ryan, L. M., Weinstein, R. S., et al. (1999). Alkaline phosphatase knock-out mice recapitulate the metabolic and skeletal defects of infantile hypophosphatasia. *J. Bone Miner. Res.* 14, 2015–2026. doi: 10.1359/jbmr.1999.14.12.2015

Francis, F., Strom, T. M., Hennig, S., Böddrich, A., Lorenz, B., Brandau, O., et al. (1997). Genomic organization of the human PEX gene mutated in X-linked dominant hypophosphatemic rickets. *Genome Res.* 7, 573–585. doi: 10.1101/gr.7.6.573

Kalai, M., Lamkanfi, M., Denecker, G., Boogmans, M., Lippens, S., Meeus, A., et al. (2003). Regulation of the expression and processing of caspase-12. *J. Cell Biol.* 162, 457–467. doi: 10.1083/jcb.200303157

Kratochvílová, A., Veselá, B., Ledvina, V., Švandová, E., Klepárník, K., Dadáková, K., et al. (2020). Osteogenic impact of pro-apoptotic caspase inhibitors in MC3T3-E1 cells. *Sci. Rep.* 10, 1–8. doi: 10.1038/s41598-020-64294-9

Liu, L., Zhang, Y., Gu, H., Zhang, K., and Ma, L. (2015). Fluorosis induces endoplasmic reticulum stress and apoptosis in osteoblasts in vivo. *Biol. Trace Elem. Res.* 164, 64–71. doi: 10.1007/s12011-014-0192-4

Lorenz-Depiereux, B., Bastepe, M., Benet-Pagès, A., Amyere, M., Wagenstaller, J., Müller-Barth, U., et al. (2006). DMP1 mutations in autosomal recessive hypophosphatemia implicate a bone matrix protein in the regulation of phosphate homeostasis. Nat. Genet. 38, 1248–1250. doi: 10.1038/ng1868

Minaříková, M., Oralová, V., Veselá, B., Radlanski, R. J., and Matalová, E. (2015). Osteogenic profile of mesenchymal cell populations contributing to alveolar bone formation. *Cells Tissues Organs* 200, 339–348. doi: 10.1159/000439165

Mogi, M., and Togari, A. (2003). Activation of caspases is required for osteoblastic differentiation. *J. Biol. Chem.* 278, 47477–47482. doi: 10.1074/jbc.M307055200

Nakagawa, T., and Yuan, J. (2000). Cross-talk between two cysteine protease families: activation of caspase-12 by calpain in apoptosis. *J. Cell Biol.* 150, 887–894. doi: 10.1083/jcb.150.4.887

Nakagawa, T., Zhu, H., Morishima, N., Li, E., Xu, J., Yankner, B. A., et al. (2000). Caspase-12 mediates endoplasmic-reticulum-specific apoptosis and cytotoxicity by amyloid-β. *Nature* 403, 98–103. doi: 10.1038/47513

Nakajima, Y. I., and Kuranaga, E. (2017). Caspase-dependent non-apoptotic processes in development. *Cell Death Differ.* 24, 1422–1430. doi: 10.1038/cdd.2017.36

Rao, R. V., Hermel, E., Castro-Obregon, S., Del Rio, G., Ellerby, L. M., Ellerby, H. M., et al. (2001). Coupling endoplasmic reticulum stress to the cell death program. Mechanism of caspase activation. *J. Biol. Chem.* 276, 33869–33874. doi: 10.1074/jbc.M102225200

Roy, S., Sharom, J. R., Houde, C., Loisel, T. P., Vaillancourt, J. P., Shao, W., et al. (2008). Confinement of caspase-12 proteolytic activity to autoprocessing. *Proc. Natl. Acad. Sci. U.S.A.* 105, 1433–1438. doi: 10.1073/pnas.0706658105

Saleh, M., Mathison, J. C., Wolinski, M. K., Bensinger, S. J., Fitzgerald, P., Droin, N., et al. (2006). Enhanced bacterial clearance and sepsis resistance in caspase-12-deficient mice. *Nature* 440, 1064–1068. doi: 10.1038/nature04656

Saleh, M., Vaillancourt, J. P., Graham, R. K., Huyck, M., Srinivasula, S. M., Alnemri, E. S., et al. (2004). Differential modulation of endotoxin responsiveness by human caspase-12 polymorphisms. *Nature* 429, 75–79. doi: 10.1038/nature02451

Salvamoser, R., Brinkmann, K., O'Reilly, L. A., Whitehead, L., Strasser, A., and Herold, M. J. (2019). Characterisation of mice lacking the inflammatory caspases-1/11/12 reveals no contribution of caspase-12 to cell death and sepsis. *Cell Death Differ.* 26, 1124–1137. doi: 10.1038/s41418-018-0188-2

Shalini, S., Dorstyn, L., Dawar, S., and Kumar, S. (2015). Old, new and emerging functions of caspases. *Cell Death Differ.* 22, 526–539. doi: 10.1038/cdd.2014.216

Shiraishi, H., Okamoto, H., Yoshimura, A., and Yoshida, H. (2006). ER stress-induced apoptosis and caspase-12 activation occurs downstream of mitochondrial apoptosis involving Apaf-1. *J. Cell Sci.* 119, 3958–3966. doi: 10.1242/jcs.03160

Sudo, H., Kodama, H. A., Amagai, Y., Yamamoto, S., and Kasai, S. (1983). *In vitro* differentiation and calcification in a new clonal osteogenic cell line derived from newborn mouse calvaria. *J. Cell Biol.* 96, 191–198. doi: 10.1083/jcb.96.1.191

Svandova, E., Lesot, H., Vanden Berghe, T., Tucker, A. S., Sharpe, P. T., Vandenabeele, P., et al. (2014). Non-apoptotic functions of caspase-7 during osteogenesis. *Cell Death Dis.* 5:e1366. doi: 10.1038/cddis.2014.330

Svandova, E., Vesela, B., Tucker, A. S., and Matalova, E. (2018). Activation of pro-apoptotic caspases in non-apoptotic cells during odontogenesis and related osteogenesis. *Front. Physiol.* 9:174. doi: 10.3389/fphys.2018.00174

Tsapras, P., and Nezis, I. P. (2017). Caspase involvement in autophagy. *Cell Death Differ.* 24, 1369–1379. doi: 10.1038/cdd.2017.43

Van Opdenbosch, N., and Lamkanfi, M. (2019). Caspases in cell death, inflammation, and disease. *Immunity* 50, 1352–1364. doi: 10.1016/j.immuni.2019.05.020

Vande Walle, L., Jiménez Fernández, D., Demon, D., Van Laethem, N., Van Hauwermeiren, F., Van Gorp, H., et al. (2016). Does caspase-12 suppress inflammasome activation? *Nature* 534, E1–E4. doi: 10.1038/nature17649

Veselá, B., and Matalová, E. (2015). Expression of apoptosis-related genes in the mouse skin during the first postnatal catagen stage, focused on localization of Bnip3L and caspase-12. *Connect. Tissue Res.* 56, 326–335. doi: 10.3109/03008207.2015.1040546

Veselá, B., Švandová, E., Bobek, J., Lesot, H., and Matalová, E. (2019). Osteogenic and angiogenic profiles of mandibular bone-forming cells. *Front. Physiol.* 10:124. doi: 10.3389/fphys.2019.00124

9

Sonic Hedgehog Signaling in Cranial Neural Crest Cells Regulates Microvascular Morphogenesis in Facial Development

*Miranda R. Sun[1], Hannah M. Chung[1,2], Veronika Matsuk[1,2], Dustin M. Fink[1], Matthew J. Stebbins[3], Sean P. Palecek[3], Eric V. Shusta[3,4] and Robert J. Lipinski[1,2]**

[1] *Department of Comparative Biosciences, School of Veterinary Medicine, University of Wisconsin–Madison, Madison, WI, United States,* [2] *Molecular and Environmental Toxicology Center, University of Wisconsin–Madison, Madison, WI, United States,* [3] *Department of Chemical and Biological Engineering, University of Wisconsin–Madison, Madison, WI, United States,* [4] *Department of Neurological Surgery, University of Wisconsin–Madison, Madison, WI, United States*

Correspondence:
Robert J. Lipinski
robert.lipinski@wisc.edu

Sonic hedgehog (Shh) pathway disruption causes craniofacial malformations including orofacial clefts (OFCs) of the lip and palate. In normal craniofacial morphogenesis, Shh signals to multipotent cranial neural crest cells (cNCCs) and was recently discovered to regulate the angiogenic transcriptome, including expression markers of perivascular cells and pericytes. The mural cells of microvasculature, pericytes in the brain and face differentiate from cNCCs, but their role in facial development is not known. Here, we examined microvascular morphogenesis in a mouse model of Shh pathway antagonist-induced cleft lip and the impact of cNCC-specific Shh pathway activation in a cNCC-endothelial cell co-culture system. During cleft pathogenesis *in vivo*, disrupted microvascular morphogenesis localized with attenuated tissue outgrowth in the medial nasal processes that form the upper lip. *In vitro*, we found that human umbilical vein endothelial cell (HUVEC) cord formation was not affected by direct Shh pathway perturbation. However, in a co-culture system in which cNCCs directly interact with endothelial cells, cNCC-autonomous Shh pathway activity significantly prolonged endothelial cord network stability. Taken together, these findings support the premise that Shh pathway activation in cNCCs promotes pericyte-like function and microvascular stability. In addition to suggesting a previously unrecognized role for Shh signaling in facial development, these studies also identify perivascular differentiation and microvascular morphogenesis as new focuses for understanding normal and abnormal craniofacial development.

Keywords: perivascular, pericyte, cranial neural crest, Sonic hedgehog, orofacial clefting, microvascular morphogenesis

INTRODUCTION

Orofacial clefts (OFCs) of the lip and palate are among the most common human birth defects and impose a substantial burden on the health and well-being of affected individuals (Wehby and Cassell, 2010; Watkins et al., 2014). OFCs are etiologically complex, and the cellular processes and molecular mechanisms underlying normal and abnormal craniofacial morphogenesis are incompletely understood, hindering the development of effective prevention strategies. Sonic hedgehog (Shh) signaling is required for normal facial morphogenesis and plays a critical role in the outgrowth of the facial processes that form the upper lip and palate (Bush and Jiang, 2012; Kurosaka, 2015). Disruption of the Shh pathway causes OFCs in animal models and is linked to OFC pathogenesis in humans (Roessler et al., 1996, 2003; Heyne et al., 2015a; Yu et al., 2017). However, a cohesive cellular mechanism explaining the role of Shh signaling in normal and abnormal facial development has yet to be established.

Recently, we found that Shh signaling regulates the angiogenic and perivascular transcriptomes in a mouse model of cleft lip (Everson et al., 2018). While Shh signaling has previously been shown to affect angiogenesis and vascular development, the underlying mechanisms are not well defined (Chapouly et al., 2019). Some studies suggest that Shh signaling acts directly on endothelial cells to promote vascular function (Renault et al., 2010; Alvarez et al., 2011). One of these studies has reported canonical pathway activation in endothelial cells after SHH ligand stimulation (Alvarez et al., 2011), but whether Shh signaling promotes angiogenesis and vascular development directly through endothelial cells remains controversial.

Other lines of investigation have linked Shh signaling to pericytes, the mural cells of the microvasculature, which signal to adjacent endothelial cells to promote proliferation, angiogenesis, and microvascular stability (Armulik et al., 2005, 2011; Chapouly et al., 2019). Pericytes have received resurgent interest as they have been identified to play important roles in development, wound healing, tissue regeneration, and disease pathogenesis (Armulik et al., 2011). Shh signaling has been shown to regulate pericyte biology in the liver and may also promote pericyte recruitment in several organs (Armulik et al., 2011; Machado and Diehl, 2018). Craniofacial pericytes are derived from multipotent cranial neural crest cells (cNCCs), which also form most of the cartilage and bone of the head (Etchevers et al., 2001; Jiang et al., 2002; Stebbins et al., 2019). While cNCC-derived pericytes have been less-studied than the mesoderm-derived pericytes of the trunk, their involvement in blood-brain barrier development and maintenance as well as retina development and disease has received substantial recent attention (Trost et al., 2016; Santos et al., 2018; Brown et al., 2019). In contrast, our understanding of the signaling pathways that drive cNCC-to-pericyte differentiation and the role of pericyte-endothelial cell interactions in normal and abnormal craniofacial and upper lip morphogenesis is extremely limited.

In this study, we use *in vivo* and *in vitro* models to investigate the effect of Shh signaling on microvasculature in the developing upper lip. A mouse model of Shh pathway antagonist-induced cleft lip is used to examine microvascular morphogenesis during normal and abnormal upper lip development. We then establish an *in vitro* co-culture model using cNCC-derived pericytes and endothelial cells to dissect the individual cell-type contributions of Shh pathway perturbation on microvascular stability. Our findings suggest a previously unrecognized role for Shh signaling in facial development and identify perivascular differentiation and microvascular morphogenesis as new focuses for understanding normal and abnormal craniofacial development.

MATERIALS AND METHODS

Animal Studies

All studies were conducted in strict accordance with the recommendations in the Guide for the Care and Use of Laboratory Animals of the National Institutes of Health. The protocol was approved by the University of Wisconsin–Madison, School of Veterinary Medicine Institutional Care and Use Committee (Protocol No. 13–081.0). Male and female C57BL/6J mice (*Mus musculus*, Jackson Laboratory strain 00664) were housed under specific-pathogen-free conditions in disposable, ventilated cages (Innovive). Rooms were maintained at 22 ± 2°C and 30–70% humidity with a 12-h light, 12-h dark cycle. Mice were fed Irradiated Soy Protein-Free Extruded Rodent Diet (Catalog No. 2920x; Envigo Teklad Global) until day of copulation plug when dams were switched to Irradiated Teklad Global 19% Protein Extruded Rodent Diet (Catalog No. 2919; Envigo Teklad Global).

One to two nulliparous female mice were placed with a single male for 1–2 h and subsequently examined for the presence of copulation plugs. The beginning of the mating period was designated as gestational day (GD)0. Pregnancy was confirmed by assessing weight gain at GD7, as previously described (Heyne et al., 2015b). Pregnant dams were administered 90 or 120 mg/kg/day cyclopamine (LC Laboratories, CAS #4449-51-8) or vehicle alone from GD8.25 to approximately GD9.375 by subcutaneous infusion exposure using ALZET 2001D micro-osmotic pumps (Cupertino, CA, United States) as previously described (Lipinski et al., 2008, 2010; Everson et al., 2017; Ansen-Wilson et al., 2018). Pregnant dams were euthanized by carbon dioxide inhalation followed by cervical dislocation for embryo collection at GD9.25 or GD11 ± 1 h.

Light Imaging

GD11 embryos for light imaging were fixed in Bouin's solution, and representative images were taken using a MicroPublisher 5.0 camera (QImaging) mounted on an Olympus SZX-10 stereomicroscope. A single litter each of vehicle- and 120 mg/kg/day cyclopamine-exposed embryos was collected for imaging.

PECAM1 Whole-Mount Immunohistochemistry for Quantitative Analysis

GD11 embryos exposed to vehicle or 90 mg/kg/day cyclopamine were fixed in 4% paraformaldehyde (PFA) in PBS for 6 h before dehydration through a graded series into 100% methanol for storage at −20°C. After rehydration, embryos were hemisected, and one half of each embryo was embedded in 4% agarose in PBS. A vibrating microtome was used to make a single 400-μm section of the lambdoidal junction, the rostral-most aspect of the developing facial processes containing the medial nasal, lateral nasal, and maxillary processes (MNP, LNP, and MxP, respectively). Sections were blocked in PBS with 0.3% Triton X, 0.2% BSA, and 5% goat serum for 1 h at room temperature followed by incubation with an antibody against PECAM1 (1:200 dilution, BD Pharmingen 557355) overnight at 4°C. A goat anti-rat secondary antibody conjugated with Alexa Fluor 488 (1:200 dilution, Jackson ImmunoResearch 112-546-003) and 60 nM DAPI were incubated with the sections at room temperature for 2 h. Sections were mounted on microscope slides with Vectashield mounting medium (Vector Laboratories) and imaged using a Leica SP8 confocal microscope. Four vehicle-treated litters and four cyclopamine-treated litters were collected, and 1–4 embryos from each litter were selected for analysis based on phenotype (cleft and non-cleft in the cyclopamine group) and proper staging (total $n = 10$ vehicle-exposed embryos, $n = 12$ cyclopamine-exposed embryos).

Image Processing and Microvasculature Analysis

Z-stacks from confocal imaging of PECAM1-stained lambdoidal junction sections were imported into ImageJ, and image stacks for all samples were three-dimensionally rotated for consistent orientation. A maximum projection of the rostral-most 50 μm of each re-oriented stack was used for subsequent analysis. A standard-size square region of interest (ROI) was drawn within the vascularized mesenchymal tissue of the MNP and analyzed using AngioTool software. Lambdoidal sections from embryos exposed to 90 mg/kg/day cyclopamine were classified as having either a non-clefted (NC) or cleft lip (CL) phenotype. Samples were considered NC if the MNP was touching or fused with the MxP, and samples were considered CL if the MNP was not touching the MxP. Analysis was carried out by a single investigator blinded to sample treatment group.

PECAM1 and Laminin Immunohistochemistry

For qualitative *in vivo* PECAM1 and Laminin co-immunostaining, a PFA-fixed control GD11 embryo was coronally sectioned into 50-μm sections using a vibrating microtome and subsequently immunostained following the above protocol for whole-mount immunohistochemistry. Primary antibodies against PECAM1 (1:200 dilution, BD Pharmingen 557355) and Laminin (1:1000 dilution, Sigma-Aldrich L9393) were used to stain for microvasculature. A goat anti-rat secondary antibody conjugated with Alexa Fluor 488 (1:200 dilution, Jackson ImmunoResearch 112-546-003) and a goat anti-rabbit secondary antibody conjugated with DyLight 594 (1:200 dilution, Thermo Scientific 35560) were used. Sections were imaged on a Keyence BZ-X700 fluorescent microscope.

Cell Culture

Human umbilical vein endothelial cells (HUVECs) were purchased from Lonza, cultured in EGM-2 according to manufacturer recommendations, and used for experiments at passage 5. O9-1 cells, a mouse cNCC line, were cultured as described previously (Ishii et al., 2012). O9-1 cNCCs stably expressing a mutated constitutively activated form of Smoothened (SMO^{M2}) along with GFP (cNCC-SMO), or GFP alone as a control (cNCC-GFP), were generated as previously described (Everson et al., 2017). To differentiate O9-1 cNCCs into pericytes, cells were cultured in E6 media with 10% FBS, following a previously described protocol (Stebbins et al., 2019). Pericyte-differentiated cNCC-GFP and cNCC-SMO were designated as cNCC-GFP-PC and cNCC-SMO-PC, maintained in E6 media with 10% FBS, and used for experiments at passages 8–11. Five biological replicates of cNCC-GFP-PC and cNCC-SMO-PC were collected for gene expression analyses.

For SHH ligand treatment, parent O9-1 cNCCs were plated at 5×10^5 cells/ml (0.4 ml per well in a 24-well plate) and allowed to attach in complete medium for 24 h before media were replaced with DMEM containing 1% FBS and recombinant human SHH ligand (0.4 μg/ml final concentration, R&D Systems 1845-SH), made in a stock solution at 100 μg/ml in sterile-filtered 5 mg/ml bovine serum albumin (BSA) in PBS, or equivalent volume of BSA vehicle. After 48 h, cells were harvested for RNA isolation. Five biological replicates were collected for gene expression analyses.

Matrigel Cord Formation Assay

For cord formation assays, 100 μl of Matrigel (Corning) was added to the wells of a chilled 48-well plate and incubated at 37°C for at least 30 min according to manufacturer recommendations. In the HUVEC-alone experiments, cells were trypsinized, and 1.58×10^4 HUVECs were resuspended in 300 μl EGM-2 per well with 0.4 μg/ml SHH ligand or BSA vehicle and 200 nM vismodegib (dissolved in 100% DMSO) or DMSO vehicle and plated into wells containing Matrigel. A total of 12 biological replicates per treatment group were plated for phase contrast imaging. For RNA extraction, four wells were pooled for each experimental group 12 h after plating, and a total of five biological replicates were plated.

For the cNCC-endothelial cell co-culture experiments, cells were trypsinized, and 1.4×10^4 HUVECs and 0.18×10^4 cNCC-GFP-PC or cNCC-SMO-PC (8:1 ratio, based on not shown preliminary optimization) were resuspended in 300 μl EGM-2 per well and plated into wells containing Matrigel. Pericyte-differentiated cNCCs were switched to EGM-2 media 24 h before plating. A total of 12 biological replicates per treatment group were plated for phase contrast imaging (one well had a tear in the Matrigel within the imaging field; therefore, that replicate was excluded, and a total of 11 biological replicates were used for analysis).

Matrigel Cord Formation Assay Analysis

Phase contrast images were taken with a MicroPublisher 5.0 camera (QImaging) mounted on a Nikon Eclipse TS100 with a 4x objective at 12 and 22 h after cells were plated for cord formation assays. Images were imported into ImageJ and analyzed using the Angiogenesis plugin. ImageJ was used to modify cord network schematics generated by the Angiogenesis plugin for better visibility in representative images.

Immunocytochemistry and Imaging

At 6–8 h after plating, cells in cord formation assays were fixed in 4% PFA in PBS for 15 min at room temperature. Cords were blocked in PBS with 0.3% Triton X, 0.2% BSA, and 5% goat serum for 1 h at room temperature and then incubated overnight at 4°C with primary antibodies against PECAM1 (1:200 dilution, Proteintech 66065-1-Ig) or Laminin (1:1000 dilution, Sigma-Aldrich L9393). Cords were incubated with a goat anti-rabbit or anti-mouse secondary antibody conjugated to DyLight 594 (1:200, Thermo Scientific 35560 and 35511) and 60 nM DAPI for 1 h at room temperature for detection. A Keyence BZ-X700 was used for fluorescent imaging.

RNA Extraction, Reverse Transcription, and qPCR

A GE Illustra RNA spin mini kit was used for RNA extraction according to manufacturer protocols. A total of 100–500 ng of RNA was used for cDNA synthesis using GoScript reverse transcription reaction kits (Promega). Singleplex quantitative real-time PCR (qPCR) was performed on a Bio-Rad CFX96 system using SsoFast EvaGreen Supermix (Bio-Rad), and primers were designed using the IDT PrimerQuest tool. qPCR primer sequences are shown in **Table 1**. Target gene and species specificity was confirmed using NCBI Primer-BLAST. Mouse *Gapdh* or human *GAPDH* was used as the housekeeping gene, and analyses were conducted using the $2^{-\Delta\Delta Ct}$ method.

Statistics

Graphpad Prism 8 was used for all statistical analysis. Results from *in vivo* experiments were analyzed using unpaired statistical tests. Two-tailed *t*-tests were used to analyze the differences between proximal and distal microvasculature. Ordinary one-way analysis of variance (ANOVA) with Tukey's *post hoc* test for multiple comparisons was used for analyses of microvasculature between vehicle and cyclopamine-exposed groups. *In vitro* experiments were run in pairwise manner and paired statistical tests were used. Ordinary one-way ANOVA with Tukey's *post hoc* test for multiple comparisons was used for cord formation assays and Shh pathway gene expression in HUVEC-alone experiments. Two-tailed *t*-tests were used to analyze differences in gene expression in parent cNCCs and pericyte-differentiated cNCCs as well as in co-culture cord formation between groups. An alpha value of 0.05 was maintained for determination of significance for all experiments.

TABLE 1 | Primer sequences used for qPCR.

Primer	Species	Sequence
GAPDH forward	human	CCACATCGCTCAGACACCAT
GAPDH reverse	human	GCAACAATATCCACTTACCAGAGTTAA
GLI1 forward	human	AATGCTGCCATGGATGCTAGA
GLI1 reverse	human	GAGTATCAGTAGGTGGGAAGTCCATAT
PTCH1 forward	human	CGCTGGGACTGCTCCAAGT
PTCH1 reverse	human	GAGTTGTTGCAGCGTTAAAGGAA
Angpt1 forward	mouse	CCATTCCAGCAGCAAGTGGTTA
Angpt1 reverse	mouse	TGAAGTGCAGCAAGCTGAGAAG
Angpt2 forward	mouse	CCACATTCCTCTAAGCACGGTTTC
Angpt2 reverse	mouse	TAACCTGTGCCCACCACTTAGA
Cd248 forward	mouse	GTTGCTGGATGATGGAGAAGAAGG
Cd248 reverse	mouse	GCCAAAGTCAGGTGGATGTGTAG
Cspg4 forward	mouse	CAAATGCTCCCGTCCTCACTAAC
Cspg4 reverse	mouse	AGGCTGCTCCATCACCTCATA
Edn1 forward	mouse	CCAAGCGCTGTTCCTGTTCTT
Edn1 reverse	mouse	TGGAAGAACCTCCCAGTCCATAC
Foxc1 forward	mouse	TTCTTGCGTTCAGAGACTCG
Foxc1 reverse	mouse	TCTTACAGGTGAGAGGCAAGG
Foxd1 forward	mouse	CGTTTCTAGATTCTCACTCCTC
Foxd1 reverse	mouse	TCCACTGTGGTCCCTTTA
Foxf2 forward	mouse	TTCTCTAGTTCCCTGGCTCAGTAG
Foxf2 reverse	mouse	TGTTCTTTGGCACCTGTATCCG
Gapdh forward	mouse	AGCCTCGTCCCGTAGACAAAAT
Gapdh reverse	mouse	CCGTGAGTGGAGTCATACTGGA
Gli1 forward	mouse	GGAAGTCCTATTCACGCCTTGA
Gli1 reverse	mouse	CAACCTTCTTGCTCACACATGTAAG
Lama2 forward	mouse	CGCACCTTGAATGCAGACTTGA
Lama2 reverse	mouse	GCACATCCCGCCAACTGAAATA
Ptch1 forward	mouse	CTCTGGAGCAGATTTCCAAGG
Ptch1 reverse	mouse	TGCCGCAGTTCTTTTGAATG
Tbx18 forward	mouse	ACGAAATAGGCACCGAGATG
Tbx18 reverse	mouse	ATTGCTGGTGAGGGTCTAATC

RESULTS

Microvascular Density Is Increased at the Distal Tip of the Medial Nasal Processes

The midface forms through precisely coordinated growth and fusion of three bilaterally paired facial growth centers, the medial nasal, lateral nasal, and maxillary processes (MNP, LNP, and MxP, respectively). We visualized vasculature in these growth centers when the MNP and MxP begin to fuse bilaterally to close the upper lip at gestational day (GD)11.0 in the mouse. Staining for the endothelial marker PECAM1 revealed a network of microvasculature with a dense plexus apparent in the distal aspect of the MNP that extends to make contact and subsequently fuse with the MxP (**Figures 1A,A'**). AngioTool software was then used to quantitatively compare microvascular characteristics between selected regions of interest (ROIs) representing proximal (**Figures 1B,B'**) and distal (**Figures 1C,C'**) regions of the MNP. Vessel area and number of junctions were not significantly different between the proximal and distal regions, but the average vessel length was significantly decreased and the number of endpoints was significantly increased in the distal region, suggesting an increase in the number and therefore density of vessels at the distal tip of the MNP (**Figures 1D–G**).

Microvascular Patterning Is Disrupted in Cleft Lip Pathogenesis

Next, we tested whether microvascular morphogenesis was altered in animals with cleft lip using a well-characterized model of Shh pathway inhibition via targeted maternal exposure to the Smoothened antagonist cyclopamine (Lipinski et al., 2008;

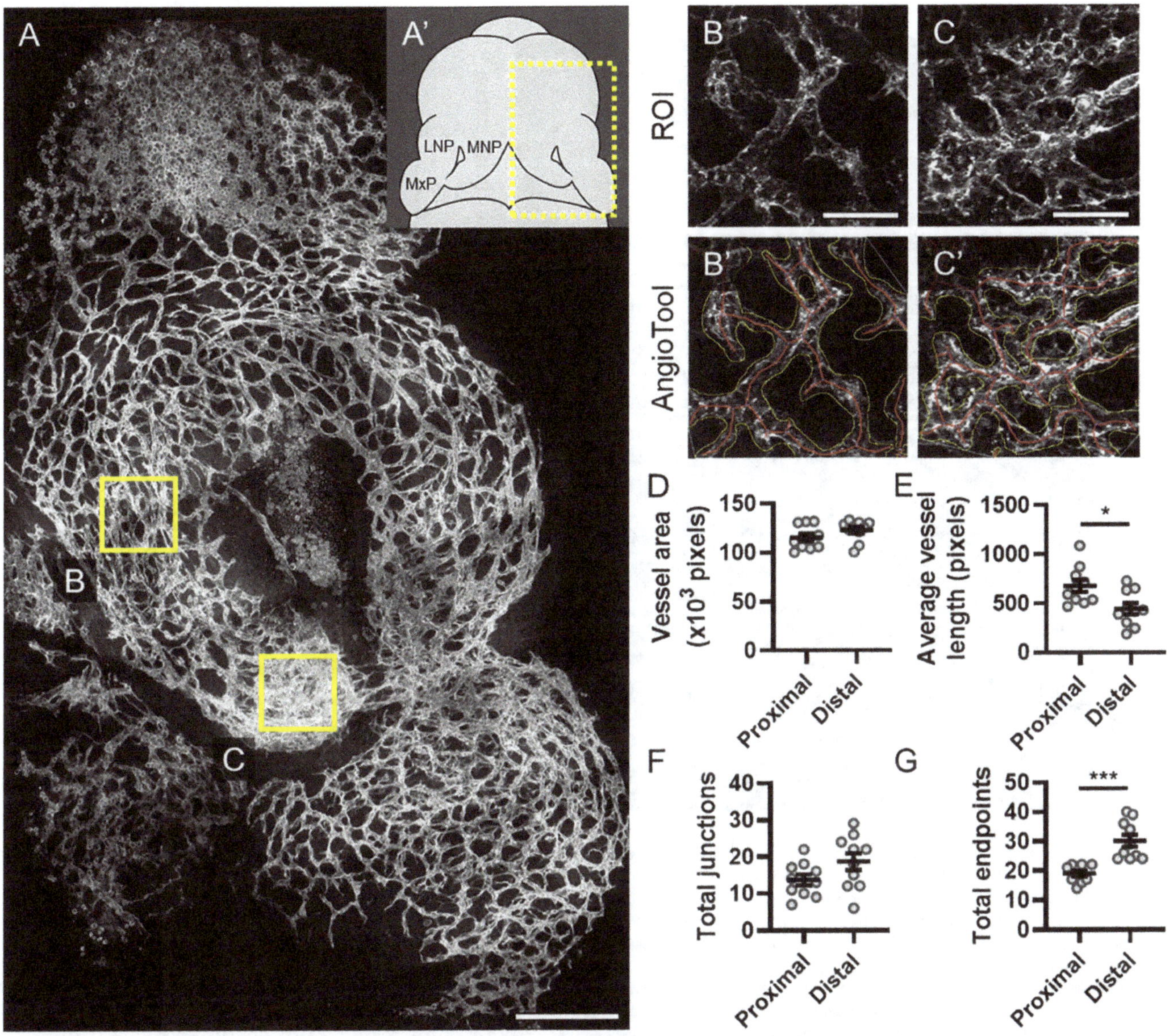

FIGURE 1 | Microvascular density is increased in the distal medial nasal process. **(A)** A representative maximum projection of a 180-μm z-stack of the lambdoidal junction stained for PECAM1 of a vehicle-exposed GD11 embryo is shown with the proximal **(B)** and distal **(C)** regions of the medial nasal process (MNP) indicated. Scale bar is 200 μm. **(A')** Schematic of a GD11 embryo head with the MNP, lateral nasal process (LNP), and maxillary process (MxP) labeled. Representative regions of interest (ROIs) of the microvasculature of the proximal **(B)** and distal **(C)** MNP from a maximum projection of the rostral-most 50 μm of each section are shown. Scale bars are 50 μm. The vascular networks identified by AngioTool are shown in **(B')** and **(C')**. Vessel areas are outlined in yellow and the vessels lengths are in red. **(D–G)** The vessel area, average vessel lengths, number of junctions, and number of endpoints in the microvasculature from 10 vehicle-exposed embryos were analyzed by AngioTool. Measurements for individual embryos are indicated by the icons, and the means ± SEM are shown. $^*p < 0.05$ and $^{***}p < 0.001$ between the indicated groups.

Heyne et al., 2015a). Smoothened is a G protein-coupled receptor that is necessary for Shh signaling transduction. As previously described, cyclopamine exposure resulted in animals with cleft lip (CL) and without cleft lip (no cleft; NC), which were compared against vehicle-treated control embryos (**Figures 2A–C**) using the same approach described for **Figure 1** (**Figures 2D–F"**). In the proximal region of the MNP, no significant differences were observed between the vehicle- or cyclopamine-exposed groups in all measured parameters (**Supplementary Figure 1**). In the distal MNP, however, vessel area and number of junctions were significantly lower in cyclopamine-exposed embryos with cleft lip compared to control embryos or cyclopamine-exposed embryos without clefts (**Figures 2G,I**). No significant differences were observed between vehicle controls and cyclopamine-exposed embryos without clefts in any measured parameter, and no significant differences in average vessel length or total endpoints were detected between any of the groups (**Figures 2G–J**).

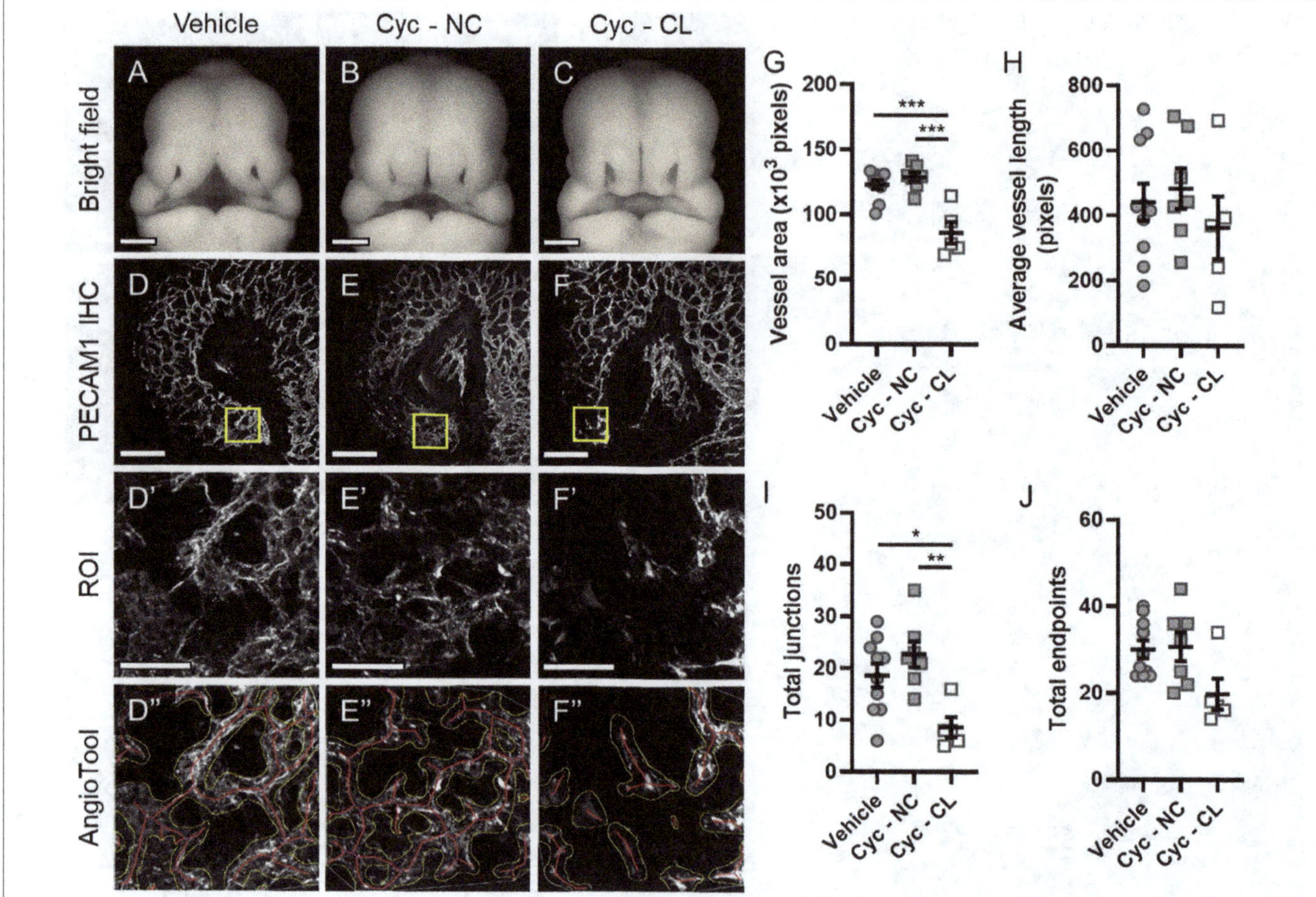

FIGURE 2 | Microvascular patterning is disrupted in cyclopamine-exposed embryos with cleft lip phenotype. **(A–C)** Representative phenotypes in GD11 embryos transiently exposed to vehicle and cyclopamine (cyc) and fixed in Bouin's solution were imaged. Cyclopamine-exposed embryos were classified as having a non-clefted (NC) or cleft lip (CL) phenotype for analysis. Scale bars are 500 μm. **(D–F)** One lambdoidal junction of each vehicle- and cyclopamine-exposed embryo fixed in 4% PFA was sectioned by vibrating microtome at 400-μm thickness and stained for PECAM1 by whole-mount immunohistochemistry (IHC) to visualize the microvasculature. Maximum projections of the rostral-most 50 μm of the resulting 3D confocal images are shown. Scale bars are 200 μm. **(D'–F')** Regions of interest (ROIs) were defined at the distal end of the medial nasal process (MNP) as indicated by the boxes in **(D–F)**. Scale bars are 50 μm. **(D"–F")** An overlay of vessels identified by AngioTool is shown for each ROI in **(D'–F')**. The vessel areas are outlined in yellow and the vessels lengths are in red. Images are representative of 5–10 embryos per analysis group. **(G–J)** Vessel area, average vessel length, total junctions, and total endpoints in the ROIs were measured by AngioTool. Measurements for individual embryos are indicated by the icons, and the means ± SEM for each group are shown. **$p < 0.05$*, ***$p < 0.01$*, and ****$p < 0.001$* between indicated treatment groups.

Shh Pathway Modulation in Endothelial Cells Does Not Affect Cord Formation

To interrogate the mechanism by which Shh signaling regulates microvascular morphogenesis, we cultured HUVECs, which form networks of endothelial cords *in vitro*. HUVECs plated on Matrigel were treated with SHH ligand and/or the potent Smoothened inhibitor vismodegib, and cord networks imaged at 12 and 22 h (**Supplementary Figure 2**) were analyzed using the Angiogenesis plugin for ImageJ (**Figures 3A–H**). While there were significant differences within treatment groups from 12 to 22 h, no treatment-dependent differences were detected at either time point (**Figures 3I–L**). qPCR analysis of a parallel cohort demonstrated no treatment-dependent differences in expression of the conserved Shh pathway target genes *GLI1* and *PTCH1* (**Figures 3M,N**).

cNCC-Derived Pericytes Interact With Endothelial Cell Cords

While Shh pathway modulation did not impact endothelial cord formation directly, we previously observed that Shh signaling altered the angiogenic transcriptome in cultured multipotent cNCCs (Everson et al., 2018). Among the derivatives of cNCCs are pericytes, the mural cells of microvessels that actively signal with endothelial cells. We therefore sought to establish an *in vitro* culture in which cNCC-derived pericytes interact with HUVEC cords in a manner that approximates the *in vivo* pericyte-endothelial relationship. cNCCs were cultured according to a recently described protocol for differentiation of pericytes from human pluripotent stem cell-derived cNCCs (Stebbins et al., 2019), which were then cultured with HUVECs at a 1:8 ratio on Matrigel. By 8 h, cNCC-HUVEC co-cultures formed networks

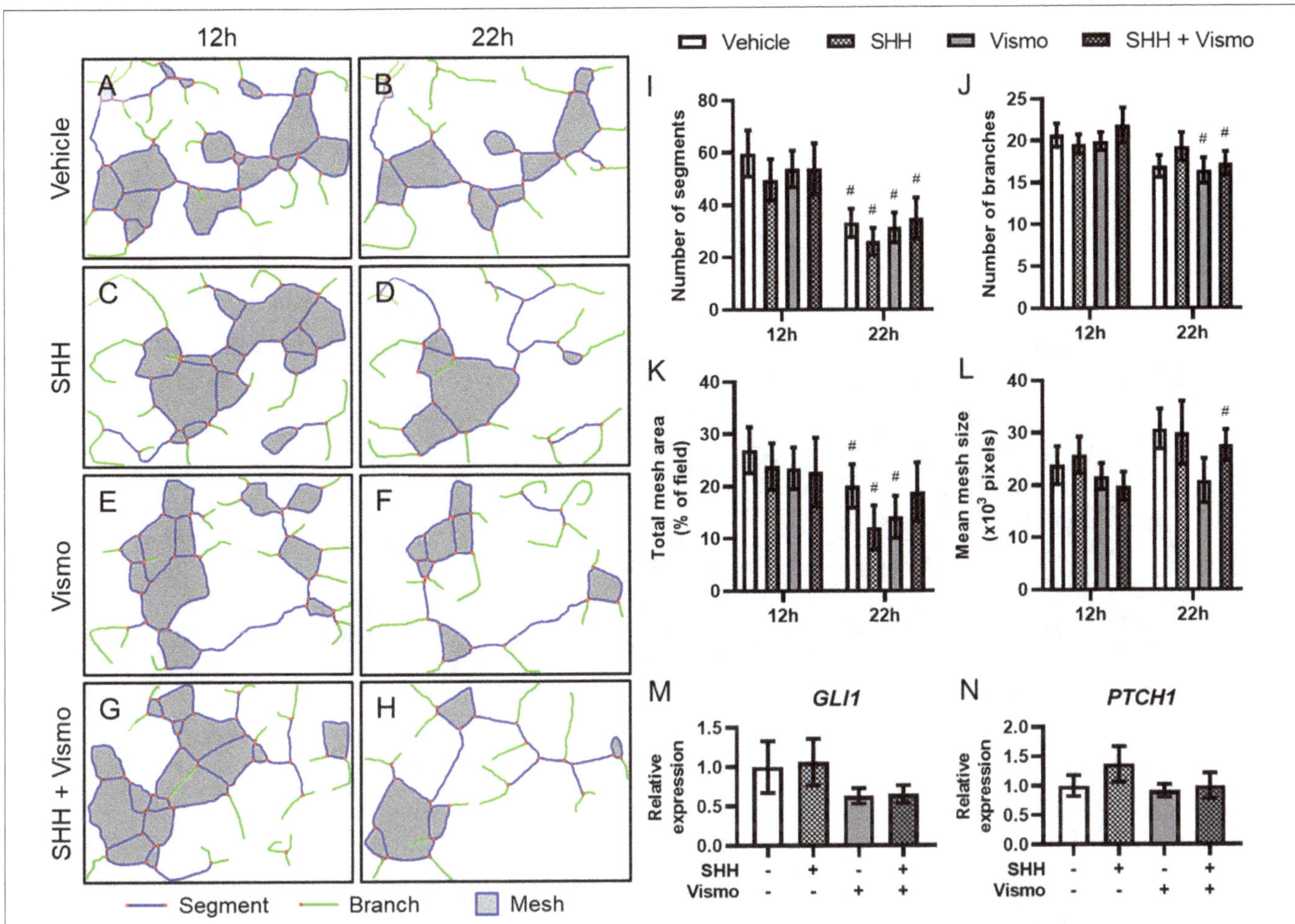

FIGURE 3 | Shh pathway perturbation in endothelial cells does not affect cord formation or downstream Shh pathway targets. **(A–H)** Cord network schematics of HUVECs ± 0.4 μg/ml SHH ligand ± 200 nM vismodegib (vismo) plated on Matrigel were generated from images taken at 12 and 22 h. Blue lines are segments, green lines are branches, red dots are junctions, and filled gray areas are meshes. Images are representative of 12 biological replicates per treatment group. **(I–L)** Number of segments, number of branches, total mesh area, and mean mesh size as measured by the Angiogenesis plugin for ImageJ are shown for the indicated groups at 12 and 22 h. $^{\#}p < 0.05$ of the indicated treatment group compared to the same group at 12 h. **(M,N)** Canonical Shh pathway targets *GLI1* and *PTCH1* were assayed for gene expression by qPCR in HUVEC cords treated with SHH and/or vismodegib and harvested at 12 h. Five biological replicates were harvested for gene expression.

similar to HUVECs alone but with apparently thicker cords (**Figures 4A,B**). Examination by fluorescent microscopy revealed that GFP-expressing pericyte-differentiated cNCCs approximate and appear to wrap around PECAM1-expressing HUVEC cords (**Figures 4C,D**). The extracellular matrix protein family of Laminins, an integral component of the basement membrane of vasculature, was found to surround cords formed by HUVECs alone and cNCC-HUVEC co-cultures (**Figures 4E,F**), resembling the Laminin staining observed in the microvasculature of the MNP *in vivo* (**Figures 4G,G'**).

cNCC-Autonomous Shh Pathway Activation Increases Pericyte-Associated Gene Expression

Having established an *in vitro* model of direct cNCC-pericyte/HUVEC interaction, we next sought to test the impact of cNCC-specific Shh pathway activation. From parent cNCCs, we generated lines expressing a mutated constitutively active form of Smoothened (SMO^{M2}) and GFP, or GFP alone for control. qPCR analysis showed increased expression of Shh target genes *Gli1* and *Ptch1* in SMO^{M2}-expressing cNCCs that approximated the level of induction achieved by treating parent cells with SHH ligand (**Figures 5A,B**). Both SHH ligand stimulation and SMO^{M2} expression also resulted in increased expression of *Foxd1* and *Foxf2* (**Figures 5C,D**), which have been demonstrated to be Shh target genes and required for brain or kidney pericyte differentiation and function (Jeong et al., 2004; Gomez and Duffield, 2014; Reyahi et al., 2015; Everson et al., 2017, 2018; Fink et al., 2018). We next assessed pericyte-differentiated GFP- or SMO^{M2}-expressing cNCCs by qPCR. Relative to GFP controls, SMO^{M2}-expressing cNCCs exhibited increased expression of multiple pericyte-associated genes, including *Foxc1*, *Foxd1*, *Foxf2*, *Cd248*, *Cspg4*, *Lama2*,

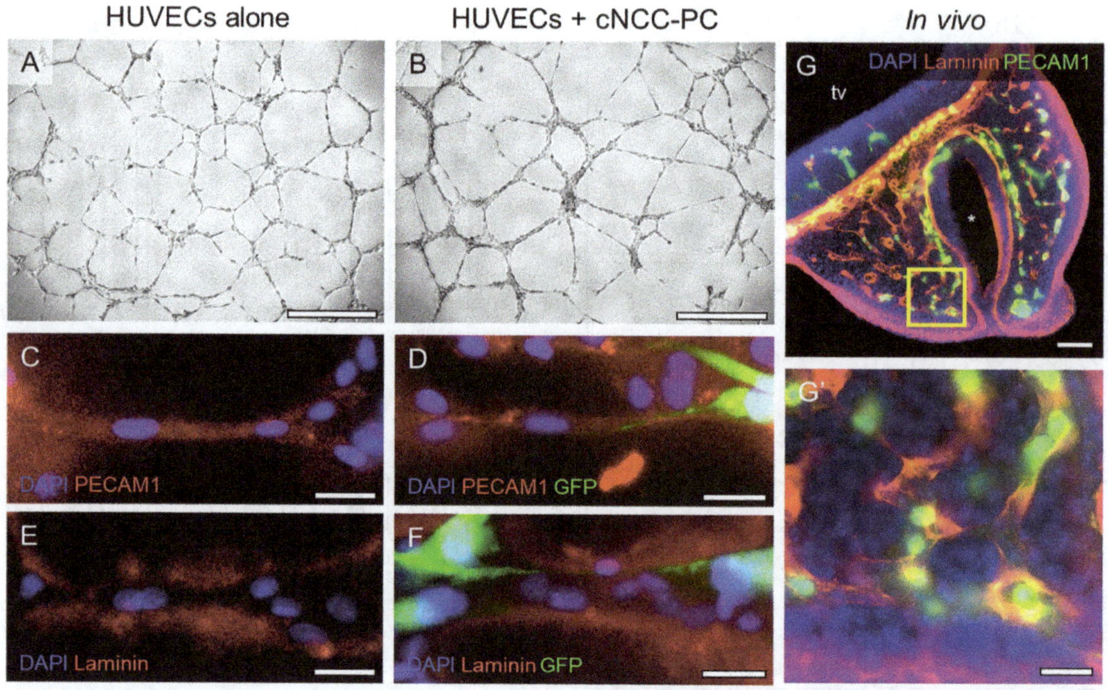

FIGURE 4 | cNCC-derived pericytes interact with endothelial cell cords. **(A,B)** Phase contrast images of HUVECs alone or HUVECs with GFP-expressing pericyte-differentiated cNCCs (cNCC-PC) plated at a ratio of 8:1 on Matrigel for 8 h. Scale bar is 500 μm. **(C–F)** Cords were stained for PECAM1 to mark endothelial cells or for the extracellular matrix protein Laminin. GFP marks cNCC-PC, and DAPI was used to stain nuclei. Scale bars are 25 μm. **(G)** A 50-μm coronal section from a control GD11 embryo head was stained for PECAM1 and Laminin to visualize the microvasculature. tv, telencephalic vesicle, * indicates the nasal pit. Scale bar is 100 μm. **(G')** A higher magnification image of the field indicated by the box in the medial nasal process in **(G)**. Scale bar is 25 μm.

and *Tbx18*. SMO^{M2}-expressing pericyte-differentiated cNCCs also exhibited increased expression of pro-angiogenic factor *Angpt1* and decreased expression of anti-angiogenic factor *Edn1* (**Figure 5E**).

cNCC-Autonomous Shh Pathway Activation Promotes Cord Stability

We next examined whether pericyte-differentiated cNCC-autonomous Shh pathway activation impacts endothelial cord formation or stability. HUVECs were co-cultured on Matrigel with control cNCC-GFP-PC or Shh pathway-activated cNCC-SMO-PC and imaged at 12 and 22 h (**Supplementary Figure 3**). At 12 h, there was a significant difference in only the number of segments between the two co-cultures (**Figure 6E**). By 22 h, however, the cord networks in the control co-culture had begun to dissociate while the cord networks in Shh-pathway-activated co-culture remained mostly intact (**Figures 6A–D**). At 22 h, the number of segments, number of branches, total mesh area, and mean mesh size were significantly greater in co-cultures with cNCC-SMO-PC compared to co-cultures with cNCC-GFP-PC (**Figures 6E–H**).

DISCUSSION

Attenuated outgrowth of the midfacial primordia has long been recognized as a morphological mechanism of OFCs. However, relatively little attention has been given to understanding the role of angiogenesis and microvascular biology in facial morphogenesis and cleft pathogenesis. Here, we present evidence suggesting that Shh signaling promotes pericyte-like function in cNCCs and that this activity is necessary for microvascular stability and proper facial morphogenesis. We found that outgrowth of the MNPs is accompanied by dense microvasculature and that both microvascular patterning and outgrowth are disrupted by Shh pathway inhibition in a mouse model of cleft lip. In an *in vitro* co-culture model recapitulating direct interaction of cNCC-derived pericytes and endothelial cells, we found that cNCC-autonomous Shh pathway activation was sufficient to promote cord stability. Together, these findings suggest a previously unrecognized role for Shh signaling in facial development and highlight pericyte-endothelial signaling and microvascular biology as new areas of investigation in OFC etiology and pathogenesis.

Disruption of angiogenesis, which is required for tissue outgrowth by providing oxygen and nutrients, has previously been linked to birth defect pathogenesis. For example, thalidomide-induced limb truncations have been reported to result from direct disruption of angiogenesis, where the perturbation of microvascular morphogenesis was found to precede changes in tissue patterning, cell proliferation, and cell death, during proximal-distal limb outgrowth (Therapontos et al., 2009). More recently, conditional deletion of *Vegfa* in cNCCs was shown to cause cleft palate in the mouse, supporting

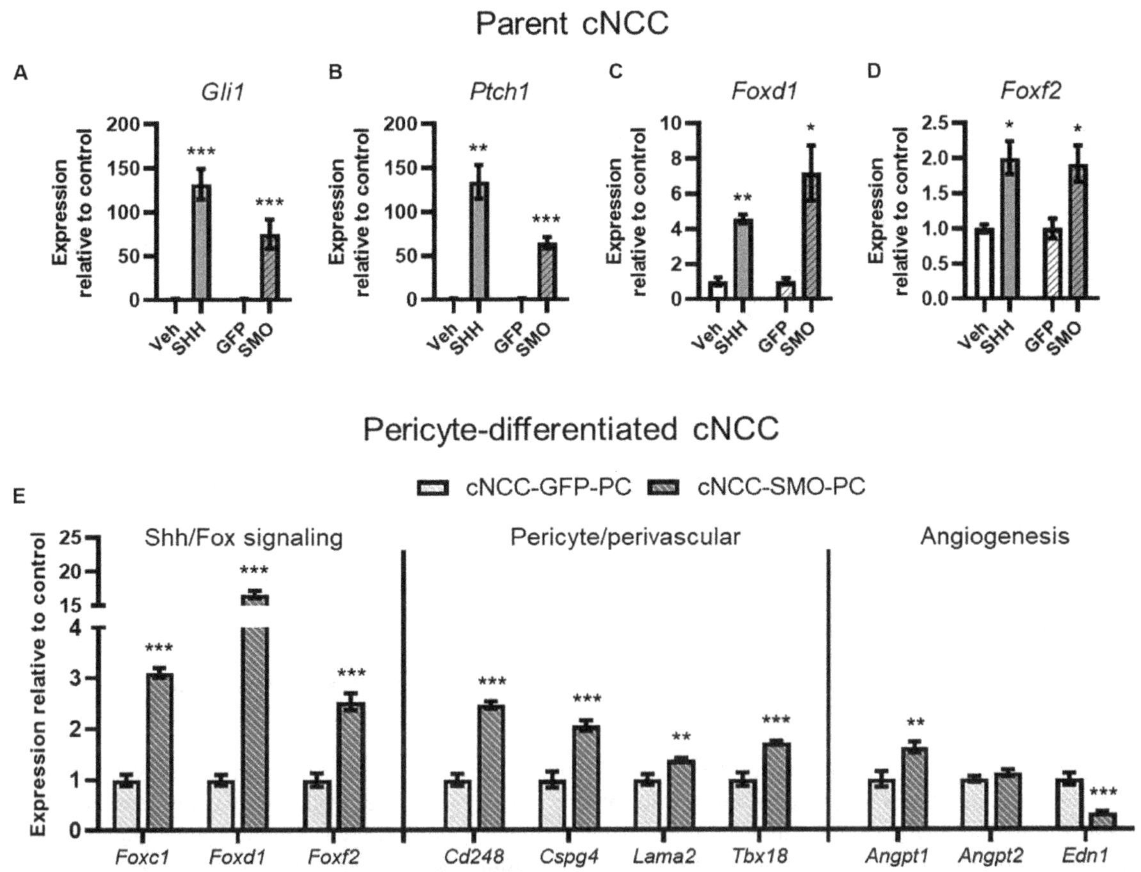

FIGURE 5 | cNCC-autonomous Shh pathway activation increases pericyte-associated gene expression. **(A–D)** SHH ligand treatment or expression of the constitutively active SMO^{M2} (SMO) induces expression of Shh target genes *Gli1* and *Ptch1* in addition to Shh pathway-regulated Forkhead box transcription factor (Fox) genes. **(E)** Shh/Fox genes, pericyte/perivascular genes, and angiogenic genes are regulated by cNCC-autonomous Shh pathway activation in pericyte-differentiated cNCCs. Five biological replicates were analyzed for all groups. $^{*}p < 0.05$, $^{**}p < 0.01$, and $^{***}p < 0.001$ compared to respective control group.

the premise that disrupted angiogenesis can specifically cause OFCs (Hill et al., 2015). In addition, angiogenic gene expression has been found to be altered in animal models and in patients with OFCs (François-Fiquet et al., 2014; Francois et al., 2017; Everson et al., 2018). The high frequency of cardiovascular abnormalities in patients with OFCs may also support the relevance of angiogenic and vascular dysfunction as an underlying mechanism (Milerad et al., 1997; Sekhon et al., 2011).

During upper lip morphogenesis, we identified a dense microvascular plexus at the distal end of the MNP, which normally extends to make contact and fuse with the MxP to close the upper lip (**Figure 1**). Using an inducible lineage tracing model, we found previously that SHH-responsive cells during the critical period for cleft lip (GD8.75) populate this distal aspect of the MNP (**Supplementary Figure 4**; Ansen-Wilson et al., 2018). Here, we show that the microvasculature in this region of the MNP is also disrupted after Shh pathway inhibition (**Figure 2**). This effect on the microvasculature appeared specific to the distal aspect of the MNP and exclusive to animals with cleft lip resulting from attenuated outgrowth of the MNP. These observations link Shh signaling to both microvascular morphogenesis and tissue outgrowth during upper lip development. Notably, disrupted microvasculature and tissue deficiency identified at GD11 follow Shh pathway inhibition and disruption of the angiogenic transcriptome previously identified at GD9.25 (Everson et al., 2018). However, elucidating whether microvascular defects are the primary cause of the Shh-mediated craniofacial malformation will require further investigation.

The Shh pathway is known to regulate vasculogenesis, angiogenesis, and vascular stability in various aspects of development, wound healing, and tumor formation (Chapouly et al., 2019). During facial development, we propose that, rather than acting directly on endothelial cells, Shh signals through cNCC-derived pericytes, which interact with endothelial cells and maintain microvascular stability. Our results indicate that HUVECs, a cell type commonly used to model endothelial cell function, do not respond directly to Shh pathway modulation. However, cNCC-autonomous Shh pathway activation led to increased expression of pericyte-associated genes and other pro-angiogenic transcriptional responses (**Figure 5**) and significantly delayed the degeneration of microvessel-like cords in culture (**Figure 6**).

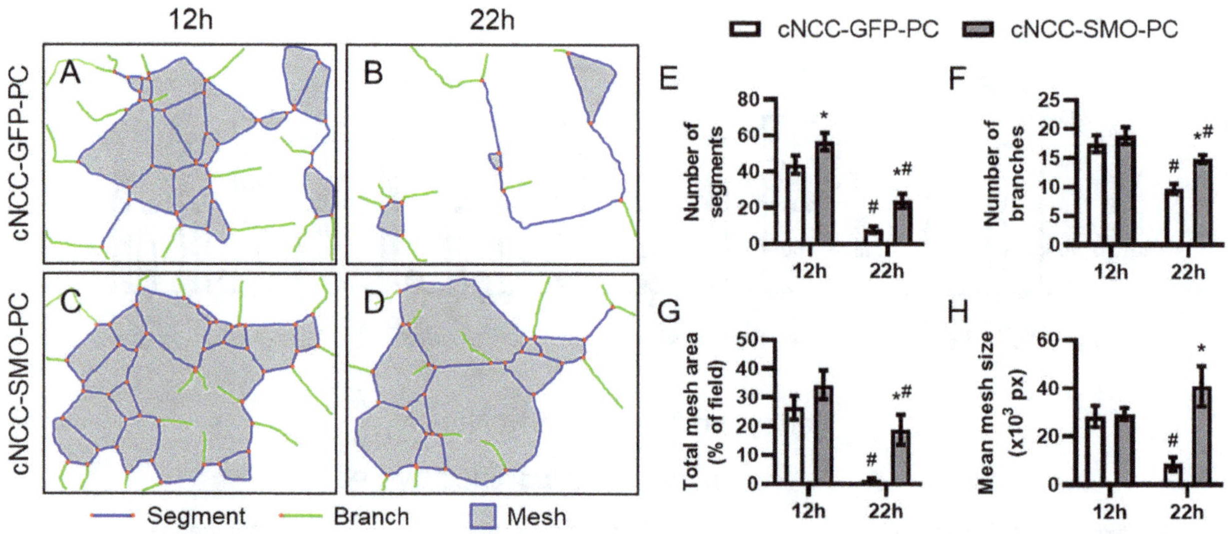

FIGURE 6 | Cell-autonomous Shh pathway activation in cNCC-derived pericytes promotes endothelial cord stability. **(A–D)** Cord network schematics of HUVEC and control cNCC-GFP-PC or Shh pathway-activated cNCC-SMO-PC co-cultures were generated from images taken at 12 and 22 h. Blue lines are segments, green lines are branches, red dots are junctions, and filled gray areas are meshes. Images are representative of 11 biological replicates per group. **(E–H)** Number of segments, number of branches, total mesh area, and mean mesh size were measured by the Angiogenesis plugin for ImageJ for the indicated groups at 12 and 22 h. $^{*}p < 0.05$ between co-cultures at the same time point, $^{\#}p < 0.05$ of the indicated co-culture at 22 h compared to the same co-culture at 12 h.

Pericytes have been increasingly recognized to play a critical role in regulating endothelial cell biology as well as microvascular morphology and homeostasis (Armulik et al., 2011). Lineage tracing studies have shown that, while trunk pericytes are mesoderm-derived, pericyte populations in the head are derived from cNCCs (Etchevers et al., 2001). Although cNCC-derived pericytes of the blood-brain barrier and retina have received substantial research attention, little is known about the molecular drivers of their differentiation in the facial primordia and the role that pericytes play in facial morphogenesis. Expression of the Forkhead box transcription factor (Fox) family genes *Foxc1* and *Foxf2* has been found in brain pericytes and has been shown to be critical for pericyte differentiation and function (Siegenthaler et al., 2013; Reyahi et al., 2015), while lineage tracing has found that *Foxd1*-expressing cells give rise to pericytes in the developing kidney (Gomez and Duffield, 2014). In craniofacial morphogenesis, SHH peptide secreted from the facial ectoderm produces a gradient of target gene expression, including *Foxd1* and *Foxf2*, in the cNCC mesenchyme, with strong and apparent ubiquitous expression nearest the ectoderm (Everson et al., 2017; Fink et al., 2018). Here, we found that Shh pathway activation in cNCCs leads to increased expression of *Foxc1*, *Foxd1*, and *Foxf2* and promotion of pericyte-like activity. Activation of Fox transcription factors in cNCCs may therefore be common drivers of pericyte differentiation and/or function, though it is likely that they act in concert with additional factors secreted by endothelial cells – a premise supported by recent findings that signaling from the endothelium also drive pericyte differentiation (Brandt et al., 2019; Niimi et al., 2019).

Our limited knowledge of pericyte-endothelial biology in facial development stems, at least in part, from paucity of reliable pericyte markers. Pericytes and pericyte-like cells have been reported to express numerous gene products that are classically associated with vascular homeostasis as well as other genes that may serve as important endothelial-pericyte signals including *Pdgfrβ*, *Cspg4*, *Tbx18*, *Rgs5*, *Nestin*, *Lama2*, and *Cd248* (Cho et al., 2003; MacFadyen et al., 2005; Murfee et al., 2005; Armulik et al., 2011; Menezes et al., 2014; De La Fuente et al., 2017; Guimarães-Camboa et al., 2017). However, the most commonly employed marker for pericyte populations, *Pdgfrβ*, is ubiquitously expressed in cNCCs, and several of these markers are expressed in other cell populations, including vascular smooth muscle and even endothelial cells themselves (Guimarães-Camboa et al., 2017; Stebbins et al., 2019). We show that Shh pathway activation in cNCCs leads to increased expression of several presumptive pericyte markers, including *Cspg4*, *Cd248*, *Lama2*, and *Tbx18* (**Figure 5**). Determining the fidelity and specificity of these genes as markers of cNCC-derived pericytes is an important area of future investigation that could drive new approaches to examining the role of pericytes in craniofacial morphogenesis, tissue healing, and repair.

The study of cleft lip pathogenesis has historically focused on proliferation and apoptosis during tissue outgrowth and fusion. Here, we provide evidence that microvascular morphogenesis may be an underlying OFC mechanism and warrants further investigation. While Shh signaling is known to be crucial in craniofacial morphogenesis, our findings point to a previously unrecognized role for Shh signaling in pericyte-endothelial cell interaction where perivascular Shh signaling promotes microvascular stability. Disruption of Shh signaling may therefore interfere with pericyte differentiation and function, leading to microvascular dysfunction, a lack of tissue outgrowth, and cleft of the upper lip. These findings support microvascular morphogenesis as a novel focus for the role of Shh in birth defects as well as for understanding the etiology of structural birth defects more generally.

ETHICS STATEMENT

The animal study was reviewed and approved by the University of Wisconsin–Madison, School of Veterinary Medicine Institutional Care and Use Committee.

AUTHOR CONTRIBUTIONS

RL and MRS conceived the studies and wrote the manuscript. MRS, HC, MJS, SP, ES, and RL designed the methodology. MRS, HC, VM, and DF conducted the experiments and acquired and analyzed the data. All authors contributed to the article and approved the submitted version.

ACKNOWLEDGMENTS

The authors are grateful to Benjamin Gastfriend for sharing technical expertise and review of the manuscript. The authors also thank Kenneth Rivera-González, Austin Steward, and Tyler Beames for their critical review of the manuscript.

REFERENCES

Alvarez, J. I., Dodelet-Devillers, A., Kebir, H., Ifergan, I., Fabre, P. J., Terouz, S., et al. (2011). The Hedgehog pathway promotes blood-brain barrier integrity and CNS immune quiescence. *Science* 334, 1727–1731. doi: 10.1126/science.1206936

Ansen-Wilson, L. J., Everson, J. L., Fink, D. M., Kietzman, H. W., Sullivan, R., and Lipinski, R. J. (2018). Common basis for orofacial clefting and cortical interneuronopathy. *Transl. Psychiatry* 8, 8.

Armulik, A., Abramsson, A., and Betsholtz, C. (2005). Endothelial/pericyte interactions. *Circ. Res.* 97, 512–523. doi: 10.1161/01.res.0000182903.16652.d7

Armulik, A., Genové, G., and Betsholtz, C. (2011). Pericytes: developmental, physiological, and pathological perspectives, problems, and promises. *Dev. Cell* 21, 193–215. doi: 10.1016/j.devcel.2011.07.001

Brandt, M., van Dijk, C., Maringanti, R., Chrifi, I., Kramann, R., Verhaar, M., et al. (2019). Transcriptome analysis reveals microvascular endothelial cell-dependent pericyte differentiation. *Sci. Rep.* 9:15586.

Brown, L., Foster, C., Courtney, J., King, N., Howells, D., and Sutherland, B. (2019). Pericytes and neurovascular function in the healthy and diseased brain. *Front. Cell. Neurosci.* 13:282. doi: 10.3389/fncel.2019.00282

Bush, J. O., and Jiang, R. (2012). Palatogenesis: morphogenetic and molecular mechanisms of secondary palate development. *Development* 139, 231. doi: 10.1242/dev.067082

Chapouly, C., Guimbal, S., Hollier, P. L., and Renault, M. A. (2019). Role of hedgehog signaling in vasculature development, differentiation, and maintenance. *Int. J. Mol. Sci.* 20:3076. doi: 10.3390/ijms20123076

Cho, H., Kozasa, T., Bondjers, C., Betsholtz, C., and Kehrl, J. H. (2003). Pericyte-specific expression of Rgs5: implications for PDGF and EDG receptor signaling during vascular maturation. *FASEB J.* 17, 440–442.

De La Fuente, A. G., Lange, S., Silva, M. E., Gonzalez, G. A., Tempfer, H., van Wijngaarden, P., et al. (2017). Pericytes stimulate oligodendrocyte progenitor cell differentiation during CNS remyelination. *Cell Rep.* 20, 1755–1764. doi: 10.1016/j.celrep.2017.08.007

Etchevers, H. C., Vincent, C., Le Douarin, N. M., and Couly, G. F. (2001). The cephalic neural crest provides pericytes and smooth muscle cells to all blood vessels of the face and forebrain. *Development* 128, 1059–1068.

Everson, J. L., Fink, D. M., Chung, H. M., Sun, M. R., and Lipinski, R. J. (2018). Identification of sonic hedgehog-regulated genes and biological processes in the cranial neural crest mesenchyme by comparative transcriptomics. *BMC Genomics* 19:497. doi: 10.1186/s12864-018-4885-5

Everson, J. L., Fink, D. M., Yoon, J. W., Leslie, E. J., Kietzman, H. W., Ansen-Wilson, L. J., et al. (2017). Sonic hedgehog regulation of Foxf2 promotes cranial neural crest mesenchyme proliferation and is disrupted in cleft lip morphogenesis. *Development* 144, 2082–2091. doi: 10.1242/dev.149930

Fink, D. M., Sun, M. R., Heyne, G. W., Everson, J. L., Chung, H. M., Park, S., et al. (2018). Coordinated d-cyclin/Foxd1 activation drives mitogenic activity of the Sonic Hedgehog signaling pathway. *Cell. Signal.* 44, 1–9. doi: 10.1016/j.cellsig.2017.12.007

Francois, C., Poli-Merol, M. L., Tournois, C., Cornillet-Lefebvre, P., Guillard, T., Djerada, Z., et al. (2017). New in vivo model to analyse the expression of angiogenic genes in the borders of a cleft lip. *Br. J. Oral Maxillofac. Surg.* 55, 488–495. doi: 10.1016/j.bjoms.2017.01.018

François-Fiquet, C., Poli-Merol, M. L., Nguyen, P., Landais, E., Gaillard, D., and Doco-Fenzy, M. (2014). Role of angiogenesis-related genes in cleft lip/palate: review of the literature. *Int. J. Pediatr. Otorhinolaryngol.* 78, 1579–1585. doi: 10.1016/j.ijporl.2014.08.001

Gomez, I. G., and Duffield, J. S. (2014). The FOXD1 lineage of kidney perivascular cells and myofibroblasts: functions and responses to injury. *Kidney Int. Suppl.* 4, 26–33. doi: 10.1038/kisup.2014.6

Guimarães-Camboa, N., Cattaneo, P., Sun, Y., Moore-Morris, T., Gu, Y., Dalton, N. D., et al. (2017). Pericytes of multiple organs do not behave as mesenchymal stem cells in vivo. *Cell Stem Cell* 20, 345.e–359.e.

Heyne, G. W., Melberg, C. G., Doroodchi, P., Parins, K. F., Kietzman, H. W., Everson, J. L., et al. (2015a). Definition of critical periods for Hedgehog pathway antagonist-induced holoprosencephaly, cleft lip, and cleft palate. *PLoS One* 10:e0120517. doi: 10.1371/journal.pone.0120517

Heyne, G. W., Plisch, E. H., Melberg, C. G., Sandgren, E. P., Peter, J. A., and Lipinski, R. J. (2015b). A simple and reliable method for early pregnancy detection in inbred mice. *J. Am. Assoc. Lab. Anim. Sci.* 54, 368–371.

Hill, C., Jacobs, B., Kennedy, L., Rohde, S., Zhou, B., Baldwin, S., et al. (2015). Cranial neural crest deletion of VEGFa causes cleft palate with aberrant vascular and bone development. *Cell Tissue Res.* 361, 711–722. doi: 10.1007/s00441-015-2150-7

Ishii, M., Arias, A. C., Liu, L., Chen, Y. B., Bronner, M. E., and Maxson, R. E. (2012). A stable cranial neural crest cell line from mouse. *Stem Cells Dev.* 21, 3069–3080. doi: 10.1089/scd.2012.0155

Jeong, J., Mao, J., Tenzen, T., Kottmann, A. H., and McMahon, A. P. (2004). Hedgehog signaling in the neural crest cells regulates the patterning and growth of facial primordia. *Genes Dev.* 18, 937–951. doi: 10.1101/gad.1190304

Jiang, X., Iseki, S., Maxson, R. E., Sucov, H. M., and Morriss-Kay, G. M. (2002). Tissue origins and interactions in the mammalian skull vault. *Dev. Biol.* 241, 106–116. doi: 10.1006/dbio.2001.0487

Kurosaka, H. (2015). The roles of hedgehog signaling in upper lip formation. *Biomed. Res. Int.* 2015:901041.

Lipinski, R. J., Hutson, P. R., Hannam, P. W., Nydza, R. J. I, Washington, M., Moore, R. W., et al. (2008). Dose-and route-dependent teratogenicity, toxicity, and pharmacokinetic profiles of the hedgehog signaling antagonist cyclopamine in the mouse. *Toxicol. sci.* 104, 189–197. doi: 10.1093/toxsci/kfn076

Lipinski, R. J., Song, C., Sulik, K. K., Everson, J. L., Gipp, J. J., Yan, D., et al. (2010). Cleft lip and palate results from Hedgehog signaling antagonism in the mouse:

phenotypic characterization and clinical implications. *Birth Defects Res. A Clin. Mol. Teratol.* 88, 232–240.

MacFadyen, J. R., Haworth, O., Roberston, D., Hardie, D., Webster, M. T., Morris, H. R., et al. (2005). Endosialin (TEM1, CD248) is a marker of stromal fibroblasts and is not selectively expressed on tumour endothelium. *FEBS Lett.* 579, 2569–2575. doi: 10.1016/j.febslet.2005.03.071

Machado, M. V., and Diehl, A. M. (2018). Hedgehog signalling in liver pathophysiology. *J. Hepatol.* 68, 550–562. doi: 10.1016/j.jhep.2017.10.017

Menezes, M. J., McClenahan, F. K., Leiton, C. V., Aranmolate, A., Shan, X., and Colognato, H. (2014). The extracellular matrix protein laminin α2 regulates the maturation and function of the blood–brain barrier. *J. Neurosci.* 34, 15260–15280. doi: 10.1523/jneurosci.3678-13.2014

Milerad, J., Larson, O., PhD, D., Hagberg, C., and Ideberg, M. (1997). Associated malformations in infants with cleft lip and palate: a prospective, population-based study. *Pediatrics* 100, 180–186. doi: 10.1542/peds.100.2.180

Murfee, W. L., Skalak, T. C., and Peirce, S. M. (2005). Differential arterial/venous expression of NG2 proteoglycan in perivascular cells along microvessels: identifying a venule-specific phenotype. *Microcirculation* 12, 151–160. doi: 10.1080/10739680590904955

Niimi, K., Adachi, Y., Ishikawa, H., Yamaguchi, W., Kubota, Y., Inagaki, S., et al. (2019). Endothelial specific deletion of FOXO1 alters pericyte coverage in the developing retina. *Biochem. Biophys. Res. Commun.* 520, 304–310. doi: 10.1016/j.bbrc.2019.10.040

Renault, M. A., Roncalli, J., Tongers, J., Thorne, T., Klyachko, E., Misener, S., et al. (2010). Sonic hedgehog induces angiogenesis via Rho kinase-dependent signaling in endothelial cells. *J. Mol. Cell Cardiol.* 49, 490–498. doi: 10.1016/j.yjmcc.2010.05.003

Reyahi, A., Nik, A. M., Ghiami, M., Gritli-Linde, A., Pontén, F., Johansson, B. R., et al. (2015). Foxf2 is required for brain pericyte differentiation and development and maintenance of the blood-brain barrier. *Dev. Cell* 34, 19–32. doi: 10.1016/j.devcel.2015.05.008

Roessler, E., Belloni, E., Gaudenz, K., Jay, P., Berta, P., Scherer, S. W., et al. (1996). Mutations in the human sonic hedgehog gene cause holoprosencephaly. *Nat. Genet.* 14, 357–360. doi: 10.1038/ng1196-357

Roessler, E., Du, Y. Z., Mullor, J. L., Casas, E., Allen, W. P., Gillessen-Kaesbach, G., et al. (2003). Loss-of-function mutations in the human GLI2 gene are associated with pituitary anomalies and holoprosencephaly-like features. *Proc. Natl. Acad. Sci. U.S.A.* 100, 13424–13429. doi: 10.1073/pnas.2235734100

Santos, G., Prazeres, P., Mintz, A., and Birbrair, A. (2018). Role of pericytes in the retina. *Eye* 32, 483–486. doi: 10.1038/eye.2017.220

Sekhon, P. S., Ethunandan, M., Markus, A. F., Krishnan, G., and Rao, C. B. (2011). Congenital anomalies associated with cleft lip and palate-an analysis of 1623 consecutive patients. *Cleft. Palate. Craniofac. J.* 48, 371–378. doi: 10.1597/09-264

Siegenthaler, J. A., Choe, Y., Patterson, K. P., Hsieh, I., Li, D., Jaminet, S. C., et al. (2013). Foxc1 is required by pericytes during fetal brain angiogenesis. *Biol. Open* 2, 647–659. doi: 10.1242/bio.20135009

Stebbins, M. J., Gastfriend, B. D., Canfield, S. G., Lee, M.-S., Richards, D., Faubion, M. G., et al. (2019). Human pluripotent stem cell–derived brain pericyte–like cells induce blood-brain barrier properties. *Sci. Adv.* 5:eaau7375. doi: 10.1126/sciadv.aau7375

Therapontos, C., Erskine, L., Gardner, E. R., Figg, W. D., and Vargesson, N. (2009). Thalidomide induces limb defects by preventing angiogenic outgrowth during early limb formation. *Proc Natl Acad Sci U S A.* 106, 8573–8578. doi: 10.1073/pnas.0901505106

Trost, A., Lange, S., Schroedl, F., Bruckner, D., Motloch, K. A., Bogner, B., et al. (2016). Brain and retinal pericytes: origin, function and role. *Front. Cell Neurosci.* 10:20. doi: 10.3389/fncel.2016.00020

Watkins, S. E., Meyer, R. E., Strauss, R. P., and Aylsworth, A. S. (2014). Classification, epidemiology, and genetics of orofacial clefts. *Clin. Plast. Surg.* 41, 149–163. doi: 10.1016/j.cps.2013.12.003

Wehby, G. L., and Cassell, C. H. (2010). The impact of orofacial clefts on quality of life and healthcare use and costs. *Oral Dis.* 16, 3–10. doi: 10.1111/j.1601-0825.2009.01588.x

Yu, Y., Zuo, X., He, M., Gao, J., Fu, Y., Qin, C., et al. (2017). Genome-wide analyses of non-syndromic cleft lip with palate identify 14 novel loci and genetic heterogeneity. *Nat. Commun.* 8:14364.

10

Association Study of Genetic Variants in Autophagy Pathway and Risk of Non-syndromic Cleft Lip with or without Cleft Palate

Shu Lou[1,2†], Lan Ma[1,3†], Shiyi Kan[1,2†], Xin Yu[1,2], Yuting Wang[1,2], Fan Yang[1,2], Guirong Zhu[1,2], Liwen Fan[1,2], Dandan Li[1,2], Hua Wang[1,2], Wei Wang[1,2], Weibing Zhang[1,2], Lin Wang[1,2,4*] and Yongchu Pan[1,2,4*]

[1] Jiangsu Key Laboratory of Oral Diseases, Nanjing Medical University, Nanjing, China, [2] Department of Orthodontics, Affiliated Hospital of Stomatology, Nanjing Medical University, Nanjing, China, [3] Department of Environmental Genomics, School of Public Health, Nanjing Medical University, Nanjing, China, [4] State Key Laboratory of Reproductive Medicine, Nanjing Medical University, Nanjing, China

***Correspondence:**
Lin Wang
lw603@njmu.edu.cn
Yongchu Pan
panyongchu@njmu.edu.cn

† These authors have contributed equally to this work

Although genetic variants in autophagy pathway genes were associated with the risk of oral cancers and early development in embryos, their associations with non-syndromic cleft lip with or without cleft palate (NSCL/P) risk remained unclear. A two-stage case-control study (2,027 NSCL/P cases and 1,843 controls) was performed to investigate the associations between single nucleotide polymorphisms (SNPs) in 23 autophagy pathway genes and NSCL/P susceptibility. The logistic regression model was used to calculate effects of SNPs on NSCL/P susceptibility. Gene-based analysis was performed via the sequence kernel association test (SKAT) and multi-marker analysis of genomic annotation (MAGMA) methods. Expression quantitative trait loci (eQTL) analysis was conducted using NSCL/P lip tissue samples. Gene expression during embryonic development was evaluated using RNA-Seq. Functional roles were explored by luciferase activity assay, cell apoptosis, proliferation, and cycle *in vitro*. Rs2301104 in *HIF1A* was significantly associated with NSCL/P susceptibility in the combined analysis (OR: 1.29, 95% CI: 1.09–1.29, $P = 3.39 \times 10^{-03}$), and showed strong evidence of association heterogeneity ($P = 9.06 \times 10^{-03}$) with obvious association in the female (OR: 1.80; 95% CI: 1.32–2.45; $P = 1.79 \times 10^{-04}$). The G allele of rs2301104 was associated with enhanced transcription activity and high expression of *HIF1A* compared with that of C allele. Moreover, rs2301104 exhibited an eQTL effect for *HIF1A* with its GC/CC genotypes associated with decreased *HIF1A* expression compared with those with GG genotypes ($P = 3.1 \times 10^{-2}$). Knockdown of *HIF1A* induced cell apoptosis and inhibited cell proliferation in human embryonic palate mesenchyme (HEPM) and human oral epithelium cells (HOEC). This study demonstrated that rs2301104 in autophagy pathway gene *HIF1A* was associated with susceptibility of NSCL/P.

Keywords: autophagy, non-syndromic cleft lip with or without cleft palate, single nucleotide polymorphism, molecular genetics, *HIF1A*

INTRODUCTION

Non-syndromic cleft lip with or without cleft palate (NSCL/P) is one of the most common human birth defects contributing huge health and financial burdens to the affected individuals, families, and societies (Mangold et al., 2010; Heike and Evans, 2016). It occurs in ~1 in 700 live births worldwide, with prevalence varying by population (Birnbaum et al., 2009).

The occurrence of NSCL/P results from failure of the facial processes to grow or fuse appropriately during early embryologic development (between the 4th and 12th week of gestation) (Beaty et al., 2016; Li et al., 2017). Signaling pathways, including Bmp, Fgf, Shh, and Wnt signaling pathways, are critical for proper lip fusion (Jiang et al., 2006). Similarly, the growth of the palatal shelves is also mediated by epithelial-mesenchymal interactions regulated by multiple signaling pathways and transcriptional factors (Lan et al., 2015). Cell migration, proliferation, and apoptosis in both epithelial cells and cranial neural crest (CNC)-derived mesenchymal cells are involved in mechanisms leading to cleft lip and palate (Tian et al., 2017).

The underlying etiology is complex and multifactorial with a wide range of influences including genetic and environmental factors. Extensive human genetic studies and animal studies have attempted to identify the genetic variants associated with NSCL/P risk (Leslie et al., 2016; Hammond et al., 2018; Reynolds et al., 2019). For instance, Leslie et al. (2016) conducted a multiethnic genome-wide association study in 6480 participants and revealed novel associations on 2p24 near *FAM49A*, and 19q13 near *RHPN2*. Hammond et al. demonstrated that ectopic Hh-Smo signaling downregulates Wnt/BMP pathways, resulting in cleft palate and defective osteogenesis (Hammond et al., 2018).

As a conserved lysosomal degradation process in eukaryotes, autophagy prevents cells from different kinds of stress, such as starvation, hypoxia, or exposure to toxic molecules (Huang and Klionsky, 2007). Defective autophagy is related to physiological and pathological conditions, such as cancer, metabolic, neurodegenerative disease, and aging (Netea-Maier et al., 2016). In the early development stage, autophagy has been shown to be essential in the transition of oocytes to embryos, postpartum survival, development, differentiation and aging in mouse models (Hale et al., 2013). Additionally, autophagy degrades cytoplasmic components, which is vital for embryonic development and human health (Fenouille et al., 2017). Susceptible genes may play essential roles in cell death and inflammation by influencing autophagy in neighboring cells during developmental periods (Lin et al., 2017). Previous studies showed that single nucleotide polymorphisms (SNPs) in autophagy pathway genes were related to the risk of melanoma, neck squamous cell carcinoma, and early embryo development (Capela et al., 2016; White et al., 2016; Fernandez-Mateos et al., 2017), however, their associations with the risk of NSCL/P have never been explored.

Highlighting these bases, with the aim of exploring associations between genetic variants in autophagy pathway and the risk of NSCL/P, we conducted a two-stage case-control study with 2,027 NSCL/P cases and 1,843 controls in the present study. We finally found that rs2301104 in autophagy pathway gene *HIF1A* was associated with susceptibility of NSCL/P. Moreover, we explored the functional roles of the SNP and the gene with *in vivo* and *in vitro* experiments. Our study provides a deeper insight into the roles of autophagy pathway-related genetic variants in the development of NSCL/P.

MATERIALS AND METHODS

Selection of Genes and SNPs From the Autophagy Pathway

The key autophagy associated genes were selected from the Kyoto Encyclopedia of Genes and Genomes (KEGG) and published studies. We obtained 109 genes from the autophagy pathway included in KEGG (map04140), and the following key words were used to search PubMed for publications on or before September 30th, 2018: gene name and craniofacial, craniofacial development, or facial development. Finally, 23 genes related to autophagy and craniofacial development were kept for further analysis (**Supplementary Figure 1** and **Supplementary Table 1**).

The flow chart of selecting putative functional SNPs based on 23 genes we selected is shown in **Figure 1**. First, a total of 27,240 SNPs in gene regions was selected using the CHB data from the 1000 Genomes Project (Phase I, March 2012) and 3,156 SNPs remained after the following quality control criteria (Wang et al., 2019; Zhu et al., 2019): (a) minor allele frequency (MAF) $\geq$ 0.05, (b) Hardy-Weinberg equilibrium (HWE) $\geq$ 0.05, and (c) call rate $\geq$ 95%. Second, we used RegulomeDB and HaploReg to predict SNP functions. SNPs with Regulome DB Score below five and predicted to hit eQTL effects or bind transcription factors from HaploReg database were retained. Besides, SNPs with pairwise linkage disequilibrium (LD) $r^2 \geq 0.5$ were excluded using PLINK 1.09. Finally, a total of 146 putative functional SNPs in 23 autophagy pathway genes were identified and further explored in a two-stage case-control study.

Study Participants

We performed a two-stage case-control analysis of NSCL/P in the Chinese Han population. Two stages were totally independent from each other: the stage I was comprised of 504 NSCL/P cases, and 455 newborn controls who were recruited from West China Hospital of Stomatology Sichuan University and the stage II included 1,523 NSCL/P cases and 1,388 controls who were recruited from Affiliated Stomatological Hospital of Nanjing Medical University, Nanjing Children's Hospital, Xuzhou First People's Hospital, and Huai'an First People's Hospital (**Supplementary Table 2**).

All patients were interviewed and clinically evaluated by an experienced oral surgeon based on detailed diagnostic information from medical records and physical examinations to ensure that individuals with other congenital anomalies, identified CL/P syndromes or developmental delays were excluded from this study. Venous blood samples were collected from all subjects for genetic analysis. The present study was approved by the Ethics Committee of Nanjing Medical University [NJMUERC (2008) No. 20]. At recruitment, informed written consent was obtained from all the participants or their guardians.

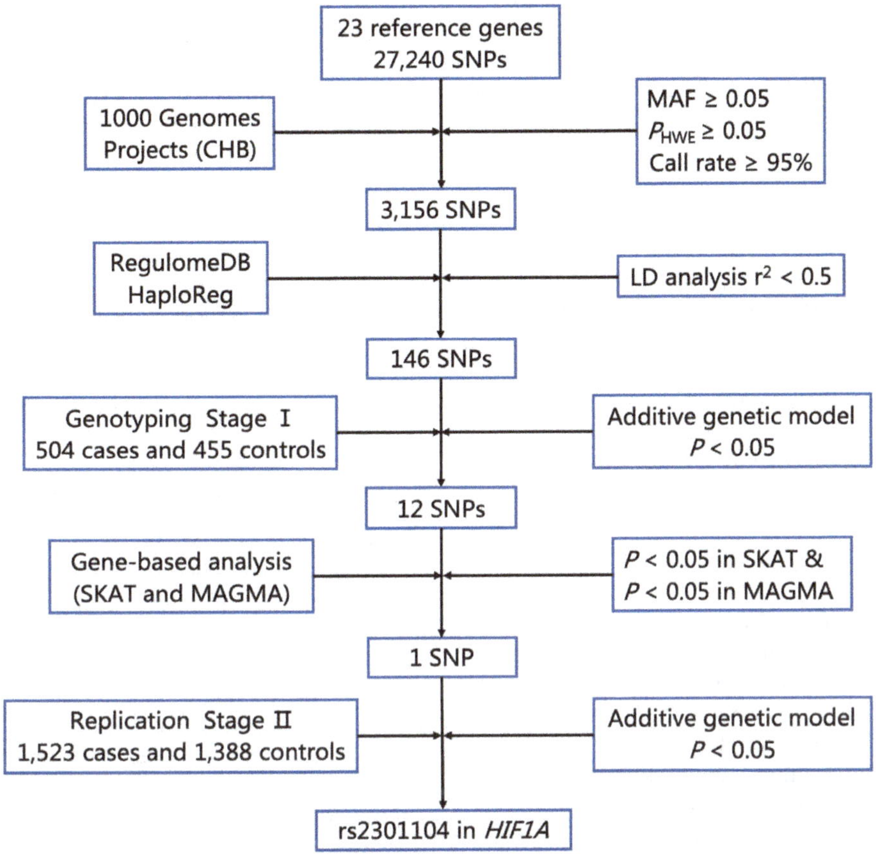

FIGURE 1 | Flow chart for selecting putative functional SNP in autophagy pathway genes. MAF, minor allele frequency; HWE, Hardy–Weinberg Equilibrium; LD, linkage disequilibrium.

Genotyping

All samples in stage I were genotyped using Affymetrix Axiom CHB1 & CHB2 arrays. Systematic quality control (Wang et al., 2019; Zhu et al., 2019) was performed to filter SNPs, including $P_{HWE} \geq 0.05$, MAF ≥ 0.05, and call rate $\geq 95\%$. Genotyping in stage II was performed by TaqMan-MGB assays on an ABI-Prism 7900 instrument (Applied Biosystems, Foster City, CA). The primers of the Taqman probes are listed in **Supplementary Table 3**.

Annotations for Candidate SNPs

SNPs were annotated for potential regulatory functions using RegulomeDB[1] and HaploReg v4.1[2]. We also evaluated the SNPs in the integrative analysis of 127 reference human epigenomes based on NIH Roadmap Epigenomics database[3].

Extraction of Mouse Embryo Tissues and RNA-Seq

We purchased six adult male and twelve adult female C57BL/6 mice from Animal Center of Yangzhou University. Two female mice and one male mouse were placed together in the same cage at 8 p.m. and separated at 8 a.m. the next morning. Embryos were counted as E0.5d in the morning that vaginal plug was checked. Lip and palate tissues of E10.5d, E11.5d, E12.5d, E13.5d, E14.5d, and E15.5d embryos were collected. Total RNA was extracted with TRIzol reagent (Invitrogen, Carlsbad, CA, United States) from embryonic tissues of mice, which were approved in quantity and quality by Nanodrop and 1% agarose electrophoresis. mRNA sequencing was performed on Hiseq3000 platform in 10M and 6G depth, respectively. RNA reads were aligned to the mouse genome (MM10) by gSNAP, and the average fragments per kilobase of exon model per million fragments mapped (FPKM) value of all samples was used to normalize mRNA expression.

In silico Gene Expression During Mouse Craniofacial Development and in Human Samples

RNA-Seq data on craniofacial structures during mouse embryo development were downloaded from the FaceBase consortium at FaceBase.org[4], an online database that describes the overall

[1]http://www.regulomedb.org

[2]http://www.broadinstitute.org/mammals/haploreg/haploreg.php

[3]http://www.roadmapepigenomics.org/

[4]https://www.facebase.org/, GSE67985.

gene expression during mouse craniofacial development. Count data were normalized using the regularized logarithmic transformation in the DESeq2 R package.

Gene expression in NSCL/P cases and controls of dental pulp stem cells (DPSCs), and mesenchymal stem cells (MSCs) in lip muscle were obtained from Gene Expression Omnibus (GEO) repository (GSE42589 and GSE85748, respectively).

Cell Culture

The human embryonic palatal mesenchymal (HEPM) cell lines were purchased from American Type Culture Collection (ATCC, Manassas, VA, United States), and cultured in Eagle's Minimum Essential Medium (ATCC), supplemented with 10% fetal bovine serum (FBS, Gibco), 100 units/ml antibiotics at 37°C under 5% CO_2. The human oral epithelial cells (HOEC) were obtained from BeNa Culture Collection (Beijing, China), and cultured in Dulbecco's Modified Eagle Medium (Gibco) supplemented with 10% FBS (Gibco) and 100 units/ml antibiotics and maintained at 37°C under 5% CO_2.

Luciferase Activity Assay

In order to evaluate whether there is a difference in the enhancer activity in *HIF1A* of different alleles, we performed the luciferase activity assay. A sequence of 1,000-bp containing rs2301104 G or C allele and *HIF1A* promoter region were synthesized and cloned into the *Nhe*I and *Xho*I restriction sites of the pGL3-basic vector (Promega). HEPM and HOEC cells were seeded at in 24-well culture plates, and each well was transiently transfected with reporter plasmids using Lipofectamine 2000 (Invitrogen, Carlsbad, CA, United States) according to the manufacturer's instructions. All plasmids were co-transfected with 10 ng pRL-SV40, which contained the *Renilla* luciferase gene. The luciferase activities were measured 48 h after transfection with a dual-luciferase reporter assay system (Promega). The ratio of Firefly luciferase to *Renilla* luciferase activity was assessed. The transfection experiments were performed in triplicate.

RNA Extraction and Quantitative Real-Time PCR

To compare gene expression of cells and tissues with different genotypes, we constructed the pcDNA3.1-rs2301104 G and pcDNA3.1-rs2301104 C vectors, which were transfected into cells and harvested for 48 h. Total RNA was extracted from cells and 68 NSCL/P lip tissue samples to reverse transcription and PCR reactions using PrimeScript™ RT-PCR kit (TaKaRa, Shiga, Japan). The relative mRNA expression level of *HIF1A* and the internal control *GAPDH* were quantified using ABI 7900 Real-Time PCR system (Applied Biosystems). The primers were listed as follows: *HIF1A* (forward: TCAGGACACAGATTTAGACTTGGAG, reverse: AGTGGTAG TGGTGGCATTAGCA) and *GAPDH* (forward: GGACCTGAC CTGCCGTCTAG, reverse: GTAGCCCAGGATGCCCTTGA). All reactions were conducted in triplicate, and the data were analyzed by the $2^{-\Delta\Delta Ct}$ method. Data are shown as the mean ± standard deviations (SD).

Small Interference RNA (siRNA) Constructs and Transfection

The small interference RNA (siRNA) oligonucleotides including *HIF1A* siRNA-378 (5′-CCAGAUCUCGGCGAAGUAATT-3′, 5′-UUACUUCGCCGAGAUCUGGTT-3′), *HIF1A* siRNA-2107 (5′-CCAGCAGACUCAAAUACAATT-3′, 5′-UUGUAUUUGAG UCUGCUGGTT-3′), *HIF1A* siRNA-2637 (5′-GCUACUACAUC ACUUUCUUTT-3′, 5′-AAGAAAGUGAUGUAGUAGCTT-3′) and control siRNA (5′-UUCUCCGAACGUGUCACGUTT-3′, 5′-ACGUGACACGUUCGGAGAATT-3′) were designed and purchased from GenePharma (Shanghai, China). Transfection of siRNAs with final concentration 100 nM was performed with Lipofectamine 2000 (Invitrogen, Carlsbad, CA, United States) following the manufacturer's instructions. Cells were harvested 48 h later for further experiments.

Cell Apoptosis, Cell Cycle, and Cell Proliferation Assay

Cells were treated with trypsin-EDTA (Gibco) and resuspended as single-cell suspension 48 h after transfection. We stained cells with Annexin V:PE Apoptosis Detection Kit (BD Biosciences, San Jose, CA, United States) for cell apoptosis analysis and analyzed using a Fluorescence Activated Cell Sorting (FACS) System by BD Biosciences (San Jose, CA, United States). As for cell cycle analysis, cells were then fixed in 70% ethanol overnight at 4°C after digested. Propidium iodide (PI)/RNase staining was conducted on fixed cells for flow cytometric analysis. Data were analyzed with FlowJo software (TreeStar, Ashland, OR, United States). Cell proliferation was assessed by absorbance using a Cell Counting Kit-8 assay (CCK8, Dojindo, Kumamoto, Japan) according to the manufacturer's instructions. Cells were seeded in 96-well plates at a density of 3×10^3 cells per well, approximately. CCK-8 reaction solution was added into each well for 2 h incubation in new medium containing. The absorbance was measured on a spectrophotometer microplate reader (Multiskan MK3, Thermo) at a wavelength of 450 nm. All data are shown as the mean ± SD.

Statistical Analysis

For evaluating the association between NSCL/P risk and genetic variants, logistic regression analysis under additive model with adjustment for gender was implemented to calculate the crude and adjusted odds ratios (ORs) and their 95% confidence intervals (CIs) (Wang et al., 2016; Zhu et al., 2019). Haplotype analysis were performed using Haploview software with parameters of MAF $\geq$ 5% and pairwise r^2 threshold of 0.8 (Barrett et al., 2005). The epistasis test between SNPs in the candidate gene was performed using R software, which was computed by an unconditional logistic regression model specifies the log-odds as: $\text{logit(P)} = \beta_0 + \beta_G(G_i) + \beta_{G\times G}(G_i{*}G_j)$. Goodness-of-fit Chi-square test was performed to test HWE in control groups. We used the sequence kernel association test (SKAT) (Timbers et al., 2016) and Multi-marker Analysis of GenoMic Annotation (MAGMA) tool (de Leeuw et al., 2015) for gene-based analysis. Combined analysis of two stages was performed using a fixed-effect model in R software (Dai et al., 2019). The measure of heterogeneity was tested using Cochran's Q statistics and I^2. Gene-by-sex (G × S) interaction was computed by an unconditional logistic regression model specifies the log-odds as: $\text{logit}(P) = \beta_0 + \beta_G(G_i) + \beta_{G\times E}(G_i{*}E_i)$. For all graphs, statistical analyses were carried out using two-tailed, unpaired Student' s *t*-test. Before *t*-test, normal distribution of all the data were checked using normality test and equality of variances were checked using *F*-test. All statistical analyses were performed by R software 3.4.2[5] and PLINK 1.09. Data were considered statistically significant when *P*-value < 0.05.

RESULTS

Association Between Genetic Variants of Autophagy Pathway Genes With the Risk of NSCL/P

As shown in **Figure 1**, 27,240 SNPs in 23 genes related to autophagy pathway were identified. Among them, 146 putative functional SNPs were picked out, and their associations with risk of NSCL/P were examined in the stage I that was comprised of 504 NSCL/P cases and 455 newborn controls. Twelve SNPs (rs77141447, rs16822638, rs7625881, rs14016, rs12813551, rs147920828, rs2301104, rs4776786, rs80225705, rs3784605, rs7182342, and rs2283791) were significantly associated with the risk of NSCL/P in additive logistic model with the adjustment of gender (**Table 1**).

Gene-Based Analysis With the Risk of NSCL/P

To evaluate the joint effects of common SNPs in a gene unit, we further performed gene-based analysis using SKAT and MAGMA methods to identify potentially associated genes and found that *HIF1A* ($P_{SKAT} = 9.42 \times 10^{-03}$, $P_{MAGMA} = 2.74 \times 10^{-02}$), *BCL2L1* ($P_{SKAT} = 1.05 \times 10^{-02}$) and *KRAS* ($P_{MAGMA} = 1.76 \times 10^{-02}$) were significantly associated with NSCL/P susceptibility. Only *HIF1A* achieved consistent associations in both methods (**Supplementary Table 4**); thus, rs2301104 in *HIF1A* remained for further analysis.

Replication and Combined Analysis of rs2301104 With the Risk of NSCL/P

Rs2301104 was genotyped for validation with an additional 1,523 NSCL/P case and 1f88 control subjects and showed significant association with the same direction of effect as that observed in stage I (OR: 1.39; 95% CI: 1.01–1.92; $P = 4.55 \times 10^{-02}$ in stage I, OR: 1.25; 95% CI: 1.03–1.53; $P = 2.72 \times 10^{-02}$ in stage II, **Table 2**). Similar results were also observed in the combined analysis from the two stages (OR: 1.29; 95% CI: 1.09–1.53; $P = 3.39 \times 10^{-03}$, **Table 2**). No significant heterogeneity for rs2301104 was observed among different stages ($P_{het} = 0.70$, **Table 2**). Further, to explore whether rs2301104 participated in development of NSCL/P alone or

[5]http://www.r-project.org/

TABLE 1 | The association of 12 significant SNPs with the risk of NSCL/P.

Chr	SNP	Gene	Allele[a]	Call rate (%)	MAF		Genotype distribution[b]		P_{hwe}	OR (95% CI)	P	OR (95% CI)[c]	P^c
					Case	Control	Case	Control					
2	rs77141447	*IRS1*	C/A	96.976	0.071	0.049	421/68/1	397/43/0	0.25	1.53 (1.02–2.28)	3.84E−02	1.50 (1.00–2.24)	4.91E−02
2	rs16822638	*IRS1*	A/G	100.000	0.217	0.177	303/183/18	313/123/19	1.00	1.29 (1.03–1.63)	2.70E−02	1.30 (1.04–1.64)	2.32E−02
3	rs7625881	*ATG7*	A/G	95.620	0.373	0.318	184/235/62	199/197/40	0.24	1.29 (1.06–1.58)	1.11E−02	1.29 (1.05–1.57)	1.42E−02
3	rs14016	*ATG7*	C/T	100.000	0.432	0.380	161/251/92	168/228/59	0.32	1.25 (1.04–1.50)	2.03E−02	1.25 (1.03–1.50)	2.17E−02
12	rs12813551	*KRAS*	T/C	99.896	0.194	0.244	329/153/21	270/148/37	0.57	0.76 (0.62–0.94)	1.08E−02	0.75 (0.61–0.93)	7.95E−03
12	rs147920828	*KRAS*	C/T	96.767	0.093	0.131	403/83/4	333/95/10	0.40	0.68 (0.51–0.91)	9.94E−03	0.67 (0.50–0.90)	7.67E−03
14	rs2301104	*HIF1A*	G/C	100.000	0.100	0.073	408/91/5	393/58/4	0.42	1.41 (1.03–1.95)	3.48E−02	1.39 (1.01–1.92)	4.55E−02
15	rs4776786	*MAP2K1*	T/C	98.749	0.073	0.050	427/66/3	409/39/3	0.16	1.47 (1.01–2.14)	4.64E−02	1.48 (1.02–2.17)	4.15E−02
15	rs80225705	*IGF1R*	C/T	96.976	0.090	0.065	418/81/5	396/59/0	1.00	1.44 (1.02–2.03)	3.80E−02	1.44 (1.02–2.04)	3.71E−02
15	rs3784605	*IGF1R*	T/C	100.000	0.153	0.115	370/114/20	354/97/4	0.07	1.36 (1.05–1.76)	2.06E−02	1.34 (1.04–1.75)	2.66E−02
15	rs7182342	*IGF1R*	C/G	96.976	0.314	0.367	236/220/48	187/202/66	0.57	0.79 (0.65–0.95)	1.44E−02	0.79 (0.65–0.96)	1.54E−02
22	rs2283791	*MAPK1*	C/G	99.270	0.165	0.204	342/151/7	286/148/18	0.16	0.76 (0.60–0.97)	2.64E−02	0.77 (0.61–0.99)	3.73E−02

NSCL/P, non-syndromic cleft lip with or without cleft palate; Chr, chromosome; SNP, single nucleotide polymorphism; MAF, minor allele frequency; OR, odds ratio; CI, confidence interval. [a]*Alleles: shown as major/minor allele.* [b]*Major homozygote/heterozygote/minor homozygote.* [c]*OR (95% CI) and P values were derived from logistic regression analysis with adjustment for gender under the assumption of an additive genetic model.*

not, we also performed haplotype and epistasis analysis. No significant haplotype and SNPs interacted with rs2301104 was found, which indicated rs2301104 may play an independent role in development of NSCL/P (**Supplementary Figure 2** and **Supplementary Table 5**).

Gender Stratification Analysis of rs2301104 With the Risk of NSCL/P

As shown in **Figure 2**, the association of rs2301104 with the risk of NSCL/P showed strong evidence of heterogeneity (P_{het} = 9.06 × 10^{-03}) among males and females. Significant association between rs2301104 and NSCL/P risk were observed in the female (OR: 1.80; 95% CI: 1.32–2.45; P = 1.79 × 10^{-04}), rather than in the male (OR: 1.10; 95% CI: 0.90–1.35; P = 0.362, **Figure 2**). Further, rs2301104 had a significant interaction with gender (P = 1.13 × 10^{-03}), constituting highly statistically significant evidence of the involvement of rs2301104 with gender preference in NSCL/P.

Potential Regulatory Role of rs2301104 on HIF1A

To investigate the underlying mechanisms of rs2301104, we conducted functional annotation analysis on it. It was found that rs2301104 resided within chromatin regions expressing marks indicative of enhancer activity, promoter activity, transcription regulatory by predictions from Haploreg, RegulomeDB, UCSC Genome Browser, and Roadmap Epigenomics Project (**Supplementary Table 6** and **Supplementary Figure 3**).

We thereby constructed enhancer luciferase reporter vectors containing the rs2301104-centered region and the *HIF1A* promoter and then tested the luciferase activity 48 h after transfecting different plasmids in HEPM and HOEC cells. The rs2301104 G allele revealed a significantly increased enhancer activity compared with that of C allele (**Figures 3A,B**). This result was also supported in HEPM and HOEC cells that the mRNA expression of *HIF1A* was lower with C allele constructs, compared with G allele constructs (**Figures 3C,D**).

To evaluate the effect on rs2301104 in *HIF1A*, we further performed an eQTL analysis in lip tissue samples from 68 NSCL/P patients and found that rs2301104 was significantly associated with the expression of *HIF1A* (P = 3.1 × 10^{-2}). Expression of *HIF1A* was higher in samples of GG genotypes compared with those of GC/CC genotypes (**Figure 3E**).

HIF1A Expression During Mouse Craniofacial Development and in Human Samples

We detected continuous expression of *HIF1A* in the mouse lip and palate development during E10.5d to E15.5d as well as craniofacial structures from E10.5d to E14.5d (**Supplementary Figure 4**), implicating its essential role in the craniofacial development. In addition, we found that the expression of *HIF1A* was decreased in the DPSCs, and MSCs in lip muscle of NSCL/P cases, compared with those in controls (P = 8.37 × 10^{-2} and P = 3.74 × 10^{-1}, respectively, **Supplementary Figure 5**).

Functional Analyses of *HIF1A in vitro*

To further address the function of *HIF1A*, we knocked down the expression of *HIF1A* in HEPM and HOEC cells through the transfection of *HIF1A* siRNA-2107 given its highest efficiency (**Figures 4A,B**). Flow cytometric analysis revealed a significantly increased apoptosis rate in cells transfected with *HIF1A* siRNA-2107 (**Figures 4E–H**). The results of CCK-8 assays showed that knockdown of *HIF1A* significantly inhibited cell proliferation (**Figures 4C,D**). Moreover, the cell cycle assay showed that knockdown of *HIF1A* increased the number of G0/G1 phase cells, with a significant reduction in the number of S phase cells (**Figures 4I,J**).

DISCUSSION

Autophagy participates in many pathological conditions, such as neurodegeneration, autoimmune disease, cancer, and Crohn's disease (Nyfeler and Eng, 2016). In the present study, we evaluated the relationships between SNPs on core genes of autophagy pathway with risk of NSCL/P by a two-stage case-control study. Using association and gene-based analysis, we found that rs2301104 in *HIF1A* was significantly associated with NSCL/P risk. Notably, gender stratification analysis indicated that rs2301104 exhibited a significant association in the females but not males. Given several possible mechanisms, the underlying biochemical causes might involve sex hormones, sex-biased methylation (McCarthy et al., 2014). Moreover, autophagy is differentially regulated by sex, and the interaction between sex, sex-hormones, and tissue variability in regulating the heat shock response pathway was also observed (Tower et al., 2020).

TABLE 2 | Association between rs2301104 in *HIF1A* and the risk of NSCL/P.

Loci	SNP	Position (hg19)	Gene	Alleles[a]	Stage	Call rate (%)	MAF (Case/Control)	GG/GC/CC		OR (95% CI)[b]	P^b	$P_{het}{}^c$
								Case	Control			
14q23.2	rs2301104	62165028	*HIF1A*	G/C	Stage I	100.000	0.100/0.073	408/91/5	393/58/4	1.39 (1.01–1.92)	4.55E−02	–
					Stage II	98.111	0.075/0.060	1256/201/11	1240/129/19	1.25 (1.03–1.53)	2.72E−02	–
					Combine	–	–	–	–	1.29 (1.09–1.29)	3.39E−03	0.70

NSCL/P, non-syndromic cleft lip with or without cleft palate; SNP, single-nucleotide polymorphism; MAF, minor allele frequency; OR, odds ratio; CI, confidence interval.
[a]Alleles: shown as major/minor allele. [b]OR (95% CI) and P values were derived from logistic regression analysis with adjustment for gender under the assumption of an additive genetic model. [c]P-value of heterogeneity test.

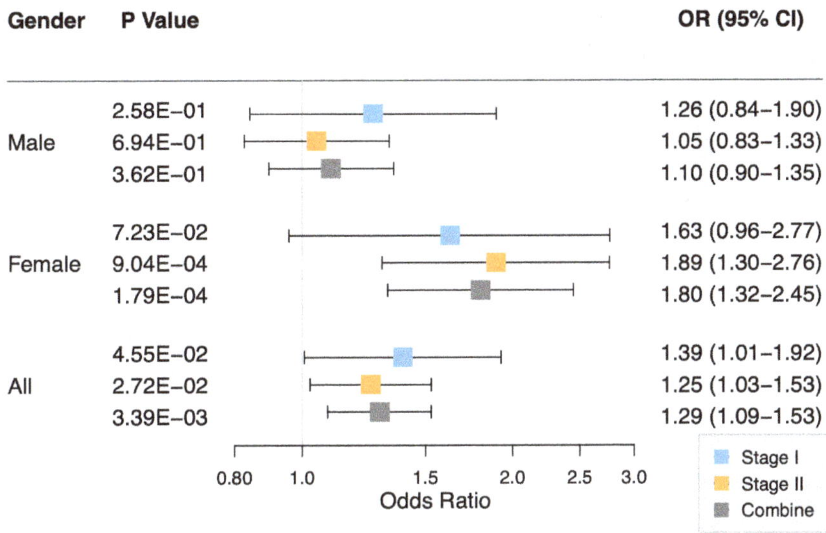

FIGURE 2 | Forest plot of the association between rs2301104 with risk of NSCL/P in stage I, stage II, and combined analysis, stratified according to the gender of study participants.

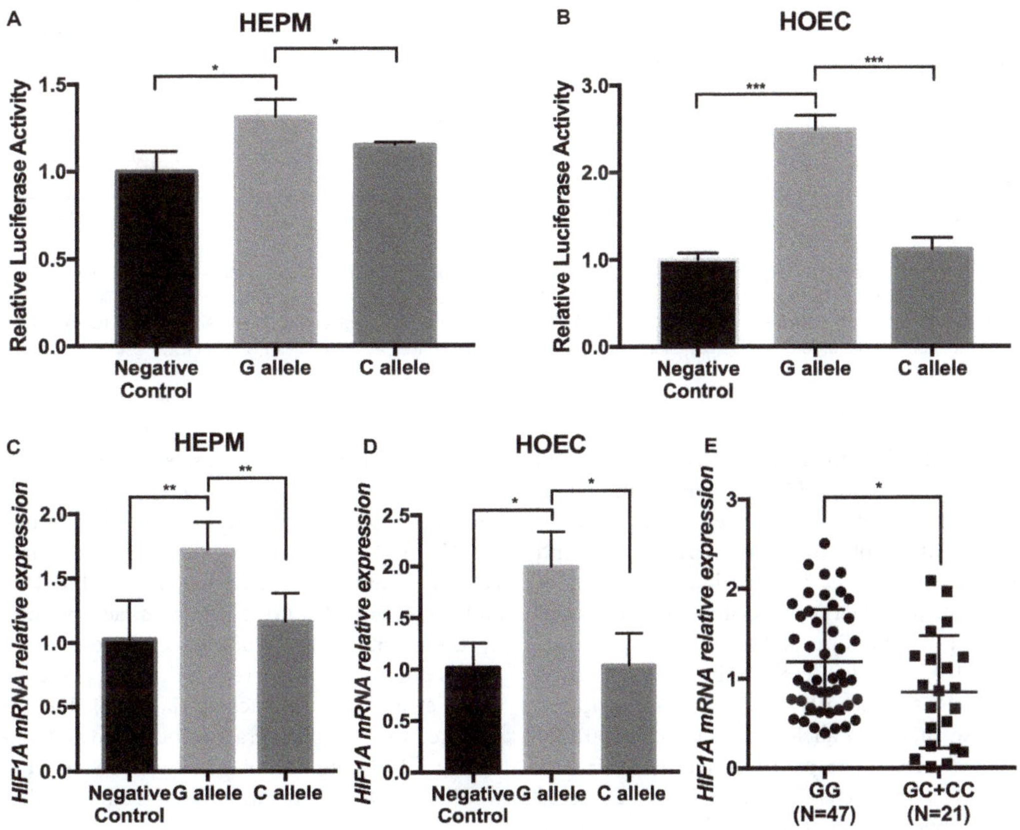

FIGURE 3 | The rs2301104 alleles affect the enhancer activity and expression of *HIF1A*. **(A)** HEPM and **(B)** HOEC cells were transiently transfected with rs2301104 [G], rs2301104 [C], and *HIF1A* promoter with PGL3-basic luciferase reporter vector. pRL-SV40 was co-transfected into cells. The activity of luciferase was assayed 48h later. qRT-PCR analysis of *HIF1A* expression at 48 h after plasmids transfection in **(C)** HEPM and **(D)** HOEC cells. It was indicated that the expression of *HIF1A* was lower with C allele constructs, compared with G allele constructs. Results are shown as mean values with the standard deviation (SD) normalized to *GAPDH*. **(E)** *HIF1A* mRNA expression was detected by qRT-PCR in 68 NSCL/P lip tissue samples. The *HIF1A* expression was significantly lower in samples with GC/CC genotypes than those with GG genotypes. The results were normalized to *GAPDH*. The *P*-value was calculated with two-side *t*-test ($n = 6$; $^{*}P < 0.05$, $^{**}P < 0.01$, $^{***}P < 0.001$).

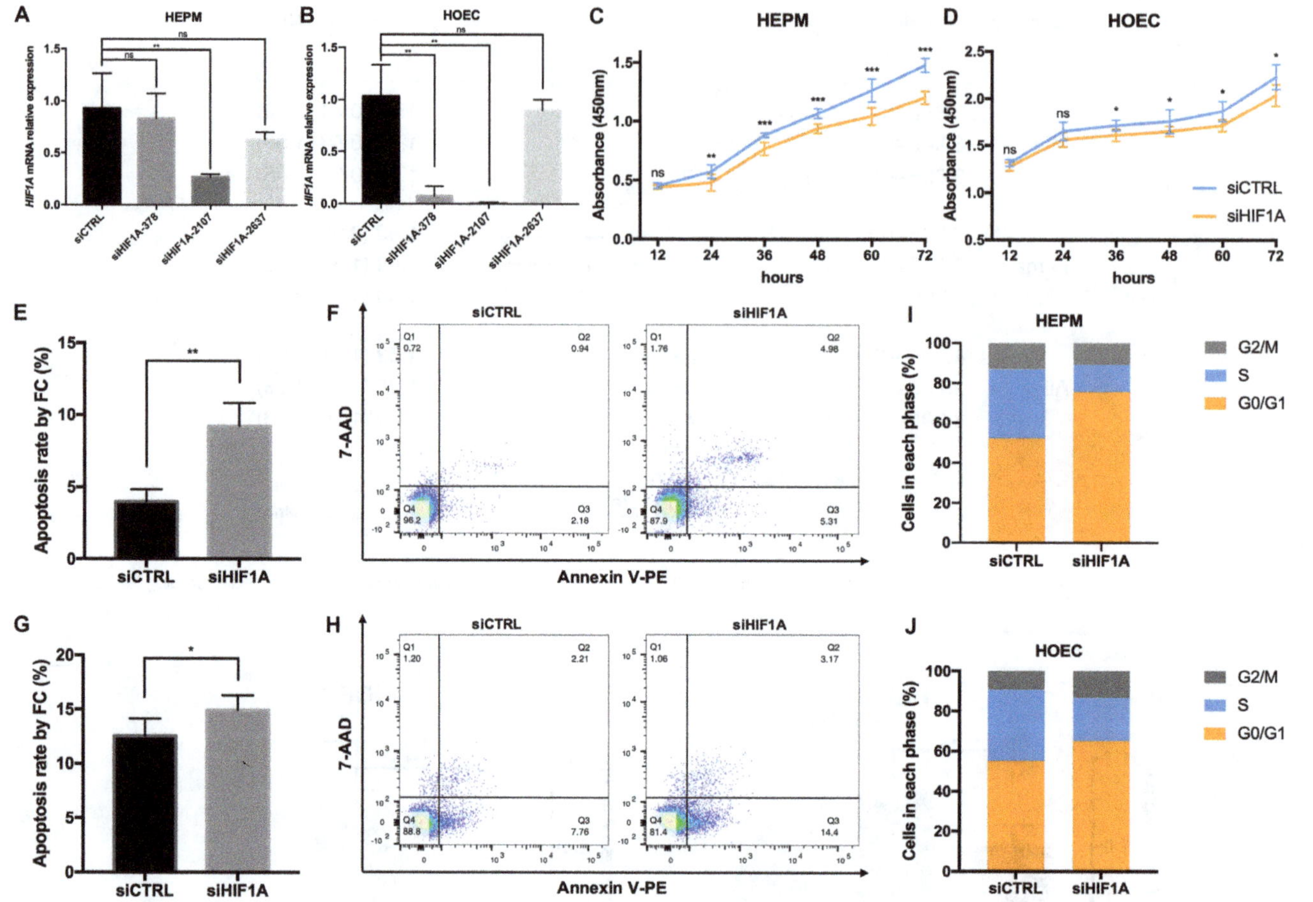

FIGURE 4 | *In vitro* functional roles of *HIF1A* in HEPM and HOEC. **(A,B)** qRT-PCR analysis of the *HIF1A* knockdown efficiency in HEPM and HOEC cells, respectively (n = 6). **(C,D)** Cell counting kit-8 assay was used to assess the proliferation of HEPM and HOEC cells after transfection with *HIF1A* siRNAs (n = 6). **(E–H)** Quantitative analysis of cell apoptosis by flow cytometry between the two groups (n = 6). The rate of apoptosis is higher in **(E,F)** HEPM cells, and **(G,H)** HOEC cells with *HIF1A* knockdown than in the corresponding negative controls. **(I,J)** Effects of *HIF1A* knockdown on the cell cycle in HEPM and HOEC cells (n = 6). (ns, no significance, *P < 0.05, **P < 0.01, ***P < 0.001).

Rs2301104 located in the first intron of *HIF1A* with enriched enhancer histone marks (including H3K4me1, H3K4me3, and H3K27ac) and previous studies had proven that SNPs in this region played essential roles in gene transcription and expression. For instance, Wang et al. identified a variant at 12p13.2 with enriched histone marks associated with colorectal cancer risk by affecting the binding affinity of transcriptional factor (Wang et al., 2016). Here, luciferase activity assay showed that rs2301104 C allele significantly decreased transcription activity, compared with that of G allele. Further, the rs2301104 C allele was associated with lower expression level of *HIF1A* mRNA in HEPM and HOEC cells. These findings suggested that rs2301104 was involved in transcriptional regulation of *HIF1A*.

We observed expression of *HIF1A* during mouse craniofacial development from E10.5d to E14.5d, implicating its involvement in the development of lip and palate. Notably, individuals carrying rs2301104 GC/CC genotypes (risk genotype) showed significantly lower expression of *HIF1A* than GG genotypes in lip tissue samples and a similar trend was also observed in DPSCs, and MSCs in lip muscle of NSCL/P cases and controls, highlighting the association between low expression of *HIF1A* and increased susceptibility of NSCL/P. We further knockdown of *HIF1A* to evaluate its role in the function of HOEC and HEPM. Promoted cell apoptosis, inhibited cell proliferation, and increase in G0/G1 phase cells, accompanied by a decrease in the number of S phase cells were detected and all of events commonly occurred during the development of NSCL/P (Tian et al., 2017; Lukacs et al., 2019). For instance, Lu et al. reported that cell proliferation increased and apoptosis decreased in the E13d mutant rabbit model related to NSCL/P, which would lead to the persistence of seams in the facial processes (Lu et al., 2019).

HIF1A played an important role in terms of embryo development. Severe congenital malformations including heart defects, retinopathy, brain lesions could be detected by culturing embryos at an inappropriate oxygen concentration level, which is mainly regulated by hypoxia-inducible factors (HIFs) (Bohuslavova et al., 2013; Feliciano et al., 2013; Nunes et al., 2015). *Hif1a*-deficient mice exhibited abnormal development of heart morphology and embryonic lethality between E11.0d and E12.0d (Krishnan et al., 2008; Forristal et al., 2010). According to the DECIPHER database, deletion of *HIF1A* resulted in congenital developmental defects, including microcephaly, aplasia of the tongue, and facial asymmetry (Firth et al., 2009).

The exact reason that *HIF1A* contributed to these developmental anomalies remained obscure. However, autophagy, induced by hypoxia whose activation was dependent on *HIF1A* (Liu et al., 2017), may be a possible way. Lu et al. demonstrated that the inhibition of autophagy might cause delayed development by affecting the epithelial-mesenchymal transitions process during chick development (Lu et al., 2014). Previous study showed that the loss of autophagy function in both osteoblasts and osteocytes might lead to a decrease in craniofacial bone mass in mouse models (Thomas et al., 2019). It had been reported that impaired autophagy could cause the loss of the protein quality control mechanism that is at the basis of inherited cardiomyopathies (Dorsch et al., 2019). Based on these studies, we hypothesized that decreased expression of *HIF1A* might break the oxygen homeostatic response during embryonic development, thereby inhibit autophagy and further exacerbate susceptibility to various developmental anomalies, including NSCL/P. A schematic model is shown in **Supplementary Figure 6**.

Taken together, we identified rs2301104 in autophagy pathway genes *HIF1A* that contributed to the risk of NSCL/P, providing further knowledge about the etiology of the disease. Further studies were warranted to explore the underlying mechanisms.

ETHICS STATEMENT

The studies involving human participants were reviewed and approved by the Ethics Committee of Nanjing Medical University. Written informed consent to participate in this study was provided by the participants' legal guardian/next of kin. The animal study was reviewed and approved by the Ethics Committee of Nanjing Medical University.

AUTHOR CONTRIBUTIONS

SL analyzed the data, drafted the manuscript, and performed *in vivo* and *in vitro* experiments with SK. LM, WZ, YP, and LW designed and directed the study, obtained the financial support, and critically revised the manuscript. XY performed the genotyping in stage II. YW, LF, and DL were responsible for sample processing. FY and GZ performed the statistical analysis. HW and WW were responsible for subject recruitment and sample collection. All authors read and approved the final manuscript.

ACKNOWLEDGMENTS

We thank all the study participants, research staff, and students who contributed to this study.

REFERENCES

Barrett, J. C., Fry, B., Maller, J., and Daly, M. J. (2005). Haploview: analysis and visualization of LD and haplotype maps. *Bioinformatics* 21, 263–265. doi: 10.1093/bioinformatics/bth457

Beaty, T. H., Marazita, M. L., and Leslie, E. J. (2016). Genetic factors influencing risk to orofacial clefts: today's challenges and tomorrow's opportunities. *F1000Research* 5:2800. doi: 10.12688/f1000research.9503.1

Birnbaum, S., Ludwig, K. U., Reutter, H., Herms, S., Steffens, M., Rubini, M., et al. (2009). Key susceptibility locus for nonsyndromic cleft lip with or without cleft palate on chromosome 8q24. *Nat. Genet.* 41, 473–477. doi: 10.1038/ng.333

Bohuslavova, R., Skvorova, L., Sedmera, D., Semenza, G. L., and Pavlinkova, G. (2013). Increased susceptibility of HIF-1alpha heterozygous-null mice to cardiovascular malformations associated with maternal diabetes. *J. Mol. Cell. Cardiol.* 60, 129–141. doi: 10.1016/j.yjmcc.2013.04.015

Capela, C., Dossou, A. D., Silva-Gomes, R., Sopoh, G. E., Makoutode, M., Menino, J. F., et al. (2016). Genetic variation in autophagy-related genes influences the risk and phenotype of buruli ulcer. *PLoS Negl. Trop. Dis.* 10:e0004671. doi: 10.1371/journal.pntd.0004671

Dai, J., Lv, J., Zhu, M., Wang, Y., Qin, N., Ma, H., et al. (2019). Identification of risk loci and a polygenic risk score for lung cancer: a large-scale prospective cohort study in Chinese populations. *Lancet Respir. Med.* 7, 881–891. doi: 10.1016/S2213-2600(19)30144-4

de Leeuw, C. A., Mooij, J. M., Heskes, T., and Posthuma, D. (2015). MAGMA: generalized gene-set analysis of GWAS data. *PLoS Comput. Biol.* 11:e1004219. doi: 10.1371/journal.pcbi.1004219

Dorsch, L. M., Schuldt, M., Knezevic, D., Wiersma, M., Kuster, D. W. D., van der Velden, J., et al. (2019). Untying the knot: protein quality control in inherited cardiomyopathies. *Pflugers Arch.* 471, 795–806. doi: 10.1007/s00424-018-2194-0

Feliciano, D. M., Zhang, S., Quon, J. L., and Bordey, A. (2013). Hypoxia-inducible factor 1a is a Tsc1-regulated survival factor in newborn neurons in tuberous sclerosis complex. *Hum. Mol. Genet.* 22, 1725–1734. doi: 10.1093/hmg/ddt018

Fenouille, N., Nascimbeni, A. C., Botti-Millet, J., Dupont, N., Morel, E., and Codogno, P. (2017). To be or not to be cell autonomous? Autophagy says both. *Essays Biochem.* 61, 649–661. doi: 10.1042/EBC20170025

Fernandez-Mateos, J., Seijas-Tamayo, R., Klain, J. C. A., Borgonon, M. P., Perez-Ruiz, E., Mesia, R., et al. (2017). Analysis of autophagy gene polymorphisms in Spanish patients with head and neck squamous cell carcinoma. *Sci. Rep.* 7:6887. doi: 10.1038/s41598-017-07270-0

Firth, H. V., Richards, S. M., Bevan, A. P., Clayton, S., Corpas, M., Rajan, D., et al. (2009). DECIPHER: database of chromosomal imbalance and phenotype in humans using ensembl resources. *Am. J. Hum. Genet.* 84, 524–533. doi: 10.1016/j.ajhg.2009.03.010

Forristal, C. E., Wright, K. L., Hanley, N. A., Oreffo, R. O., and Houghton, F. D. (2010). Hypoxia inducible factors regulate pluripotency and proliferation in human embryonic stem cells cultured at reduced oxygen tensions. *Reproduction* 139, 85–97. doi: 10.1530/REP-09-0300

Hale, A. N., Ledbetter, D. J., Gawriluk, T. R., and Rucker, E. B. III (2013). Autophagy: regulation and role in development. *Autophagy* 9, 951–972. doi: 10.4161/auto.24273

Hammond, N. L., Brookes, K. J., and Dixon, M. J. (2018). Ectopic hedgehog signaling causes cleft palate and defective osteogenesis. *J. Dent. Res.* 97, 1485–1493. doi: 10.1177/0022034518785336

Heike, C. L., and Evans, K. N. (2016). Evaluation of adults born with an oral cleft: aren't adults just big kids? *JAMA Pediatr.* 170, 1045–1046. doi: 10.1001/jamapediatrics.2016.2639

Huang, J., and Klionsky, D. J. (2007). Autophagy and human disease. *Cell Cycle* 6, 1837–1849. doi: 10.4161/cc.6.15.4511

Jiang, R., Bush, J. O., and Lidral, A. C. (2006). Development of the upper lip: morphogenetic and molecular mechanisms. *Dev. Dyn.* 235, 1152–1166. doi: 10.1002/dvdy.20646

Krishnan, J., Ahuja, P., Bodenmann, S., Knapik, D., Perriard, E., Krek, W., et al. (2008). Essential role of developmentally activated hypoxia-inducible factor 1alpha for cardiac morphogenesis and function. *Circ. Res.* 103, 1139–1146. doi: 10.1161/01.RES.0000338613.89841.c1

Lan, Y., Xu, J., and Jiang, R. (2015). Cellular and molecular mechanisms of palatogenesis. *Curr. Top. Dev. Biol.* 115, 59–84. doi: 10.1016/bs.ctdb.2015.07.002

Leslie, E. J., Carlson, J. C., Shaffer, J. R., Feingold, E., Wehby, G., Laurie, C. A., et al. (2016). A multi-ethnic genome-wide association study identifies novel loci for non-syndromic cleft lip with or without cleft palate on 2p24.2, 17q23 and 19q13. *Hum. Mol. Genet.* 25, 2862–2872. doi: 10.1093/hmg/ddw104

Li, C., Lan, Y., and Jiang, R. (2017). Molecular and cellular mechanisms of palate development. *J. Dent. Res.* 96, 1184–1191. doi: 10.1177/0022034517703580

Lin, L., Rodrigues, F., Kary, C., Contet, A., Logan, M., Baxter, R. H. G., et al. (2017). Complement-related regulates autophagy in neighboring cells. *Cell* 170, 158.e8–171.e8. doi: 10.1016/j.cell.2017.06.018

Liu, H., Zhang, Z., Xiong, W., Zhang, L., Xiong, Y., Li, N., et al. (2017). Hypoxia-inducible factor-1alpha promotes endometrial stromal cells migration and invasion by upregulating autophagy in endometriosis. *Reproduction* 153, 809–820. doi: 10.1530/REP-16-0643

Lu, W. H., Wang, G., Li, Y., Li, S., Song, X. Y., Wang, X. Y., et al. (2014). Autophagy functions on EMT in gastrulation of avian embryo. *Cell Cycle* 13, 2752–2764. doi: 10.4161/15384101.2015.945850

Lu, Y., Liang, M., Zhang, Q., Liu, Z., Song, Y., Lai, L., et al. (2019). Mutations of GADD45G in rabbits cause cleft lip by the disorder of proliferation, apoptosis and epithelial-mesenchymal transition (EMT). *Biochim. Biophys. Acta Mol. Basis Dis.* 1865, 2356–2367. doi: 10.1016/j.bbadis.2019.05.015

Lukacs, M., Roberts, T., Chatuverdi, P., and Stottmann, R. W. (2019). Glycosylphosphatidylinositol biosynthesis and remodeling are required for neural tube closure, heart development, and cranial neural crest cell survival. *eLife* 8:45248. doi: 10.7554/eLife.45248

Mangold, E., Ludwig, K. U., Birnbaum, S., Baluardo, C., Ferrian, M., Herms, S., et al. (2010). Genome-wide association study identifies two susceptibility loci for nonsyndromic cleft lip with or without cleft palate. *Nat. Genet.* 42, 24–26. doi: 10.1038/ng.506

McCarthy, N. S., Melton, P. E., Cadby, G., Yazar, S., Franchina, M., Moses, E. K., et al. (2014). Meta-analysis of human methylation data for evidence of sex-specific autosomal patterns. *BMC Genomics* 15:981. doi: 10.1186/1471-2164-15-981

Netea-Maier, R. T., Plantinga, T. S., van de Veerdonk, F. L., Smit, J. W., and Netea, M. G. (2016). Modulation of inflammation by autophagy: consequences for human disease. *Autophagy* 12, 245–260. doi: 10.1080/15548627.2015.1071759

Nunes, D. N., Dias-Neto, E., Cardo-Vila, M., Edwards, J. K., Dobroff, A. S., Giordano, R. J., et al. (2015). Synchronous down-modulation of miR-17 family members is an early causative event in the retinal angiogenic switch. *Proc. Natl. Acad. Sci. U.S.A.* 112, 3770–3775. doi: 10.1073/pnas.1500008112

Nyfeler, B., and Eng, C. H. (2016). Revisiting autophagy addiction of tumor cells. *Autophagy* 12, 1206–1207. doi: 10.1080/15548627.2016.1170265

Reynolds, K., Kumari, P., Sepulveda Rincon, L., Gu, R., Ji, Y., Kumar, S., et al. (2019). Wnt signaling in orofacial clefts: crosstalk, pathogenesis and models. *Dis. Model. Mech.* 12:dmm037051. doi: 10.1242/dmm.037051

Thomas, N., Choi, H. K., Wei, X., Wang, L., Mishina, Y., Guan, J. L., et al. (2019). Autophagy regulates craniofacial bone acquisition. *Calcif. Tissue Int.* 105, 518–530. doi: 10.1007/s00223-019-00593-2

Tian, H., Feng, J., Li, J., Ho, T. V., Yuan, Y., Liu, Y., et al. (2017). Intraflagellar transport 88 (IFT88) is crucial for craniofacial development in mice and is a candidate gene for human cleft lip and palate. *Hum. Mol. Genet.* 26, 860–872. doi: 10.1093/hmg/ddx002

Timbers, T. A., Garland, S. J., Mohan, S., Flibotte, S., Edgley, M., Muncaster, Q., et al. (2016). Accelerating gene discovery by phenotyping whole-genome sequenced multi-mutation strains and using the sequence kernel association test (SKAT). *PLoS Genet.* 12:e1006235. doi: 10.1371/journal.pgen.1006235

Tower, J., Pomatto, L. C. D., and Davies, K. J. A. (2020). Sex differences in the response to oxidative and proteolytic stress. *Redox Biol.* 31:101488. doi: 10.1016/j.redox.2020.101488

Wang, M., Gu, D., Du, M., Xu, Z., Zhang, S., Zhu, L., et al. (2016). Common genetic variation in ETV6 is associated with colorectal cancer susceptibility. *Nat. Commun.* 7:11478. doi: 10.1038/ncomms11478

Wang, M. H., Cordell, H. J., and Van Steen, K. (2019). Statistical methods for genome-wide association studies. *Semin. Cancer Biol.* 55, 53–60. doi: 10.1016/j.semcancer.2018.04.008

White, K. A. M., Luo, L., Thompson, T. A., Torres, S., Hu, C.-A. A., Thomas, N. E., et al. (2016). Variants in autophagy-related genes and clinical characteristics in melanoma: a population-based study. *Cancer Med.* 5, 3336–3345. doi: 10.1002/cam4.929

Zhu, M., Xu, K., Chen, Y., Gu, Y., Zhang, M., Luo, F., et al. (2019). Identification of novel T1D risk loci and their association with age and islet function at diagnosis in autoantibody-positive T1D individuals: based on a two-stage genome-wide association Study. *Diabetes Care* 42, 1414–1421. doi: 10.2337/dc18-2023

11

Dental Characteristics of Different Types of Cleft and Non-cleft Individuals

Mohammad Khursheed Alam[1†] and Ahmed Ali Alfawzan[2†]*

[1] Orthodontic Division, Department of Preventive Dental Science, College of Dentistry, Jouf University, Sakaka, Saudi Arabia,
[2] Department of Preventive Dentistry, College of Dentistry in Ar Rass, Qassim University, Ar Rass, Saudi Arabia

***Correspondence:**
Mohammad Khursheed Alam
dralam@gmail.com;
mkalam@ju.edu.sa

†These authors have contributed equally to this work

Objective: The objective of this study was to compare the novel artificial intelligence (A.I.)-driven lateral cephalometric (Late. Ceph.) analysis of 14 different dental characteristics (DC) among different types of cleft lip and palate (CLP) and non-cleft (NC) individuals.

Materials and Methods: A retrospective study was conducted on 123 individuals [31 = NC, 29 = BCLP (bilateral cleft lip and palate), 41 = UCLP (unilateral cleft lip and palate), 9 = UCLA (unilateral cleft lip and alveolus), and 13 = UCL (unilateral cleft lip)] with an average age of 14.77 years. Demographic details were gathered from the clinical records. A novel artificial intelligence-driven Webceph software has been used for the Late. Ceph. analysis. A total of 14 different types of angular and linear DC measurements were analyzed and compared among groups. Two-way ANOVA and multiple-comparison statistics tests were applied to see the differences between gender and among different types of CLP versus NC subjects.

Results: Of the 14 DC tested, no significant gender disparities were found ($p > 0.05$). In relation to different types of CLP versus NC subjects, 8 over 14 DC were statistically significant ($p <$ 001 to $p = 0.03$). Six other DC variables show insignificant ($p > 0.05$) noteworthy alterations in relation to type of CLP.

Conclusion: Based on the results, type of CLP revealed significantly altered DC compared to NC. Among different types of CLP, BCLP exhibited a maximum alteration in different DC.

Keywords: non-syndromic cleft lip and palate, bilateral cleft lip and palate, unilateral cleft lip and palate, dental characteristics, overjet, overbite, incisal display

INTRODUCTION

Any deformations (anatomical or chromosomal) that start during pregnancy and their belongings identified after birth are considered intrinsic oddities (Sekhon et al., 2011). Among them, cleft lip and palate (CLP) is one of the most widely recognized and major inherent craniofacial peculiarities in humans, brought about by strange facial development during embryogenesis that presents during childbirth and portrayed by halfway or complete clefting of the upper lip, with or without clefting of the alveolar edge or the hard or soft palate (Erverdi and Motro, 2015). Cleft can happen along with

CLP or independently like a detached cleft lip and or isolated cleft palate. The point when cleft lip and palate emerge together is named as CLP. The highlights of CLP went from the least serious to the most extreme structure with a unilateral or bilateral manner. CLP can be syndromic or non-syndromic. Clinically, when CLP shows up with other deformities (normally at least two or more), for an inconspicuous example, it is delegated syndromic CLP. In the event that it shows up as a secluded deformity or if the disorder cannot be recognized, the term non-syndromic CLP (NSCLP) is utilized (Kohli and Kohli, 2012).

The etiology of CLP is still controversial. According to previous studies, it is to be thought that both genetic and environmental factors are responsible for CLP (Alam et al., 2012; Berkowitz, 2013; Haque et al., 2015; Haque and Alam, 2015a,c). Studies of the etiology of non-syndromic clefts pivot on candidate genes associated with craniofacial development, genes influenced by environmental teratogens or deficiencies, and genes associated with syndromic clefts (Murray, 2002; Haque et al., 2015). CLP shows significant heterogeneity among different ethnic groups.

Numerous strategies for the evaluation of the craniofacial characteristics, dental relationship, and maxillary morphometry measurement of CLP individuals have been depicted already (Alam et al., 2008, 2013, 2019; Kajii et al., 2013; Asif et al., 2016; Arshad et al., 2017a,b, 2018; Haque et al., 2017a,b, 2018). The result of the craniofacial characteristics of CLP can be evaluated from multifacets of factors, for example, dental relationship (Haque et al., 2018), cephalogram (Alam et al., 2013, 2019; Wu et al., 2013; Batwa et al., 2018; Alam and Alfawzan, 2020), cone-beam computed tomography (Parveen et al., 2018), and maxillary morphometry (Haque et al., 2020). Oral clefts show an assortment of clinical inconsistencies (Batwa et al., 2018). Lee et al. (2020) and Kunz et al. (2020) uncovered artificial intelligence (A.I.) into dentistry, particularly in orthodontics ready to break down obscure Late. Ceph. at nearly a similar quality level as the ongoing highest-quality level estimated by a calibrated specialist. Lee et al. (2020) used A.I.-driven profound convolutional neural system-based assessment of Late. Ceph. for the sign of orthognathic surgery cases of differential determination and discovered 95.6% exactness.

This first-in-human study in a Saudi Arabian population, among different types of NSCLP and NC individuals, is yet to be investigated in regard to different dental characteristics (DC). Hence, in the present study an attempt is made to contribute a novel A.I.-driven analysis of different DC in multiple types of NSCLP and to compare the findings with gender- and age-matched NC individuals. Hence, this study aimed to investigate (1) how the DC are different among gender, (2) how the disparities in DC exist in multiple types of NSCLP and NC individuals, and (3) how the disparities exist in gender times multiple types of NSCLP and NC individuals. The hypothesis of this study is as follows: types of DC are different in relation to gender, type of NSCLP, and NC subjects.

MATERIALS AND METHODS

All the records (clinical and demographic details, X-rays) were collected from Saudi Board of dental residents. The research protocol was arranged by one calibrated orthodontist, and the data was stored. The research protocol was presented to the Ethical Committee of Al rass Dental Research Center, Qassim University. Full Ethical approval was obtained with the code #: DRC/009FA/20. The following inclusion and exclusion criteria are followed, non-syndromic cleft subjects with good-quality x-ray images. There was no history of craniofacial surgical treatment besides cleft lip and palate surgery. No orthodontic treatment was done. A match with healthy control without any craniofacial deformity was found.

Digital Late. Ceph. X-rays were used to investigate 14 different DC of 123 NC and cleft subjects based on convenient sampling

TABLE 1 | Dental characteristic measured in NSCLP and NC individuals.

Variables	Short form	Details
Overjet	OJ	Extent of horizontal (anterior-posterior) overlap of the maxillary central incisors over the mandibular central incisors
Overbite	OB	Extent of vertical (superior-inferior) overlap of the maxillary central incisors over the mandibular central incisors
Upper 1 to Frankfort horizontal plane	U1 to FH	Angle between long axis of upper incisor and Frankfort horizontal plane
Upper 1 to sella-nasion plane	U1 to SN	Angle between long axis of upper incisor and sella-nasion plane
Upper 1 to upper occlusal plane	U1 to UOP	Angle between long axis of upper incisor and upper occlusal plane
Incisor mandibular plane angle	IMPA	Angle between long axis of lower incisor and mandibular plane angle
Lower 1 to lower occlusal plane	L1 to LOP	Angle between long axis of lower incisor and lower occlusal plane
Inter-incisor angle	IIA	Angle between long axis of upper and lower incisor
Cant of occlusal plane	COP	Occlusal plane to FH plane
Upper 1 to nasion and point A	U1 to NA (mm)	Distance from upper incisor edge to nasion to point A plane
Upper 1 to nasion and point A	U1 to NA (degree)	Angle between long axis of upper incisor and nasion to point A plane
Lower 1 to nasion and point B	L1 to NB (mm)	Distance from lower incisor edge to nasion to point B plane
Lower 1 to nasion and point B	L1 to NB (degree)	Angle between long axis of lower incisor and nasion to point B plane
Upper incisal display	UID	Maxillary incisal display is one of the most important attributes of smile esthetics. The maximum distance from the lowest point of upper lip to the incisal edge of any of the upper incisor

following inclusion and exclusion criteria. Among them, 31 NC subjects and 92 cleft subjects [29 had BCLP (bilateral cleft lip and palate), 41 had UCLP (unilateral cleft lip and palate), 9 had UCLA (unilateral cleft lip and alveolus), and 13 had UCL (unilateral cleft lip)]. According to gender, male = 14 NC + 19 BCLP + 26 UCLP + 3 UCLA + 7 UCL and female = 17 NC + 10 BCLP + 15 UCLP + 6 UCLA + 6 UCL. Ages of the subjects were 13.29 ± 3.52 NC, 14.07 ± 4.73 BCLP, 14.32 ± 4.46 UCLP, 12.78 ± 4.09 UCLA, and 13.31 ± 4.46 UCL. In this retrospective study, clinical and radiographic details were used. Fourteen (14) different DC were measured by one examiner using automated A.I.-driven Webceph software (South Korea). The angular and linear measurements used in this study are detailed in **Table 1** and **Figure 1**.

Statistical Analyses

To survey the estimation mistake, 20 Late. Ceph. cases were arbitrarily chosen and the means of A.I.-driven investigation were rehashed by one analyst following 2 weeks of first examination. Intra-class correlation coefficients were performed to evaluate the unwavering quality for the two arrangements of estimations. The estimations of coefficients of unwavering quality were seen as more prominent than 0.95 and 0.91 for all linear and angular variables, respectively. Data were analyzed in SPSS (SPSS Inc., Chicago, IL, United States). The Kolmogorov–Smirnov test was utilized to check the normality of the estimations. A two-way ANOVA examination was utilized for gender orientation, types of cleft and gender*types of cleft. A *p*-esteem < 0.05 was considered as significant statistically.

RESULTS

Tables 2–8 show the details of the analyzed results of 14 different DC among gender, types of cleft and gender*types of cleft. **Figures 2A–C** show the profile plot of estimated marginal means of types of cleft and gender*types of cleft.

In **Table 2A**, overjet DC is presented, which shows no significant gender disparities and highly significant disparities among NC and different types of clefts (BCLP

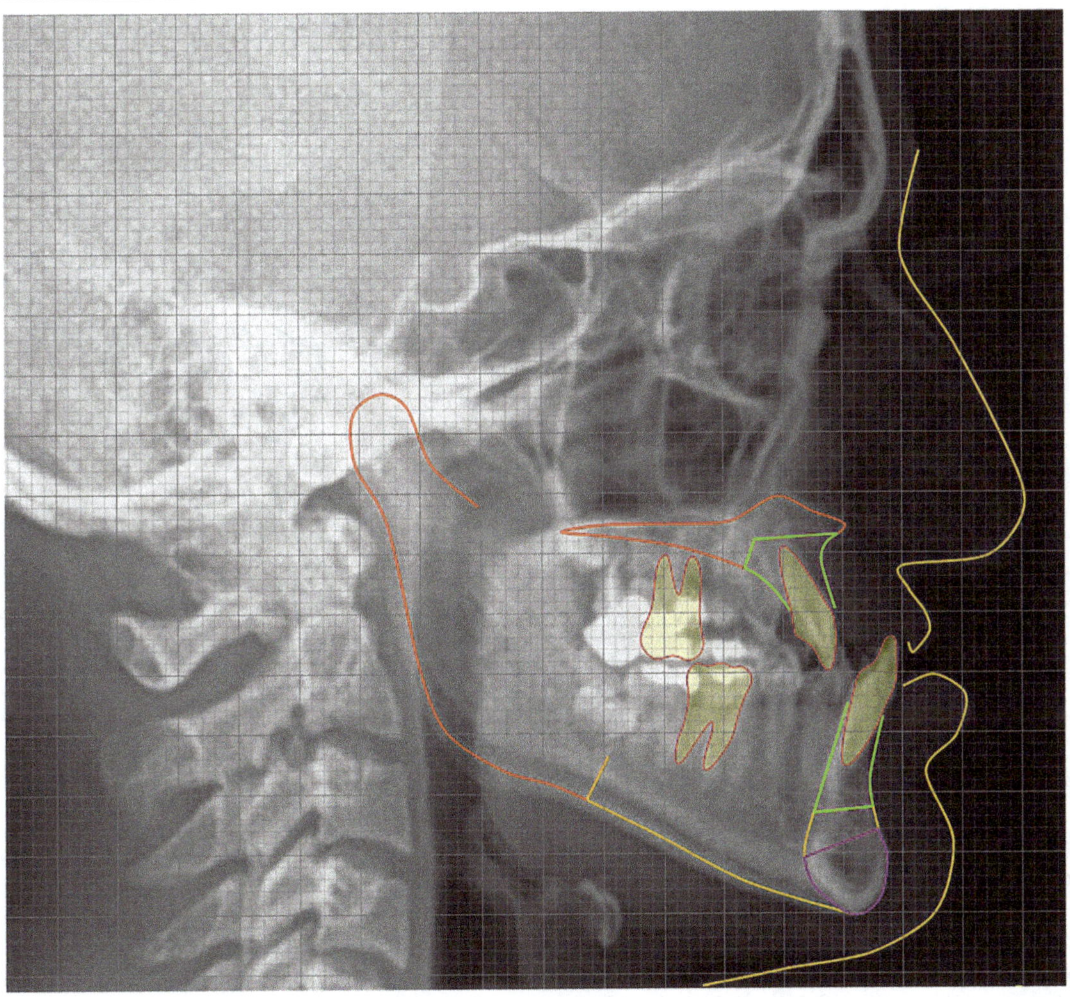

FIGURE 1 | Artificial intelligence-driven lateral cephalometric analysis.

TABLE 2 | Dental characteristics – **(A)** Overjet and **(B)** Overbite: Gender, types of cleft and gender times types of cleft two-way ANOVA analysis results.

Gender	Type	Mean	SD	Cleft Type	Mean	Multiple comparison			SE	*p*-value	95% CI	
											Lower bound	Upper bound
(A) Overjet												
Male	NC	4.449	2.016	NC	4.429	NC	vs	BCLP	11.573*	1.144	0.000	8.299
	BCLP	−5.801	5.104	BCLP	−7.144		vs	UCLP	8.064*	0.992	0.000	5.224
	UCLP	−4.098	5.299	UCLP	−3.635		vs	UCL	4.359*	1.378	0.020	0.413
	UCL	0.021	5.147	UCL	0.071		vs	UCLA	4.548	1.650	0.068	−0.176
	UCLA	−0.523	4.547	UCLA	−0.118	BCLP	vs	UCLP	−3.509*	1.080	0.015	−6.602
	Total	−2.153	5.960				vs	UCL	−7.215*	1.443	0.000	−11.346
Female	NC	4.410	2.602				vs	UCLA	−7.026*	1.704	0.001	−11.905
	BCLP	−8.486	5.485			UCLP	vs	UCL	−3.706	1.326	0.061	−7.502
	UCLP	−3.173	3.342				vs	UCLA	−3.517	1.606	0.306	−8.116
	UCL	0.120	1.266			UCL	vs	UCLA	0.189	1.870	1.000	−5.164
	UCLA	0.287	2.725									
	Total	−1.015	5.506									
Total	NC	4.427	2.317									
	BCLP	−6.542	5.256									
	UCLP	−3.646	4.423									
	UCL	0.067	3.730									
	UCLA	−0.253	3.866									
	Total	−1.653	5.770									

	p-value	PES
Gender	0.846	0.000
Cleft Type	0.000	0.512
Gender * Cleft Type	0.566	0.026

Gender	Type	Mean	SD	Cleft Type	Mean	Multiple comparison			SE	*p*-value	Lower bound	Upper bound
(B) Overbite												
Male	NC	1.237	2.441	NC	1.571	NC	vs	BCLP	0.764	1.000	−2.271	2.107
	BCLP	1.638	3.978	BCLP	1.653		vs	UCLP	0.663	1.000	−1.921	1.876
	UCLP	1.643	3.147	UCLP	1.593		vs	UCL	0.921	1.000	−1.170	4.104
	UCL	1.159	1.650	UCL	0.104		vs	UCLA	1.103	1.000	−3.022	3.292
	UCLA	1.470	1.972	UCLA	1.437	BCLP	vs	UCLP	0.722	1.000	−2.008	2.127
	Total	1.495	3.045				vs	UCL	0.964	1.000	−1.212	4.310
Female	NC	1.905	1.240				vs	UCLA	1.139	1.000	−3.045	3.478
	BCLP	1.669	3.872			UCLP	vs	UCL	0.886	0.957	−1.048	4.027
	UCLP	1.544	2.381				vs	UCLA	1.074	1.000	−2.917	3.231
	UCL	−0.950	0.856			UCL	vs	UCLA	1.250	1.000	−4.910	2.246
	UCLA	1.403	1.270									
	Total	1.391	2.309									
Total	NC	1.604	1.875									
	BCLP	1.646	3.879									
	UCLP	1.595	2.766									
	UCL	0.185	1.692									
	UCLA	1.448	1.684									
	Total	1.449	2.736									

	p-value	PES
Gender	0.607	0.002
Cleft Type	0.510	0.028
Gender * Cleft Type	0.683	0.020

SD, standard deviation; MD, mean difference; SE, standard error; CI, confidence interval; and PES, partial eta square.

$p < 0.001$, UCLP $p < 0.001$ and UCL, $p = 0.020$). UCLP $p = 0.015$, UCL $p < 0.001$, and UCLA, $p = 0.001$, showed a significant difference in comparison with BCLP. In relation to overbite DC, no significant disparities were observed (**Table 2B**).

Tables 3A,B shows U1 to FH and U1 to SN DC with no significant gender disparities and highly significant disparities among NC and different types of clefts (BCLP $p < 0.001$ and UCLP $p < 0.001$) in comparison with NC. UCLP $p = 0.015$, UCL $p < 0.001$, and UCLA, $p = 0.002$, showed significant difference in comparison with BCLP in relation to U1 to FH DC. Moreover, UCLP $p = 0.009$, UCL $p < 0.001$, and UCLA, $p = 0.001$, showed a significant difference in comparison with BCLP in relation to U1 to SN DC.

TABLE 3 | Dental characteristics – **(A)** U1 to FH and **(B)** U1 to SN: Gender, types of cleft and gender times types of cleft two-way ANOVA analysis results.

Gender	Type	Mean	SD	Cleft type	Mean	Multiple comparison			SE	*p*-value	95% CI	
											Lower bound	Upper bound
(A) U1 to FH												
Male	NC	116.074	8.465	NC	115.416	NC	vs	BCLP	2.988	0.000	17.360	34.473
	BCLP	86.171	11.990	BCLP	89.500		vs	UCLP	2.592	0.000	9.285	24.128
	UCLP	99.056	14.532	UCLP	98.710		vs	UCL	3.601	0.381	−2.753	17.867
	UCL	103.914	12.800	UCL	107.860		vs	UCLA	4.311	0.470	−3.684	21.001
	UCLA	107.443	5.413	UCLA	106.758	BCLP	vs	UCLP	2.823	0.015	−17.292	−1.128
	Total	99.809	15.927				vs	UCL	3.770	0.000	−29.155	−7.564
Female	NC	114.759	4.750				vs	UCLA	4.453	0.002	−30.009	−4.508
	BCLP	92.829	13.762			UCLP	vs	UCL	3.465	0.094	−19.070	0.771
	UCLP	98.365	9.516				vs	UCLA	4.198	0.577	−20.067	3.971
	UCL	111.805	10.308			UCL	vs	UCLA	4.886	1.000	−12.887	15.090
	UCLA	106.073	10.698									
	Total	104.627	12.382									
Total	NC	115.353	6.597									
	BCLP	88.008	12.618									
	UCLP	98.719	12.195									
	UCL	107.556	11.956									
	UCLA	106.987	6.885									
	Total	101.925	14.620									

	p-value	PES
Gender	0.352	0.008
Cleft Type	0.000	0.432
Gender * Cleft Type	0.482	0.030

Gender	Type	Mean	SD	Cleft type	Mean	Multiple comparison			SE	*p*-value	95% CI Lower bound	95% CI Upper bound
(B) U1 to SN												
Male	NC	106.671	8.479	NC	105.731	NC	vs	BCLP	3.172	0.000	17.509	35.673
	BCLP	76.177	13.008	BCLP	79.140		vs	UCLP	2.751	0.000	8.487	24.242
	UCLP	90.420	15.290	UCLP	89.367		vs	UCL	3.822	0.945	−4.498	17.389
	UCL	95.234	13.826	UCL	99.285		vs	UCLA	4.576	0.987	−5.482	20.719
	UCLA	99.395	6.536	UCLA	98.113	BCLP	vs	UCLP	2.996	0.009	−18.805	−1.648
	Total	90.651	16.695				vs	UCL	4.002	0.000	−31.604	−8.687
Female	NC	104.792	5.593				vs	UCLA	4.727	0.001	−32.506	−5.439
	BCLP	82.104	15.417			UCLP	vs	UCL	3.678	0.081	−20.448	0.611
	UCLP	88.314	9.676				vs	UCLA	4.455	0.521	−21.502	4.011
	UCL	103.337	10.000			UCL	vs	UCLA	5.186	1.000	−13.674	16.020
	UCLA	96.830	10.398									
	Total	94.724	12.985									
Total	NC	105.640	6.982									
	BCLP	77.812	13.695									
	UCLP	89.393	12.748									
	UCL	98.974	12.447									
	UCLA	98.540	7.441									
	Total	92.439	15.256									

	p-value	PES
Gender	0.556	0.003
Cleft Type	0.000	0.416
Gender * Cleft Type	0.456	0.031

SD, standard deviation; MD, mean difference; SE, standard error; CI, confidence interval; and PES, partial eta square.

Tables 4A,B shows U1 to UOP and IMPA DC with significant disparities among NC and different types of clefts (BCLP < 0.001 and p = 0.001 and UCLP < 0.001 and p = 0.009, respectively).

In relation to L1 to LOP DC, no significant disparities were observed (**Table 5A**). **Table 5B** shows inter-incisor angle DC with highly significant disparities among NC and different types of clefts (BCLP < 0.001, UCLP < 0.001, and UCLA < 0.001). UCL < 0.001 and UCLA < 0.001 showed a significant difference in comparison with BCLP. UCL p = 0.03 showed a significant difference in comparison with UCLP.

In relation to Cant of occlusal plane, upper incisal display DC, and U1 to NA (mm), no significant disparities were observed

TABLE 4 | Dental characteristics – **(A)** U1 to UOP and **(B)** IMPA: Gender, types of cleft and gender times types of cleft two-way ANOVA analysis results.

Gender	Type	Mean	SD	Cleft type	Mean	Multiple comparison			SE	*p*-value	95% CI	
											Lower bound	Upper bound
(A) U1 to UOP												
Male	NC	54.119	6.073	NC	54.075	NC	vs	BCLP	2.658	0.000	−24.426	−9.207
	BCLP	73.341	12.229	BCLP	70.891		vs	UCLP	2.305	0.000	−21.969	−8.768
	UCLP	70.295	12.922	UCLP	69.443		vs	UCL	3.202	0.033	−18.783	−0.444
	UCL	65.503	7.232	UCL	63.688		vs	UCLA	3.834	0.740	−17.890	4.063
	UCLA	60.197	3.379	UCLA	60.988	BCLP	vs	UCLP	2.510	1.000	−5.740	8.636
	Total	66.576	12.636				vs	UCL	3.353	0.338	−2.398	16.804
Female	NC	54.030	4.391				vs	UCLA	3.961	0.138	−1.437	21.243
	BCLP	68.441	11.177			UCLP	vs	UCL	3.081	0.644	−3.067	14.578
	UCLP	68.592	10.414				vs	UCLA	3.733	0.254	−2.234	19.144
	UCL	61.873	3.587			UCL	vs	UCLA	4.345	1.000	−9.741	15.140
	UCLA	61.780	5.103									
	Total	62.860	10.280									
Total	NC	54.070	5.125			*p*-value	PES					
	BCLP	71.990	11.959		Gender	0.412	0.006					
	UCLP	69.464	11.651		Cleft Type	0.000	0.338					
	UCL	63.828	5.921		Gender * Cleft Type	0.878	0.010					
	UCLA	60.724	3.778									
	Total	64.945	11.761									
(B) IMPA												
Male	NC	91.971	8.365	NC	92.173	NC	vs	BCLP	2.051	0.001	2.380	14.127
	BCLP	81.274	8.759	BCLP	83.920		vs	UCLP	1.779	0.009	0.969	11.159
	UCLP	84.625	8.473	UCLP	86.109		vs	UCL	2.472	1.000	−3.376	10.779
	UCL	87.520	4.118	UCL	88.472		vs	UCLA	2.959	1.000	−5.819	11.126
	UCLA	89.982	4.400	UCLA	89.519	BCLP	vs	UCLP	1.938	1.000	−7.737	3.359
	Total	85.855	8.741				vs	UCL	2.588	0.813	−11.963	2.859
Female	NC	92.374	6.227				vs	UCLA	3.057	0.696	−14.352	3.153
	BCLP	86.565	2.899			UCLP	vs	UCL	2.378	1.000	−9.173	4.447
	UCLP	87.593	7.980				vs	UCLA	2.882	1.000	−11.661	4.840
	UCL	89.423	7.148			UCL	vs	UCLA	3.354	1.000	−10.650	8.555
	UCLA	89.057	5.356									
	Total	89.230	6.841									
Total	NC	92.192	7.144			*p*-value	PES					
	BCLP	82.734	7.918		Gender	0.242	0.012					
	UCLP	86.073	8.270		Cleft Type	0.001	0.147					
	UCL	88.398	5.545		Gender * Cleft Type	0.755	0.016					
	UCLA	89.673	4.414									
	Total	87.337	8.109									

SD, standard deviation; MD, mean difference; SE, standard error; CI, confidence interval; and PES, partial eta square.

(**Tables 6A,B, 7A**). **Table 7B** shows U1 to NA (degree) DC with significant disparities among NC and different types of clefts (BCLP $p = 0.001$ and UCLP $p = 0.009$).

Table 8A shows L1 to NB (mm) DC, no significant disparities were observed. L1 to NB (degree) DC show significant disparities among NC and different types of clefts (BCLP $p = 0.017$ and UCLP $p = 0.009$) (**Table 8B**).

DISCUSSION

Fourteen (14) distinctive DC of five unique groups of individuals are researched in the present study. As far as we could possibly know, A.I.-driven computerized Late. Ceph. examination in such gatherings and populace is yet to be researched. Irrelevant mistake in the estimations; exact, automated, basic, brisk, savvy,

TABLE 5 | Dental characteristics – **(A)** L1 to LOP and **(B)** inter-incisor angle: Gender, types of cleft and gender times types of cleft two-way ANOVA analysis results.

Gender	Type	Mean	SD	Cleft type	Mean	Multiple comparison			SE	*p*-value	95% CI	
											Lower bound	Upper bound
(A) L1 to LOP												
Male	NC	67.216	7.982	NC	67.133	NC	vs	BCLP	1.991	0.029	−11.757	−0.355
	BCLP	77.005	8.648	BCLP	73.189		vs	UCLP	1.727	0.081	−9.599	0.292
	UCLP	72.454	6.708	UCLP	71.786		vs	UCL	2.399	1.000	−9.007	4.733
	UCL	69.199	5.452	UCL	69.270		vs	UCLA	2.872	1.000	−8.782	7.666
	UCLA	66.292	3.959	UCLA	67.691	BCLP	vs	UCLP	1.881	1.000	−3.982	6.788
	Total	71.910	8.208				vs	UCL	2.512	1.000	−3.274	11.112
Female	NC	67.050	7.733				vs	UCLA	2.967	0.665	−2.998	13.994
	BCLP	69.374	6.580			UCLP	vs	UCL	2.309	1.000	−4.094	9.126
	UCLP	71.119	7.269				vs	UCLA	2.797	1.000	−3.913	12.104
	UCL	69.342	3.906			UCL	vs	UCLA	3.255	1.000	−7.741	10.900
	UCLA	69.090	6.946									
	Total	69.269	6.989									
Total	NC	67.125	7.714			*p*-value	PES					
	BCLP	74.900	8.734		Gender	0.438	0.005					
	UCLP	71.803	6.932		Cleft Type	0.017	0.100					
	UCL	69.265	4.607		Gender * Cleft Type	0.271	0.044					
	UCLA	67.224	4.880									
	Total	70.751	7.778									
(B) Inter-incisor angle												
Male	NC	124.194	13.399	NC	124.704	NC	vs	BCLP	3.828	0.000	−43.443	−21.523
	BCLP	160.287	13.646	BCLP	157.186		vs	UCLP	3.320	0.000	−31.953	−12.939
	UCLP	147.191	19.669	UCLP	147.149		vs	UCL	4.613	0.951	−20.971	5.443
	UCL	137.156	14.119	UCL	132.468		vs	UCLA	3.828	0.000	21.523	43.443
	UCLA	132.308	4.941	UCLA	132.786	BCLP	vs	UCLP	3.616	0.064	−0.316	20.390
	Total	144.198	20.123				vs	UCL	4.830	0.000	10.890	38.547
Female	NC	125.214	10.023				vs	UCLA	5.705	0.000	8.067	40.734
	BCLP	154.086	13.486			UCLP	vs	UCL	4.438	0.013	1.974	27.389
	UCLP	147.108	13.318				vs	UCLA	5.377	0.087	−1.032	29.759
	UCL	127.780	5.060			UCL	vs	UCLA	6.258	1.000	−18.236	17.601
	UCLA	133.263	13.700									
	Total	138.332	16.224									
Total	NC	124.753	11.474			*p*-value	PES					
	BCLP	158.576	13.654		Gender	0.373	0.007					
	UCLP	147.150	16.664		Cleft Type	0.000	0.441					
	UCL	132.828	11.576		Gender * Cleft Type	0.721	0.018					
	UCLA	132.627	7.900									
	Total	141.623	18.671									

SD, standard deviation; MD, mean difference; SE, standard error; CI, confidence interval; and PES, partial eta square.

future orthodontic computerized apparatuses; and different types of cleft examples are the novelty of the current examination (Lee et al., 2020; Kunz et al., 2020). The current investigation results may help the clinician in approaching where the impacts of essential CLP medical procedures are on various DC, supporting the restoration procedure in subjects with various sorts of NSCLP in building up a positive administration convention.

Batwa et al. (2018) recommended broadly that analysts in the CLP field should embrace exhaustive activities to survey a wide range of CLP. Longitudinal and extensive examination studies will empower social insurance suppliers to actualize substantial treatment conventions that are suitable for the extraordinary nature and intricacy of the CLP populace. The unilateral complete type of CLP subjects with multiple missing

TABLE 6 | Dental characteristics – **(A)** Cant of occlusal plane and **(B)** Upper incisal display: Gender, types of cleft and gender times types of cleft two-way ANOVA analysis results.

Gender	Type	Mean	SD	Cleft type	Mean	Multiple comparison			SE	*p*-value	95% CI	
											Lower bound	Upper bound
(A) Cant of occlusal plane												
Male	NC	8.480	3.892	NC	124.704	NC	vs	BCLP	1.433	1.000	−3.378	4.829
	BCLP	12.146	4.315	BCLP	157.186		vs	UCLP	1.243	1.000	−2.576	4.543
	UCLP	8.377	5.113	UCLP	147.149		vs	UCL	1.727	1.000	−5.118	4.771
	UCL	9.430	5.911	UCL	132.468		vs	UCLA	2.067	1.000	−6.661	5.178
	UCLA	7.943	3.873	UCLA	132.786	BCLP	vs	UCLP	1.354	1.000	−3.618	4.134
	Total	9.614	4.818				vs	UCL	1.808	1.000	−6.076	4.278
Female	NC	9.334	3.494				vs	UCLA	2.136	1.000	−7.582	4.648
	BCLP	4.216	7.823			UCLP	vs	UCL	1.662	1.000	−5.914	3.601
	UCLP	7.470	6.710				vs	UCLA	2.013	1.000	−7.489	4.039
	UCL	8.730	5.553			UCL	vs	UCLA	2.343	1.000	−7.277	6.140
	UCLA	11.353	5.241									
	Total	7.930	5.948									
Total	NC	8.948	3.642									
	BCLP	9.959	6.451									
	UCLP	7.934	5.888									
	UCL	9.107	5.518									
	UCLA	9.080	4.376									
	Total	8.875	5.387									

	p-value	PES
Gender	0.359	0.007
Cleft Type	0.857	0.012
Gender * Cleft Type	0.018	0.099

Gender	Type	Mean	SD	Cleft type	Mean	Multiple comparison			SE	*p*-value	Lower bound	Upper bound
(B) Upper incisal display												
Male	NC	3.750	3.093	NC	3.982	NC	vs	BCLP	0.792	0.607	−0.767	3.770
	BCLP	2.640	3.650	BCLP	2.480		vs	UCLP	0.687	0.215	−0.365	3.570
	UCLP	2.579	2.497	UCLP	2.379		vs	UCL	0.955	0.232	−0.536	4.932
	UCL	2.560	2.290	UCL	1.784		vs	UCLA	1.143	0.803	−1.255	5.290
	UCLA	1.525	2.960	UCLA	1.964	BCLP	vs	UCLP	0.749	1.000	−2.042	2.244
	Total	2.741	3.007				vs	UCL	1.000	1.000	−2.166	3.559
Female	NC	4.214	2.099				vs	UCLA	1.181	1.000	−2.865	3.897
	BCLP	2.321	3.649			UCLP	vs	UCL	0.919	1.000	−2.035	3.226
	UCLP	2.180	2.806				vs	UCLA	1.113	1.000	−2.772	3.602
	UCL	1.008	1.927			UCL	vs	UCLA	1.296	1.000	−3.889	3.529
	UCLA	2.403	2.680									
	Total	2.723	2.778									
Total	NC	4.004	2.560									
	BCLP	2.552	3.587									
	UCLP	2.384	2.627									
	UCL	1.844	2.195									
	UCLA	1.818	2.732									
	Total	2.733	2.897									

	p-value	PES
Gender	0.770	0.001
Cleft Type	0.081	0.070
Gender * Cleft Type	0.833	0.013

SD, standard deviation; MD, mean difference; SE, standard error; CI, confidence interval; and PES, partial eta square.

teeth had the significantly smallest overjet (−3.89 ± 2.75 mm) among the three groups (without missing teeth, with only one missing tooth, and with two or more missing teeth). In the current study, overjet in NC = 4.429, BCLP = −7.144, UCLP = −3.635, UCL = 0.071, and UCLA = −0.118 exhibits significant disparities. Maximum alterations are found in the BCLP group. UCLP results almost coincide with the results of Batwa et al. (2018) in which the smallest overjet was found in the unilateral complete type of CLP subjects with multiple missing teeth.

These disparities may be due to multiple-factor relations. When a patient is born with CLP, a number of surgeries take

TABLE 7 | Dental characteristics – **(A)** U1 to NA (mm) and **(B)** U1 to NA (degree): Gender, types of cleft and gender times types of cleft two-way ANOVA analysis results.

Gender	Type	Mean	SD	Cleft type	Mean	Multiple comparison			SE	*p*-value	95% CI	
											Lower bound	Upper bound
(A) U1 to NA (mm)												
Male	NC	4.823	2.557	NC	4.645	NC	vs	BCLP	0.699	1.000	−1.007	2.996
	BCLP	3.907	2.706	BCLP	3.650		vs	UCLP	0.606	0.059	−0.033	3.439
	UCLP	3.792	3.049	UCLP	2.942		vs	UCL	0.842	1.000	−1.223	3.600
	UCL	3.646	2.417	UCL	3.456		vs	UCLA	1.008	1.000	−1.410	4.365
	UCLA	3.032	2.393	UCLA	3.167	BCLP	vs	UCLP	0.660	1.000	−1.183	2.599
	Total	3.955	2.706				vs	UCL	0.882	1.000	−2.332	2.719
Female	NC	4.466	1.927				vs	UCLA	1.042	1.000	−2.501	3.465
	BCLP	3.393	3.429			UCLP	vs	UCL	0.811	1.000	−2.835	1.806
	UCLP	2.092	1.715				vs	UCLA	0.982	1.000	−3.037	2.586
	UCL	3.267	2.428			UCL	vs	UCLA	1.143	1.000	−2.984	3.561
	UCLA	3.303	3.260									
	Total	3.230	2.381									
Total	NC	4.627	2.201			***p*-value**	**PES**					
	BCLP	3.765	2.868		Gender	0.340	0.008					
	UCLP	2.963	2.605		Cleft Type	0.091	0.068					
	UCL	3.471	2.328		Gender * Cleft Type	0.729	0.018					
	UCLA	3.122	2.501									
	Total	3.637	2.584									
(B) U1 to NA (degree)												
Male	NC	27.376	8.148	NC	25.938	NC	vs	BCLP	1.584	0.000	3.903	12.974
	BCLP	16.857	4.241	BCLP	17.499		vs	UCLP	1.374	0.000	3.807	11.675
	UCLP	19.793	5.928	UCLP	18.197		vs	UCL	1.909	1.000	−2.642	8.289
	UCL	22.557	5.638	UCL	23.114		vs	UCLA	2.285	0.659	−2.300	10.785
	UCLA	20.850	5.838	UCLA	21.695	BCLP	vs	UCLP	1.496	1.000	−4.982	3.586
	Total	20.810	6.925				vs	UCL	1.999	0.058	−11.338	.107
Female	NC	24.500	3.660				vs	UCLA	2.361	0.782	−10.955	2.563
	BCLP	18.141	5.246			UCLP	vs	UCL	1.837	0.085	−10.176	.341
	UCLP	16.601	5.426				vs	UCLA	2.225	1.000	−9.869	2.873
	UCL	23.672	9.276			UCL	vs	UCLA	2.590	1.000	−5.996	8.834
	UCLA	22.540	5.545									
	Total	20.431	6.371									
Total	NC	25.799	6.167			***p*-value**	**PES**					
	BCLP	17.211	4.480		Gender	0.755	0.001					
	UCLP	18.236	5.845		Cleft Type	0.000	0.274					
	UCL	23.072	7.217		Gender * Cleft Type	0.417	0.034					
	UCLA	21.413	5.450									
	Total	20.644	6.663									

SD, standard deviation; MD, mean difference; SE, standard error; CI, confidence interval; and PES, partial eta square.

place in the 1st 2 years of life. One study used the presurgical orthopedic feeding plate after birth (Haque and Alam, 2015b); at 3–6 months of age, the patients underwent cheiloplasty (Haque and Alam, 2014), and at 9–18 months of age they underwent palatoplasty (Haque and Alam, 2015c). There was a formation of excessive scar tissues, and the undermining of soft tissue was observed after these surgeries, which may have resulted in maxillary contracture which finally leads to class III malocclusion. Maxillary growth retardation is often observed in patients with repaired unilateral cleft lip and palate (UCLP) (Alam et al., 2008; Kajii et al., 2013). Altered craniofacial morphology was also observed in relation to postnatal treatment factors and congenital factors in the Japanese population (Alam et al., 2013, 2019).

TABLE 8 | Dental characteristics – **(A)** L1 to NB (mm) and **(B)** L1 to NB (degree): Gender, types of cleft and gender times types of cleft two-way ANOVA analysis results.

Gender	Type	Mean	SD	Cleft type	Mean	Multiple comparison			SE	*p*-value	95% CI	
											Lower bound	Upper bound
(A) L1 to NB (mm)												
Male	NC	5.654	3.036	NC	25.938	NC	vs	BCLP	0.721	0.447	−0.601	3.530
	BCLP	3.811	2.436	BCLP	17.499		vs	UCLP	0.626	0.187	−0.299	3.285
	UCLP	4.660	2.710	UCLP	18.197		vs	UCL	0.869	1.000	−2.716	2.262
	UCL	5.397	1.772	UCL	23.114		vs	UCLA	1.041	1.000	−3.474	2.486
	UCLA	6.062	1.504	UCLA	21.695	BCLP	vs	UCLP	0.681	1.000	−1.922	1.980
	Total	4.800	2.597				vs	UCL	0.910	0.658	−4.297	0.915
Female	NC	5.930	3.053				vs	UCLA	1.075	0.712	−5.036	1.120
	BCLP	4.844	2.575			UCLP	vs	UCL	0.836	0.421	−4.115	0.675
	UCLP	3.938	2.126				vs	UCLA	1.013	0.524	−4.889	0.914
	UCL	6.640	2.782			UCL	vs	UCLA	1.179	1.000	−3.644	3.110
	UCLA	6.510	4.526									
	Total	5.142	2.817									
Total	NC	5.805	2.998			*p*-value	PES					
	BCLP	4.096	2.473		Gender	0.431	0.005					
	UCLP	4.308	2.440		Cleft Type	0.030	0.090					
	UCL	5.971	2.283		Gender * Cleft Type	0.666	0.021					
	UCLA	6.211	2.566									
	Total	4.950	2.690									
(B) L1 to NB (degree)												
Male	NC	24.875	6.460	NC	25.582	NC	vs	BCLP	1.993	0.017	0.708	12.120
	BCLP	17.726	7.604	BCLP	19.168		vs	UCLP	1.729	0.009	0.920	10.819
	UCLP	19.421	8.771	UCLP	19.712		vs	UCL	2.401	1.000	−6.173	7.578
	UCL	22.524	4.887	UCL	24.880		vs	UCLA	2.875	1.000	−7.664	8.798
	UCLA	24.787	4.940	UCLA	25.015	BCLP	vs	UCLP	1.882	1.000	−5.934	4.846
	Total	20.793	7.755				vs	UCL	2.514	0.250	−12.911	1.488
Female	NC	26.289	6.619				vs	UCLA	2.970	0.514	−14.350	2.656
	BCLP	20.610	5.193			UCLP	vs	UCL	2.311	0.273	−11.783	1.448
	UCLP	20.004	7.808				vs	UCLA	2.799	0.607	−13.318	2.712
	UCL	27.235	6.745			UCL	vs	UCLA	3.258	1.000	−9.464	9.193
	UCLA	25.243	8.616									
	Total	23.167	7.466									
Total	NC	25.650	6.478			*p*-value	PES					
	BCLP	18.522	7.054		Gender	0.210	0.014					
	UCLP	19.705	8.216		Cleft Type	0.002	0.141					
	UCL	24.698	6.072		Gender * Cleft Type	0.905	0.009					
	UCLA	24.939	5.820									
	Total	21.835	7.690									

SD, standard deviation; MD, mean difference; SE, standard error; CI, confidence interval; and PES, partial eta square.

Wu et al. (2013) proposed that further investigations are expected to investigate the skeletal and dental attributes of individuals with CLP in other ethnic gatherings, especially in the Middle Eastern region. They assessed only individuals with unilateral complete CLP among various kinds of CLP. They found various cephalometric characteristics present in Taiwanese people with unilateral complete CLP and found a general decrease in their skeletal vertical measurements and a decrease in the overjet. The current study also revealed a significant alteration in overjet. However, overbite, which determines the vertical dental relationship, shows no significant alterations. Five other DC—L1 to LOP, Cant of occlusal plane, U1 to NA (mm), L1 to NB (mm), and upper incisal display DC—also showed no significant disparities among genders, types of CLP, and NC individuals.

Alam et al. (2019), Alam and Alfawzan (2020) investigated the craniofacial morphology of Japanese UCLP patients and investigated the association with congenital (2019) and postnatal treatment factors (2013). Among congenital factors, gender and DC (U1-SN) showed insignificant disparities, which coincide with the results of the present study. Among postnatal treatment factors, significantly larger U1-SN measurements are found in subjects that underwent preoperative orthopedic treatment with a Hotz plate in comparison with the subjects that underwent no preoperative orthopedic treatment (HOTZ plate) or an active plate. These investigations are researched in UCLP subjects only. The current study compared four types of NSCLP and NC individuals. These disparities may be due to the fact that the management protocol of a patient with cleft is complex and requires a lengthy procedure. The involvement of multi-specialties working in tandem is suggested to bring out physical, psychological, and social rehabilitation. Likewise, maxillary arch constriction (maxillary growth retardation) is a common dental problem of CLP patients, resulting in a concave facial profile (Alam et al., 2019), class III malocclusion (Alam et al., 2013), midfacial growth deficiency (Alam et al., 2013, 2019), and congenitally missing and malformed teeth. Orthodontic anomalies like crowding, rotation, and malposition of teeth are also commonly observed (Haque and Alam, 2015a; Haque et al., 2018; Adetayo et al., 2019). In the current study, maximum alterations in 8 different DC were found to be mostly altered in relation to upper incisors [U1-FH, U1-SN, U1-UOP, IIA, and U1-NA (degree)]. Our results clearly indicate that NSCLP subjects exhibit a class III malocclusion pattern based on investigated multiple DC. Also, the results are more prominent in BCLP individuals.

Batwa et al. (2018) found U1-SN values of 85.04 ± 12.13 and 91.63 ± 10.62 (mean ± SD) in the control and case groups (UCCLP), respectively. Utilizing the mean ± SD values

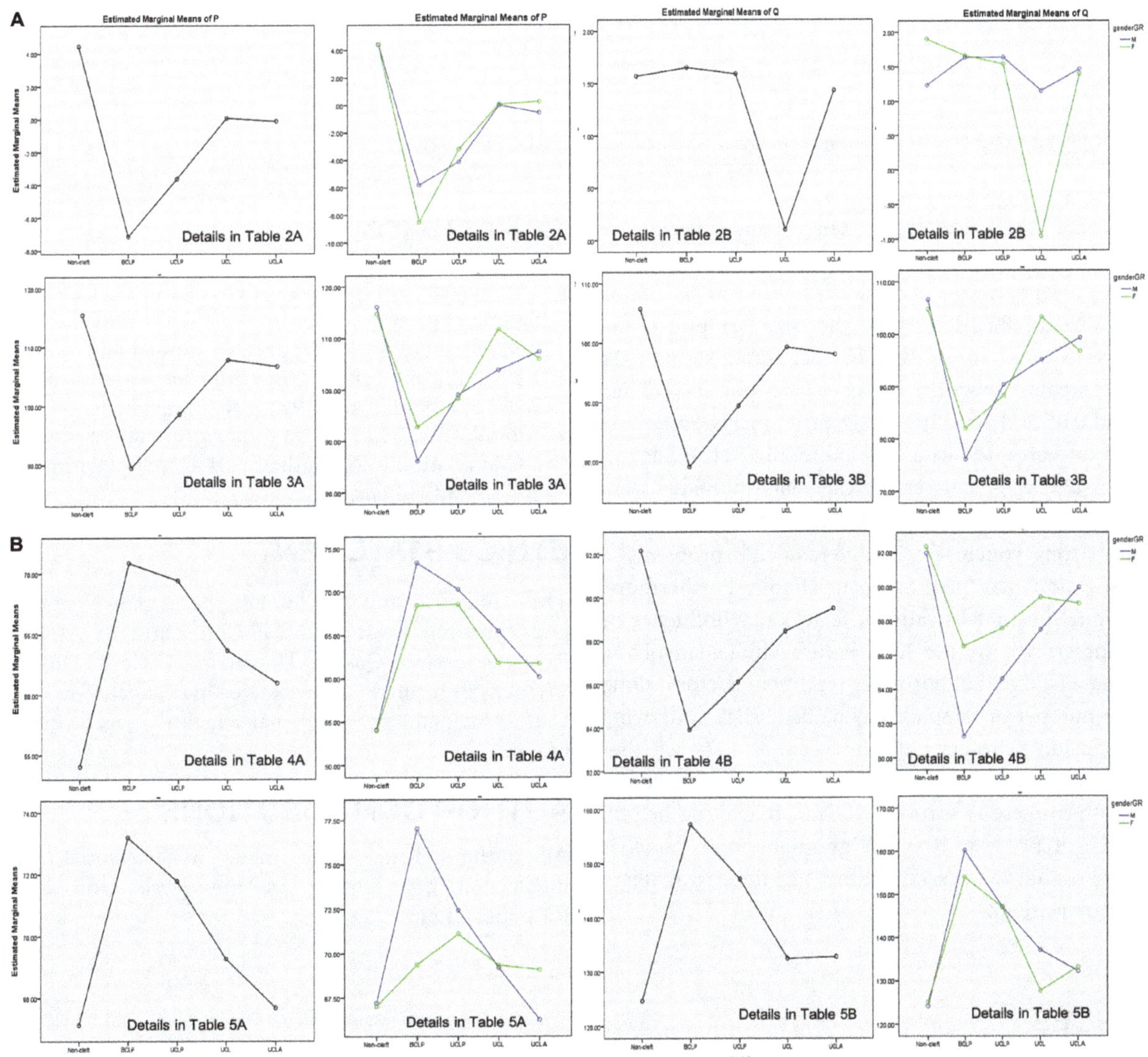

FIGURE 2 | Continued

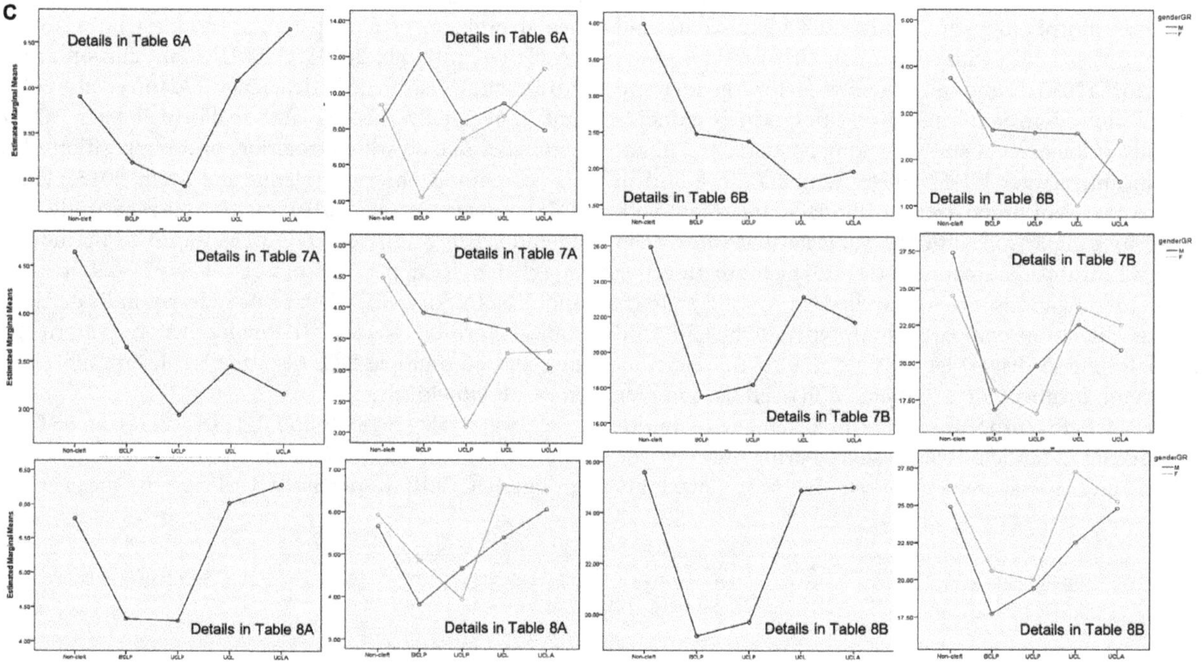

FIGURE 2 | (A–C) Profile plot of the estimated marginal means of types of cleft and gender*types of cleft.

of the two groups, the calculated Cohen's d and effect-size r were 0.578 and 0.277, respectively. Sample power analysis was done using G*Power software, and the effect size was calculated (Batwa et al., 2018). Based on this, the total sample in the five groups is required to be 103. In each group, 20 or 21 individuals are required with α err prob and power (1-β err prob) values of 0.05 and 80, respectively. Strict inclusion criteria were followed to recruit the data. A good number of BCLP and UCLP samples and age- and sex-matched NC individuals are recruited; however, the sample size of UCLA and UCL is lacking. To draw any strong conclusion in different CLP problems, a genetic investigation may play a beneficial role. Furthermore, genetic/congenital/postnatal treatment factors may influence or alter the shape/growth of the DC. Future studies involving effects of genetic/congenital/postnatal treatment factors along with a greater number of samples may be beneficial in drawing a strong conclusion. The current study cannot state whether comparative discoveries may have been obtained from different individuals with numerous sorts of NSCLP. It may be helpful to do this type of two-way ANOVA examination in bunches from different hospitals/clinics. Future investigations with bigger example sizes are justified.

CONCLUSION

- The current study investigated 14 different DC. Among 14 different DC, 8 variables showed a significant alteration among different types of NSCLP and NC individuals.
- No significant gender disparities were found in relation to types of different NSCLP and NC individuals.
- Among CLP, BCLP showed maximum alterations in different DC in relation to NC individuals as well as within other types of CLP individuals.

ETHICS STATEMENT

The studies involving human participants were reviewed and approved by the Ethical Committee of Al Rass Dental Research Center, Qassim University, Code #: DRC/009FA/20. Written informed consent to participate in this study was provided by the participants' legal guardian/next of kin.

AUTHOR CONTRIBUTIONS

All authors listed have made a substantial, direct and intellectual contribution to the work, and approved it for publication.

REFERENCES

Adetayo, A. M., Adetayo, M. O., Adeyemo, W. L., James, O. O., and Adeyemi, M. O. (2019). Unilateral cleft lip: evaluation and comparison of treatment outcome with two surgical techniques based on qualitative (subject/guardian and professional) assessment. *J. Korean Assoc. Oral. Maxillofac. Surg.* 45, 141–151.

Alam, M. K., and Alfawzan, A. A. (2020). Evaluation of sella turcica bridging and morphology in different types of cleft patients. *Front. Cell Dev. Biol.* 8:656. doi: 10.3389/fcell.2020.00656

Alam, M. K., Iida, J., Sato, Y., and Kajii, T. S. (2013). Postnatal treatment factors affecting craniofacial morphology of unilateral cleft lip and palate (UCLP) patients in a Japanese population. *Br. J. Oral. Maxillofac. Surg.* 51, 205–210.

Alam, M. K., Kajii, T. S., and Iida, J. (2012). "Spectrum of factors affecting dental arch relationships in japanese unilateral cleft lip and palate patients," in *Orthodontics-Basic Aspects and Clinical Considerations* ed. F. Bourzgui, (London: Intech Open). 13, 301–324.

Alam, M. K., Kajii, T. S., Matsuno, M. K., Kato, Y. S., and Iida, J. (2008). Multivariate analysis of factors affecting dental arch relationships in Japanese unilateral cleftlip and palate patients at Hokkaido University Hospital. *Orthod. Waves.* 67, 45–53. doi: 10.1016/j.odw.2007.12.001

Alam, M. K., Kajii, T. S., Sato, Y., and Iida, J. (2019). Clinical investigation of congenital factor affecting craniofacial morphology of unilateral cleft lip and palate in japanese patients. *Pesqui Bra. Odontopediatria Clín. Integr.* 19:4642.

Arshad, A. I., Alam, M. K., and Khamis, M. F. (2017a). Assessment of complete unilateral cleft lip and palate patients: determination of factors effecting dental arch relationships. *Int. J. Paed. Otorihnolaryng.* 92, 70–74. doi: 10.1016/j.ijporl.2016.11.006

Arshad, A. I., Alam, M. K., and Khamis, M. F. (2017b). Assessment of complete unilateral cleft lip and palate treatment outcome using EUROCRAN index and associated factors. *Int. J. Paed. Otorihnolaryng.* 100, 91–95. doi: 10.1016/j.ijporl.2017.06.025

Arshad, A. I., Alam, M. K., and Khamis, M. F. (2018). Dentoalveolar cleft treatment outcome using modified Huddart-Bodenham index and regression analysis of associated factors. *Cleft. Palate. Craniofac. J.* 55, 682–687. doi: 10.1177/1055665618758278

Asif, J. A., Alam, M. K., Haque, S., and Pohchi, A. (2016). Treatment outcome and factors affecting dental arch relationship in Malay children with unilateral cleft lip and palate (UCLP). *J. Hard. Tissue Biolog.* 25, 371–376. doi: 10.2485/jhtb.25.371

Batwa, W., Almarhoon, H. A., Almoammar, K. A., Alqahtani, N., Albarakati, S. F., and Al-Jewair, T. (2018). Dento-skeletal characteristics of cleft patients with missing teeth. *Clin., Cosmet. Investig. Dent.* 10, 237–244. doi: 10.2147/ccide.s170717

Berkowitz, S. (2013). *Cleft Lip and Palate: Diagnosis and Management.* Berlin: Springer.

Erverdi, N., and Motro, M. eds. (2015). "Cleft lip and palate treatment," in, *Alveolar Distraction Osteogenesis.* Berlin: Springer, 7–17.

Haque, S., Alam, M. K., and Basri, R. (2015). Gene involvement in cleft lip and palate (CLP) patients. *Bangladesh J. Med. Sci.* 14, 113–116. doi: 10.3329/bjms.v14i1.20928

Haque, S., Alam, M. K., and Khamis, M. F. (2017a). Factors responsible for unfavorable dental arch relationship in non syndromic unilateral cleft lip and palate children. *J. Clin. Pediatr. Dent.* 41, 236–242. doi: 10.17796/1053-4628-41.3.236

Haque, S., Alam, M. K., and Khamis, M. F. (2017b). The effect of various factors on the dental arch relationship in non-syndromic unilateral cleft lip and palate children assessed by new approach: a retrospective study. *BMC Pediatr.* 17:119. doi: 10.1186/s12887-017-0870-4

Haque, S., Alam, M. K., and Khamis, M. F. (2018). Treatment outcome of Bangladeshi UCLP patients based on both phenotype and postnatal treatment factors using modified Huddart Bodenham (mHB) index. *Cleft. Palate. Craniofac. J.* 55, 966–973. doi: 10.1597/15-293

Haque, S., and Alam, M. K. (2014). Spectrum of cheiloplasty has detrimental effect on maxillary growth: myth or fact? *Bangladesh J. Med. Sci.* 13, 473–476. doi: 10.3329/bjms.v13i4.20653

Haque, S., and Alam, M. K. (2015a). Common dental anomalies in cleft lip and palate patients. *Malaysian J. Med. Sci.* 22, 55–60.

Haque, S., and Alam, M. K. (2015b). Pre-surgical orthopedic treatment using Hotz plate: an update. *Int. J. Pharm. Bio. Sci.* 6, 318–327.

Haque, S., and Alam, M. K. (2015c). Spectrum of palatoplasty has detrimental effect on: myth or fact? *Bangladesh J. Med. Sci.* 14, 109–110. doi: 10.3329/bjms.v14i1.20926

Haque, S., Khamis, M. F., Alam, M. K., and Ahmed, W. M. A. W. (2020). Effects of multiple factors on treatment outcome in the 3d maxillary arch morphometry of unilateral cleft lip and palate children. *J. Craniofac. Surg.* doi: 10.1097/SCS.0000000000006464 Online ahead of print

Kajii, T. S., Alam, M. K., Milkoya, T., Oyama, A., Matsuno, M. K., Kato, Y. S., et al. (2013). Congenital and postnatal factors including malocclusion in Japanese unilateral cleft lip and patient- determination using logistic regression analysis. *Cleft. Palate. Craniofac. J.* 50, 466–472. doi: 10.1597/11-150

Kohli, S. S., and Kohli, V. S. (2012). A comprehensive review of the genetic basis of cleft lip and palate. *J. Oral. Maxillofac. Pathol.* 16, 64–72.

Kunz, F., Stellzig-Eisenhauer, A., Zeman, F., and Boldt, J. (2020). Evaluation of a fully automated cephalometric analysis using a customized convolutional neural network. *J. Orofac. Orthop.* 81, 52–68. doi: 10.1007/s00056-019-00203-8

Lee, K. S., Ryu, J. J., Jang, H. S., Lee, D. Y., and Jung, S. K. (2020). Deep convolutional neural networks based analysis of cephalometric radiographs for differential diagnosis of orthognathic surgery indications. *Appl. Sci.* 10:2124. doi: 10.3390/app10062124

Murray, J. C. (2002). Gene/environment causes of cleft lip and/or palate. *Clin. Genet.* 61, 248–256. doi: 10.1034/j.1399-0004.2002.610402.x

Parveen, S., Shetty. R., Husain, A., Mascarenhas, R., D'Souza, N., and Shetty, N. K. (2018). Three-dimensional assessment of alveolar bone thickness in individuals with nonsyndromic unilateral complete cleft lip and palate. *J. Cleft Lip Palate Craniofac. Anomal.* 5, 106–112. doi: 10.4103/jclpca.jclpca_11_18

Sekhon, P. S., Ethunandan, M., Markus, A. F., Krishnan, G., and Rao, C. B. (2011). Congenital anomalies associated with cleft lip and palate-an analysis of 1623 consecutive patients. *Cleft. Palate. Craniofac. J.* 48, 371–378. doi: 10.1597/09-264

Wu, T. T., Ko, E. W., Chen, P. K., and Huang, C. S. (2013). Craniofacial characteristics in unilateral complete cleft lip and palate patients with congenitally missing teeth. *Am. J. Orthod. Dentofacial Orthop.* 144, 381–390. doi: 10.1016/j.ajodo.2013.04.019

12

Evaluation of Sella Turcica Bridging and Morphology in Different Types of Cleft Patients

Mohammad Khursheed Alam[1]* and Ahmed Ali Alfawzan[2]

[1] Orthodontic Division, Department of Preventive Dental Science, College of Dentistry, Jouf University, Sakaka, Saudi Arabia,
[2] Department of Preventive Dentistry, College of Dentistry in Ar Rass, Qassim University, Ar Rass, Saudi Arabia

****Correspondence:***
Mohammad Khursheed Alam
dralam@gmail.com;
mkalam@ju.edu.sa

Objectives: To evaluate sella turcica (ST) bridging, associated anomalies, and morphology, in subjects with four different types of clefts, and compare them with non-cleft (NC) subjects.

Materials and Methods: A total of 123 (31 NC and 92 cleft) Saudi subjects who had their lateral cephalogram (Late. Ceph.), orthopantomogram (OPG), and clinical details for ordinary diagnosis were included in the study. Among 92 cleft subjects, 29 had bilateral cleft lip and palate (BCLP), 41 had unilateral cleft lip and palate (UCLP), nine had unilateral cleft lip and alveolus (UCLA), and 13 with unilateral cleft lip (UCL). ST bridging and seven parameters related to ST morphology and skeletal malocclusion were analyzed using Late. Ceph. Associated dental anomalies in ST bridging subjects were investigated using OPG. The images were investigated using artificial intelligence driven Webceph software. Multiple statistical tests were applied to see the differences between gender and among cleft vs NC subjects.

Results: ST bridging was found to be higher in cleft subjects (22.82%). Most of the cleft subjects had severe skeletal Class III malocclusion associated with multiple types of dental anomalies (impacted canines, congenital missing, and presence of supernumerary teeth). No significant gender disparities in all seven parameters of ST morphology were found between NC and cleft groups. However, there were significant differences when compared among four different types of cleft individuals vs NC subjects.

Conclusion: ST bridging is more prevalent in cleft subjects along with Class III malocclusion and associated dental anomalies. ST morphometry differs significantly between cleft vs NC subjects. BCLP exhibits smaller values of all seven parameters as compared to all other groups.

Keywords: sella turcica, sella turcica bridging, morphometry, bilateral cleft lip and palate, unilateral cleft lip and palate

INTRODUCTION

Lateral cephalogram (Late. Ceph.) uses a number of landmarks as reference points for analysis/study of craniofacial structures. Sella turcica (ST) serves as one such important landmark in the cranium on Late. Ceph. The sella point or the center of the ST is a point in the cranial base which is situated at the midpoint of ST that accommodates the pituitary gland (Celik-Karatas et al., 2015). It plays an important role in cephalometric analysis and helps us identify pathologies related to pituitary gland and hence becomes an exceptional source of information, specifically those syndromes that affect craniofacial region. A thorough knowledge of its radiological anatomy and variations may help us evaluate the growth and recognize any deviation in a variety of anomalies or pathological situations, and the possible outcome of the orthodontic treatment in such situations.

Congenital anomalies, though identified at birth often, get initiated during pregnancy due to chromosomal abnormalities. A gamut of congenital anomalies occurs in the craniofacial region, cleft lip and palate (CLP) being the most common anomaly in the head and neck region, only second to congenital heart disease in the whole body. Hence, cleft deformities have been included in their Global Burden of Disease initiative, by World Health Organization (WHO). CLP is quite variable in its presentation and affects about 1.17/1000 birth overall 1.30 of every 1000 live births in Saudi (Sabbagh et al., 2015) and Asian populations (Cooper et al., 2006). CLP has a multifactorial etiology with genetics and environmental factors to be the major contributing factors (Mars and Houston, 1990). The clefts have been classified depending upon the extent of involvement and their location as cleft palate, cleft lip, unilateral cleft lip (UCL), unilateral cleft lip and alveolus (UCLA), unilateral cleft lip and palate (UCLP), bilateral cleft lip and palate (BCLP), etc. The affected children may have retarded maxillary growth (Alam et al., 2013), malposed teeth, crowding and rotation of teeth, and a high incidence of class III malocclusion (Haque and Alam, 2015).

Most of the previous studies relating to craniofacial anomalies have used 2D imaging, such as Late. Ceph. which was cost-effective with low radiation exposure and the study of various landmarks were done efficiently by linear and angular measurements (Alkofide, 2008). The morphology of ST can be efficiently measured with Late. Ceph. With the advancement in radiographic techniques and imaging, there is a shift toward 3D imaging techniques, particularly 3D imaging using CT scan (Hasan et al., 2016a,b, 2019; Islam et al., 2017) and CBCT (Yasa et al., 2017) as they give a better and accurate extent of the lesions in a 3D view and hence play a key role in the diagnosis and treatment of craniofacial malformations.

Extensive search of literature relating to the measurement of ST revealed that there was only one study on clefts in Saudi population with little or no focus on its relation to ST (Alkofide, 2008). Very few studies have evaluated the postnatal development and structure of ST and its relation to clefts (Alkofide, 2008; Yasa et al., 2017) which measured only three parameters to establish the morphology of ST. Due to limited research in this area and alarming number of individuals with clefts without the syndrome in Saudi Arabia with this genotype, the current investigation was undertaken to calculate the seven parameters of morphology of the ST, and to compare the findings with non-cleft (NC) healthy subjects with the following aims:

1. Investigation of ST bridging, type of skeletal malocclusion, and different dental anomalies.
2. Gender disparities of seven parameters of morphology of the ST among cleft and NC subjects.
3. Multiple comparisons of seven parameters of morphology of the ST among four different types of cleft and NC subjects.

MATERIALS AND METHODS

In this retrospective study, clinical and radiographic details of 31 NC subjects and 92 cleft subjects were used. All the records were collected from Saudi board Dental residents. The research protocol was prepared by one calibrated specialist orthodontist and the data were stored. The protocol was submitted for ethical board review. After approval, data investigations and analysis were completed. The details of ethical approval number are shown in **Table 1**. Out of 92 cleft subjects, 29 had BCLP, 41 had UCLP, nine had UCLA, and 13 had UCL as per cleft classification details from the clinical records. The details of age and gender distribution, demographic details, and inclusion and exclusion criteria are presented in **Table 1**.

Lateral cephalogram X-rays were used to investigate of ST bridging by two observers and the data were recorded after agreement by both the observers and analyzed. In a similar manner, each orthopantomogram (OPG) was investigated and dental anomalies are listed after agreement by both the observers in cases with ST bridging. Late. Ceph. X-ray was also used for skeletal class of malocclusion assessment (based on ANB and Wits measurement) only in cases with ST bridging and seven parameters of ST morphology in all subjects (Hasan et al., 2016a,b, 2019; Islam et al., 2017) were measured by one examiner using artificial intelligence driven Webceph software (Korea). The details of the seven parameters measurements are presented in **Table 1** (Hasan et al., 2016a,b, 2019; Islam et al., 2017) and shown in **Figure 1** (Hasan et al., 2016a,b, 2019; Islam et al., 2017).

Statistical Analyses

After a 2-week interval, 20 randomly selected X-rays were used for re-measurement in a similar fashion. For ST bridging and dental anomalies results were tested using Kappa test for intra and inter-examiner reliability. Error testing in the investigation of ST morphology based on seven parameters measurements were tested by intra-class correlation co-efficient (ICC) test. Total investigated data were analyzed using version 26.0 SPSS software (IBM, Armonk, NY, United States). Normality of the measured seven parameters of ST morphology data was assessed using Kolmogorov–Smirnov test. Descriptive statistics were calculated for each parameter and presented in a tabulated format. Independent *t*-test was used for gender disparities and ANOVA test used for multiple comparison among NC and all four types of cleft groups.

TABLE 1 | Demographic details and methods.

Population	**Saudi subjects**					
Inclusion and exclusion criteria	Non syndromic cleft subjects with good quality x-ray images. No history of craniofacial surgical treatment besides lip and palate surgery. No orthodontic treatment has been done. No anatomical variation in the ST and sphenoidal regions. Matched with healthy control without any craniofacial deformity. Subjects using hormonal medications or corticosteroids were excluded from the study.					
Sampling	Convenient sampling following inclusion and exclusion criteria.					
Type of cleft		**Non-cleft**	**BCLP**	**UCLP**	**UCLA**	**UCL**
Subjects distribution	Male	14	19	26	3	7
	Female	17	10	15	6	6
	Total (N = 123)	31	29	41	9	13
Age		13.29 ± 3.52	14.07 ± 4.73	14.32 ± 4.46	12.78 ± 4.09	13.31 ± 4.46
Data used	Digital lateral cephalogram, orthopantomogram, and clinical record details.					
Ethical clearance	Protocol has been presented to the ethical board of Alrass Dental Research Center, Qassim University. Ethical clearance has been obtained with the Code #: DRC/009FA/20.					
Method	**Artificial intelligence driven technique using Webceph software (Korea)**					
Landmarks used and the details	TS	Tuberculum sella	The most anterior point of the contour of the sella turcica			
	DS	Dorsum sellae	The posterior wall of the sella turcica			
	SF	Sella floor	The deepest point on the floor of pituitary fossa			
	Pclin	Posterior clenoid	The most anterior point of the PClin process			
	SA	Sella anterior	The most anterior point of the sella			
	SP	Sella posterior	The most posterior point of the sella			
	SM	Sella median	A point midway between PClin and TS			
Measurements (seven parameters)			**Significance/importance**			
a	Sella length	TS-Pclin	Changes in the size of sella turcica are often identified with the pathology of pituitary gland and may have an undetected hidden disease; hence, sella length is one of the parameters to determine the sella size.			
b	Sella width	SA-SP	Utilized clinically for pubertal growth phase determination, would be increased by advanced age, it has strong correlation with age.			
c	Sella diameter	TS-DS	Growth of an individual can be assessed based on the diameter of the sella turcica at different age periods.			
d	Sella height anterior	TS-SF	As the anterior part of the sella turcica is believed to develop mainly from neural crest cell, so we need to measure the sella height anterior. So that, we can assume or determine any structural deviation in the anterior wall which are believed to be associated with the specific deviation in the facial structure.			
e	Sella height posterior	PClin-SF	The posterior part of the sella turcica develops from the para-axial-mesoderm, which develops approximately 7 weeks of gestation. If any disturbance occurs in this area it remains throughout the life, as the time of formation of sella closely associated with the development of maxilla. So that, it may be assumed that any aberration leading to cleft may be associated with some fault at the level of sella turcica.			
f	Sella height median	SM-SF	Utilized clinically for pubertal growth phase determination, would be increased with age.			
g	Sella area	TS-SA-SF-SP-Pclin	During embryological development of the sella area is the key point for the migration of the neural crest cells to the fronto nasal and maxillary developmental fields. Pituitary fossa increased in size with age and found a positive correlation of the area of the sella to age.			

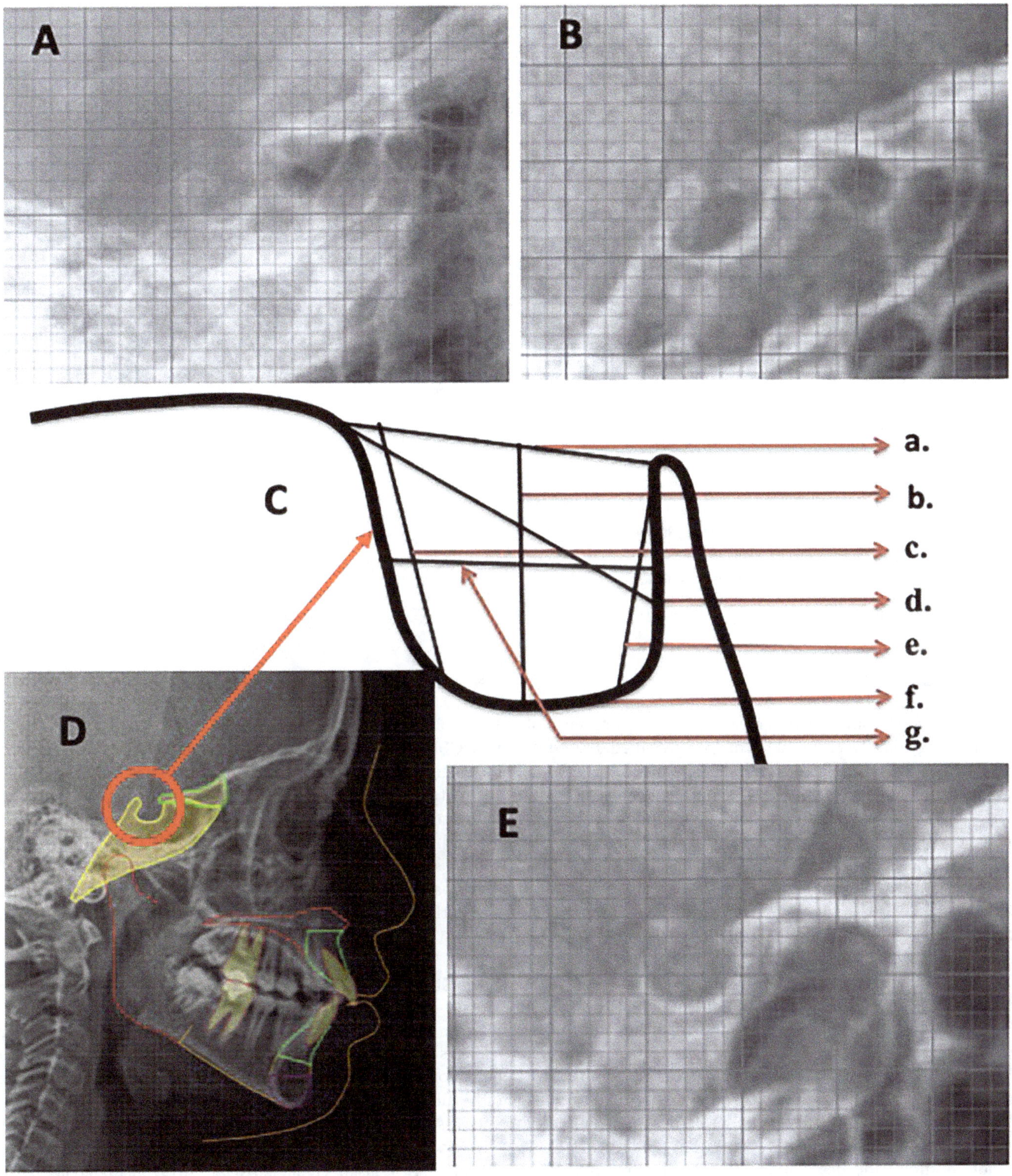

FIGURE 1 | Lateral cephalogram view of sella turcica in **(A)** BCLP, **(B)** UCLP, **(C)** sella turcica parameters: **(a)** TS-Pclin; **(b)** SA-SP; **(c)** TS-DS; **(d)** TS-SF; **(e)** PClin-SF; **(f)** SM-SF; and **(g)** sella area, **(D)** Control, and **(E)** UCLA subjects.

TABLE 2 | Sella turcica bridging, type of malocclusion and associated anomalies.

Gender	Sella bridging	Subject	Skeletal malocclusion	Dental anomalies	Prevalence
F	Complete	Non-cleft	Class I	IC	Non-cleft = 6.45%
M	Partial	Non-cleft	Class II	IC	
F	Partial	Bilateral Cleft Lip and Palate	Class III	CM + IC	BCLP = 20.69%
M	Partial	Bilateral Cleft Lip and Palate	Class III	CM	
M	Partial	Bilateral Cleft Lip and Palate	Class III	None	
M	Partial	Bilateral Cleft Lip and Palate	Class III	CM	
M	Partial	Bilateral Cleft Lip and Palate	Class III	CM + IC	
M	Partial	Bilateral Cleft Lip and Palate	Class III	None	
M	Partial	Unilateral Cleft Lip and Palate Lt Side	Class III	CM	UCLP = 24.39%
F	Partial	Unilateral Cleft Lip and Palate Lt Side	Class III	IC	
M	Partial	Unilateral Cleft Lip and Palate Lt Side	Class III	CM	
F	Complete	Unilateral Cleft Lip and Palate Lt Side	Class III	CM + IC	
F	Partial	Unilateral Cleft Lip and Palate Lt Side	Class III	CM + IC	
M	Partial	Unilateral Cleft Lip and Palate Lt Side	Class III	IC	
F	Complete	Unilateral Cleft Lip and Palate Lt Side	Class III	CM + IC + Dilaceration	
M	Partial	Unilateral Cleft Lip and Palate Rt Side	Class I	CM	
M	Partial	Unilateral Cleft Lip and Palate Rt Side	Class III	CM + IC	
M	Complete	Unilateral Cleft Lip and Palate Rt Side	Class I	CM	
F	Partial	Unilateral Cleft Lip and Alveolus Rt Side	Class III	CM	UCLA = 11.11%
F	Complete	Unilateral Cleft Lip Lt Side	Class III	CM	UCL = 30.77%
M	Partial	Unilateral Cleft Lip Rt Side	Class III	SN	
M	Partial	Unilateral Cleft Lip Rt Side	Class II	CM + IC	
F	Complete	Unilateral Cleft Lip Rt Side	Class III	CM	

Non-cleft = M, male; F, female; IC, impacted canine; CM, congenital missing; SN, supernumerary tooth.

RESULTS

Using Kolmogorov–Smirnov test, measured seven parameters of ST morphology data were found normally distributed. Error test results of the ST bridging and dental anomalies investigation showed excellent intra and inter-examiner reliability. ICC results for all seven parameters of ST morphology ranged from 0.86 to 0.94.

Prevalence of ST bridging, type of malocclusion involved, and associated dental anomalies are listed in **Table 2**. Overall, 6.45 and 22.82% ST bridging was found in NC and cleft individuals, respectively. Among four types of clefts, ST bridging found, UCL > UCLP > BCLP > UCLA. Highest % in UCL (30.77%). Skeletal Class III malocclusion was found to be more prevalent in ST bridging individuals. Among dental anomalies, impacted canine, congenital missing, and supernumerary teeth were found to be common.

Table 3 shows the details of descriptive and comparative gender disparities results among NC and different types of clefts (NC, BCLP, UCLP, UCLA, and UCL). Overall ST morphometry has been presented which shows no significant gender disparities.

Table 4 shows the description total details among all five groups (NC, BCLP, UCLP, UCLA, and UCL) subjects. Multiple comparison results are presented in **Table 5**. Significantly larger TS-Pclin has been found in NC group in comparison to all four-cleft group ($p < 0.001$). However, there are no significant differences within the cleft group found. Smallest value found in BCLP group was 7.884 mm. Sa-SP value shows significant disparities between NC vs BCLP ($p < 0.001$), NC vs UCLP ($p < 0.001$), and NC vs UCL ($p = 0.012$) groups. When TS-DS values were compared, NC vs BCLP ($p < 0.001$), BCLP vs UCLP ($p = 0.018$) and UCL ($p = 0.037$) showed significant disparities. There were significant disparities between NC vs BCLP ($p < 0.001$) and BCLP vs UCL ($p = 0.019$) in PClin-SF parameter. And, when compared the parameters of SM-SF and TS-SA-SF-SP-PClin, NC vs BCLP and NC vs UCLP shows significant disparities. In BCLP group, values of all seven parameters of ST morphometry showed smallest values in comparison with all four groups.

DISCUSSION

Unique quality of this study is that five different groups of subjects were investigated. Only one study has been found based on literature search and used three groups of subjects of Saudi population. ST bridging, type of skeletal malocclusion, and associated dental anomalies at time in a single study have not been investigated before. All seven parameters of ST morphology (Hasan et al., 2016a,b, 2019; Islam et al., 2017) are investigated in this study. Previous studies measured three parameters of ST morphology and ST bridging only (Alkofide, 2008; Yasa et al., 2017).

A thorough knowledge of ST and its variations is very important to identify it from medically compromised patients such as spina bifida or craniofacial deviations (Axelsson et al., 2004).

TABLE 3 | Gender disparities of all sella turcica morphomometric parameters among all five groups.

Group	Variables	Gender	Mean	SD	95% CI		p
					Lower	Upper	
Control	A	Male	11.164	1.690	−0.685	1.369	0.501
		Female	10.822	1.090			
	B	Male	9.669	1.466	−1.105	1.123	0.987
		Female	9.659	1.544			
	C	Male	10.925	3.296	−1.489	2.966	0.503
		Female	10.187	2.771			
	D	Male	8.210	1.461	−0.649	1.708	0.366
		Female	7.681	1.698			
	E	Male	7.779	0.911	−1.049	1.329	0.812
		Female	7.639	2.007			
	F	Male	8.746	1.131	−0.531	1.355	0.379
		Female	8.335	1.385			
	G	Male	77.133	22.446	−9.325	23.683	0.381
		Female	69.954	22.288			
BCLP	A	Male	8.075	0.989	−0.390	1.495	0.239
		Female	7.522	1.480			
	B	Male	7.422	1.289	−0.520	1.639	0.297
		Female	6.862	1.455			
	C	Male	7.663	2.258	−1.330	2.366	0.570
		Female	7.145	2.398			
	D	Male	6.254	1.487	−0.897	1.452	0.632
		Female	5.977	1.420			
	E	Male	6.229	1.142	−0.876	1.083	0.829
		Female	6.125	1.368			
	F	Male	7.210	1.308	−0.928	1.365	0.699
		Female	6.991	1.650			
	G	Male	49.767	17.188	−9.614	18.425	0.525
		Female	45.362	18.076			
UCLP	A	Male	8.223	1.266	−0.381	1.308	0.273
		Female	7.759	1.324			
	B	Male	7.774	1.492	−1.081	1.018	0.951
		Female	7.806	1.778			
	C	Male	9.392	2.418	−1.659	1.480	0.908
		Female	9.481	2.348			
	D	Male	6.903	1.227	−1.034	0.513	0.499
		Female	7.164	1.089			
	E	Male	6.895	1.054	−0.798	0.549	0.710
		Female	7.019	0.977			
	F	Male	7.278	1.158	−0.872	0.582	0.689
		Female	7.423	1.013			
	G	Male	57.560	12.685	−6.058	10.327	0.601
		Female	55.425	12.139			
UCL	A	Male	8.873	1.495	−0.940	2.356	0.365
		Female	8.165	1.141			
	B	Male	8.034	1.636	−1.968	2.016	0.979
		Female	8.010	1.616			
	C	Male	9.739	2.744	−3.412	2.480	0.734
		Female	10.205	1.923			
	D	Male	7.199	1.377	−2.404	0.968	0.369
		Female	7.917	1.378			
	E	Male	7.543	0.845	−1.474	1.400	0.956
		Female	7.580	1.474			

(Continued)

TABLE 3 | Continued

Group	Variables	Gender	Mean	SD	95% CI		*p*
					Lower	Upper	
	F	Male	7.711	1.692	−2.626	1.652	0.626
		Female	8.198	1.810			
	G	Male	62.428	21.557	−29.800	19.872	0.669
		Female	67.392	18.638			
UCLA	A	Male	8.303	1.414	−2.153	1.033	0.433
		Female	8.863	0.686			
	B	Male	8.120	1.026	−3.044	2.150	0.696
		Female	8.567	1.719			
	C	Male	10.167	0.257	−3.081	4.514	0.669
		Female	9.450	2.683			
	D	Male	6.823	0.770	−2.662	2.129	0.800
		Female	7.090	1.624			
	E	Male	6.923	1.822	−3.178	3.048	0.962
		Female	6.988	1.878			
	F	Male	7.040	1.574	−3.876	2.599	0.655
		Female	7.678	2.064			
	G	Male	54.233	10.970	−39.066	31.380	0.804
		Female	58.076	23.940			

**$p < 0.05$ considered statistically significant.*

TABLE 4 | Descriptive results of all sella turcica morphomometric parameters among all five groups.

	TS-PClin		SA-SP		TS-DS		TS-SF		PClin-SF		SM-SF		TS-SA-SF-SP-PClin	
	Mean	SD	Mean	SD	Mean	SD	Mean	SD	Mean	SD	Mean	SD	Mean	SD
Control	10.976	1.379	9.664	1.484	10.520	2.991	7.920	1.592	7.702	1.585	8.521	1.273	73.196	22.281
BCLP	7.884	1.185	7.229	1.350	7.484	2.278	6.159	1.445	6.193	1.201	7.134	1.409	48.248	17.306
UCLP	8.053	1.291	7.786	1.580	9.424	2.363	6.999	1.172	6.940	1.016	7.331	1.096	56.779	12.378
UCL	8.546	1.340	8.023	1.557	9.954	2.316	7.530	1.370	7.560	1.124	7.936	1.691	64.720	19.589
UCLA	8.677	0.934	8.418	1.470	9.689	2.155	7.001	1.347	6.967	1.742	7.466	1.839	56.795	19.799

In a study by Alkofide (2008), the morphological variations of ST were assessed in CLP patients and it was found that most of the patients had morphological deviations such as irregular posterior wall and double contour of the floor as compared to normally formed ST. Second, in the NC subjects included in the study, the morphology of ST was normal as compared to the people with clefts. In the earlier study, it was shown that ST bridging was 5.5–22% in normal person, while it was 6.45% in the NC individuals. In the present study, it is 22.82% overall in the cleft patients. However, its occurrence was more in patients with craniofacial deviations. ST bridging was 30.77% in subjects with UCL in the present study. Under such circumstances, it draws attention and marks the direction for future research and study if ST bridge exists in normal individuals in the current population.

Various investigations have been done on the morphology of ST with varying techniques (Axelsson et al., 2004; Alkofide, 2008; Hasan et al., 2016a,b, 2019; Islam et al., 2017; Yasa et al., 2017). In the current study, no significant gender disparities of the ST morphology in all seven parameters were found. Taking into account the results of the current and the previous studies (Islam et al., 2017; Yasa et al., 2017), gender disparities were measurably insignificant for all linear and area measurements of ST. According to Weisberg et al. (1976), individuals with abnormal ST may suffer from undetected hidden disease. Hence, from an altered state of ST, pathology or anomaly can be identified that may influence the secretion of hormones such as growth hormone, prolactin, follicle stimulating hormone, and thyroid stimulating hormone (Alkofide, 2007).

The results revealed significant disparities in different parameters of the ST morphology in cleft subjects (BCLP, UCLP, UCLA, and UCL) as compared to the NC and also among different types of cleft subjects (BCLP, UCLP, UCLA, and UCL). BCLP subjects exhibited smaller measurements in all parameters compared to the other groups. Results revealed disparities in the measured three parameters of ST morphology are smaller (Alkofide, 2008) and larger (Yasa et al., 2017) between cleft subjects than in NC subjects. Alkofide (2008) found smaller measurements in UCLP subjects. Yasa at al. found larger values in all three measured parameters in cleft group, only length showed highly significant disparities, however, the type of cleft was not mentioned. In another study, data of 62 subjects with palatally impacted canine revealed significant disparities in ST bridging

TABLE 5 | Multiple comparison of all sella turcica morphomometric parameters among all five groups.

Variables	Multiple comparison			MD	SE	95% CI		p-Value
						Lower bound	Upper bound	
TS-PClin	Control	vs	BCLP	3.09199*	0.329	2.150	4.034	0.000
			UCLP	2.92271*	0.303	2.055	3.790	0.000
			UCL	2.42998*	0.421	1.226	3.634	0.000
			UCLA	2.29946*	0.482	0.919	3.680	0.000
	BCLP	vs	UCLP	−0.16928	0.309	−1.054	0.715	1.000
			UCL	−0.66202	0.425	−1.879	0.555	1.000
			UCLA	−0.79253	0.486	−2.183	0.598	1.000
	UCLP	vs	UCL	−0.49274	0.406	−1.653	0.667	1.000
			UCLA	−0.62325	0.469	−1.965	0.718	1.000
	UCL	vs	UCLA	−0.13051	0.552	−1.711	1.450	1.000
SA-SP	Control	vs	BCLP	2.43493*	0.386	1.331	3.539	0.000
			UCLP	1.87769*	0.356	0.860	2.895	0.000
			UCL	1.64047*	0.494	0.228	3.053	0.012
			UCLA	1.24577	0.566	−0.373	2.864	0.296
	BCLP	vs	UCLP	−0.55723	0.363	−1.594	0.480	1.000
			UCL	−0.79446	0.499	−2.221	0.632	1.000
			UCLA	−1.18916	0.570	−2.820	0.442	0.391
	UCLP	vs	UCL	−0.23722	0.476	−1.598	1.123	1.000
			UCLA	−0.63192	0.550	−2.205	0.941	1.000
	UCL	vs	UCLA	−0.3947	0.648	−2.248	1.459	1.000
TS-DS	Control	vs	BCLP	3.03586*	0.646	1.187	4.885	0.000
			UCLP	1.09561	0.595	−0.608	2.799	0.683
			UCL	0.56615	0.827	−1.799	2.931	1.000
			UCLA	0.83111	0.947	−1.879	3.541	1.000
	BCLP	vs	UCLP	−1.94025*	0.607	−3.677	−0.204	0.018
			UCL	−2.46971*	0.835	−4.858	−0.081	0.037
			UCLA	−2.20475	0.955	−4.936	0.526	0.226
	UCLP	vs	UCL	−0.52946	0.796	−2.807	1.749	1.000
			UCLA	−0.2645	0.921	−2.899	2.370	1.000
	UCL	vs	UCLA	0.26496	1.085	−2.838	3.368	1.000
TS-SF	Control	vs	BCLP	1.76106*	0.358	0.737	2.785	0.000
			UCLP	0.92114	0.330	−0.022	1.864	0.061
			UCL	0.38968	0.458	−0.920	1.699	1.000
			UCLA	0.91857	0.525	−0.582	2.419	0.825
	BCLP	vs	UCLP	−0.83992	0.336	−1.801	0.122	0.138
			UCL	−1.37138*	0.462	−2.694	−0.049	0.037
			UCLA	−0.84249	0.529	−2.355	0.670	1.000
	UCLP	vs	UCL	−0.53146	0.441	−1.793	0.730	1.000
			UCLA	−0.00257	0.510	−1.461	1.456	1.000
	UCL	vs	UCLA	0.52889	0.601	−1.190	2.247	1.000
PClin-SF	Control	vs	BCLP	1.50883*	0.333	0.555	2.463	0.000
			UCLP	0.76169	0.307	−0.117	1.640	0.146
			UCL	0.14194	0.426	−1.078	1.362	1.000
			UCLA	0.73527	0.489	−0.663	2.133	1.000
	BCLP	vs	UCLP	−0.74714	0.313	−1.643	0.149	0.186
			UCL	−1.36690*	0.431	−2.599	−0.135	0.019
			UCLA	−0.77356	0.492	−2.182	0.635	1.000
	UCLP	vs	UCL	−0.61976	0.411	−1.795	0.555	1.000
			UCLA	−0.02642	0.475	−1.385	1.333	1.000
	UCL	vs	UCLA	0.59333	0.560	−1.008	2.194	1.000

(Continued)

TABLE 5 | Continued

Variables	Multiple comparison			MD	SE	95% CI		*p*-Value
						Lower bound	Upper bound	
SM-SF	Control	vs	BCLP	1.38651*	0.348	0.392	2.381	0.001
			UCLP	1.18991*	0.320	0.274	2.106	0.003
			UCL	0.58449	0.445	−0.688	1.857	1.000
			UCLA	1.05509	0.510	−0.403	2.513	0.406
	BCLP	vs	UCLP	−0.19659	0.327	−1.131	0.738	1.000
			UCL	−0.80202	0.449	−2.087	0.483	0.767
			UCLA	−0.33142	0.513	−1.800	1.138	1.000
	UCLP	vs	UCL	−0.60542	0.428	−1.831	0.620	1.000
			UCLA	−0.13482	0.495	−1.552	1.282	1.000
	UCL	vs	UCLA	0.4706	0.584	−1.199	2.140	1.000
TS-SA-SF-SP-PClin	Control	vs	BCLP	24.94809*	4.584	11.835	38.061	0.000
			UCLP	16.41760*	4.223	4.336	28.499	0.002
			UCL	8.4768	5.863	−8.295	25.249	1.000
			UCLA	16.40092	6.718	−2.819	35.621	0.161
	BCLP		UCLP	−8.53049	4.305	−20.847	3.786	0.499
			UCL	−16.4713	5.922	−33.414	0.471	0.063
			UCLA	−8.54716	6.770	−27.915	10.821	1.000
	UCLP		UCL	−7.9408	5.648	−24.097	8.216	1.000
			UCLA	−0.01667	6.531	−18.702	18.668	1.000
	UCL		UCLA	7.92413	7.694	−14.087	29.935	1.000

$^*p < 0.05$ considered statistically significant.

and three parameters of ST morphology as compared to the control in Saudi population (Baidas et al., 2018).

Studies in the past have shown that patients with disorders or syndromes such as holoprosencephaly (Kjær et al., 2002), Down syndrome (Hasan et al., 2019), spina bifida (Kjær et al., 1999), CLP (Alkofide, 2008; Yasa et al., 2017), fragile X syndrome (Kjær et al., 2001), Williams syndrome (Axelsson et al., 2004), and severe craniofacial deformities (Becktor et al., 2000) have craniofacial malformations which affect the size and/or morphology of ST.

It is well established that the anatomy of ST is variable, and it is of remarkable importance in orthodontics. The anterior form of ST may aid in predicting the patient growth and in surveying craniofacial morphology (Bishara and Athanasiou, 1995). An orthodontist should be aware of the normal variations in the ST which might help in identifying any pathology associated with it (Du Boulay and Trickey, 1967). The outcomes suggest that ST bridging and altered ST morphology in CLP subjects required careful monitoring of skeletal malocclusion, dental anomalies, and canine eruption are required to diagnosed and guide for better management at an early age.

CONCLUSION

ST bridging, type of skeletal malocclusion, and associated dental anomalies are common in cleft subjects compared to NC subjects. No significant gender disparities were found in four different types of cleft vs NC subjects. All seven parameters of ST morphology are smaller in NC subjects compared to those with clefts. BCLP subjects had smaller measurements in all seven parameters of ST morphology as compared to NC and all other types of cleft subjects.

ETHICS STATEMENT

The studies involving human participants were reviewed and approved by the Ethical Board of Alrass Dental Research Center, Qassim University. Ethical clearance has been obtained with the Code #: DRC/009FA/20. Written informed consent to participate in this study was provided by the participants' legal guardian/next of kin.

AUTHOR CONTRIBUTIONS

Both authors contributed to the article and approved the submitted version.

REFERENCES

Alam, M. K., Iida, J., Sato, Y., and Kajii, T. S. (2013). Postnatal treatment factors affecting craniofacial morphology of unilateral cleft lip and palate (UCLP) patients in a Japanese population. *Br. J. Oral Maxillofac. Surg.* 51, e205–e210. doi: 10.1016/j.bjoms.2012.10.001

Alkofide, E. (2007). The shape and size of sella turcica in skeletal class I, class II, and class III Saudi subjects. *Eur. J. Orthod.* 29, 457–463. doi: 10.1093/ejo/cjm049

Alkofide, E. A. (2008). Sella turcica morphology and dimensions in cleft subjects. *Cleft Palate Craniofac J.* 45, 647–653. doi: 10.1597/07-058.1

Axelsson, S., Storhaug, K., and Kjaer, I. (2004). Post-natal size and morphology of the sella turcica. Longitudinal cephalometric standards for Norwegians between 6 and 21 years of age. *Eur. J. Orthod.* 26, 597–604. doi: 10.1093/ejo/26.6.597

Baidas, L. F., Al-Kawari, H. M., Al-Obaidan, Z., Al-Marhoon, A., and Al-Shahrani, S. (2018). Association of sella turcica bridging with palatal canine impaction in skeletal Class I and Class II. *Clin. Cosmet Investig Dent.* 10, 179–187. doi: 10.2147/ccide.s161164

Becktor, J. P., Einersen, S., and Kjaer, I. (2000). A sella turcica bridge in subjects with severe craniofacial deviations. *Eur. J. Orthod.* 22, 69–74. doi: 10.1093/ejo/22.1.69

Bishara, S., and Athanasiou, A. (1995). "Cephalometric methods for assessment of dentofacial changes," in *Orthodontic Cephalometry*, ed. A. E. Athanasiou (St Louis, MO: Mosby-Wolfe), 105–124.

Celik-Karatas, R. M., Kahraman, F. B., and Akin, M. (2015). The shape and size of the sella turcica in turkish subjects with different skeletal patterns. *Eur. J. Med. Sci.* 2, 65–71.

Cooper, M. E., Ratay, J. S., and Marazita, M. L. (2006). Asian oral-facial cleft birth prevalence. *Cleft Palate Craniofac J.* 43, 580–589. doi: 10.1597/05-167

Du Boulay, G., and Trickey, S. (1967). The choice of radiological investigations in the management of tumours around the sella. *Clin. Radiol.* 18, 349–365. doi: 10.1016/s0009-9260(67)80035-7

Haque, S., and Alam, M. K. (2015). Common dental anomalies in cleft lip and palate patients. *Malays J. Med. Sci.* 22, 55–60.

Hasan, H. A., Alam, M. K., Abdullah, Y. J., Nakano, J., Yusa, T., Yusof, A., et al. (2016a). 3DCT morphometric analysis of sella turcica in Iraqi population. *J. Hard. Tissue Biol.* 25, 227–232. doi: 10.2485/jhtb.25.227

Hasan, H. A., Alam, M. K., Yusof, A., Mizushima, H., Kida, A., and Osuga, N. (2016b). Size and morphology of sella turcica in Malay populations: a 3D CT study. *J. Hard. Tissue Biol.* 25, 313–320. doi: 10.2485/jhtb.25.313

Hasan, H. A., Hameed, H. A., Alam, M. K., Yusof, A., Murakami, H., Kubo, K., et al. (2019). Sella turcica morphology phenotyping in Malay subjects with down's syndrome. *J. Hard. Tissue Biol.* 28, 259–264. doi: 10.2485/jhtb.28.259

Islam, M., Alam, M. K., Yusof, A., Kato, I., Honda, Y., Kubo, K., et al. (2017). 3D CT study of morphological shape and size of sella turcica in Bangladeshi population. *J. Hard. Tissue Biol.* 26, 1–6. doi: 10.2485/jhtb.26.1

Kjær, I., Fischer Hansen, B., Reintoft, I., and Keeling, J. (1999). Pituitary gland and axial skeletal malformation in human fetuses with spina bifida. *Eur. J. Pediatr. Surg.* 9, 354–358. doi: 10.1055/s-2008-1072282

Kjær, I., Hjalgrim, H., and Russell, B. G. (2001). Cranial and hand skeleton in fragile X syndrome. *Am. J. Med. Genet.* 100, 156–161. doi: 10.1002/ajmg.1226

Kjær, I., Keeling, J. W., Fischer, H. B., and Becktor, K. B. (2002). Midline skeletodental morphology in holoprosencephaly. *Cleft Palate Craniofacial J.* 39, 357–363. doi: 10.1597/1545-1569_2002_039_0357_msmih_2.0.co_2

Mars, M., and Houston, W. J. (1990). A preliminary study of facial growth and morphology in unoperated male unilateral cleft lip and palate subjects over 13 years of age. *Cleft Palate J.* 27, 7–10. doi: 10.1597/1545-1569_1990_027_0007_apsofg_2.3.co_2

Sabbagh, H. J., Innes, N. P., Sallout, B. I., Peter, A. M., Nasir, A., Al-Khozami, A. I., et al. (2015). Birth prevalence of non-syndromic orofacial clefts in Saudi Arabia and the effects of parental consanguinity. *Saud. Med. J.* 36, 1076–1083. doi: 10.15537/smj.2015.9.11823

Weisberg, L. A., Zimmerman, E. A., and Frantz, A. G. (1976). Diagnosis and evaluation of patients with an enlarged sella turcica. *Am. J. Med.* 61, 590–596. doi: 10.1016/0002-9343(76)90136-4

Yasa, Y., Bayrakdar, I. S., Ocak, A., Duman, S. B., and Dedeoglu, N. (2017). Evaluation of sella turcica shape and dimensions in cleft subjects using cone-beam computed tomography. *Med. Princ. Pract.* 26, 280–285. doi: 10.1159/000453526

13

New Insights Into Cranial Synchondrosis Development

Noriko Funato*[1,2]

[1] Department of Signal Gene Regulation, Tokyo Medical and Dental University, Tokyo, Japan,

[2] Research Core, Tokyo Medical and Dental University, Tokyo, Japan

****Correspondence:***
Noriko Funato
noriko-funato@umin.ac.jp

The synchondroses formed via endochondral ossification in the cranial base are an important growth center for the neurocranium. Abnormalities in the synchondroses affect cranial base elongation and the development of adjacent regions, including the craniofacial bones. In the central region of the cranial base, there are two synchondroses present—the intersphenoid synchondrosis and the spheno-occipital synchondrosis. These synchondroses consist of mirror image bipolar growth plates. The cross-talk of several signaling pathways, including the parathyroid hormone-like hormone (PTHLH)/parathyroid hormone-related protein (PTHrP), Indian hedgehog (Ihh), Wnt/β-catenin, and fibroblast growth factor (FGF) pathways, as well as regulation by cilium assembly and the transcription factors encoded by the *RUNX2*, *SIX1*, *SIX2*, *SIX4*, and *TBX1* genes, play critical roles in synchondrosis development. Deletions or activation of these gene products in mice causes the abnormal ossification of cranial synchondrosis and skeletal elements. Gene disruption leads to both similar and markedly different abnormalities in the development of intersphenoid synchondrosis and spheno-occipital synchondrosis, as well as in the phenotypes of synchondroses and skeletal bones. This paper reviews the development of cranial synchondroses, along with its regulation by the signaling pathways and transcription factors, highlighting the differences between intersphenoid synchondrosis and spheno-occipital synchondrosis.

Keywords: cranial base, cartilage, mesoderm, neural crest, spheno-occipital synchondrosis, intersphenoid synchondrosis, *RUNX2*

INTRODUCTION

In vertebrates, the cranial base lies below the brain and forms a central bone structure of the skull. Within the cranial base, synchondroses play a critical role in the longitudinal growth of the skull (McBratney-Owen et al., 2008; Wei et al., 2017). Precocious ossification and/or malformation of cranial synchondroses can induce the fusion of adjacent bones and subsequent cranium deformities, such as microcephaly and midface hypoplasia (Goldstein et al., 2014; Funato et al., 2020). In order to understand the nature of craniofacial development and related congenital anomalies, identifying the signaling molecules that regulate synchondrosis development is necessary.

Cartilaginous segments that persist between the ossification centers in the cranial base represent various synchondroses, such as the sphenoethmoidal synchondrosis, intersphenoid synchondrosis (ISS), spheno-occipital synchondrosis (SOS), and intraoccipital synchondrosis (**Figure 1A**). The ISS is located between the presphenoid and basisphenoid bones in the central region of the cranial base, while the SOS is located between the basisphenoid and basioccipital bones (**Figures 1A,B**). The medial line of the cranial base is originally composed of the hypophyseal, acrochordal, and parachordal cartilages (McBratney-Owen et al., 2008). Subsequently, the hypophyseal cartilage and acrochordal cartilage develop into the ISS and SOS, respectively (McBratney-Owen et al., 2008). The cartilage primordium of the ISS is derived from the neural crest, whereas the SOS has a more complex origin, wherein its cartilage primordium is derived from the neural crest as well as the cranial mesoderm (**Figure 1C**; McBratney-Owen et al., 2008). The SOS contributes to the embryonic and postnatal elongation of the cranial base, until its ossification between the ages of 16 and 18 years in humans, whereas complete ossification of the ISS occurs between 2 and 3 years of age (Madeline and Elster, 1995), suggesting that the role of the SOS, in particular, is important in the postnatal stage.

The cranial base is formed by endochondral ossification, which begins with the formation of a cartilage primordium from condensed mesenchymal cells (McBratney-Owen et al., 2008). Chondrocyte proliferation maintains the synchondroses and leads to elongation of the cranial base (Matsushita et al., 2009). Immature chondrocytes undergo hypertrophy and subsequent apoptosis, followed by the formation of ossification centers after the invasion of osteoblasts from the perichondrium (St-Jacques et al., 1999). Endochondral ossification of the cranial synchondroses is different from that of skeletal bones in several ways. The synchondrosis is composed of bipolar growth plates with resting, proliferating, pre-hypertrophic, and hypertrophic zones that produce growth in opposing directions, whereas long bones are composed of a unipolar growth plate (Wei et al., 2016). This review presents new insights on the signaling pathways and transcription factors involved in the regulation of synchondrosis development, highlighting the differences and similarities between synchondroses present in the cranial base.

SIGNALING PATHWAYS IN SYNCHONDROSIS DEVELOPMENT

For the normal progression of the development of synchondroses, stringent regulation of chondrocyte differentiation in the cranial synchondroses is crucial. To find the relationship between genetic or molecular interaction networks in the synchondroses, genetically modified mice associated with abnormal synchondroses were investigated. Using the Mouse Genome Informatics[1] database and PubMed[2], 31 mouse genes with abnormal annotations in SOS and/or ISS were discovered (**Table 1**). These genes indicated that the regulation of synchondrosis development involves the interaction of several signaling pathways, including the parathyroid hormone-like hormone (PTHLH)/parathyroid hormone-related protein (PTHrP), Indian hedgehog (Ihh), Wnt/β-catenin, and fibroblast growth factor (FGF) pathways, as well as control by cilium assembly and by transcription factors encoded by specific genes (**Figure 1D**). This review focuses on the genes listed in **Table 1**.

[1]http://www.informatics.jax.org

[2]http://www.ncbi.nlm.nih.gov/pubmed

Runt-Related Transcription Factor 2

Runt-Related Transcription Factor 2 (*RUNX2*), a gene implicated in cleidocranial dysplasia (Online Mendelian Inheritance in Man; OMIM #119600), is a crucial transcription factor of osteoblast and chondrocyte differentiation (Ducy et al., 1997; Komori et al., 1997; Yoshida et al., 2004). Skull radiography of patients with cleidocranial dysplasia caused by *RUNX2* haploinsufficiency showed persistent synchondroses primarily associated with defective development of membranous bones (Kreiborg et al., 1999; Al Kaissi et al., 2013). Chondrocyte-specific constitutive *Runx2* expression in mice has also been shown to induce precocious endochondral ossification in the cranial cartilage (Takeda et al., 2001).

RUNX2 and histone deacetylase 4 (HDAC4) are expressed in prehypertrophic and hypertrophic chondrocytes present in developing cartilages. HDAC4 regulates chondrocyte differentiation and endochondral bone formation by interacting with and inhibiting the activity of RUNX2 (Inada et al., 1999; Enomoto et al., 2000; Vega et al., 2004). Furthermore, *Hdac4*-deletion mice exhibit precocious endochondral ossification of cranial synchondrosis (Vega et al., 2004). Myocyte enhancer factor 2C (MEF2C) regulates a *Runx2* enhancer in chondrocytes, and an activating form of MEF2C in mice causes precocious chondrocyte hypertrophy as well as ossification in SOS (Arnold et al., 2007). *Runx2* expression has been detected in the cartilaginous condensation of the cranial cartilages at embryonic day 13.5 (Funato et al., 2020), yet ossification of synchondroses did not occur in the wild-type embryos. This time lag between *Runx2* expression and execution of chondrocyte differentiation in the synchondroses implies that multiple layers of regulation are required in synchondrosis development and that HDAC4 and MEF2C could be the regulators involved in this process.

T-Box Transcription Factor Family 1

T-box Transcription Factor Family 1 (*TBX1*) is the candidate gene of DiGeorge (OMIM #188400), velocardiofacial (OMIM #192430), and conotruncal anomaly face (OMIM #217095) syndromes. *Tbx1*-deficient mice exhibit most features similar to the human syndromes, including microcephaly (Jerome and Papaioannou, 2001; Lindsay et al., 2001; Funato et al., 2012, 2015). Mice lacking *Chrd*—which encodes chordin, i.e., an antagonist of bone morphogenetic proteins (BMPs)—exhibit recapitulating phenotypes of DiGeorge syndrome and *Tbx1*-deletion mice (Bachiller et al., 2003). Recently, we reported that TBX1 is a specific and essential regulator of chondrocyte differentiation and subsequent ossification at the SOS (Funato et al., 2020). By inhibiting the activity of RUNX2 and the expression of RUNX2 target genes, TBX1 negatively regulates chondrocyte differentiation and subsequent ossification in the SOS (**Figure 1E**).

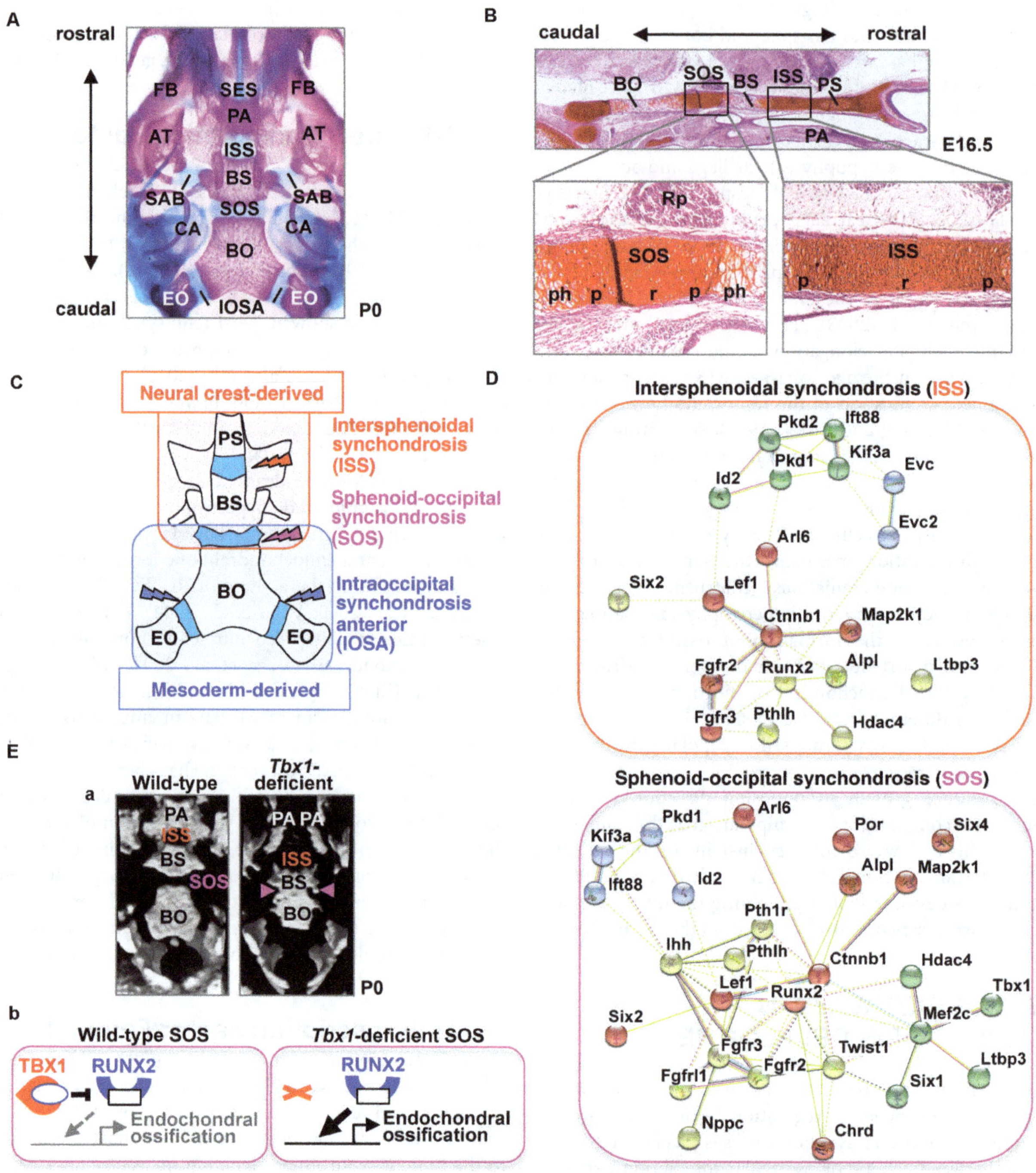

FIGURE 1 | The cranial base and synchondroses. **(A)** Ventral view of bone staining of the mouse cranial base at postnatal day (P) 0. The middle line of the cranial base is formed by the presphenoid, basisphenoid (BS), and basioccipital (BO) bones. Between the mineralized bones, there are two cartilaginous synchondroses, the intersphenoid synchondrosis (ISS) and the spheno-occipital synchondrosis (SOS). Please note that the presphenoid bone is invisible because of the palatine process (PA). AT, ala temporalis (greater wing) of the basisphenoid bone; CA, canalicular part of auditory capsule; EO, exoccipital bone; FB, facial bone; IOSA, intraoccipital synchondrosis; SAB, synchondrosis, alar-basisphenoidalis; SES, spheno-ethmoidal synchondrosis. **(B)** Safranin-O staining of the mouse cranial base at embryonic day (E) 16.5. The presphenoid (PS), basisphenoid (BS), and basioccipital (BO) bones are separated by two synchondroses, the intersphenoid synchondrosis (ISS) and spheno-occipital synchondrosis (SOS). The synchondrosis is composed of bipolar growth plates with a central resting (r), proliferating (p), and prehypertrophic (ph) zones. PA, palate; Rp, Rathke's pouch. **(C)** Schematic illustration of the tissue origins of the cranial base derived from the neural crest shown in red and those derived from the mesoderm in blue (McBratney-Owen et al., 2008). BS, basisphenoid bone; BO, basioccipital bone; EO, exoccipital bone; PS, presphenoid bone. **(D)** STRING protein-protein interaction network of mouse genes involved in abnormal synchondroses. The network was constructed using

(Continued)

FIGURE 1 | Continued
the STRING tool[3], with mouse genes involved in abnormal synchondroses (**Table 1**) used as input. Different colors represent different kinds of evidence of connection between proteins. **(E) (a)** Skulls from wild-type and *Tbx1*-deficient mice at birth were analyzed by micro-computed tomography and are shown in a "bird's eye view." In *Tbx1*-deficient mice, the spheno-occipital synchondrosis (SOS) was completely mineralized (Funato et al., 2020). BO, basioccipital bone; BS, basisphenoid bone; ISS, intersphenoid synchondrosis; PA, palatine process. **(b)** A predicted model for TBX1-mediated regulation of endochondral ossification of SOS. By inhibiting the activity of RUNX2 and the expression of RUNX2 target genes, TBX1 negatively regulates chondrocyte differentiation as well as subsequent endochondral ossification in the SOS.

TABLE 1 | Mouse genes involved in abnormal development of the cranial synchondroses.

Gene	Protein	Induced mutation type	SOS/ISS	Age	Ossification	References
Tbx1	T-box 1	Deletion (*Mesp1-Cre*)	SOS	E15.5	Partially increased	Funato et al., 2020
Fgfrl1	FGF receptor like 1	Deletion	SOS	E18.5	Increased	Catela et al., 2009
Ihh	Indian hedgehog	Deletion (*Col2a1-Cre*)	SOS	E18.5	Increased	Razzaque et al., 2005
Mef2c	myocyte enhancer factor 2C	Activation	SOS	E18.5	Increased	Arnold et al., 2007
Pth1r	parathyroid hormone 1 receptor	Deletion	SOS	E18.5	Increased	Lanske et al., 1996
Six1; Six4	sine oculis-related homeobox 1; sine oculis-related homeobox 4	Deletion	SOS	E18.5	Partially increased	He et al., 2010
Chrd	chordin	Deletion	SOS	P1	Partially increased	Bachiller et al., 2003
Por	P450 oxidoreductase	Deletion (*Dermo1-Cre*)	SOS	P4	Partially increased	Panda et al., 2013
Nppc	natriuretic peptide type C	Deletion	SOS	P14	Decreased	Nakao et al., 2013
Twist1	twist bHLH transcription factor 1	Deletion (heterozygous)	SOS	P25-30	Increased	Hermann et al., 2012
Evc	EvC ciliary complex subunit 1	Deletion	ISS	E18.5	Increased	Pacheco et al., 2012
Evc2	EvC ciliary complex subunit 2	Deletion	ISS	E18.5	Increased	Caparrós-Martín et al., 2013
Pkd2	polycystin 2	Deletion (*Wnt1-Cre*)	ISS	P14	Increased	Khonsari et al., 2013
Lef1	lymphoid enhancer binding factor 1	Activation	ISS, SOS	E17.5	Increased	Nagayama et al., 2008
Ctnnb1	catenin beta 1	Deletion (*Col2a1-Cre*)	ISS, SOS	E17.5	Decreased	Nagayama et al., 2008
Arl6/Bbs3	ADP-ribosylation factor-like 6	Deletion	ISS, SOS	E18.5	Decreased	Kawasaki et al., 2017
Pthlh/Pthrp	parathyroid hormone-like peptide	Deletion	ISS, SOS	P1	Increased	Ishii-Suzuki et al., 1999
Runx2	runt-related transcription factor 2	Activation	ISS, SOS	P1	Increased	Takeda et al., 2001
Six2	sine oculis-related homeobox 2	Deletion	ISS, SOS	P1	Increased	He et al., 2010
Fgfr2	fibroblast growth factor receptor 2	Activation	ISS, SOS	P1 (SOS) P28 (ISS)	Increased	Nagata et al., 2011
Pkd1	polycystin 1	Deletion (*Dermo1-Cre*)	ISS, SOS	P5	Partially increased	Kolpakova-Hart et al., 2008
Kif3a	kinesin family member 3A	Deletion (*Col2a1-Cre*)	ISS, SOS	P7	Partially increased	Koyama et al., 2007
Hdac4	histone deacetylase 4	Deletion	ISS, SOS	P8	Increased	Vega et al., 2004
Map2k1	mitogen-activated protein kinase kinase 1	Activation	ISS, SOS	P11	Increased	Matsushita et al., 2009
Id2	inhibitor of DNA binding 2	Deletion	ISS, SOS	P14	Growth defects	Sakata-Goto et al., 2012
Ift88	intraflagellar transport 88	Deletion (*Col2a1-Cre*)	ISS, SOS	P14	Partially increased	Ochiai et al., 2009
Alpl	alkaline phosphatase, liver/bone/kidney	Deletion	ISS, SOS	P20	Increased	Liu et al., 2014; Nam et al., 2017
Ltbp3	latent transforming growth factor beta binding protein 3	Deletion	ISS, SOS	P21	Increased	Dabovic et al., 2002
Fgfr3	fibroblast growth factor receptor 3	Activation	ISS, SOS	P21	Increased	Chen et al., 1999
Pfas	Phosphoribosyl-formylglycinamidine synthase	Mutation (heterozygous)	n/a	P84	Increased	Palmer et al., 2016

E, embryonic day; P, postnatal day; SOS, spheno-occipital synchondrosis; ISS, intersphenoid synchondrosis; n/a, not available.

FGF Pathway

The FGF receptor (FGFR) family is a subfamily of receptor tyrosine kinases. Dominant gain-of-function mutations of *FGFR2* induce craniofacial dysmorphology in Apert (OMIM #101200), Crouzon (OMIM #123500), Pfeiffer (OMIM #101600), Jackson-Weiss (OMIM #123150), and Antley-Bixler (OMIM #207410) syndromes. Mice carrying the *Fgfr2* mutation exhibit accelerated chondrocyte maturation, accompanied by precocious ossification in the SOS and ISS synchondroses, at birth and 4 week-old stage, respectively (Nagata et al., 2011). A patient with Antley-Bixler syndrome was also identified to be harboring a mutation in *FGFRL1* (Rieckmann et al., 2009). *Fgfrl1*-deficient

[3]http://string-db.org

mice showed precocious ossification in the SOS at E18.5 (Catela et al., 2009). Homozygous mutations in the *POR* gene, encoding cytochrome P450 oxidoreductase, induce midface hypoplasia and craniosynostosis in Antley-Bixler syndrome, accompanied by genital anomalies and disordered steroidogenesis (OMIM #201750). Conditional deletion of *Por* in osteoprogenitors with *Dermo1-Cre* affects synchondrosis and long bone development in mice recapitulating Antley-Bixler syndrome (Panda et al., 2013). Although the craniofacial dysmorphology caused by *POR* mutations and by *FGFR2* mutations overlap, the pathogenesis underlying the skeletal malformation in *POR* deficiency remains to be elucidated.

Gain-of-function mutation of *FGFR3* is reported in most cases of achondroplasia (OMIM #100800) and Muenke syndrome (OMIM #602849), which are associated with craniofacial and skeletal abnormalities. Targeted mutations in *Fgfr3* in mice carrying the equivalent human syndromes lead to decreased chondrocyte proliferation along with accelerated osteoblast differentiation, resulting in precocious ossification of synchondroses (Chen et al., 1999, 2001; Matsushita et al., 2009; Laurita et al., 2011). Additionally, chondrocyte-specific expression of constitutively active mitogen-activated protein kinase 1 (MAP2K1)/MEK1 causes precocious ossification of cranial synchondroses and effectively rescues the *Fgfr3*-deficient mouse phenotype (Matsushita et al., 2009).

PTHLH/PTHrP Pathway

PTHLH, also known as PTHrP, maintains chondrocyte proliferation in conjunction with parathyroid hormone 1 receptor (PTH1R). PTHLH/PTHrP impedes chondrocyte differentiation through the inhibition of *Runx2* expression (Li et al., 2004). In *Pthlh/Pthrp*-deletion mice, chondrocyte differentiation is accelerated in both the SOS as well as the ISS (Ishii-Suzuki et al., 1999). Moreover, PTHLH/PTHrP promotes dephosphorylation and nuclear localization of HDAC4, subsequently inhibiting MEF2C transcription (Kozhemyakina et al., 2009). *Pth1r*-deletion mice are shown to exhibit abnormal neurocranium morphology due to excessive mineralization of synchondroses present between the basioccipital, exoccipital, and basisphenoid bones (Lanske et al., 1996).

Ihh Pathway

The Ihh pathway coordinates diverse aspects of bone morphogenesis via PTHLH/PTHrP-dependent and independent processes (St-Jacques et al., 1999). Ihh is expressed in the synchondroses within the prehypertrophic chondrocytes via RUNX2 regulation and promotes chondrocyte proliferation as well as differentiation (Young et al., 2006; Nagayama et al., 2008; Ushijima et al., 2014). In *Ihh*-deficient synchondroses, chondrocyte proliferation is decreased, and their differentiation is initially delayed (Razzaque et al., 2005; Young et al., 2006). Furthermore, conditional deletion of *Ihh* with *Col2a1-Cre* results in loss of the SOS at E18.5 (Razzaque et al., 2005).

Cilium Assembly

The hedgehog signaling pathway requires cilium assembly. Kinesin family member 3A (KIF3A) is an intraflagellar transport (IFT) motor protein essential for the formation of cilia (Huangfu et al., 2003). Conditional deletion of *Kif3a* with *Col2a1-Cre* results in precocious ossification of synchondroses, by disrupting the expression pattern of *Ihh* in synchondroses (Koyama et al., 2007). Conditional deletion of *Ift88*, which encodes IFT88/polaris, ultimately results in a deformed basicranium, along with precocious ossification of synchondroses due to disruption of the Ihh signaling pathway (Ochiai et al., 2009). Polycystin-1 and polycystin-2, which are encoded by *Pkd1* and *Pkd2*, form a protein complex and localize to the primary cilium. Conditional deletion of *Pkd1* with *Dermo1-Cre* exhibits a premature closure of both the ISS and SOS (Kolpakova-Hart et al., 2008), whereas conditional deletion of *Pkd2* in neural crest with *Wnt1-Cre* exhibits abnormal ossification of neural crest-derived ISS (Khonsari et al., 2013).

EVC and *EVC2* are the disease genes implicated in Ellis-van Creveld syndrome (OMIM #225500) as well as Weyers acrofacial dysostosis (OMIM #193530). EvC ciliary complex subunit 1 (EVC) and EVC2 localize at the base of chondrocyte cilia and function as positive regulators of Ihh-mediated bone development (Takeda et al., 2002; Ruiz-Perez et al., 2007; Caparrós-Martín et al., 2013). Both *Evc*- and *Evc2*-deficient mice exhibit precocious ossification of the ISS at E18.5 (Pacheco et al., 2012; Caparrós-Martín et al., 2013).

ADP-ribosylation factor-like 6, which is encoded by *ARL6/BBS3*, regulates intracellular traffic. Mutations in *ARL6/BBS3* account for Bardet-Biedl syndrome-3 (OMIM #600151), which is characterized by retinal dystrophy, renal structural abnormalities, history of obesity, and skeletal abnormalities. *Arl6/Bbs3*-deficient mice are shown to exhibit hypomorphic cranial synchondroses at E18.5 (Kawasaki et al., 2017).

Wnt/β-Catenin Pathway

The Wnt/β-catenin and Ihh signaling pathways interact with one another to regulate the development of the endochondral bones (Mak et al., 2006). Conditional deletion of *Ctnnb1*, which encodes CTNNB1/β-catenin, with *Col2a1-Cre* results in abnormal bone formation (Day et al., 2005; Nagayama et al., 2008). β-catenin and T-cell factor/lymphoid enhancer factor 1 (TCF/LEF1) are transcriptional mediators of the Wnt/β-catenin signaling pathway that directly interact with the *Ihh* promoter in chondrocytes *in vivo*, suggesting that the Wnt/β-catenin signaling pathway regulates *Ihh* expression (Später et al., 2006). Cartilage overexpression of a constitutively active form of LEF1 causes accelerated chondrocyte hypertrophy, topographical disorganization, and excessive bone collar formation in the ISS and SOS (Nagayama et al., 2008). Interestingly, LEF1 is reported to interact with and consequently inhibit the activity of RUNX2 (Kahler and Westendorf, 2003), suggesting that LEF1 might regulate RUNX2 activity during the development of synchondroses.

SIX Homeobox Family

The sine oculis homeobox (SIX) family of transcription factors regulates the embryonic development of the ears and kidneys. *Six2*-deficient mice display precocious ossification of synchondroses at birth due to disruptions in chondrocyte differentiation, in conjunction with reduced proliferation and accelerated terminal differentiation of the cells (He et al., 2010). *SIX1* is implicated in Branchiootic syndrome 3 (OMIM #608389) and deafness (OMIM #605192). Double knockout mice of *Six1* and *Six4* genes show a precocious partial ossification of the SOS at E18.5 (He et al., 2010).

DISCUSSION

During synchondrosis development, the cross-talk between several signaling pathways, including PTHLH/PTHrP, FGF, Ihh, and Wnt/β-catenin, and control by cilium assembly and by transcription factors, play critical roles. Since the cranial abnormalities in female carriers of the P250R mutation in FGFR3 are more severe than those of the male carriers (Lajeunie et al., 1999), it would be interesting to study whether the onset and complete ossification of synchondroses vary based on gender in wild-type and genetically modified mice. Histological analysis of precocious ossification of synchondroses indicated that the deletion of the RUNX2 inhibitors HDAC4, MEF2C, and TBX1 in mice resulted in accelerated chondrocyte differentiation and, consequently, precocious endochondral ossification of cranial synchondroses (Vega et al., 2004; Arnold et al., 2007; Funato et al., 2020). Consistent with the precocious ossification of the synchondroses in these genetically modified mice, chondrogenic markers were ectopically expressed during synchondrosis formation. Since bone collar ossification occurs secondary to chondrocyte hypertrophy during endochondral bone formation (Chung et al., 2001; Arnold et al., 2007), precocious ossification of synchondroses in these genetically modified mice could occur when chondrocyte hypertrophy is accelerated. The accelerated chondrocyte hypertrophy may also result in a shortage of the reserves of resting and proliferating chondrocytes.

Phenotypic Differences Between SOS and ISS

The synchondrosis phenotype is different among genetically modified mice. Deletion of *Pthlh/Pthrp* or *Six2* or overexpression of *Runx2* in chondrocytes resulted in precocious ossification both in the ISS and the SOS. Precocious ossification is specific to the SOS in *Tbx1*-, *Fgfrl1*-, *Ihh*-, and *Pth1r*-deficient mice and *Mef2c*-superactivating mice, whereas it is specific to the ISS in *Arl6/Bbs3*-, *Evc*-, and *Evc2*-deficient mice (**Table 1**). Phenotypic differences among the synchondroses may be due to varying origins of the ISS and SOS (**Figure 1C**). The cartilage primordium of the ISS is derived from the neural crest, whereas the SOS has a more complex origin, comprising the cartilage primordium derived from the neural crest along with the cranial mesoderm (McBratney-Owen et al., 2008). TBX1 is a specific regulator of SOS development. Since TBX1 is expressed in the mesoderm-derived primordium cartilage of the SOS, differences in the expression pattern of TBX1 likely contribute to the discordant abnormalities between the ISS and SOS (Funato et al., 2020). A consequence of functional redundancy of family genes might also contribute to the same. In the synchondroses of *Ihh*-deficient mice, the hypertrophic chondrocytes in the ISS are more affected than those in the SOS (Young et al., 2006). The remnants of the notochord express Sonic hedgehog (Shh) near the primordium of the SOS but not in the ISS. Since Shh has a redundant interaction with Ihh (Zhang et al., 2001), Shh may induce the milder phenotype of the SOS than the ISS of *Ihh*-deficient mice (Young et al., 2006).

Phenotypic Differences Between the Growth Plate and Synchondroses

The growth plates of cranial synchondroses and long bones contribute to bone elongation as well as shaping of the mature bone via endochondral ossification. However, the growth plate of synchondrosis and the long bone are histologically, environmentally, and developmentally different in the following aspects: (1) the mirror image growth plates of synchondrosis produce longitudinal bone growth in bipolar directions, but the growth plate of long bones produces growth in unipolar direction; (2) the long bones are overlaid by articular synovial layers, which are absent in the synchondrosis; (3) the growth plate in developing long bones present the secondary ossification center, which is absent in the synchondrosis; (4) mechanical stress influences the growth of long bones (Sharir et al., 2011); and (5) the ISS originates from the neural crest, while the SOS has a complex unique contribution of both the neural crest and cranial mesoderm, and long bones are derived from mesoderm. Therefore, discordant abnormalities in the growth plates of the long bones and synchondroses are likely attributable to the differences in location-specific downstream signaling targets and the expression patterns of the signaling factors, which differ according to the unique origins and anatomical structures.

RUNX2, HDAC4, and MEF2C control endochondral ossification in the growth plates of both synchondroses and long bones (Takeda et al., 2001; Vega et al., 2004; Arnold et al., 2007). However, in other mutant mice, discordant abnormalities between long bones and synchondroses have been reported. Zinc finger transcriptional coregulator 521 (ZFP521), whose expression is regulated by PTHLH/PTHrP, associates with and antagonizes RUNX2 activity in chondrocytes via an HDAC4-dependent mechanism (Correa et al., 2010). Deletion of *Zfp521* in chondrocytes does not affect the synchondrosis development; however, long bones appear to be hypomorphic (Correa et al., 2010). Deletion of *Tbx1* results in precocious endochondral ossification of the SOS, but not in the skeletal cartilages despite TBX1 expression in immature chondrocytes (Funato et al., 2015, 2020).

In the synchondroses of *Pthlh/Pthrp*-deletion mice, chondrocyte differentiation is significantly accelerated compared with those chondrocytes present in long bones (Ishii-Suzuki et al., 1999). Ihh is expressed in prehypertrophic chondrocytes and stimulates *Pthlh/Pthrp* expression in periarticular chondrocytes in long bones. In the synchondrosis, an overlaid periarticular layer is absent, and the Ihh signaling relays cross-talks between Ihh-producing prehypertrophic chondrocytes and PTHLH/PTHrP-producing proliferating chondrocytes

(Young et al., 2006). Since PTHLH/PTHrP is expressed in both the resting and the proliferating chondrocytes in the synchondroses and in the resting chondrocytes of long bones, varied distribution of PTHLH/PTHrP-expressing chondrocytes may contribute to the discordant phenotypes between the synchondrosis and long bones of *Pthlh/Pthrp*-deficient mice (Young et al., 2006; Nagayama et al., 2008).

CONCLUSION

Synchondroses are formed through endochondral ossification and play a critical role in the elongation of the basicranium. Deletions or activation of genes can cause the precocious ossification or hypoplasia of synchondroses, suggesting that stringent regulation of signaling pathways is crucial for proper synchondrosis development. The disruption of genes leads to both similar and distinctly different abnormalities in the development of the two synchondroses and also between the growth plates of synchondrosis and skeletal bones. Despite its importance, few studies have addressed the molecular mechanisms that regulate the endochondral ossification of synchondroses. It is important to fully elucidate the interaction of signaling pathways for the regulation of synchondrosis development. In addition, the detailed molecular mechanisms that mark the differences between the synchondroses and the skeletal bones should be deciphered. Hopefully, these insights from future studies will provide possible strategies for biologics-based therapies to treat synchondrosis anomalies.

AUTHOR CONTRIBUTIONS

NF contributed to the conceptual idea, performed the database searches, analyzed the data, and wrote the manuscript.

ACKNOWLEDGMENTS

I would like to thank Editage (www.editage.com) for English language editing.

REFERENCES

Al Kaissi, A., Ben Chehida, F., Kenis, V., Ganger, R., Radler, C., Hofstaetter, J. G., et al. (2013). Broad spectrum of skeletal malformation complex in patients with cleidocranial dysplasia syndrome: radiographic and tomographic study. *Clin. Med. Insights Arthritis Musculoskelet. Disord.* 6, 45–55. doi: 10.4137/CMAMD.S11933

Arnold, M. A., Kim, Y., Czubryt, M. P., Phan, D., McAnally, J., Qi, X., et al. (2007). transcription factor controls chondrocyte hypertrophy and bone development. *Dev. Cell* 12, 377–389. doi: 10.1016/j.devcel.2007.02.004

Bachiller, D., Klingensmith, J., Shneyder, N., Tran, U., Anderson, R., Rossant, J., et al. (2003). The role of chordin/Bmp signals in mammalian pharyngeal development and DiGeorge syndrome. *Development* 130, 3567–3578. doi: 10.1242/dev.00581

Caparrós-Martín, J. A., Valencia, M., Reytor, E., Pacheco, M., Fernandez, M., Perez-Aytes, A., et al. (2013). The ciliary Evc/Evc2 complex interacts with smo and controls hedgehog pathway activity in chondrocytes by regulating Sufu/Gli3 dissociation and Gli3 trafficking in primary cilia. *Hum. Mol. Genet.* 22, 124–139. doi: 10.1093/hmg/dds409

Catela, C., Bilbao-Cortes, D., Slonimsky, E., Kratsios, P., Rosenthal, N., and Te Welscher, P. (2009). Multiple congenital malformations of Wolf-Hirschhorn syndrome are recapitulated in Fgfrl1 null mice. *Dis. Model. Mech.* 2, 283–294. doi: 10.1242/dmm.002287

Chen, L., Adar, R., Yang, X., Monsonego, E. O., Li, C., Hauschka, P. V., et al. (1999). Gly369Cys mutation in mouse FGFR3 causes achondroplasia by affecting both chondrogenesis and osteogenesis. *J. Clin. Invest.* 104, 1517–1525. doi: 10.1172/JCI6690

Chen, L., Li, C., Qiao, W., Xu, X., and Deng, C. (2001). A Ser365Cys mutation of fibroblast growth factor receptor 3 in mouse downregulates Ihh/PTHrP signals and causes severe achondroplasia. *Hum. Mol. Genet.* 10, 457–465. doi: 10.1093/hmg/10.5.457

Chung, U. I., Schipani, E., McMahon, A. P., and Kronenberg, H. M. (2001). Indian hedgehog couples chondrogenesis to osteogenesis in endochondral bone development. *J. Clin. Invest.* 107, 295–304. doi: 10.1172/JCI11706

Correa, D., Hesse, E., Seriwatanachai, D., Kiviranta, R., Saito, H., Yamana, K., et al. (2010). Zfp521 is a target gene and key effector of parathyroid hormone-related peptide signaling in growth plate chondrocytes. *Dev. Cell* 19, 533–546. doi: 10.1016/j.devcel.2010.09.008

Dabovic, B., Chen, Y., Colarossi, C., Obata, H., Zambuto, L., Perle, M. A., et al. (2002). Bone Abnormalities in latent TGF-β binding protein (Ltbp)-3-null mice indicate a role for Ltbp-3 in modulating TGF-β bioavailability. *J. Cell Biol.* 156, 227–232. doi: 10.1083/jcb.200111080

Day, T. F., Guo, X., Garrett-Beal, L., and Yang, Y. (2005). Wnt/β-Catenin signaling in mesenchymal progenitors controls osteoblast and chondrocyte differentiation during vertebrate skeletogenesis. *Dev. Cell* 8, 739–750. doi: 10.1016/J.DEVCEL.2005.03.016

Ducy, P., Zhang, R., Geoffroy, V., Ridall, A. L., and Karsenty, G. (1997). Osf2/Cbfa1: a transcriptional activator of osteoblast differentiation. *Cell* 89, 747–754. doi: 10.1016/s0092-8674(00)80257-3

Enomoto, H., Enomoto-Iwamoto, M., Iwamoto, M., Nomura, S., Himeno, M., Kitamura, Y., et al. (2000). Cbfa1 is a positive regulatory factor in chondrocyte maturation. *J. Biol. Chem.* 275, 8695–8702. doi: 10.1074/jbc.275.12.8695

Funato, N., Nakamura, M., Richardson, J. A., Srivastava, D., and Yanagisawa, H. (2012). Tbx1 regulates oral epithelial adhesion and palatal development. *Hum. Mol. Genet.* 21, 2524–2537. doi: 10.1093/hmg/dds071

Funato, N., Nakamura, M., Richardson, J. A., Srivastava, D., and Yanagisawa, H. (2015). Loss of Tbx1 induces bone phenotypes similar to cleidocranial dysplasia. *Hum. Mol. Genet.* 24, 424–435. doi: 10.1093/hmg/ddu458

Funato, N., Srivastava, D., Shibata, S., and Yanagisawa, H. (2020). TBX1 regulates chondrocyte maturation in the spheno-occipital synchondrosis. *J. Dent. Res.* 99, 1182–1191. doi: 10.1177/0022034520925080

Goldstein, J. A., Paliga, J. T., Wink, J. D., Bartlett, S. P., and Nah, H. D. (2014). Earlier evidence of spheno-occipital synchondrosis fusion correlates with severity of midface hypoplasia in patients with syndromic craniosynostosis. *Plast. Reconstr. Surg.* 134, 504–510. doi: 10.1097/PRS.0000000000000419

He, G., Tavella, S., Hanley, K. P., Self, M., Oliver, G., Grifone, R., et al. (2010). Inactivation of Six2 in mouse identifies a novel genetic mechanism controlling development and growth of the cranial base. *Dev. Biol.* 344, 720–730. doi: 10.1016/j.ydbio.2010.05.509

Hermann, C. D., Lee, C. S. D., Gadepalli, S., Lawrence, K. A., Richards, M. A., Olivares-Navarrete, R., et al. (2012). Interrelationship of cranial suture fusion, basicranial development, and resynostosis following suturectomy in Twist1+/- mice, a murine model of Saethre-Chotzen syndrome. *Calcif. Tissue Int.* 91, 255–266. doi: 10.1007/s00223-012-9632-3

Huangfu, D., Liu, A., Rakeman, A. S., Murcia, N. S., Niswander, L., and Anderson, K. V. (2003). Hedgehog signalling in the mouse requires intraflagellar transport proteins. *Nature* 426, 83–87. doi: 10.1038/nature02061

Inada, M., Yasui, T., Nomura, S., Miyake, S., Deguchi, K., Himeno, M., et al. (1999). Maturational disturbance of chondrocytes in Cbfa1-deficient mice. *Dev. Dyn.* 214, 279–290. doi: 10.1002/(sici)1097-0177(199904)214:4<279::aid-aja1>3.0.co;2-w

Ishii-Suzuki, M., Suda, N., Yamazaki, K., Kuroda, T., Senior, P. V., Beck, F., et al. (1999). Differential responses to parathyroid hormone-related protein (PTHrP) deficiency in the various craniofacial cartilages. *Anat. Rec.* 255, 452–457. doi: 10.1002/(sici)1097-0185(19990801)255:4<452::aid-ar10>3.0.co;2-e

Jerome, L. A., and Papaioannou, V. E. (2001). DiGeorge syndrome phenotype in mice mutant for the T-Box gene, Tbx1. *Nat. Genet.* 27, 286–291. doi: 10.1038/85845

Kahler, R. A., and Westendorf, J. J. (2003). Lymphoid enhancer factor-1 and β-catenin inhibit Runx2-dependent transcriptional activation of the osteocalcin promoter. *J. Biol. Chem.* 278, 11937–11944. doi: 10.1074/jbc.M211443200

Kawasaki, M., Izu, Y., Hayata, T., Ideno, H., Nifuji, A., Sheffield, V. C., et al. (2017). Bardet-Biedl syndrome 3 regulates the development of cranial base midline structures. *Bone* 101, 179–190. doi: 10.1016/j.bone.2016.02.017

Khonsari, R. H., Ohazama, A., Raouf, R., Kawasaki, M., Kawasaki, K., Porntaveetus, T., et al. (2013). Multiple postnatal craniofacial anomalies are characterized by conditional loss of polycystic kidney disease 2 (Pkd2). *Hum. Mol. Genet.* 22, 1873–1885. doi: 10.1093/hmg/ddt041

Kolpakova-Hart, E., McBratney-Owen, B., Hou, B., Fukai, N., Nicolae, C., Zhou, J., et al. (2008). Growth of cranial synchondroses and sutures requires polycystin-1. *Dev. Biol.* 321, 407–419. doi: 10.1016/j.ydbio.2008.07.005

Komori, T., Yagi, H., Nomura, S., Yamaguchi, A., Sasaki, K., Deguchi, K., et al. (1997). Targeted Disruption of Cbfa1 results in a complete lack of bone formation owing to maturational arrest of osteoblasts. *Cell* 89, 755–764. doi: 10.1016/s0092-8674(00)80258-5

Koyama, E., Young, B., Nagayama, M., Shibukawa, Y., Enomoto-iwamoto, M., Iwamoto, M., et al. (2007). Conditional Kif3a ablation causes abnormal hedgehog signaling topography, growth plate dysfunction, and excessive bone and cartilage formation during mouse skeletogenesis. *Development* 2169, 2159–2169. doi: 10.1242/dev.001586

Kozhemyakina, E., Cohen, T., Yao, T. P., and Lassar, A. B. (2009). Parathyroid hormone-related peptide represses chondrocyte hypertrophy through a protein phosphatase 2A/histone deacetylase 4/MEF2 Pathway. *Mol. Cell. Biol.* 29, 5751–5762. doi: 10.1128/mcb.00415-09

Kreiborg, S., Jensen, B. L., Larsen, P., Schleidt, D. T., and Darvann, T. (1999). Anomalies of craniofacial skeleton and teeth in cleidocranial dysplasia. *J. Craniofac. Genet. Dev. Biol.* 19, 75–79.

Lajeunie, E., El Ghouzzi, V., Le Merrer, M., Munnich, A., Bonaventure, J., and Renier, D. (1999). Sex related expressivity of the phenotype in coronal craniosynostosis caused by the recurrent P250R FGFR3 mutation. *J. Med. Genet.* 36, 9–13.

Lanske, B., Karaplis, A. C., Lee, K., Luz, A., Vortkamp, A., Pirro, A., et al. (1996). PTH/PTHrP receptor in early development and indian hedgehog-regulated bone growth. *Science* 273, 663–666. doi: 10.1126/science.273.5275.663

Laurita, J., Koyama, E., Chin, B., Taylor, J. A., Lakin, G. E., Hankenson, K. D., et al. (2011). The Muenke syndrome mutation (FgfR3 P244R) causes cranial base shortening associated with growth plate dysfunction and premature perichondrial ossification in murine basicranial synchondroses. *Dev. Dyn.* 240, 2584–2596. doi: 10.1002/dvdy.22752

Li, T. F., Dong, Y., Ionescu, A. M., Rosier, R. N., Zuscik, M. J., Schwarz, E. M., et al. (2004). Parathyroid hormone-related peptide (PTHrP) inhibits Runx2 expression through the PKA signaling pathway. *Exp. Cell Res.* 299, 128–136. doi: 10.1016/j.yexcr.2004.05.025

Lindsay, E. A., Vitelli, F., Su, H., Morishima, M., Huynh, T., Pramparo, T., et al. (2001). Tbx1 haploinsufficiency in the DiGeorge syndrome region causes aortic arch defects in mice. *Nature* 410, 97–101. doi: 10.1038/35065105

Liu, J., Nam, H. K., Campbell, C., Gasque, K. C. S., Millán, J. L., and Hatch, N. E. (2014). Tissue-nonspecific alkaline phosphatase deficiency causes abnormal craniofacial bone development in the Alpl-/- mouse model of infantile hypophosphatasia. *Bone* 67, 81–94. doi: 10.1016/j.bone.2014.06.040

Madeline, L. A., and Elster, A. D. (1995). Postnatal development of the central skull base: normal variants. *Radiology* 196, 757–763. doi: 10.1148/radiology.196.3.7644640

Mak, K. K., Chen, M. H., Day, T. F., Chuang, P. T., and Yang, Y. (2006). Wnt/beta-catenin signaling interacts differentially with Ihh signaling in controlling endochondral bone and synovial joint formation. *Development* 133, 3695–3707. doi: 10.1242/dev.02546

Matsushita, T., Wilcox, W. R., Chan, Y. Y., Kawanami, A., Bükülmez, H., Balmes, G., et al. (2009). FGFR3 promotes synchondrosis closure and fusion of ossification centers through the MAPK pathway. *Hum. Mol. Genet.* 18, 227–240. doi: 10.1093/hmg/ddn339

McBratney-Owen, B., Iseki, S., Bamforth, S. D., Olsen, B. R., and Morriss-Kay, G. M. (2008). Development and tissue origins of the mammalian cranial base. *Dev. Biol.* 322, 121–132. doi: 10.1016/j.ydbio.2008.07.016

Nagata, M., Nuckolls, G. H., Wang, X., Shum, L., Seki, Y., Kawase, T., et al. (2011). The Primary site of the acrocephalic feature in Apert syndrome is a dwarf cranial base with accelerated chondrocytic differentiation due to aberrant activation of the FGFR2 signaling. *Bone* 48, 847–856. doi: 10.1016/j.bone.2010.11.014

Nagayama, M., Iwamoto, M., Hargett, A., Kamiya, N., Tamamura, Y., Young, B., et al. (2008). Wnt/β-catenin signaling regulates cranial base development and growth. *J. Dent. Res.* 87, 244–249. doi: 10.1177/154405910808700309

Nakao, K., Okubo, Y., Yasoda, A., Koyama, N., Osawa, K., Isobe, Y., et al. (2013). The effects of C-type natriuretic peptide on craniofacial skeletogenesis. *J. Dent. Res.* 92, 58–64. doi: 10.1177/0022034512466413

Nam, H. K., Sharma, M., Liu, J., and Hatch, N. E. (2017). Tissue nonspecific alkaline phosphatase (TNAP) regulates cranial base growth and synchondrosis maturation. *Front. Physiol.* 8:161. doi: 10.3389/fphys.2017.00161

Ochiai, T., Nagayama, M., Nakamura, T., Morrison, T., Pilchak, D., Kondo, N., et al. (2009). Roles of the primary cilium component polaris in synchondrosis development. *J. Dent. Res.* 88, 545–550. doi: 10.1177/0022034509337775

Pacheco, M., Valencia, M., Caparrós-Martín, J. A., Mulero, F., Goodship, J. A., and Ruiz-Perez, V. L. (2012). Evc works in chondrocytes and osteoblasts to regulate multiple aspects of growth plate development in the appendicular skeleton and cranial base. *Bone* 50, 28–41. doi: 10.1016/j.bone.2011.08.025

Palmer, K., Fairfield, H., Borgeia, S., Curtain, M., Hassan, M. G., Dionne, L., et al. (2016). Discovery and characterization of spontaneous mouse models of craniofacial dysmorphology. *Dev. Biol.* 415, 216–227. doi: 10.1016/j.ydbio.2015.07.023

Panda, S. P., Guntur, A. R., Polusani, S. R., Fajardo, R. J., Gakunga, P. T., Roman, L. J., et al. (2013). Conditional deletion of cytochrome P450 reductase in osteoprogenitor cells affects long bone and skull development in mice recapitulating Antley-Bixler syndrome: role of a redox enzyme in development. *PLoS One* 8:75638. doi: 10.1371/journal.pone.0075638

Razzaque, M. S., Soegiarto, D. W., Chang, D., Long, F., and Lanske, B. (2005). Conditional deletion of indian hedgehog from collagen type 2alpha1-expressing cells results in abnormal endochondral bone formation. *J. Pathol.* 207, 453–461. doi: 10.1002/path.1870

Rieckmann, T., Zhuang, L., Flück, C. E., and Trueb, B. (2009). Characterization of the first FGFRL1 mutation identified in a craniosynostosis patient. *Biochim. Biophys. Acta Mol. Basis Dis.* 1792, 112–121. doi: 10.1016/j.bbadis.2008.11.006

Ruiz-Perez, V. L., Blair, H. J., Rodriguez-Andres, M. E., Blanco, M. J., Wilson, A., Liu, Y. N., et al. (2007). Evc Is a positive mediator of Ihh-regulated bone growth that localises at the base of chondrocyte cilia. *Development* 134, 2903–2912. doi: 10.1242/dev.007542

Sakata-Goto, T., Takahashi, K., Kiso, H., Huang, B., Tsukamoto, H., Takemoto, M., et al. (2012). Id2 controls chondrogenesis acting downstream of BMP signaling during maxillary morphogenesis. *Bone* 50, 69–78. doi: 10.1016/j.bone.2011.09.049

Sharir, A., Stern, T., Rot, C., Shahar, R., and Zelzer, E. (2011). Muscle force regulates bone shaping for optimal load-bearing capacity during embryogenesis. *Development* 138, 3247–3259. doi: 10.1242/dev.063768

Später, D., Hill, T. P., O'Sullivan, R. J., Gruber, M., Conner, D. A., and Hartmann, C. (2006). Wnt9a signaling is required for joint integrity and regulation of Ihh during chondrogenesis. *Development* 133, 3039–3049. doi: 10.1242/dev.02471

St-Jacques, B., Hammerschmidt, M., and McMahon, A. P. (1999). Indian hedgehog signaling regulates proliferation and differentiation of chondrocytes and is essential for bone formation. *Genes Dev.* 13, 2072–2086. doi: 10.1101/gad.13.16.2072

Takeda, H., Takami, M., Oguni, T., Tsuji, T., Yoneda, K., Sato, H., et al. (2002). Positional cloning of the gene LIMBIN responsible for bovine chondrodysplastic dwarfism. *Proc. Natl. Acad. Sci. U.S.A.* 99, 10549–10554. doi: 10.1073/pnas.152337899

Takeda, S., Bonnamy, J. P., Owen, M. J., Ducy, P., and Karsenty, G. (2001). Continuous Expression of Cbfa1 in nonhypertrophic chondrocytes uncovers its ability to induce hypertrophic chondrocyte differentiation and partially rescues Cbfa1-deficient mice. *Genes Dev.* 15, 467–481. doi: 10.1101/gad.845101

Ushijima, T., Okazaki, K., Tsushima, H., Ishihara, K., Doi, T., and Iwamoto, Y. (2014). CCAAT/enhancer binding protein β regulates expression of indian hedgehog during chondrocytes differentiation. *PLoS One* 9:104547. doi: 10.1371/journal.pone.0104547

Vega, R. B., Matsuda, K., Oh, J., Barbosa, A. C., Yang, X., Meadows, E., et al. (2004). Histone deacetylase 4 controls chondrocyte hypertrophy during skeletogenesis. *Cell* 119, 555–566. doi: 10.1016/j.cell.2004.10.024

Wei, X., Hu, M., Mishina, Y., and Liu, F. (2016). Developmental regulation of the growth plate and cranial synchondrosis. *J. Dent. Res.* 95, 1221–1229. doi: 10.1177/0022034516651823

Wei, X., Thomas, N., Hatch, N. E., Hu, M., and Liu, F. (2017). Postnatal craniofacial skeletal development of female C57BL/6NCrl mice. *Front. Physiol.* 8:697. doi: 10.3389/fphys.2017.00697

Yoshida, C. A., Yamamoto, H., Fujita, T., Furuichi, T., Ito, K., Inoue, K., et al. (2004). Runx2 and Runx3 are essential for chondrocyte maturation, and Runx2 regulates limb growth through induction of indian hedgehog. *Genes Dev.* 18, 952–963. doi: 10.1101/gad.1174704

Young, B., Minugh-Purvis, N., Shimo, T., St-Jacques, B., Iwamoto, M., Enomoto-Iwamoto, M., et al. (2006). Indian and sonic hedgehogs regulate synchondrosis growth plate and cranial base development and function. *Dev. Biol.* 299, 272–282. doi: 10.1016/j.ydbio.2006.07.028

Zhang, X. M., Ramalho-Santos, M., and McMahon, A. P. (2001). Smoothened mutants reveal redundant roles for Shh and Ihh signaling including regulation of L/R symmetry by the mouse node. *Cell* 106, 781–792. doi: 10.1016/s0092-8674(01)00385-3

14

Effect of Age and Sodium Alendronate on Femoral Fracture Repair: Biochemical and Biomechanical Study in Rats

*Luana Mordask Bonetto[1], Paola Fernanda Cotait de Lucas Corso[1], Gabrielle Grosko Kuchar[1], Jennifer Tsi Gerber[1], Leonardo Fernandes Cunha[1], Mohammed Elsalanty[2], João Cesar Zielak[1], Carla Castiglia Gonzaga[1] and Rafaela Scariot[3]**

[1] Department of Dentistry, Positivo University, Curitiba, Brazil, [2] Department of Medical Anatomical Science, Western University of Health Sciences, Pomona, CA,Unioted States, [3] Department of Dentistry, Federal University of Parana, Curitiba, Brazil

***Correspondence:**
Rafaela Scariot
rafaela_scariot@yahoo.com.br

Background: Bisphosphonates are drugs widely used to reduce bone resorption, increase bone mineral density and control age-related bone loss. Although there are studies reporting differences in bone structure between young and old adults, it is still difficult to predict changes related to bone aging. The aim of this study was to evaluate the effect of age and sodium alendronate on bone repair of femoral fractures in rats.

Methods: *Wistar* rats ($n = 40$) were allocated into groups: O (control old-rats), Y (control young-rats), OA (alendronate old-rats) and YA (alendronate young-rats). All animals underwent linear fracture surgery followed by fixation. Groups OA and YA received 1 mg/kg alendronate three times a week until euthanasia. Biochemical analysis of calcium and alkaline phosphatase was done. After euthanasia, femurs were evaluated in relation to cross-section and flexural strength, with three-point bending test. Data were submitted to statistical analysis with significance level of 0.05.

Results: There was no difference in calcium and alkaline phosphatase levels ($p > 0.05$). Young animals presented lower cross-section than older animals ($p < 0.05$). Only fractured side, young animals presented major flexural strength than older animals ($p < 0.05$). There was no difference between the animals that used or not alendronate in relation to cross-section and flexural strength ($p > 0.05$). When compared fractured and non-fractured femurs, major cross-section on fractured side was observed ($p < 0.05$). Flexural strength presented higher values in femurs on non-fractured side ($p < 0.05$). There was correlation of weight and cross-section ($R = +0.91$) and weight with flexural strength of fractured and non-fractured side, respectively ($R = -0.97$ and -0.71).

Conclusion: In short, there was no difference of calcium and alkaline phosphatase during the bone repair process. Age has influence in cross-section and flexural strength. Alendronate showed no association with these factors.

Keywords: fracture, femur, bisphosphonates, rats, bone regeneration

INTRODUCTION

Mineralized bone matrix is an important reservoir of calcium and phosphate ions (Redmond et al., 2014). Alkaline phosphatase is produced in high concentration during bone formation and is, therefore, a good indicator of bone regeneration activity (Christenson, 1997). During bone regeneration after fracture, hematopoietic precursor cells migrate to the area and differentiate into osteoclasts to digest the necrotic bone, while mesenchymal stromal cells differentiate into bone-forming osteoblasts. During the remodeling of the bone callus, catabolic and anabolic activities interact, a balance that can be modulated by different molecules (Bosemark et al., 2014). The process of bone healing and remodeling are known to occur more rapidly in young individuals (Wendeberg, 1961). Although there are studies reporting differences in bone structure between young and old adults (Akkus et al., 2004), it is still difficult to predict changes related to bone aging. Bone aging is associated with a decrease in collagen content and bone mineral density (Bailey et al., 1999). Consequently, there is a decrease in elastic capacity of bone with age and a greater difficulty in bone healing.

Several molecules have shown potential to stimulate osteogenic activity or reduce bone resorption *in vitro* and *in vivo* (Greiner et al., 2008). Bisphosphonates are examples of drugs that increase bone mineral density and control age-related bone loss (Naruse et al., 2015). There is a decrease in the osteoclastic activity, without direct effect on bone formation (Greiner et al., 2008). Bisphosphonates bind to hydroxyapatite and can remain in bone matrix for years (Silva et al., 2010). Studies indicated that a single systemic dose of alendronate significantly increased the volume of bone callus during fracture repair and increased the bone mechanical strength. When administered in the perioperative period, it induced 30% greater mechanical resistance, compared to controls. Administration of the systemic dose within one or 2 weeks after fracture increased the mechanical strength in the regenerate by 44 and 50%, respectively, confirming the effect of the drug on bone healing (Amanat et al., 2007).

The objective of this study was to evaluate the effect of age and systemic application of alendronate on the fracture resistance of bone regenerate after controlled femoral fracture. We hypothesized that fracture resistance of the regenerate will decrease with age and that alendronate treatment would, at least partially, correct such negative effect.

MATERIALS AND METHODS

Ethical Aspects

The research was carried out in the Vivarium and in the Research Laboratory at Universidade Positivo, after approval in the Ethics Committee on the Use of Animals (ECUA 393). The animals experiments were conducted in accordance to the ARRIVE guidelines, as well as the National Institutes of Health guide for the care and use of Laboratory animals.

Experimental Design

In this study, forty male Wistar rats (Rattus norvegicus) were used: 20 middle-aged rats with 1 year and 5 months of age, with approximately 500 grams and 20 young rats with 5 months of age weighing approximately 200 grams (Andreollo et al., 2012). The rats were divided into four groups: Group O (control) and Group OA (systemic alendronate application), using rats with 1 year and 5 months of age, Group Y (control) and Group YA (systemic alendronate application), using the rats with 5 months old. The dosage used of alendronate for group OA and YA was 1 mg/kg, with three times a week applications, in intraperitoneal region, until euthanasia, starting immediately after the fracture induction. The dose of choice is based on preliminary works of our team (de Oliveira et al., 2019). Subcutaneous applications were performed on the dorsal region of the rats, introducing the needle parallel to the fold of body tissue formed by digital pressure.

Considering the importance of the regulation of calcium and alkaline phosphatase for bone metabolism, blood samples were taken at three different times for biochemical analysis. From the total of 40 animals, 20% had material collected and distributed equally among the groups.

Throughout the experiment, the ambient conditions of light, temperature and humidity of the rooms were controlled in a digital panel in order to maintain the photoperiod of 12 h, with the temperature ranging from 18 to 22°C and relative humidity of 65%.

Surgical Procedure

The rats were sedated with isoflurane 3% (Cristália, Itapira, SP, Brazil), then anesthetized with 10% ketamine hydrochloride (75 mg/kg) (Vetbrands, Paulínia, SP, Brazil) with 2% (10 mg/kg) xylazine hydrochloride (Vetbrands, Paulínia, SP, Brazil), by intraperitoneal injection.

After the anesthesia, the rats were positioned in left lateral decubitus position; and the right femur trichotomy was performed with vigorous antisepsis using iodopovidone. A straight incision along the axis of the femur was made, approximately 3 cm long, with a 15C scalpel blade. With blunt scissors, the tissues were dissected into muscular planes. Next, the periosteum was incised with a scalpel and elevated with a delicate syndesmotom, thus accessing the cortical surface of the femur. A 4-hole titanium plate of 2.0 mm system with four screws of 2.0 mm system being 5 mm long, was adapted to the bone surface prior to osteotomy in order to avoid the poor positioning of the bone segments. The fracture was then performed using a reciprocating saw (NSK, Shinagawa, Tokyo, Japan) under constant irrigation. The stability of titanium plate and screws, hemostasis and abundant wound washing with saline solution were reviewed (**Figure 1**). The suture was performed in planes with isolated stitches using Vycril 4-0 (Ethicon, Johnson & Johnson, São José dos Campos, SP, Brazil) for the muscles, and nylon 4-0 (Ethicon, Johnson & Johnson, São José dos Campos, SP, Brazil) for the skin.

To avoid postoperative infections, we used 10 mg/kg of broad-spectrum antibiotic (Kinolox 2.5%, World Animal

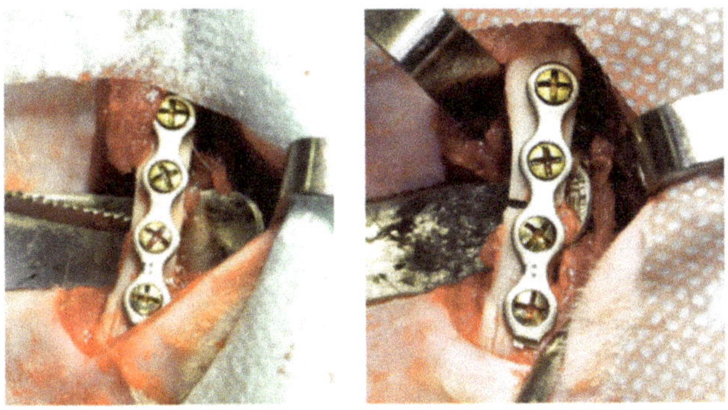

FIGURE 1 | 4-hole titanium plate of 2.0 mm system with four screws of 2.0 mm and fracture performed using a reciprocating saw.

Laboratory, Pindamonhangaba—Brazil) intraperitoneally every 24 h for 14 days. ketoprofen 50 mg/ml, at 5 mg/kg, was given intraperitoneally every 24 h for 5 days to control post-operative inflammation. For analgesia, tramadol hydrochloride 100 mg/2 ml was given intraperitoneally at the end of surgery and was maintained for 5 days, with a dosage of 7 mg/kg (União Química, Jabaquara, SP, Brazil). For gastric protection, ranitidine 15 mg/ml with a dose of 5 mg/kg, was orally administrated, every 24 h for 3 days.

In the postoperative period the animals were kept in their own cages and fed daily with heavy ration for appetite control (100 mg/day) and water at will. The surgical wound was cleaned with sterile gauze and iodopovidone, once a day, for 5 days. At the seventh day, the animals were evaluated for the presence of suture and when present was removed.

Seven days after the surgical procedure, the rats were sedated with isoflurane in order to perform the digital radiographs (Kodak x-ray sensor, Rochester, New York, United States), which were used to evaluate the positioning of the bone stumps as well as the plates and screws. After the rats were euthanized and the plates and screws removed, another digital radiograph was performed to observe the bone repair in the fracture site. Based on this exam (complete bone repair), femurs were submitted to mechanical tests.

Medication Applications

In the OA and YA groups, immediately after surgery, the application of alendronate was initiated until the day of euthanasia. The drug was administered three times a week with 1 mg/kg dosage. Groups O and Y, at the same time, received applications of saline solution at 0.9%.

Euthanasia

The animals were euthanized 90 days after the procedure, with inhalation of 3% isoflurane until complete absence of vital signs and then the fractured and non-fractured femurs were removed, clinically evaluated and stored in bottles.

Biochemical Analysis

Blood samples were collected (1 ml) by cardiac puncture, under sedation with isoflurane in three different times: after the fracture induction, after 45 days and after 90 days from the surgical procedure. Samples were sent to biochemical analysis for levels of calcium and alkaline phosphatase (VP veterinary biochemical laboratory—Curitiba—Paraná—Brazil) of groups O, Y, OA, and YA.

Mechanical Test

Three-point bending flexural tests were performed in a universal testing machine (DL2000, EMIC, São José dos Pinhais, PR, Brazil) at a crosshead speed of 1 mm/min. The distance between the supports was 16 mm. Before testing, specimens' dimensions were determined using a digital caliper with 0.01 mm accuracy. Cross-section (in mm2) was calculated using the formula CS = hb, where h corresponds to height (in mm) and b corresponds to width (in mm). Flexural strength (S, in MPa) was calculated using the following formula: S = 3Fl/2bh2, where F is the failure load (in Newtons), l is the distance between the supports, b is the width and h is the height of the specimen (all in mm).

Statistical Analysis

The variables were subjected to statistical analysis. To evaluate the association of calcium and alkaline phosphatase between groups was used the One-Way ANOVA test and to evaluate the association between serum dosages of the same group between the times was used the One-Way ANOVA of repeated measures, using the mean and standard deviation to represent the sample. To evaluate the association between cross-section of the femurs and flexural strength with the factors age and group, as well as their interactions, was used the Two-Way ANOVA test with Tukey's Posttest. To compare the cross-section and flexural strength between fractured and non-fractured femurs in animals treated with alendronate or not, was used the paired student *T* test. To evaluate the correlation of weight with cross-section and the weight with flexural strength, in femurs with and without fracture, the Pearson's correlation test was used. The statistical analysis was performed using the Statistical Packager Social Science program (SPSS, version 21.0, SPSS inc., Chicago, IL, United States), with a significance level of 0.05.

RESULTS

Tables 1, **2** outline the calcium and alkaline phosphatase levels at different time points in different groups. There were no significant differences in serum calcium and alkaline phosphatase levels evaluated at the same time and over time between the groups ($p > 0.05$).

Table 3 demonstrate the cross-sectional area and flexural strength of middle aged and young rats with and without alendronate applications. Regarding the cross-section on the fracture side, middle aged animals had higher values than young animals (53.52 versus 32.42 mm^2, respectively; $p < 0.05$). Regarding the effect of alendronate treatment, there was no difference between treated (47.50 mm^2) and untreated animals

TABLE 1 | Serum levels of calcium at different times.

Age	Alendronate	Calcium Pre-operative Mean ± SD	Calcium 45 days Mean ± SD	Calcium 90 days Mean ± SD	*P* Value Time
Middle-age	No (O)	9.40 ± 0.0	10.20 ± 0.20	14.00 ± 1.50	0.156
	Yes (OA)	10.23 ± 0.42	9.66 ± 0.75	9.73 ± 0.75	0.932
Young	No (Y)	10.55 ± 0.35	10.50 ± 0.30	9.70 ± 0.50	0.500
	Yes (YA)	11.15 ± 0.65	10.80 ± 0.90	9.70 ± 0.30	0.395
P Value Group		0.179	0.669	0.051	

One-Way ANOVA for evaluation between groups and One-Way ANOVA repeated measures for evaluation between times, with significance level of 0.05.

TABLE 2 | Serum levels of alkaline phosphatase in the groups at different times.

Age	Alendronate	Alkaline phosphatase Pre-operative Mean ± SD	Alkaline phosphatase 45 days Mean ± SD	Alkaline phosphatase 90 days Mean ± SD	*P* Value Time
Middle-age	No (O)	116.15 ± 9.35	111.15 ± 22.45	122.80 ± 5.80	0.901
	Yes (OA)	125.03 ± 39.00	110.20 ± 15.17	65.03 ± 5.57	0.525
Young	No (Y)	171.70 ± 36.60	157.15 ± 6.15	131.20 ± 30.10	0.791
	Yes (YA)	225.85 ± 47.05	93.00 ± 10.10	119.20 ± 20.80	0.173
P Value Group		0.290	0.144	0.082	

One-Way ANOVA for evaluation between groups and One-Way ANOVA repeated measures for evaluation between times, with significance level of 0.05.

TABLE 3 | Evaluation for cross-section and flexural strength related to age and presence or not of alendronate.

Age	Alendronate	Cross-section (mm2) fracture Mean ± SD	Cross-section (mm2) no fracture Mean ± SD	Flexural strength (MPa) fracture Mean ± SD	Flexural strength (MPa) no fracture Mean ± SD
Middle-age	No (O)	51.70 ± 22.37^{Aa}	20.30 ± 2.32 ^{Ab}	4.21 ± 2.87 ^{Bb}	80.43 ± 33.49 ^{Aa}
	Yes (OA)	55.35 ± 28.78 ^{Aa}	19.89 ± 4.01 ^{Ab}	13.67 ± 16.42 ^{ABb}	72.25 ± 18.03 ^{Aa}
Young	No (Y)	25.45 ± 4.33 ^{Aa}	12.87 ± 2.01 ^{Bb}	24.50 ± 9.95 ^{ABb}	112.09 ± 0.25 ^{Aa}
	Yes (YA)	37.40 ± 17.34 ^{Aa}	16.68 ± 1.89 ^{ABb}	27.37 ± 23.45 ^{Ab}	83.64 ± 25.10 ^{Aa}

Lower case letters (a, b) are used, for each group (age and use of alendronate), to indicate significant differences when comparing the conditions (fracture x no fracture) (p < 0.05). In each line, when the same lower case letter is used, the difference between the means is not statistically significant. Uppercase letters (A, B) are used, for each condition (fracture and no fracture), to indicate significant differences when comparing the groups (age and use of alendronate) (p < 0.05). In each column, when the same uppercase letter is used, the difference between the means is not statistically significant.

(42.32 mm^2). The variables alendronate and age/alendronate did not present statistically significant difference ($p > 0.05$).

Regarding the cross-section on the contralateral side, middle aged animals presented higher cross-sectional area (20.09 mm^2) that young animals (15.09 mm^2; $p < 0.05$). For the alendronate factor, there was no difference between treated (18.48 mm^2) and untreated animals (17.64 mm^2). Cross-sectional area values in old animals that were treated (19.89 mm^2) or untreated (20.30 mm^2) tended to be higher than those in young animals without the drug treatment (12.87 mm^2). However, the factors alendronate and age/alendronate did not present a statistically significant difference ($p > 0.05$).

Regarding the flexural strength on the fracture side, young animals presented higher flexural strength value (26.17 MPa) than middle aged animals (8.94 MPa; $p < 0.05$). However, there were no differences between alendronate-treated (19.66 MPa) and untreated (11.45 MPa) animals. The factors alendronate and age/alendronate did not present a statistically significant difference ($p > 0.05$).

Analyzing the flexural strength on the non-fracture side, there was no difference between young and middle aged animals $p > 0.05$). For the alendronate administration, there was no difference between treated (77.23 MPa) and untreated animals (91.73 MPa). The factors alendronate and age/alendronate did not present a statistically significant difference ($p > 0.05$).

Table 4 demonstrates the cross-sectional area and flexural strength comparison between femurs within the same animal. The fracture side had higher values of cross-sectional area compared to the non-fracture side ($p < 0.05$). However, flexural strength, were higher on the values non-fractured side, whether with or without alendronate treatment ($p < 0.05$).

In **flowchart 1**, we summarize the main findings of the study.

Correlations between weight and cross-section, and between weight and flexural strength were evaluated. Positive correlation was observed ($R = +0.91$) between cross-sectional area and weight, both on the fracture and contralateral sides (**Figure 2**). On the other hand, a negative correlation ($R = -0.91$ and $R = -0.97$) between flexural strength and weight, both for the fracture and contralateral sides (**Figure 3**).

DISCUSSION

This study examined the effect of aging on the healing of controlled femoral fracture, and whether alendronate treatment will play a role in modifying the effect of age. We found important

TABLE 4 | Comparison of cross-section and flexural strength in animals with and without alendronate treatment between the femurs on the fractured and non-fractured side.

Age	Alendronate	Cross-section (mm2)–fracture Mean ± SD	Cross-section (mm2) no fracture Mean ± SD	*P* Value	Flexural strength (MPa)–fracture Mean ± SD	Flexural strength (MPa) no fracture Mean ± SD	*P* Value
Middle-age	No (O)	51.70 ± 22.37	20.30 ± 2.32	0.002	4.21 ± 2.87	80.43 ± 33.49	<0.001
	Yes (OA)	55.35 ± 28.78	19.89 ± 4.01	0.006	13.67 ± 16.42	72.25 ± 18.03	<0.001
Young	No (Y)	25.45 ± 4.33	12.87 ± 2.01	0.008	24.50 ± 9.95	112.09 ± 0.25	0.002
	Yes (YA)	37.40 ± 17.34	16.68 ± 1.89	0.022	27.37 ± 23.45	83,64 ± 25.10	0.006

Paired T Test, with significance level 0.05.

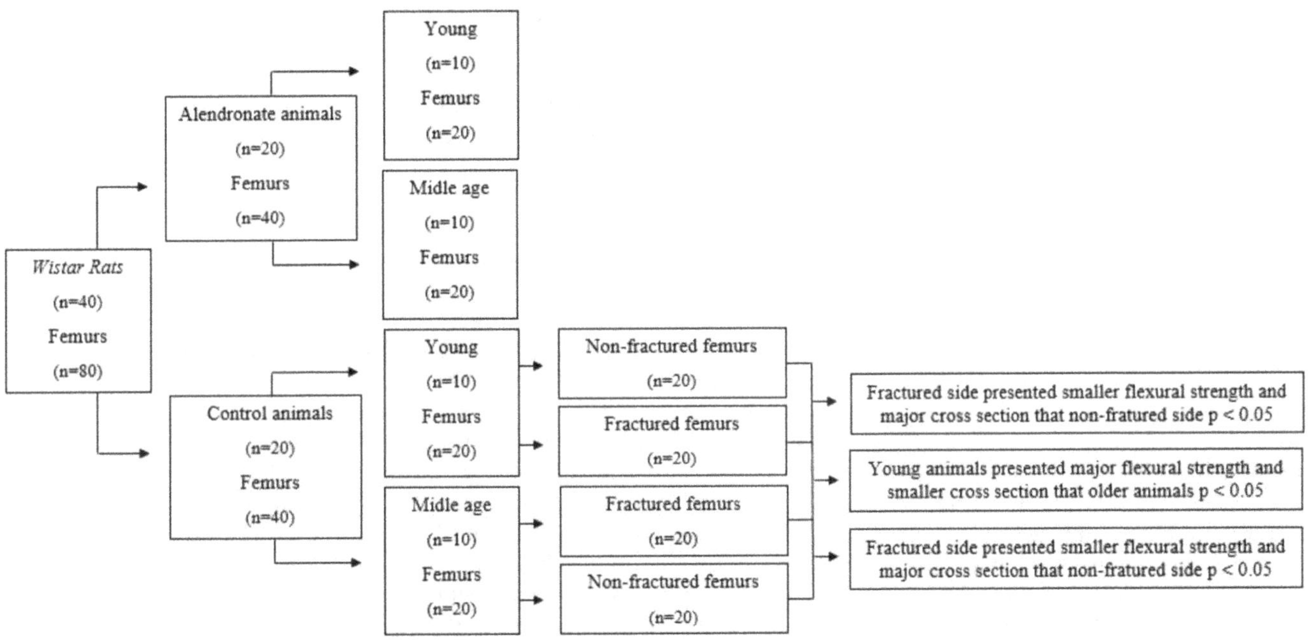

FLOWCHART 1 | Main findings of the study.

findings related to age. Young animals presented lower cross-section than older animals. Besides, on fractured side, young animals presented major flexural strength than older animals. Related to the use of alendronate, there was no difference in relation to cross-section and flexural strength.

Cross-sectional area of bone was tested as a factor of change in animal size with age. We observed that Younger animals had a smaller cross-section than middle aged animals. According to the study by Kang et al. (2016), bone mineral density is widely used in the assessment of bone strength, but it is not enough to predict the risk of fractures in an individual. Studies have reported that bone geometry is one of the major determinants of the mechanical strength and flexural strength along the cortical surfaces of the bone (Faulkner et al., 2006; Kaptoge et al., 2008; LaCroix et al., 2010). Some factors, including age, have substantial effects on bone. The velocity of bone resorption exceeds bone apposition with aging. Besides that, the weight of the animals influenced in the cross-section, as shown in the study by Ong et al. (2014), which affirms that a greater weight is associated to a higher bone density and greater bone geometry, but this do not influence in a lower risk of fracture. This was demonstrated in the present study, where there was a positive correlation of the weight with the cross-section, showing that middle aged animals, with a higher weight (mean 499.16g) presented greater cross-section and young animals with, lower weight (mean 262.50g) presented lower cross-section.

Although the non-fracture side showed smaller cross-sectional area in young versus middle aged animals, there was no difference in flexural strength in any of the groups on that side. On the other hand, the fractured side showed a difference in flexural strength, where young animals presented greater resistance than middle aged animals. Regarding the fractured side, there was no difference in flexural strength between treated and untreated animals, whether old or young Beck et al. (2001), reported that lower weight may improve the bone strength though the mechanical tensions capable of stimulating the beneficial response of the bone. Greater weight can directly influence the bone through gravitational load (Zhao et al., 2007). In addition, other studies have shown that the negative impact of greater weight on the bone may be due to increase

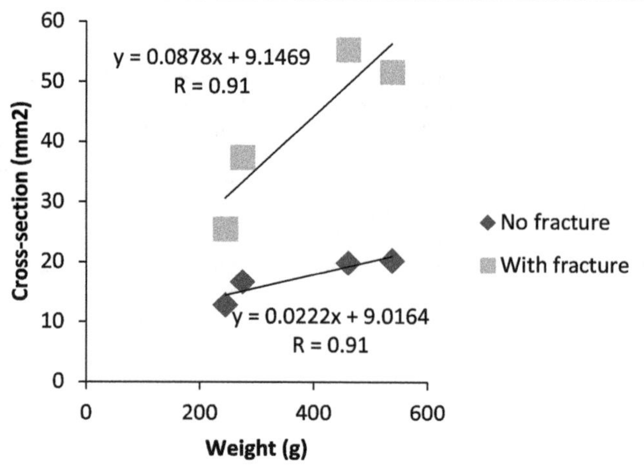

FIGURE 2 | Person's correlation test between weight and cross-section, with and without fracture.

of parathyroid hormone concentration (Pitroda et al., 2009), reduction of inflammatory cytokines (Braun and Schett, 2012) and involvement of mesenchymal stem cells in osteoblastogenic cells (Ilich et al., 2014). This affirmation corroborates with the findings of this study, that there was a negative correlation of the weight with the resistance to flexion, in which, with the increase of the weight of the animal the resistance of flexion of the femur decreases.

The process of bone healing in young and old individuals work differently. In order to this process to occur, it is necessary to balance the reabsorption of the initial callus by osteoclasts and the deposition of lamellar bone by osteoblasts, which begins around three to 4 weeks after the trauma, both in animal models and humans. This process can take years to achieve a regenerated bone structure and can occur faster in young individuals because they present a more active metabolism (Wendeberg, 1961).

In addition, according to Manalagas and Parfitt, in 2010, the aging process is related to hormonal changes, such as reduction of antioxidant capacity, sexual hormone deficiency and excess glucocorticoids, which may have influence in the healing process of tissues (Kaptoge et al., 2008).

Relate to age, it is known that in childhood and adolescence, bone formation overcomes bone resorption, reaching peak bone mass around 30 years of age. After this process, bone resorption slowly begins to overcome bone formation (Dean, 2003), in other words, aging is associated with an accelerated loss of bone mass. With this increase in bone resorption, serum calcium is reduced, and this explains the importance of correct nutrition and supplementation of calcium and vitamin D in the elderly (Bonjour et al., 2008; Reid et al., 2008). In addition to calcium, alkaline phosphatase is highly studied in research with postmenopausal women, in which the accelerated bone loss process occurs, and the serum level of alkaline phosphatase increases as a result of bone remodeling (Bhattarai et al., 2014; LeKhi et al., 2012). For these reasons, we tested serum levels of calcium and alkaline phosphatase, knowing that both markers act in the process of bone formation and remodeling.

Authors, in 2015, reported that serum calcium slightly decreased during treatment with alendronate, due to a reduction in the flow of calcium from the bone, causing an increase in parathyroid secretion, which increases bone turnover (Sakai et al., 2015). Therefore, supplementation of vitamin D and calcium are indicated during treatment with alendronate, in order to maintain the right balance of calcium levels. Our results did not corroborate with the findings of previous studies, in which the serum calcium level remained stable in the groups treated with bisphosphonate. This may be because the biochemical test was performed with only 20% of the sample, which may have weakened the statistical power of this analysis. Regarding alkaline phosphatase, there was no statistical difference between the groups. Goes et al., in 2012 evaluated the effect of alendronate on serum alkaline phosphatase levels and loss of periodontal

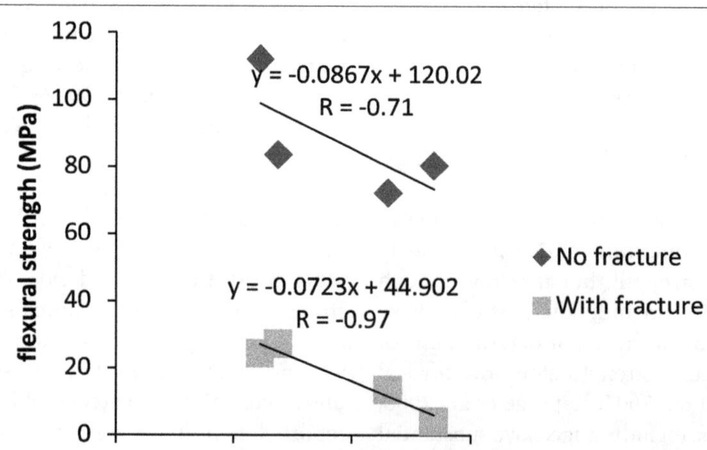

FIGURE 3 | Person's correlation test between weight and flexural strength, with and without fracture.

bone in Wistar rats. The authors concluded that the induction of periodontitis caused reduction of levels of alkaline phosphatase and severe alveolar bone loss, revealing that the serum alkaline phosphatase levels reduces with bone loss (Goes et al., 2012).

In the present study, animals treated with alendronate, middle aged or young, showed no difference in flexural strength. Researchers, in 2006, described that increases related to fracture resistance are observed after weeks or months of alendronate administration. In their studies, treatment with alendronate demonstrated increased density of bone mineral, cross-sectional area of the bone, and mechanical strength of the femur (Spadaro et al., 2006). Our results do not corroborate with these findings. It is possible that our sample was not enough to detect the significance (Type II error). It is worth mentioning that in the data analysis, we observed higher values of flexural strength in the groups treated with alendronate than in control group.

There were several limitations during the execution of this work, since the experimental design included middle aged animals. In order to perform the research, in the group with older animals, it was necessary to wait 18 months after their birth to perform the surgical procedures, that which makes the study quite long. Other point related to age is the chose for groups. In a future study, we suggest adding more age groups to analyze the influence of age throughout life. Another point worth mentioning was the use of stable internal fixation with plates and screws. In the previous work of our team (Weiss et al., 2018), we used the fixation only in young animals. With middle aged animals, often fractures of the femur occurred during the drilling of screws, because of the mineral bone density.

Other important limitation of the study is the absence of imaginological exams, like X-Ray or Micro-UT before mechanical tests. Future studies should add these exams in order to help elucidate the bone repair process in view of the age and the presence of alendronate.

In short, there was no difference of calcium and alkaline phosphatase in the study. Age has influence in cross-section and flexural strength during the bone repair process of middle aged or young rats. It was shown to negatively influence of age in flexural strength of femoral fracture callus. Smaller cross-section in young rats was associated with greater flexural strength. Finally alendronate showed no association with these factors.

ETHICS STATEMENT

The animal study was reviewed and approved by Ethics Committee on the Use of Animals (ECUA 393), Positivo University.

AUTHOR CONTRIBUTIONS

LB designed the study and prepared the first draft of the manuscript. She is guarantor. Authors PC, GK, JG, LC, ME, and JZ contributed to the experimental work and writing the manuscript. CG was responsible for statistical analysis and contribute writing the manuscript. RS designed the study, performed some surgical procedures and coordinated the research. All authors read and approved the final version of the article.

REFERENCES

Akkus, O., Adar, F., and Schaffler, M. B. (2004). Age-related changes in physicochemical properties of mineral crystals are related to impaired mechanical function of cortical bone. *Bone* 34, 443–453. doi: 10.1016/j.bone.2003.11.003

Amanat, N., McDonald, M., Godfrey, C., Bilston, L., and Little, D. (2007). Optimal timing of a single dose of zoledronic acid to increase strength in rat fracture repair. *J. Bone. Miner. Res.* 22, 867–876. doi: 10.1359/jbmr.070318

Andreollo, N. A., Santos, E. F., Araújo, M. R., and Lopes, L. R. (2012). Rat's age versus human's age: what is the relationship? *Arq. Bras. Cir. Dig.* 25, 49–51.

Bailey, A. J., Sims, T. J., Ebbesen, E. N., Mansell, J. P., Thomsen, J. S., and Mosekilde, L. (1999). Age-related changes in the biochemical properties of human cancellous bone collagen: relationship to bone strength. *Calcif. Tissue Int.* 65, 203–210.

Beck, T. J., Oreskovic, T. L., Stone, K. L., Ruff, C. B., Ensrud, K., Nevitt, M. C., et al. (2001). Structural adaptation to changing skeletal load in the progression toward hip fragility: the study of osteoporotic fractures. *J. Bone Miner.* 16, 1108–1119. doi: 10.1359/jbmr.2001.16.6.1108

Bhattarai, T., Bhattacharya, K., Chaudhuri, P., and Sengupta, P. (2014). Correlation of common bioquímica markers for bone turnover, sérico cálcio, and alcaline phosphatase in after-menopausa women. *Malays. J. Med. Sci.* 21:58.

Bonjour, J. P., Brandolini-Bunlon, M., Boirie, Y., Morel-Laporte, F., Braesco, V., Bertière, M. C., et al. (2008). Inhibition of bone turnover by milk intake in postmenopausal women. *Br. J. Nutr.* 100, 866–874.

Bosemark, P., Isaksson, H., and Tägil, M. (2014). Influence of systemic bisphosphonate treatment on mechanical properties of BMP-induced calluses in a rat fracture model: comparison of three-point bending and twisting test. *J. Orthop. Res.* 32, 721–726.

Braun, T., and Schett, G. (2012). Pathways for bone loss in inflammatory disease. *Osteoporos. Int.* 10, 101–108. doi: 10.1007/s11914-012-0104-105

Christenson, R. H. (1997). Biochemical markers of bone metabolism: an overview. *Clin. Biochem.* 30, 573–593.

de Oliveira, N., Oliveira, J., de Souza Moraes, L., Weiss, S. G., Chaves, L. H., Casagrande, T. C., et al. (2019). Bone repair in craniofacial defects treated with different doses of alendronate: a histological, histomorphometric, and immunohistochemical study. *Clin. Oral Investig.* 23, 2355–2364. doi: 10.1007/s00784-018-2670-0

Dean, J. (2003). *Oocyte-specific Gene Expression: Roles in Folliculogenesis, Fertilization and Early Development.* Cambridge: Cambridge University Press.

Faulkner, K. G., Wacker, W. K., Barden, H. S., Simonelli, C., Burke, P. K., Ragi, S., et al. (2006). Femur strength index predicts hip fracture independent of bone density and hip axis length. *Osteoporos. Int.* 17, 593–599. doi: 10.1007/s00198-005-0019-14

Goes, P., Melo, I. M., Dutra, C. S., Lima, A. P. S., and Lima, V. (2012). Effect of alendronate on bone-specific alkaline phosphatase on periodontal bone loss in rats. *Arch. Oral. Biol.* 57, 1537–1544. doi: 10.1016/j.archoralbio.2012.07.007

Greiner, S. H., Wildemann, B., Back, D. A., Alidoust, M., Schwabe, P., and Haas, N. P. (2008). Local application of zoledronic acid incorporated in a

poly (D,L-lactide)-coated implant accelerates fracture healing in rats. *Acta Orthopaedica* 79, 717–725. doi: 10.1080/17453670810016768
Ilich, J. Z., Kelly, O. J., Inglis, J. E., Panton, L. B., Duque, G., and Ormsbee, M. J. (2014). Interrelationship among muscle, fat, and bone: connecting the dots on cellular, hormonal, and whole body levels. *Ageing Res.* 15, 51–60. doi: 10.1016/j.arr.2014.02.007
Kang, H., Chen, Y. M., Han, G., Huang, H., Chen, W. Q., Wang, X., et al. (2016). Associations of age, BMI, and years of menstruation with proximal femur strength in chinese postmenopausal women: a cross-sectional study. *Int. J. Environ. Res Public Health* 13:157. doi: 10.3390/ijerph13020157
Kaptoge, S., Beck, T. J., Reeve, J., Stone, K. L., Hillier, T. A., Cauley, J. A., et al. (2008). Prediction of incident hip fracture risk by femur geometry variables measured by hip structural analysis in the study of osteoporotic fractures. *J. Bone Miner.* 23, 1892–1904. doi: 10.1359/jbmr.080802
LaCroix, A. Z., Beck, T. J., Cauley, J. A., Lewis, C. E., Bassford, T., Jackson, R., et al. (2010). Hip structural geometry and incidence of hip fracture in postmenopausal women: what does it add to conventional bone mineral density? *Osteoporos* 21, 919–929. doi: 10.1007/s00198-009-1056-1051
LeKhi, A., LeKhi, M., Sathian, B., and Mittal, A. (2012). The role of biochemical markers in the early detection of osteoporosis in women: a comparative study from the Western Region of Nepal. *J. Clin. Diag. Res.* 6, 274–277.
Naruse, K., Uchida, K., Suto, M., Miyagawa, K., Kawata, A., and Urabe, K. (2015). Alendronate does not prevent long bone fragility in an inactive rat model. *J. Bone. Miner. Metab.* 34, 615–626. doi: 10.1007/s00774-015-0714-y
Ong, T., Sahota, O., Tan, W., and Marshall, L. (2014). A United Kingdom perspective on the relationship between body mass index (BMI) and bone health: a cross sectional analysis of data from the Nottingham Fracture Liaison service. *Endocrinol. Metab.* 59, 207–210. doi: 10.1016/j.bone.2013.11.024
Pitroda, A. P., Harris, S. S., and Dawson-Hughes, B. (2009). The association of adiposity with parathyroid hormone in healthy older adults. *Endocrine* 36, 218–223. doi: 10.1007/s12020-009-9231-x
Redmond, J., Jarjou, L. M. A., Zhou, B., Prentice, A., and Schoenmakers, I. (2014). Ethnic differences in calcium, phosphate and bone metabolism. *Proc. Nutr. Soc.* 73, 340–351. doi: 10.1017/S0029665114000068
Reid, I. R., Ames, R., Mason, B., Reid, H. E., Bacon, C. J., Bolland, M. J., et al. (2008). Randomized controlled trial of calcium supplementation in healthy, nonosteoporotic, older men. *Arch. Int. Med.* 168, 2276–2282.
Sakai, A., Ito, M., Tomomitsu, T., Tsurukami, H., Ikeda, S., Fukuda, F., et al. (2015). Efficacy of combined treatment with alendronate and eldecalcitrol, a new active vitamin d analog, compared to that of concomitand alendronate, vitamin d, plus calcium treatment in japanese patients with primary osteopororosis. *Osteoporos* 26, 1193–1202. doi: 10.1007/s00198-014-2991-z
Silva, Éccd, Terreri, M. T. R. A., Castro, T. C. M. D., Barbosa, C. P. L., Fernandes, A. R. C., et al. (2010). Sclerotic metaphyseal lines in children and adolescents treated with alendronate. *Bras. J. Rheumatol.* 50, 283–290.
Spadaro, J. A., Damron, T. A., Horton, J. A., Margulies, B. S., Murray, G. M., Clemente, D. A., et al. (2006). Density and structural changes in the bone of growing rats after weekly alendronate administration with and without a methotrexate challenge. *J. Orthop. Res.* 24, 936–944.
Weiss, S. G., Kuchar, G. O., Gerber, J. T., Tiboni, F., Storrer, C. L. M., Casagrande, T. C., et al. (2018). Dose of alendronate directly increases trabeculae expansivity without altering bone volume in rat femurs. *World J. Orthop.* 9, 190–197. doi: 10.5312/wjo.v9.i10.190
Wendeberg, B. (1961). Mineral metabolism of fracture of the tibia in man studied with external counting of Sr85. *Acta Orthop. Scand.* 52, 1–79. doi: 10.3109/ort.1961.32.suppl-52.01
Zhao, L. J., Liu, Y. J., Liu, P. Y., Hamilton, J., Recker, R. R., and Deng, H. W. (2007). Relationship of obesity with osteoporosis. *J. Clin. Endocrinol. Metab.* 92, 1640–1646. doi: 10.1210/jc.2006-2572

15

Formation and Developmental Specification of the Odontogenic and Osteogenic Mesenchymes

*Eva Svandova[1], Renata Peterkova[2], Eva Matalova[1,3] and Herve Lesot[1]**

[1] Laboratory of Odontogenesis and Osteogenesis, Institute of Animal Physiology and Genetics, Academy of Sciences, Brno, Czechia, [2] Department of Histology and Embryology, Third Faculty of Medicine, Charles University, Prague, Czechia, [3] Department of Physiology, University of Veterinary and Pharmaceutical Sciences, Brno, Czechia

***Correspondence:**
Herve Lesot
Herve.Lesot@gmail.com

Within the mandible, the odontogenic and osteogenic mesenchymes develop in a close proximity and form at about the same time. They both originate from the cranial neural crest. These two condensing ecto-mesenchymes are soon separated from each other by a very loose interstitial mesenchyme, whose cells do not express markers suggesting a neural crest origin. The two condensations give rise to mineralized tissues while the loose interstitial mesenchyme, remains as a soft tissue. This is crucial for proper anchorage of mammalian teeth. The situation in all three regions of the mesenchyme was compared with regard to cell heterogeneity. As the development progresses, the early phenotypic differences and the complexity in cell heterogeneity increases. The differences reported here and their evolution during development progressively specifies each of the three compartments. The aim of this review was to discuss the mechanisms underlying condensation in both the odontogenic and osteogenic compartments as well as the progressive differentiation of all three mesenchymes during development. Very early, they show physical and structural differences including cell density, shape and organization as well as the secretion of three distinct matrices, two of which will mineralize. Based on these data, this review highlights the consecutive differences in cell-cell and cell-matrix interactions, which support the cohesion as well as mechanosensing and mechanotransduction. These are involved in the conversion of mechanical energy into biochemical signals, cytoskeletal rearrangements cell differentiation, or collective cell behavior.

Keywords: development, mouse, mandible, mesenchyme, condensation, odontogenesis, osteogenesis

INTRODUCTION

During development, epithelially derived organs (e.g., skin appendages, teeth) form from an initial epithelial bud surrounded by a condensed mass of embryonic connective tissue (mesenchyme). The mesenchyme-derived organs (e.g., bones, cartilages) develop from mesenchymal cell condensations (Hall and Miyake, 2000; Giffin et al., 2019).

The odontogenic and osteogenic jaw ecto-mesenchymes originate from cranial neural crest-derived cells (NCDCs). Their condensation takes place in two distinct regions, at about the same time in the embryonic mouse lower jaw. They later diversify into multiple cell types, along with their progressive dental or bone specification (Ruch et al., 1995; Santagati and Rijli, 2003).

Cranial neural crest cells are multipotent and differ according to distinct migratory streams and environments at a post-migratory stage (Yuan and Chai, 2019). Both the odontogenic and osteogenic condensations are progressively invaded by exogenous cells, which increases cell diversity. The cellular heterogeneity of the mesenchyme will be discussed below, as well as the mechanisms suggested to be involved in mesenchymal condensation, the progressive specification of the different mesenchymal areas, and the biological interfaces between soft and hard tissues.

The cell diversity in the three mesenchymal areas, including the participation of exogenous cells, is still under investigation in several laboratories. Comparison between situation in all three regions was discussed with regard to their ability to condense and mineralize or not. Particular attention was given to differential cell–cell and cell–matrix interactions and thus mechanosensing and mechanotransduction. All together, the sequential steps and mechanisms involved in it ultimately lead to the formation of a functional unit: a tooth firmly attached to the surrounding mandibular/alveolar bone by means of the non-mineralized periodontal ligament (PDL). Most of the data discussed here are related to the mouse first lower molar, a very common model. However, the general aspects considered here should be applicable to other models.

MESENCHYMAL CELL HETEROGENEITY IN THE MANDIBLE

In the mouse mandible at embryonic day (ED)12.5, two distant condensations are separated from each other by a looser uncondensed mesenchyme: an osteogenic one, deep in the embryonic jaw and the odontogenic one, adjacent to the thickened dental epithelium/dental lamina in the prospective first molar (M1) region (**Figures 1A–C**). At early stages, the external limits of the two condensations can hardly be determined since there is a continuous decreasing gradient in cell density toward the surrounding uncondensed mesenchyme (**Figures 1A,B**). Both the odontogenic mesenchymal condensation and the dental epithelium represent the ecto-mesenchymal and epithelial components of a developing tooth primordium, respectively.

At ED13.5, the odontogenic condensation becomes more pronounced and surrounds the dental epithelium, which acquires the shape of a tooth bud (**Figures 1D,E**). A bone matrix is already visible in the osteogenic condensation in the mouse lower jaw (**Figure 1F**). At early stages, the intramembranous bone formation is characterized by apposition only. The characteristic of intramembranous bone formation is the absence of a chondrogenic step as it exists during endochondral bone development. Progenitor cells present in the condensation

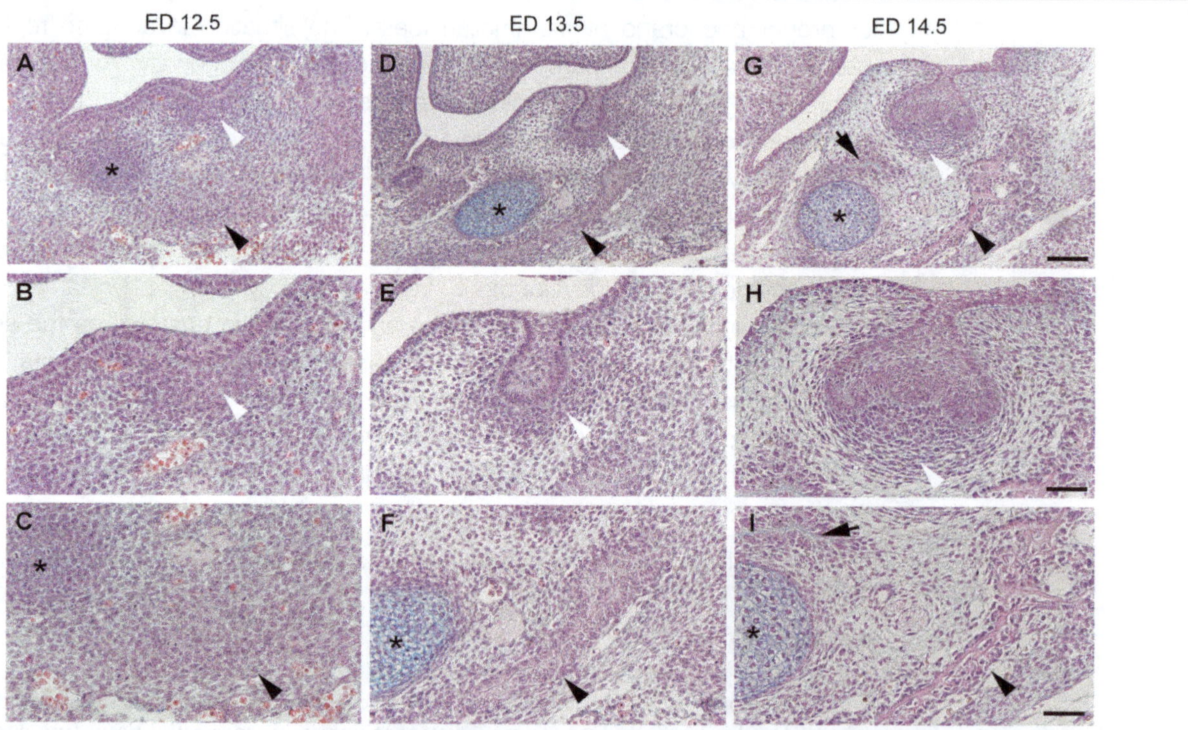

FIGURE 1 | Histological sections of the embryonic mouse lower jaw at the level of M1. The two odontogenic (white arrowhead) and osteogenic (black arrowhead) mesenchymal condensations are distant from each other being separated by a looser interstitial mesenchyme at embryonic day (ED)12.5 **(A–C)**. Jaw bone appears at ED13.5 **(D–F)**, and ED14.5 **(G–I)**, and its development is accelerated on the lateral side (black arrowhead) when compared to the medial side (black arrow). Both the bone and tooth germ grow and approach each other at the expense of the area of the interstitial mesenchyme. The dental follicle cells achieve progressively a typical pattern (compare to **Figure 2**). Although mineralization will take place in both osteogenic and odontogenic condensations, the interstitial mesenchyme (see **Figure 2**) will never mineralize in normal conditions. * Refers to the Meckel's cartilage, Bars = 100 mm **(A,D,G)** and 50 mm **(B,C,E,F,H,I)**.

differentiate directly into osteoblasts (Berendsen and Olsen, 2015). Signaling and transcriptional regulation, involved in osteoblasts differentiation, have been investigated (for review, see Huang et al., 2007; Ferguson and Atit, 2019).

Within 2 days, from ED13 to ED15, when cell differentiation occurs, the osteogenic condensation turns into a vascularized bone containing bone specific cells: (e.g., Alfaqeeh et al., 2013; Vesela et al., 2019). From ED15, the bony crypt around the dental primordia starts to be remodeled, mostly by bone resorption (Radlanski et al., 2015).

The transition from the epithelial tooth bud to cap is accompanied by the differentiation of the former odontogenic mesenchymal condensation. This condensation gives rise to two compartments: (1) the dental papilla encapsulated by the epithelial cap, and (2) the dental follicle (or dental sac), which surrounds the epithelial cap and papilla (**Figure 2**). The papilla cells are progressively specified by sequential epithelial-mesenchymal interactions, and the preodontoblasts/odontoblasts lineage will later be controlled by the inner dental epithelium (Mina and Kollar, 1987; Lumsden, 1988; Ruch et al., 1995). The cell heterogeneity in the dental papilla becomes more and more complex (Keller et al., 2012; Kokten et al., 2014b; Krivanek et al., 2017). The characteristic shape and pattern of cells within the dental follicle allows its delineation from the surrounding loose interstitial mesenchyme (**Figures 1H, 2**).

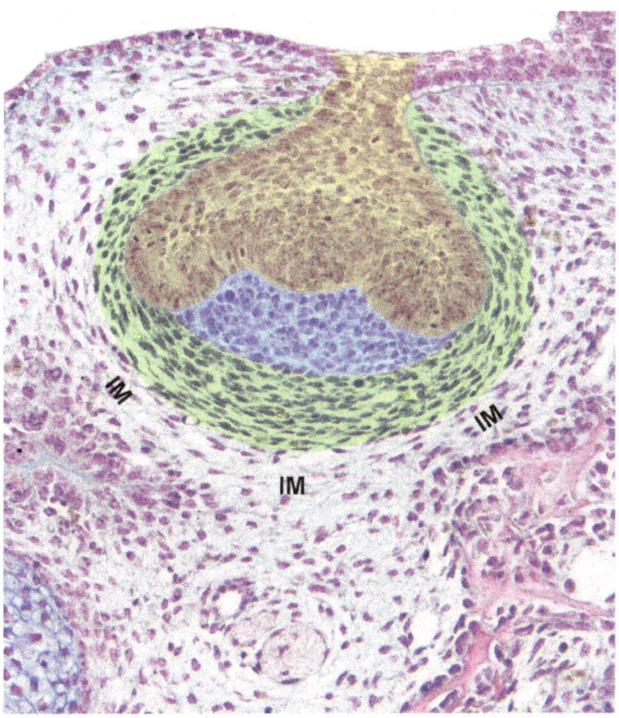

FIGURE 2 | Components of a tooth germ and surrounding tissues. Mouse first lower molar germ at ED14.5 exhibits a clear subdivision of dental mesenchyme including the dental papilla (blue) and dental follicle/dental sac (green). Cells of the dental papilla show neither specific shape nor spatial organization. Conversely, cells of the dental sac show an elongated shape being arranged in concentric rings (green). The contemporaneous presence of increased cell density, their specific shape and pattern are criteria for the determination of the dental sac boundary. The dental epithelium is at a cap stage (yellow). IM, interstitial mesenchyme.

At ED14.5, dispersed cells of the interstitial mesenchyme are interposed between the external cells of the dental follicle and the osteogenic condensation (**Figures 1G–I, 2**). Very quickly, this mesenchyme shows further peculiarity. Immunostainings for VEGFR2, CD31, CD34 showed that the interstitial mesenchyme is vascularized at ED14, slightly before the dental mesenchyme and before the forming bone itself (Nait Lechguer et al., 2008; Keller et al., 2012; Vesela et al., 2019).

This interstitial mesenchyme is maintained at ED15, when the tooth germ has reached the late cap stage and bone has developed. How far these cells will later participate to the PDL and possibly even to the osteogenic mesenchyme is unknown since cell tracing has not been performed for this population (Zhao et al., 2013), in opposition to cranial neural crest cells (Chai et al., 2000), or mesenchymal cells facing the tip of the tooth bud (Rothova et al., 2012). Dissociation-reassociation experiments were performed using dissociated papilla and follicle cells from cap stage (ED14) molar germs (see Figure 1 in Kokten et al., 2014a). When re-associated with an intact enamel organ or dissociated epithelial cells, it was possible to reconstitute a whole tooth. This showed that although all initial positional information had been lost, mesenchymal cells at this stage can reconstitute a whole tooth germ. This demonstrated a high cell plasticity (Hu et al., 2005; Kuchler-Bopp et al., 2011), which decreases at later stages (Keller et al., 2011). This was in agreement with labeling and fate-mapping experiments showing that cells from the odontogenic condensation at the bud stage could participate in the follicle at the cap stage (Rothova et al., 2012). These experiments still raise the question of understanding why do these cells migrate, when cells of the follicle are already present there at that stage (**Figure 2**). One possibility is that the migrating dental mesenchymal cells increase the heterogeneity of the dental follicle and bring new necessary cell type(s) still absent before. It would thus be of interest to investigate in more details the heterogeneity of dental follicle cells before and after cell migration. Two other questions to be addressed concern: (1) the disruption of cell-cell/cell-matrix interactions within the dental papilla to allow cell migration and (2) the nature of the signals driving such a long distance migration and mediating cell targeting.

Cells from the interstitial mesenchyme (**Figure 2**), or at least a sub-population, are particularly important as possibly contributing to the development of the future PDL. At early developmental stage, and in opposition to the dental mesenchyme and follicle cells, interstitial mesenchymal cells do not express markers for NCDCs (Chai et al., 2000). It has been proposed that gingival connective tissue fibroblasts originate from perifollicular mesenchyme, a derivative of the stomodeal mesoderm (Cho and Garant, 2000). This particular origin of least part of the PDL fibroblasts might explain their specific properties and differences with the neighboring ecto-mesenchymal odontogenic and osteogenic condensations. Among these peculiarities, interstitial mesenchymal cells produce an extracellular matrix (ECM) that will not mineralize, thus impairing tooth ankylosis during later development.

MECHANISMS INVOLVED IN MESENCHYMAL CELL CONDENSATIONS

Cell condensation is a fundamental mechanism involved in morphogenesis. Condensations of mesenchymal cells take place during the development of almost all tissues and organs, including skin appendages, primordia of sensory organs, parenchymatous organs and musculo-skeletal structures (for review, see Giffin et al., 2019). Cell condensation occurs when a population of originally dispersed cells aggregates to differentiate into a specific cell/tissue type (**Scheme 1**; Hall and Miyake, 2000). The condensation results from altered mitotic activity, absence of centrifugal cell movement and/or centripetal cell aggregation (Hall and Miyake, 1995). According to Shyer et al. (2017), mesenchymal cells have an intrinsic potential to aggregate. The increase in cell density might facilitate cell–cell communication, possibly required for subsequent lineage acquisition (McKeown et al., 2005). However, the odontogenic and osteogenic mesenchymal condensations are separated by a non-condensed region. This illustrates early differences in the characteristics of mesenchymal cells, despite they are very next to each other. Each of these three cases reflect collective cell behavior, where mechanobiology might play an important role (Ladoux and Mège, 2017). The mesenchymal cell condensation, as it appears in early stage of odontogenesis and mandibular osteogenesis, precedes blood vessels ingrowth. This might be a general situation to be considered for regenerative medicine (Takebe et al., 2015). Furthermore, during tooth development, vascularization is anticipated in the interstitial mesenchyme, and blood vessels do not enter the condensed mesenchyme before the cap stage tooth germ as stated above. Similarly, blood vessels do not enter the osteogenic condensation before ED14 (Vesela et al., 2019).

Odontogenic Condensation

Condensation of the dental mesenchyme occurs during early steps of odontogenesis. Changes in the cell shape or size were suggested to possibly mediate this phenomenon (Mammoto et al., 2011, 2013). At this stage, histology did not confirm it, but showed change in cell density (**Figures 1B,E**). A decrease in intercellular spaces was obvious, which could be related to a change in either the ECM itself, in cell–cell interactions, or both. At the bud stage, syndecan and tenascin were detected within the odontogenic mesenchymal condensation and might be involved the in condensation process (Vainio and Thesleff, 1992; Thesleff et al., 1996). Collagen type VI, also present there, has been suggested to play a key role by stabilizing odontogenic cell condensation (Mammoto et al., 2015). According to these authors, cross-linking of collagen type VI by lysyl-oxidase would be involved and interfering with it would change the size of the condensation.

The condensation of the odontogenic mesenchyme appears to be regulated by signaling from the bud epithelium (Dassule and McMahon, 1998). Little is known about this signaling. Mammoto et al. (2011) showed that during mouse tooth development, FGF8 and (semaphorin) SEMA3F, produced by early dental epithelium, were causally involved in mesenchymal cell condensation. This mechanical compaction induced changes in the expression of transcription factors (PAX9, MSX1) and a growth factor (BMP4). These authors concluded that mechanical compression of the mesenchyme is necessary to induce tooth-specific cell fate although a condensation also takes place before osteogenic markers are expressed. The fact that one is in contact with an epithelium, while the other is not, is probably much more important. This has been very precisely documented in the developing tooth at later stage. In case of odontoblasts layer versus sub-odontoblastic cells, this is determined after the last cell division. Among the two daughter cells, the one in contact with a stage-specific basement membrane will differentiate as an odontoblast and elongate, while the other one will gets a flatten shape (Ruch et al., 1982, 1995; Ruch, 1998). However, *in vitro* experiments showed that growth factors, such as TGFbeta-1 or -3, when immobilized by heparin, can replace the inner dental epithelium and basement membrane, and induce preodontoblasts to odontoblasts differentiation (Ruch et al., 1995). BMP-2, -4, and -7 can induce it as well, although in more restricted areas. This involves a change in cell shape, elongation, as well as cytological and functional differentiation (polarized secretion of predentin), as it occurs in physiological conditions (Ruch, 1998).

In case of skin and follicle patterning in avian, Shyer et al. (2017) suggested an inverse mechanism, where mesenchymal cell condensation would change the organization of adjacent epidermal cells by triggering a mechanosensitive activation of beta-catenin in these cells.

Osteogenic Condensation

During development, a pre-osteogenic phase characterized by mesenchymal cell condensation (for review, see Hall and Miyake, 2000; Jabalee et al., 2013) is followed by post-condensation stage, including osteogenic cell differentiation, vascularization, innervation and mineralization of the ECM. However, these pre- and post-condensation stages remain connected (Dunlop and Hall, 1995). Although the mechanism mediating it remains unclear, mesenchymal cell condensation represents the initial stage of osteogenic specification. Hall and Miyake (2000) have proposed a series of molecules possibly involved in it (**Scheme 1**).

Fibroblast growth factors (FGFs) as well as bone morphogenetic proteins (BMPs) have been suggested to play a role in the initiation of condensation (Wu et al., 2007; Javed et al., 2010). Tissue cultures and recombinations *in vitro* showed that mandibular osteogenesis involves post-migratory neural crest-derived ecto-mesenchymal cells and their interaction with a mandibular epithelium (Hall, 1980; MacDonald and Hall, 2001). These experimental results raise interesting questions about the signaling process, given the long distance between the initially condensing osteogenic mesenchyme and epithelial tissues *in situ*.

The process of condensation itself requires changes in the local tissue mechanical properties (Mammoto et al., 2011). The generation of contractile forces within mesenchymal cells has been suspected (Oster et al., 1983;

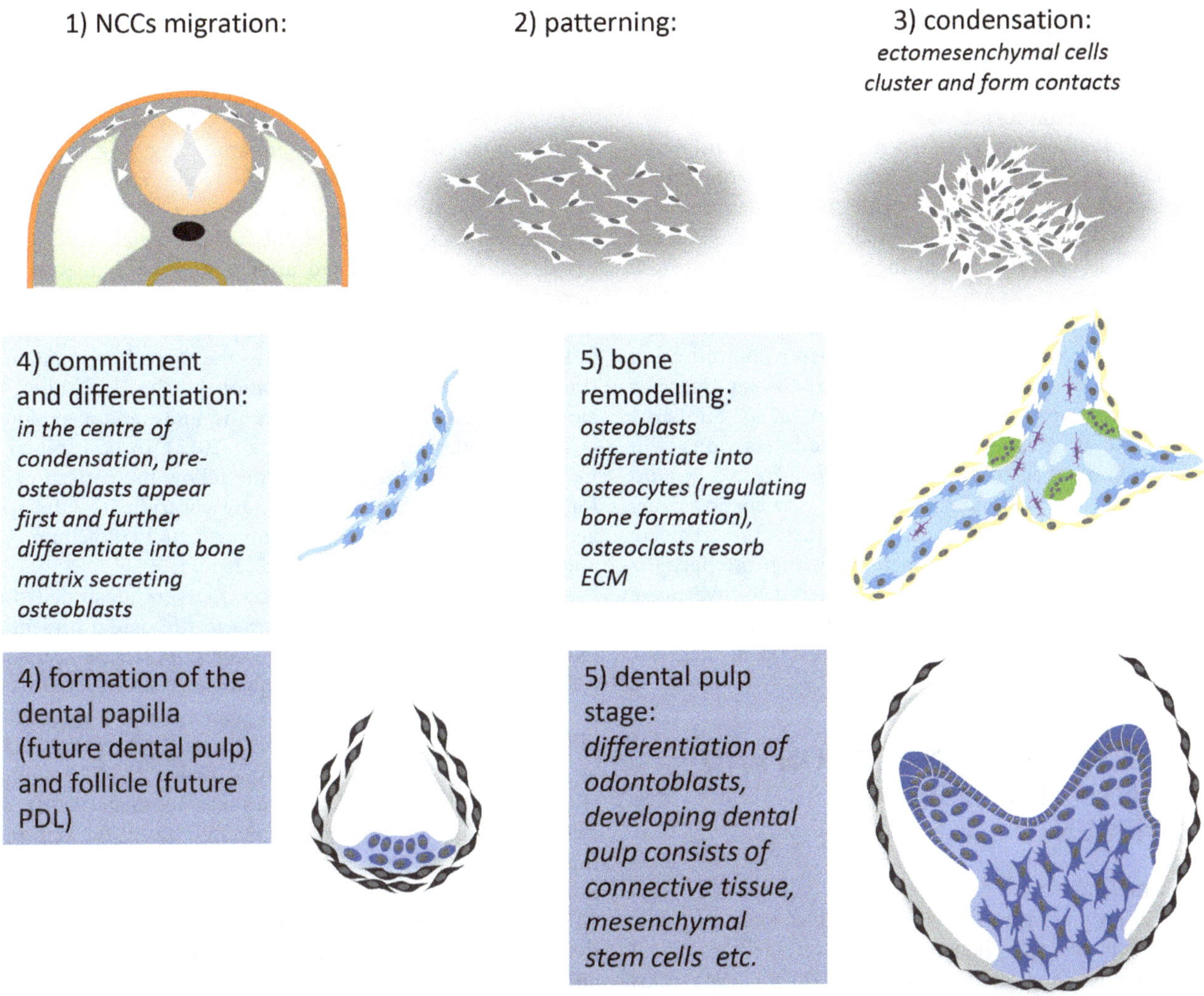

bone		tooth
Bmps, Fgfs, Tgfb2, Msx-1	2	Lhx6/7, Gli1/2/3, Msx1/2, Dlx1/2, Barx, Pax9, Bmps, activin
tenascin, fibronectin, N-cadherin, N-CAM, Cx43	3	Lhx6/7, Gli1/2/3, Msx1/2, Dlx1/2, Barx, Pax9, Lef, Runx2, Bmps, Fgfs, Wnt
commitment: Cbfa1, Osx pre-osteoblasts: Alp, Col1a1 osteoblasts: Bsp, Ocn, Rankl	4	Lhx6/7, Gli1/2/3, Msx1/2, Dlx1/2, Barx, Pax9, Lef, Runx2, Bmps, Fgfs, Wnt DFCs: Notch-1, Stro-1, CD13, CD44, CD73, CD105, CD56, CD271, HLA-ABC, Oct-4, Sox-2
osteocytes: Sost, Phex, Mepe, Dmp1, osteoclasts: TRAP, Ctsk, Mmps, Fgf23 lining cells (differentiate from osteoblasts): Stro-1, absence of Ocn	5	odontoblasts: Dmp1, Dspp, Alp, Msx2, Bmp4, Fgfs, Klf4, Mepe, Col1a1, Ocn, Colla1, Colla1a2, fibronectin, BSP, proteoglycans MSCs: CD73, CD90, CD105, Stro-1, Sca-1, Oct-4 cells of connective tissue: col12a, col14

SCHEME 1 | Crucial steps and molecules involved in the development of mesenchymal condensations. Molecular markers were summarized according to Casagrande et al. (2010), Dallas and Bonewald (2010), Everts et al. (2002), Ferguson and Atit (2019), Franz-Odendaal (2011), Giffin et al. (2019), Hall and Miyake (2000), Ledesma-Martínez et al. (2016), Lin et al., 2011, 2013; Nanci et al. (2008), Zhou et al. (2019), and Zvackova et al. (2017). Ectoderm (orange), NCCs (white), somite (light green), osteoblasts (light blue), lining cells – osteogenic cells (yellow), osteocytes (purple), osteoclasts (green), dental follicle (gray), dental papilla (dark blue), odontoblasts (dark blue-columnar).

Ray and Chapman, 2015). Most of the data to support it and their role in mechanotransduction during osteogenesis have been obtained from *in vitro* experiments (Discher et al., 2005; Komatsu et al., 2018; Giffin et al., 2019). Concerning cell–cell interactions, three connexins, involved in the formation of gap junctions have been investigated during initial mandibular osteogenesis in the chick embryo. Among these, connexin43 (Cx43) appeared to be associated with the condensation of mesenchyme and the earliest stages of osteogenesis (Minkoff et al., 1994). Cx43 gene deletion in the mouse also leads to cell autonomous osteoblast dysfunction and delayed mineralization (Lecanda et al., 2000). Cx43-containing gap junctions thus seem to play an important role in the intercellular communication between the interconnected bone cells network (osteoprogenitor cells, osteoblast, and osteocytes) (Moorer et al., 2017). Similarly, the possible role of cadherins, which mediate interactions with the cytoskeleton of adjacent cells, has been investigated *in vitro* (Griffin et al., 2017). Adhesion junctions are mechanosensing structures, which play diverse roles. Among these, they regulate the expression of transcription factors during osteogenesis (Guntur et al., 2012). It would thus be of interest to investigate the pattern of cadherins during early mandibular/alveolar bone development and to compare it with the situation in neighbor interstitial mesenchyme.

MESENCHYMES SPECIFICATION AND DIFFERENTIATION DURING DEVELOPMENT

All three mesenchymes (odontogenous, osteogenous, and intermediary) progressively consist in heterogeneous cell types, different in each case and changing during development. In all three cases, besides the presence/absence of NCDCs, exogenous cells take part in cell heterogeneity. Most of these exogenous cells enter together during vascularization, and later during innervation (**Scheme 2**).

Dental Mesenchyme

The interactions of the odontogenic neural crest-derived mesenchymal cells with the oral epithelium determine a specific fate, very different from that of the other set of condensing osteogenic mesenchymal cells.

The dental papilla ecto-mesenchyme is clearly defined from the cap stage as part of condensed mesenchyme surrounded by the dental epithelium up to cervical loop, while the rest of the odontogenous mesenchyme gives rise to the dental follicle (**Figure 2**). Several successive steps lead to the histo-differentiation of the dental papilla and follicle mesenchymes, which are controlled by time- and space-specific epithelial-mesenchymal interactions (MacNeil and Thomas, 1993; Ruch et al., 1995; Thesleff et al., 1995; Miletich and Sharpe, 2003). The first odontoblasts differentiate at ED18. At post-natal day (PN) 1, they become positive for CD73, a 5′nucleotidase, which might be related to their functional differentiation. This 5′nucleotidase as well as alkaline phosphatase use AMP as a substrate (Andrade et al., 2008; Yegutkin, 2008) and could play a role in the expression of osteocalcin, which takes place in mature odontoblasts (Bidder et al., 1998). Odontoblasts were transiently positive for CD90 at PN1 and negative again at PN4 (Keller et al., 2012).

In opposition to clearly distinct cell compartments in the enamel organ, histology does not show anything similar in the forming dental papilla, except for preodontoblast/odontoblast, sub-odontoblastic layers and blood vessels.

Immunostaining revealed the cellular heterogeneity within the dental mesenchyme and implantation experiments in GFP mice were necessary to distinguish the endogenous/exogenous origin of these cells (Kuchler-Bopp et al., 2011; Keller et al., 2012; Kokten et al., 2014b). In the first lower molar, the timing of mesenchymal specification by the epithelium varies along the antero-posterior axis of the tooth and also along the buccal-lingual one (Nakatomi et al., 2013). In both cases, these local variations in the mesenchyme follow the pattern of cusps formation and, within one cusp, are controlled by the specific geometric determination in the inner dental epithelium (Obara and Lesot, 2007; Nakatomi et al., 2013).

Immunostaining for cell surface markers illustrated the cell heterogeneity with distinct patterns in the dental mesenchyme (Keller et al., 2012). The different cell populations also showed a differential timing in their appearance. Amongst these cells some are external to the dental papilla. At the cap stage, the first blood vessels penetrate the dental mesenchyme (Nait Lechguer et al., 2008) and their mesodermal origin has been reported (Rothova et al., 2011). When cultured tooth germs or dental cell–cells re-associations were implanted under the skin in GFP mice, both were re-vascularized. GFP-positive cells from the host were associated with blood vessels (i.e., cells expressing CD34, CD146, and later alpha-SMA) (Nait Lechguer et al., 2008). Complementary experiments showed that CD90-positive cells, and blood vessels associated Sca-1-positive cells can be either GFP-positive or negative, indicating that, in both cases, they still consist of heterogeneous populations, at least regarding their origins (Keller et al., 2012). The immunodetection of CD31, 34, and 146 showed that at ED14, while blood vessels were already present in the interstitial mesenchyme, they only started to enter the dental follicle. They were detected in the whole papilla mesenchyme at ED18 up to cells underlying the odontoblasts layer (Keller et al., 2012). Microvessels reaching the odontoblast layer at PN7 were detected after staining for CD34, collagen type IV or CD146 (Kokten et al., 2014b). Multiple double stainings showed that all three antigens were co-localized. These capillaries might be involved in the transport of calcium necessary for dentin mineralization (Bishop, 1987).

At ED18 also, CD45-positive cells were detected in the dental papilla and follicle, while CD90-positive cells were restricted to the papilla. Several dendritic cell types resident or not were present in the dental mesenchyme (Zhang et al., 2006; Keller et al., 2012). They included immunocompetent cells (Okiji et al., 1992, 1997; Kaneko et al., 2008), which can be recruited to participate in reparative processes (Jontell et al., 1998; Farges et al., 2003; Goldberg et al., 2008). From PN1, Sca-1 was detected in the dental pulp but still, very few cells were visualized. At PN4, this antigen was mainly expressed by cells associated to the largest

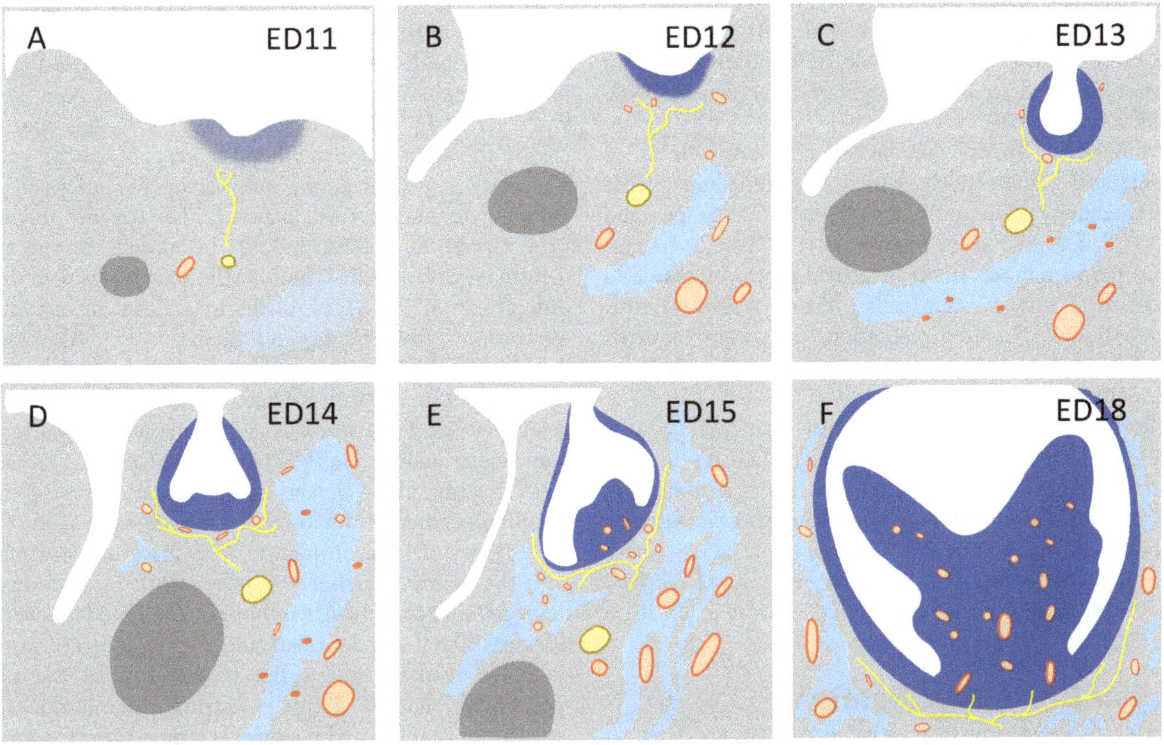

NCCs migration at ED8.25 (Nichols, 1986)

formation of the mandible at ED10.5 (Li et al., 2016)

initiation of mesenchymal condensation at ED11.5 (Hiliard e al., 2004)

condensations of mesenchyme at ED12.5 (Vesela et al., 2019)

reference	time	bone	event	tooth	time	reference
Vesela et al., 2019	ED13	osteoblasts	differentiation	odontoblasts	ED18	Ruch et al., 1995
Vesela et al., 2019	ED13	bone ECM	matrix secretion	pre-dentin	ED18.5	Ruch et al., 1995
Vesela et al., 2019	ED15	vessels in bone matrix	vascularization	vessels	ED14-18	Nait Lechguer et al., 2008
Ramaesh and Bard, 2003	ED16.5	alveolar nerve	inervation	sensory nerves sympathetic n.	P4 P9	Moe et al., 2008

SCHEME 2 | Development of mesenchymal condensations in mouse mandible. Figures show the mandible at stage ED11 **(A)**, ED12 **(B)**, ED13 **(C)**, ED14 **(D)**, ED15 **(E)**, ED18 **(F)**. Dental condensation (dark blue), bone condensation (light blue), Meckel's cartilage (dark gray), nerves (yellow), vessels (red).

blood vessels at the apical part of the papilla as also observed for alpha-SMA (Keller et al., 2012).

Sensory nerves enter the dental mesenchyme at PN3-4, while sympathetic nerves involved in vasoregulation penetrate this tissue much later, at PN9 (Tabata et al., 1998; Moe et al., 2008). Sensory and sympathetic axons can make contacts with dental pulp vessels, but most of them are sensory ones (Byers, 1984; Moe et al., 2008). In the odontoblast layer at PN7, axons were very frequently detected in close proximity with capillaries as seen after double staining for peripherin and either CD34 or collagen IV, or CD146 and confirmed by transmission electron microscopy (Kokten et al., 2014b). At PN7, when reached by axons, odontoblasts could function as mechanosensory cells (Allard et al., 2006; Magloire et al., 2009, 2010). Using confocal laser scanning microscopy, Farahani et al. (2012) showed that the heterogeneity of odontoblasts-associated cells increased precisely at that time.

Double staining for S100-beta and GFAP, two markers for glial cells, did not completely overlap, showing the existence of distinct glial cell types. S100-beta positive cells also showed more proximity with microvessels than GFAP-positive ones. Glial cells reached odontoblasts at PN7 (Kokten et al., 2014b). Schwann cells were present near the basal pole of odontoblasts from PN9, but not detected in the odontoblast layer before PN60 (Corpron and Avery, 1973).

Several different stem cell populations have been identified in the papilla and dental follicle, which also contribute to the cellular heterogeneity of these tissues (Shi et al., 2005; Yen and Sharpe, 2008; Yu et al., 2015; Sharpe, 2016). Genetic lineage tracing was performed to better understand the origin and properties of mesenchymal stem cells (MSCs) *in vivo* (Sharpe, 2016). When tested after transplantation, they were reported to exhibit different phenotypic and functional properties (for review, see Volponi and Sharpe, 2013).

Altogether, these results exemplify very dynamic changes in the heterogeneity of dental mesenchymal cells during odontogenesis. This illustrates a further progressive specification of papilla cells and the contribution of exogenous cells entering this mesenchyme from about ED14 (Moe et al., 2008; Keller et al., 2012; Krivanek et al., 2017), after it became vascularized (Chai et al., 2000; Nait Lechguer et al., 2008; Rothova et al., 2011; Feng et al., 2011).

Mandibular Bone Specification

Amongst bone cells, osteocalcin-positive osteoblasts are detected in the osteogenic condensation already at ED13 in mouse embryos. Osteoblasts directly differentiate from condensed ecto-mesenchymal cells and give rise to osteocytes. Parathormone (PTH) shares its membrane-bound parathyroid hormone 1 receptor (PTH1r) with parathyroid hormone-related protein (PTHrP). PTH1r and PTHrP are involved in osteoblast maturation in the mandibular/alveolar bone by stimulating osteocalcin expression (Martin, 2005; Bobek et al., 2020). At ED15, these osteocytes are PTH1r- and VDR-positive. Glucocorticoids are involved in the control of osteocyte differentiation (Alemi et al., 2018). Osteocytes, as forming a canalicular network, are thought to constitute a mechanosensory network, involved in mechanotransduction (Burger and Klein-Nulend, 1999; Bonewald and Johnson, 2008). LRP5, a co-receptor of Wnt, is essential for mechanotransduction, a mechanism by which cells convert mechanical energy into biochemical signals (Sawakami et al., 2006). Alveolar bone is a highly mechanoresponsive tissue. Primary cilia act as mechano- and chemosensors, transferring signals from the extracellular to intracellular compartments. Cilia also modulate the non-canonical Wnt signaling (Yavropoulou and Yovos, 2016).

Osteoclasts, responsible for bone resorption have precursors in the bone marrow. The migration of these precursors is thus associated to the vascularization. TRAP-positive mononucleated cells were detected when blood vessels start to penetrate the osteogenic condensation, at ED14 (Bobek et al., 2020). TRAP-positive osteoclasts are detected at ED14, and multinucleated osteoclasts at E15 (Bobek et al., 2020). Protocadherin-7 is involved in osteoclastogenesis by promoting cell-cell fusion (Nakamura et al., 2014). The activation of osteoclasts is mediated by RANKL produced by PTH-stimulated osteoblasts (Boyce and Xing, 2007). RANKL-RANK-OPG is an essential signaling network for osteoblast-osteoclast cross-talk (Nakagawa et al., 1998).

Besides bone cells *stricto sensu*, blood vessels penetrate the osteogenous condensation at ED14, and the bone structure is vascularized by ED15 (Vesela et al., 2019). As reported in the case of the dental papilla, blood vessels play a major role in bone homeostasis, in regulating the osteogenic microenvironment, bringing minerals, growth factors, and osteogenic progenitor cells (e.g., Grosso et al., 2017). Endothelial cells secrete osteogenic factors, such as BMP-2 and BMP-4, which support osteoblast differentiation. VEGF regulates in a dose dependent way the expression SEMA3A in endothelial cells. SEMA3A inhibits osteoclasts differentiation, thus stimulating bone development (Hayashi et al., 2012; Kenan et al., 2019). Conversely, the deletion of Vegf in Osterix-positive osteoblast precursors reduces mandibular ossification (Wang et al., 2007; Hill et al., 2015).

In human, the alveolar nerve issued from the trigeminal ganglion extends in the lower jaw before bone tissue forms and early stages of bone formation take place in close relationship with the mandibular nerve (Kjaer, 1990). Interactions between neurons and bone tissue have been documented in several models during skeletal development and repair. However, only scarce data are available about the innervation of the developing mandibular/alveolar bone. During development, CGRP (calcitonin gene-related peptide) is required for the formation of mandibular bone. When associated with blood vessels, it controls local blood flow (Hill and Elde, 1991). ISH showed that at ED14.5, Cgrp is expressed by mesenchymal cells surrounding the bone matrix and blood vessels (Maeda et al., 2017). Nerves, bone cells, and immune cells, influence bone homeostasis through a local secretion SEMA3A, which is involved in the regulation of osteoblastogenesis and osteoclastogenesis (Jabalee et al., 2013; Xu, 2014).

Schwann cells can play an active role in osteogenesis in the mandibular bone, but all studies were performed in case of distraction osteogenesis, a surgical separation of the jaw bone to elicit new bone growth in the gap (Farhadieh et al., 2003; Byun et al., 2008). It would thus be of interest to investigate the innervation during mandibular/alveolar bone formation in the mouse embryo, and compare what happens during distraction osteogenesis with what can be observed during development. A mouse model has been set up to investigate the nerve dependency of the mouse skeletal stem cell (mSSC), progenitor cells responsible for skeletal development and repair (Jones et al., 2019). According to these authors, the mandibular bone repair is compromised after inferior alveolar nerve disruption and denervation, as a result of functional deficiencies of mSSCs. A partial rescue of the denervated phenotype has been observed after Schwann cell transplantation and by Schwann cell-derived growth factors, suggesting that mSSCs would be dependent on paracrine factors secreted by Schwann cells (Jones et al., 2019).

Jaw bones contain very limited quantities of orofacial bone/bone-marrow-derived MSCs. Their isolation thus requires a specific methodology. When compared to long bone marrow-derived MSCs, orofacial bone/bone-marrow-derived MSCs demonstrated specific immunomodulatory properties and different capacities *in vitro*, thus appearing as a unique population of MSCs (Yamaza et al., 2011). *In vitro* experiments showed that Wnt/β-catenin signaling pathway is involved in the regulation of MSCs migration (He et al., 2018). *In vitro* experiments showed that the chemical and physical properties of the microenvironment modulate the commitment and fate of mesenchymal stromal/stem cells (MSSCs). Intermittent fluid shear stress, a potent and physiologically relevant mechanical stimulus, regulates osteogenic differentiation of MSCs through a transient receptor potential melastatin 7 (TRPM7). TRPM7 is a member of a family of TRP mechanosensitive cation channels with a cytosolic α-kinase domain that interferes with cytoskeletal rearrangements (Clark et al., 2006; Liu et al., 2015). TRP responds to intracellular and extracellular stimuli. Liu et al. (2015) suggested that TRPM7 has differential roles in endochondral and intramembranous ossification.

From the Dental Follicle to the Periodontal Ligament

Although the dental follicle and dental papilla have the same ecto-mesenchymal origin (Ten Cate, 1997), they soon diverge, showing distinct cell shape and arrangement (**Figure 2**). Cells initially located in the interstitial mesenchyme (**Figure 2**) participate in the formation of the PDL. Progenitor cells present in the dental follicle then give rise to cementoblasts, and possibly contribute to the alveolar bone osteoblasts (Diekwisch, 2002 and references therein; Diep et al., 2009; Dangaria et al., 2011).

Progressive Cell Heterogeneity in the Interstitial Mesenchyme

As stated above, cells from the odontogenic condensation at the bud stage later form the dental papilla in the epithelial cap. Some have been suggested to migrate and participate in the follicle at the cap and bell stages (Osborn and Price, 1988; Rothova et al., 2012). The interstitial mesenchyme is highly vascularized already at ED14 (Nait Lechguer et al., 2008; Keller et al., 2012). It also starts to be innervated at the cap stage (**Scheme 2**; Luukko and Kettunen, 2014). This very complex heterogeneous cell population is progressively set up from ED14. At the same time and later, several distinct stem cells have been described, which play complementary roles (Luan et al., 2006). SEMA3A has been detected in the dental follicle from ED15 (Wada et al., 2014). These authors suggested that, besides its important role in innervation (Moe et al., 2012; Luukko and Kettunen, 2014), SEMA3A might also induce the conversion of PDL cells into mesenchymal-stem-like cells (Wada et al., 2014; Tomokiyo et al., 2019).

Periodontal Ligament

The PDL forms and differentiates quite late postnatally. At PN4 (**Figures 3A, A1, A2**). Even at PN7 (**Figures 3B, B1, B2**), the developing PDL does not yet show any characteristic organization (Keller et al., 2015, Figure 28.3a).

The PDL consists of heterogeneous cell populations (e.g., Fleischmannova et al., 2010). These include fibroblasts (Lekic and McCulloch, 1996), vascular endothelial cells (Saghiri et al., 2018) and associated pericytes (Roguljic et al., 2013), macrophages (Epelman et al., 2014) and dendritic cells, acting as immunocompetent cells (Kaneko et al., 2008). Using the rat as a model, Kaneko et al. (2008) observed that the molecular phenotype of resident dendritic cells is heterogeneous, probably reflecting differences in their maturation/activation. From PN7 (**Figures 3B, B1**) to PN16 (**Figures 3C, C1, C2**) there is a striking increase in the density of PDL cells. A rapid growth of the PDL was reported to take place in between PN12 and PN16 (Lungova et al., 2011).

The ECM of the PDL consists in collagens, non-collagenous proteins and glycoproteins, enzymes such as MMPs and growth factors, such as FGFs, BMPs, platelet-derived growth factors (PDGFs). *In vitro* experiments showed that FGF2 inhibits the mineralization of the PDL matrix (Dangaria et al., 2009). The main role of the PDL is the anchoring of the tooth to the surrounding mandibular/alveolar bone and providing a space to allow tooth movement within the bone socket. This is mediated by bundles of collagen fibers ending as Sharpey's fibers embedded in the cementum on one side and bone on the other (**Figures 3D,E**; Ho et al., 2007; Lee et al., 2015; Hirashima et al., 2020a). Based on immunoelectron microscopy, Huang et al. (1991) have proposed that periodontal and Sharpey's fibers consist in co-fibrils of type I and type III collagens, which is supported by the similar flexibility of alfa-1 chains in both collagen types and their possible involvement in elastic energy storage during stretching (Silver et al., 2002). The PDL matrix also includes collagens types V, VI, and XII, as well as type XIV at late stage (Beertsen et al., 1997; Zvackova et al., 2017). Fibril-associated collagens with interrupted triple helices (FACITs) such as collagens XII and XIV are also involved in the regulation of collagen fibrillogenesis (Ricard-Blum, 2011). Transgenic mice carrying a mutation on collagen XII exhibit a disorganized arrangement of collagen fibers in the PDL (Reichenberger et al., 2000). Analyzing double KO mice, Wang et al. (2014) stressed the importance of small leucine-rich proteoglycans (SLRPs) in the maintenance of periodontal homeostasis, which involves the regulation of TGFβ/BMP signaling, matrix turnover, and collagen organization (Matheson et al., 2005; Wang et al., 2014; Zvackova et al., 2017).

The periodontal tissues are highly vascularized (Suphasiriroj et al., 2013; Lee et al., 2015) and close associations between blood vessels and sympathetic nerves allow their mediating vasoregulatory activities (Luukko and Kettunen, 2016). From PN4, immunostaining for peripherin showed the presence of axons in the PDL (Kokten et al., 2014a). Glial and Schwann cells are present in the PDL (Yamamoto et al., 2012; Kokten et al., 2014a). Phenotypic differences were also found when comparing Schwann cells in the pulp and PDL, based on their reactivity to antibodies to GFAP (Byers et al., 2004).

The PDL is exposed to various mechanical stresses associated with mastication. This leads to an active tissue remodeling, which involves progenitor cells (Hirashima et al., 2020a). Mechanical stimuli are important to orient the fate of stem cells. PDL stem cells (PDLSCs) can directly respond to mechanical forces. Both the ECM and mechanical forces can modulate the ability of PDLCs to sustain tissue development and maintenance (Nava et al., 2012; Sun et al., 2012). Heterogeneous populations of

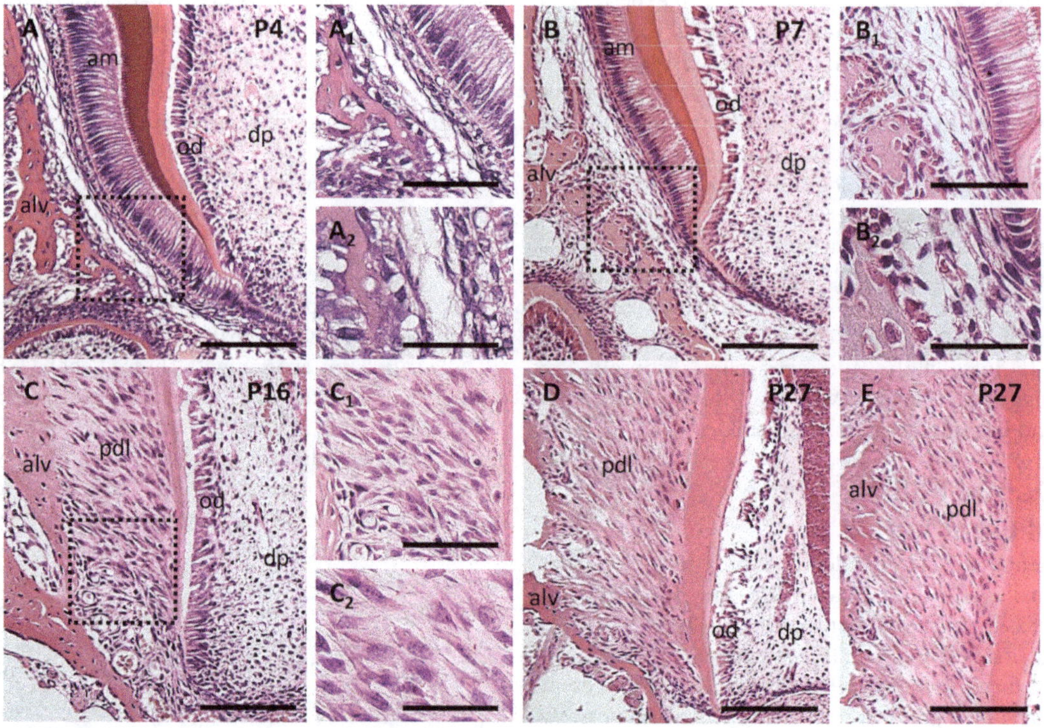

FIGURE 3 | Postnatal development of periodontal ligaments at P4 **(A,A$_1$,A$_2$)**, P7 **(B,B$_1$,B$_2$)**, P16 **(C,C$_1$,C$_2$)**, and P27 **(D,E)**. Sections were stained by hematoxylin-eosin. Alv, alveolar bone; am, ameloblasts; dp, dental pulp; od, odontoblasts; pdl, periodontal ligament. The scale bar represents: 100 μm (in figures **A–E**); 50 μm (in figures **A1,B1,C1**); 25 μm (in figures **A2,B2,C2**).

stem/progenitor cells have been identified there (Luan et al., 2006; Shinagawa-Ohama et al., 2017; Tomokiyo et al., 2018; Trubiani et al., 2019). PDLSCs showed osteogenic (Yang et al., 2017), cementogenic (Seo et al., 2004; Gauthier et al., 2017) and immunomodulatory properties (Wada et al., 2009). PDLSCs can also stimulate angiogenesis (Yeasmin et al., 2014; Amorim et al., 2016; Bae et al., 2017) or engage in neurogenesis (Ng et al., 2019). In case of angiogenesis, it seems a subset of PDLSCs (CD105+) may play a pivotal role, which would involve neuropilin-2 (NRP-2) (Amorim et al., 2016). PDLSCs can also contribute to the repair and regeneration of the periodontium (Tomokiyo et al., 2019).

BIOLOGICAL INTERFACES: SPATIAL LIMITS FOR MINERALIZATION

There are spatial limits for mineralizing areas in the tooth (predentin/dentin) as well as in the cementum/PDL and PDL/bone junctions (McKee and Nanci, 1996; Lausch et al., 2013; Foster et al., 2018). On the mesenchymal aspect of the tooth, the biological interface between predentin/dentin is controlled by the odontoblasts and this dynamic interface will be maintained all life long (Linde, 1995; Orsini et al., 2007).

Although very thin, the PDL is vascularized and innervated. Innervation is an important parameter to prevent tooth ankylosis (Fujiyama et al., 2004). As mentioned above, the PDL is a soft tissue exposed to important loadings when mediating tooth anchoring to the mandibular bone. The bone matrix, as well as the cementum, is mineralized while the PDL ECM is not. In both cases, this is controlled by specific matrix constituents (i.e., BSP, osteopontin versus PLAP1/asporin), being present or not (Steitz et al., 2002; Hakki et al., 2006; Yamada et al., 2007; Foster et al., 2018) and associated growth factors (Dangaria et al., 2009). Asporin is considered a negative regulator of mineralization (Leong et al., 2012). At their insertion sites into either the alveolar bone or cementum, the PDL fibers are mineralized (McKee et al., 2013). *In vitro* re-mineralization approaches have been designed to investigate the mechanism involved in it. These experiments showed that the ECM itself retains the necessary information to reproduce the spatial specificity of soft-mineralized tissues boundaries (Lausch et al., 2013).

These biological interfaces allow relative movements while resisting biomechanical loads (Ho et al., 2007). Their structural heterogeneity makes it difficult to investigate, and require the development of appropriated technologies together with adjusted methodologies (Boskey, 1998; Shahar and Weiner, 2018 and citations therein). For a simultaneous visualization of collagen fibrils, crystals, and intracellular components, Shahar and Weiner (2018) strongly favor 3D-imaging: complementary methods have been developed for that purpose. They include high resolution confocal light microscopy (Costello et al., 2016), high resolution Micro-CT (Burghardt et al., 2011), serial block face SEM (Denk and Horstmann, 2004), focused ion beam SEM (Hirashima et al., 2020b), each method having its own limitations. Although on a different model, backscattered electron (Kerschnitzki et al., 2011), second-harmonic generation imaging (Campagnola et al., 2002) and synchrotron small angle X-ray scattering (Groetsch et al., 2019) have been used to visualize collagen fibers crossing the soft/hard tissue junction (Paris et al., 2017). Besides structural aspects, experimental approaches allowed addressing questions about functional points of view, such as the relationship between mechanical strain amplification, mineral deposition/resorption and the dynamic correlation between these processes (Grandfield et al., 2015). In physiological conditions, mineral apposition is much more slow and regular. The transformation of amorphous to crystalline phase of mineral might allow rapid local changes, but has not yet been documented in detail.

CONCLUSION

Within the lower jaw of the mouse embryo, odontogenic and osteogenic condensations form almost simultaneously and next to each other. Although it has been published that mesenchymal cells have a natural tendency to aggregate, the two condensations remain separated by a loose interstitial mesenchyme. In opposition to the odontogenic and osteogenic ecto-mesenchymes originating from cranial NCDCs, cells from the interstitial mesenchyme do not express markers for neural crest origin. In all three zones, there is a progressive income of external cells: osteoclasts, cells mediating the vascularization or involved in the innervation, as well as stem/progenitor cells. Very soon all three mesenchymal areas show structural and physical differences. The secretion of distinct matrices will then support the different mineralization processes in odontogenic and osteogenic condensations. Besides its different origin, the interposed mesenchyme (prospective PDL) will not mineralize. This involves matrix-associated growth factors, some of which inhibit mineralization. These complementary processes lead to the formation of a functional complex: a tooth stabilized in a bone socket where movement still remains possible. While morphogenesis has been investigated in detail, mostly cellular aspects were taken into account in this review. Several questions remain, mainly concerning physical aspects within the three mesenchymes at early stages, such as the nature of differential cell-cell and cell-matrix interactions mediating cohesion as well as mechanosensing. Improving our knowledge about it would allow a better understanding of the mechanisms mediating/preventing the early mesenchymal cell segregation/compartmentalization and their condensation.

AUTHOR CONTRIBUTIONS

HL and RP contributed to the conception and writing of the manuscript. RP, ES, and EM revised it critically. ES and RP performed the illustrations. ES, RP, EM, and HL approved the content of the manuscript for publication and agreed to be accountable for all aspects of the work. All authors contributed to the article and approved the submitted version.

REFERENCES

Alemi, A. S., Mazur, C. M., Fowler, T. M., Woo, J. J., Knott, P. D., and Alliston, T. (2018). Glucocorticoids cause mandibular bone fragility and suppress osteocyte perilacunar-canalicular remodeling. *Bone Rep.* 9, 145–153. doi: 10.1016/j.bonr.2018.09.004

Alfaqeeh, S. A., Gaete, M., and Tucker, A. S. (2013). Interactions of the tooth and bone during development. *J. Dent. Res.* 92, 1129–1135. doi: 10.1177/0022034513510321

Allard, B., Magloire, H., Couble, M. L., Maurin, J. C., and Bleicher, F. (2006). Voltage-gated sodium channels confer excitability to human odontoblasts: possible role in tooth pain transmission. *J. Biol. Chem.* 281, 29002–29010. doi: 10.1074/jbc.M601020200

Amorim, B. R., Silvério, K. G., Casati, M. Z., Sallum, E. A., Kantovitz, K. R., and Nociti, F. H. Jr. (2016). Neuropilin controls endothelial differentiation by mesenchymal stem cells from the periodontal ligament. *J. Periodontol.* 87, e138–e147. doi: 10.1902/jop.2016.150603

Andrade, C. M., Roesch, G. C., Wink, M. R., Guimarães, E. L., Souza, L. F., Jardim, F. R., et al. (2008). Activity and expression of ecto-5'-nucleotidase/CD73 are increased during phenotype conversion of a hepatic stellate cell line. *Life Sci.* 82, 21–29. doi: 10.1016/j.lfs.2007.10.003

Bae, Y. K., Kim, G. H., Lee, J. C., Seo, B. M., Joo, K. M., Lee, G., et al. (2017). The significance of SDF-1α-CXCR4 axis in in vivo angiogenic ability of human periodontal ligament stem cells. *Mol. Cells* 40, 386–392. doi: 10.14348/molcells.2017.0004

Beertsen, W., McCulloch, C. A., and Sodek, J. (1997). The periodontal ligament: a unique, multifunctional connective tissue. *Periodontology* 13, 20–40. doi: 10.1111/j.1600-0757.1997.tb00094.x

Berendsen, A. D., and Olsen, B. R. (2015). Bone development. *Bone* 80, 14–18. doi: 10.1016/j.bone.2015.04.035

Bidder, M., Latifi, T., and Towler, D. A. (1998). Reciprocal temporospatial patterns of Msx2 and Osteocalcin gene expression during murine odontogenesis. *J. Bone. Miner. Res.* 13, 609–619. doi: 10.1359/jbmr.1998.13.4.609

Bishop, M. A. (1987). An investigation of pulp capillaries and tight junctions between odontoblasts in cats. *Anat. Embryol.* 177, 131–138. doi: 10.1007/BF00572537

Bobek, J., Oralova, V., Lesot, H., Kratochvilova, A., Doubek, J., and Matalova, E. (2020). Onset of calciotropic receptors during the initiation of mandibular/alveolar bone formation. *Ann. Anat.* 227:151427. doi: 10.1016/j.aanat.2019.151427

Bonewald, L. F., and Johnson, M. L. (2008). Osteocytes, mechanosensing and Wnt signaling. *Bone* 42, 606–615. doi: 10.1016/j.bone.2007.12.224

Boskey, A. L. (1998). Biomineralization: conflicts, challenges, and opportunities. *J. Cell Biochem. Suppl.* 30-31, 83–91. doi: 10.1002/(sici)1097-4644(1998)72:30/31%2B<83::aid-jcb12>3.0.co;2-f

Boyce, B. F., and Xing, L. (2007). Biology of RANK, RANKL, and osteoprotegerin. *Arthritis Res. Ther.* 9(Suppl. 1), S1. doi: 10.1186/ar2165

Burger, E. H., and Klein-Nulend, J. (1999). Mechanotransduction in bone–role of the lacuno-canalicular network. *FASEB J.* 13(Suppl.), S101–S112.

Burghardt, A. J., Link, T. M., and Majumdar, S. (2011). High-resolution computed tomography for clinical imaging of bone microarchitecture. *Clin. Orthop Relat. Res.* 469, 2179–2193. doi: 10.1007/s11999-010-1766-x

Byers, M. R. (1984). Dental sensory receptors. *Int. Rev. Neurobiol.* 25, 39–94. doi: 10.1016/s0074-7742(08)60677-7

Byers, M. R., Maeda, T., Brown, A. M., and Westenbroek, R. E. (2004). GFAP immunoreactivity and transcription in trigeminal and dental tissues of rats and transgenic GFP/GFAP mice. *Microsc. Res. Tech.* 65, 295–307. doi: 10.1002/jemt.20130

Byun, J. H., Lee, J. H., Choi, Y. J., Kim, J. R., and Park, B. W. (2008). Co-expression of nerve growth factor and p75NGFR in the inferior alveolar nerve after mandibular distraction osteogenesis. *Int. J. Oral Maxillofac. Surg.* 37, 467–472. doi: 10.1016/j.ijom.2008.01.017

Campagnola, P. J., Millard, A. C., Terasaki, M., Hoppe, P. E., Malone, C. J., and Mohler, W. A. (2002). Three-dimensional high-resolution second-harmonic generation imaging of endogenous structural proteins in biological tissues. *Biophys. J.* 82, 493–508. doi: 10.1016/S0006-3495(02)75414-3

Casagrande, L., Demarco, F. F., Zhang, Z., Araujo, F. B., Shi, S., and Nör, J. E. (2010). Dentin-derived BMP-2 and odontoblast differentiation. *J. Dent. Res.* 89, 603–608. doi: 10.1177/0022034510364487

Chai, Y., Jiang, X., Ito, Y., Bringas, P. Jr., Han, J., Rowitch, D. H., et al. (2000). Fate of the mammalian cranial neural crest during tooth and mandibular morphogenesis. *Development* 127, 1671–1679.

Cho, M. I., and Garant, P. R. (2000). Development and general structure of the periodontium. *Periodontol. 2000* 24, 9–27. doi: 10.1034/j.1600-0757.2000.2240102.x

Clark, K., Langeslag, M., van Leeuwen, B., Ran, L., Ryazanov, A. G., Figdor, C. G., et al. (2006). TRPM7, a novel regulator of actomyosin contractility and cell adhesion. *EMBO J.* 25, 290–301. doi: 10.1038/sj.emboj.7600931

Corpron, R. E., and Avery, J. K. (1973). The ultrastructure of intradental nerves in developing mouse molars. *Anat. Rec.* 175, 585–606. doi: 10.1002/ar.1091750307

Costello, M. J., Brennan, L. A., Mohamed, A., Gilliland, K. O., Johnsen, S., and Kantorow, M. (2016). Identification and ultrastructural characterization of a novel nuclear degradation complex in differentiating lens fiber cells. *PLoS One* 11:e0160785. doi: 10.1371/journal.pone.0160785

Dallas, S. L., and Bonewald, L. F. (2010). Dynamics of the transition from osteoblast to osteocyte. *Ann. N. Y. Acad. Sci.* 1192, 437–443. doi: 10.1111/j.1749-6632.2009.05246.x

Dangaria, S. J., Ito, Y., Luan, X., and Diekwisch, T. G. (2011). Differentiation of neural-crest-derived intermediate pluripotent progenitors into committed periodontal populations involves unique molecular signature changes, cohort shifts, and epigenetic modifications. *Stem Cells Dev.* 20, 39–52. doi: 10.1089/scd.2010.0180

Dangaria, S. J., Ito, Y., Walker, C., Druzinsky, R., Luan, X., and Diekwisch, T. G. H. (2009). Extracellular matrix-mediated differentiation of periodontal progenitor cells. *Differentiation* 78, 79–90. doi: 10.1016/j.diff.2009.03.005

Dassule, H. R., and McMahon, A. P. (1998). Analysis of epithelial-mesenchymal interactions in the initial morphogenesis of the mammalian tooth. *Dev. Biol.* 202, 215–227. doi: 10.1006/dbio.1998.8992

Denk, W., and Horstmann, H. (2004). Serial block-face scanning electron microscopy to reconstruct three-dimensional tissue nanostructure. *PLoS Biol.* 2:e329. doi: 10.1371/journal.pbio.0020329

Diekwisch, T. G. (2002). Pathways and fate of migratory cells during late tooth organogenesis. *Connect. Tissue Res.* 43, 245–256.

Diep, L., Matalova, E., Mitsiadis, T. A., and Tucker, A. S. (2009). Contribution of the tooth bud mesenchyme to alveolar bone. *J. Exp. Zool. B Mol. Dev. Evol.* 312B, 510–517. doi: 10.1002/jez.b.21269

Discher, D. E., Janmey, P., and Wang, Y. L. (2005). Tissue cells feel and respond to the stiffness of their substrate. *Science* 310, 1139–1143. doi: 10.1126/science.1116995

Dunlop, L. L., and Hall, B. K. (1995). Relationships between cellular condensation, preosteoblast formation and epithelial-mesenchymal interactions in initiation of osteogenesis. *Int. J. Dev. Biol.* 39, 357–371.

Epelman, S., Lavine, K. J., and Randolph, G. J. (2014). Origin and functions of tissue macrophages. *Immunity* 41, 21–35. doi: 10.1016/j.immuni.2014.06.013

Everts, V., Delaisse, J. M., Korper, W., Jansen, D. C., Tigchelaar-Gutter, W., Saftig, P., et al. (2002). The bone lining cell: its role in cleaning Howship's lacunae and initiating bone formation. *J. Bone Miner. Res.* 17, 77–90. doi: 10.1359/jbmr.2002.17.1.77

Farahani, R. M., Sarrafpour, B., Simonian, M., Li, Q., and Hunter, N. (2012). Directed glia-assisted angiogenesis in a mature neurosensory structure: pericytes mediate an adaptive response in human dental pulp that maintains blood-barrier function. *J. Comp. Neurol.* 520, 3803–3826. doi: 10.1002/cne.23162

Farges, J. C., Romeas, A., Melin, M., Pin, J. J., Lebecque, S., Lucchini, M., et al. (2003). TGF-beta1 induces accumulation of dendritic cells in the odontoblast layer. *J. Dent. Res.* 82, 652–656. doi: 10.1177/154405910308200816

Farhadieh, R. D., Nicklin, S., Yu, Y., Gianoutsos, M. P., and Walsh, W. R. (2003). The role of nerve growth factor and brain-derived neurotrophic factor in inferior alveolar nerve regeneration in distraction osteogenesis. *J. Craniofac. Surg.* 14, 859–865. doi: 10.1097/00001665-200311000-00007

Feng, J., Mantesso, A., De Bari, C., Nishiyama, A., and Sharpe, P. T. (2011). Dual origin of mesenchymal stem cells contributing to organ growth and repair. *Proc. Natl. Acad. Sci. U.S.A.* 108, 6503–6508. doi: 10.1073/pnas.1015449108

Ferguson, J. W., and Atit, R. P. (2019). A tale of two cities: the genetic mechanisms governing calvarial bone development. *Genesis* 57:e23248. doi: 10.1002/dvg.23248

Fleischmannova, J., Matalova, E., Sharpe, P. T., Misek, I., and Radlanski, R. J. (2010). Formation of the tooth-bone interface. *J. Dent. Res.* 89, 108–115. doi: 10.1177/0022034509355440

Foster, B. L., Ao, M., Salmon, C. R., Chavez, M. B., Kolli, T. N., Tran, A. B., et al. (2018). Osteopontin regulates dentin and alveolar bone development and mineralization. *Bone* 107, 196–207. doi: 10.1016/j.bone.2017.12.004

Franz-Odendaal, T. A. (2011). Induction and patterning of intramembranous bone. *Front. Biosci.* 16, 2734–2746. doi: 10.2741/3882

Fujiyama, K., Yamashiro, T., Fukunaga, T., Balam, T. A., Zheng, L., and Takano-Yamamoto, T. (2004). Denervation resulting in dento-alveolar ankylosis associated with decreased *Malassez epithelium*. *J. Dent. Res.* 83, 625–629. doi: 10.1177/154405910408300808

Gauthier, P., Yu, Z., Tran, Q. T., Bhatti, F. U., Zhu, X., and Huang, G. T. (2017). Cementogenic genes in human periodontal ligament stem cells are down-regulated in response to osteogenic stimulation while upregulated by vitamin C treatment. *Cell Tissue Res.* 368, 79–92. doi: 10.1007/s00441-016-2513-8

Giffin, J. L., Gaitor, D., and Franz-Odendaal, T. A. (2019). The forgotten skeletogenic condensations: a comparison of early skeletal development amongst vertebrates. *J. Dev. Biol.* 7:4. doi: 10.3390/jdb7010004

Goldberg, M., Farges, J. C., Lacerda-Pinheiro, S., Six, N., Jegat, N., Decup, F., et al. (2008). Inflammatory and immunological aspects of dental pulp repair. *Pharmacol. Res.* 58, 137–147. doi: 10.1016/j.phrs.2008.05.013

Grandfield, K., Herber, R. P., Chen, L., Djomehri, S., Tam, C., Lee, J. H., et al. (2015). Strain-guided mineralization in the bone-PDL-cementum complex of a rat periodontium. *Bone Rep.* 3, 20–31. doi: 10.1016/j.bonr.2015.04.002

Griffin, F. E., Schiavi, J., McDevitt, T. C., McGarry, J. P., and McNamara, L. M. (2017). The role of adhesion junctions in the biomechanical behaviour and osteogenic differentiation of 3D mesenchymal stem cell spheroids. *J. Biomech.* 59, 71–79. doi: 10.1016/j.jbiomech.2017.05.014

Groetsch, A., Gourrier, A., Schwiedrzik, J., Sztucki, M., Beck, R. J., Shephard, J. D., et al. (2019). Compressive behaviour of uniaxially aligned individual mineralised collagen fibres at the micro- and nanoscale. *Acta Biomater.* 89, 313–329. doi: 10.1016/j.actbio.2019.02.053

Grosso, A., Burger, M. G., Lunger, A., Schaefer, D. J., Banfi, A., and Di Maggio, N. (2017). It takes two to tango: coupling of angiogenesis and osteogenesis for bone regeneration. *Front. Bioeng. Biotechnol.* 5:68. doi: 10.3389/fbioe.2017.00068

Guntur, A. R., Rosen, C. J., and Naski, M. C. (2012). N-cadherin adherens junctions mediate osteogenesis through PI3K signaling. *Bone* 50, 54–62. doi: 10.1016/j.bone.2011.09.036

Hakki, S. S., Wang, D., Franceschi, R. T., and Somerman, M. J. (2006). Bone sialoprotein gene transfer to periodontal ligament cells may not be sufficient to promote mineralization *in vitro* or *in vivo*. *J. Periodontol.* 77, 167–173. doi: 10.1902/jop.2006.050057

Hall, B. K. (1980). Tissue interactions and the initiation of osteogenesis and chondrogenesis in the neural crest-derived mandibular skeleton of the embryonic mouse as seen in isolated murine tissues and in recombinations of murine and avian tissues. *J. Embryol. Exp. Morphol.* 58, 251–264.

Hall, B. K., and Miyake, T. (1995). Divide, accumulate, differentiate: cell condensation skeletal development. *Int. J. Dev. Biol.* 39, 881–893.

Hall, B. K., and Miyake, T. (2000). All for one and one for all: condensations and the initiation of skeletal development. *Bioessays* 22, 138–147. doi: 10.1002/(sici)1521-1878(200002)22:2<138::aid-bies5>3.0.co;2-4

Hayashi, M., Nakashima, T., Taniguchi, M., Kodama, T., Kumanogoh, A., and Takayanagi, H. (2012). Osteoprotection by semaphorin 3A. *Nature* 485, 69–74. doi: 10.1038/nature11000

He, J., Zhang, N., Zhang, J., Jiang, B., and Wu, F. (2018). Migration critically meditates osteoblastic differentiation of bone mesenchymal stem cells through activating canonical Wnt signal pathway. *Coll. Surf. B Biointerfaces* 171, 205–213. doi: 10.1016/j.colsurfb.2018.07.017

Hill, C., Jacobs, B., Kennedy, L., Rohde, S., Zhou, B., Baldwin, S., et al. (2015). Cranial neural crest deletion of VEGFa causes cleft palate with aberrant vascular and bone development. *Cell Tissue Res.* 361, 711–722. doi: 10.1007/s00441-015-2150-7

Hill, E. L., and Elde, R. (1991). Distribution of CGRP-, VIP-, D beta H-, SP-, and NPY-immunoreactive nerves in the periosteum of the rat. *Cell Tissue Res.* 264, 469–480. doi: 10.1007/BF00319037

Hirashima, S., Kanazawa, T., Ohta, K., and Nakamura, K. I. (2020a). Three-dimensional ultrastructural analysis and histomorphometry of collagen bundles in the periodontal ligament using focused ion beam/scanning electron microscope tomography. *J. Periodont. Res.* 55, 23–23. doi: 10.1111/jre.12592

Hirashima, S., Kanazawa, T., Ohta, K., and Nakamura, K. I. (2020b). Three-dimensional ultrastructural imaging and quantitative analysis of the periodontal ligament. *Anat. Sci. Int.* 95, 1–11. doi: 10.1007/s12565-019-00502-5

Ho, S. P., Marshall, S. J., Ryder, M. I., and Marshall, G. W. (2007). The tooth attachment mechanism defined by structure, chemical composition and mechanical properties of collagen fibers in the periodontium. *Biomaterials* 28, 5238–5245. doi: 10.1016/j.biomaterials.2007.08.031

Hu, B., Nadiri, A., Bopp-Kuchler, S., Perrin-Schmitt, F., Wang, S., and Lesot, H. (2005). Dental epithelial histo-morphogenesis in the mouse: positional information versus cell history. *Arch. Oral. Biol.* 50, 131–136. doi: 10.1016/j.archoralbio.2004.09.007

Huang, W., Yang, S., Shao, J., and Li, Y. P. (2007). Signaling and transcriptional regulation in osteoblast commitment and differentiation. *Front. Biosci.* 12, 3068–3092. doi: 10.2741/2296

Huang, Y. H., Ohsaki, Y., and Kurisu, K. (1991). Distribution of type I and type III collagen in the developing periodontal ligament of mice. *Matrix* 11, 25–35. doi: 10.1016/s0934-8832(11)80224-6

Jabalee, J., Hillier, S., and Franz-Odendaal, T. A. (2013). An investigation of cellular dynamics during the development of intramembranous bones: the scleral ossicles. *J. Anat.* 223, 311–320. doi: 10.1111/joa.12095

Javed, A., Chen, H., and Ghori, F. Y. (2010). Genetic and transcriptional control of bone formation. *Oral Maxillofac. Surg. Clin. North Am.* 22, 283–293. doi: 10.1016/j.coms.2010.05.001

Jones, R. E., Salhotra, A., Robertson, K. S., Ransom, R. C., Foster, D. S., Shah, H. N., et al. (2019). Skeletal stem cell-schwann cell circuitry in mandibular repair. *Cell Rep.* 28, 2757–2766. doi: 10.1016/j.celrep.2019.08.021

Jontell, M., Okiji, T., Dahlgren, U., and Bergenholtz, G. (1998). Immune defense mechanisms of the dental pulp. *Crit. Rev. Oral Biol. Med.* 9, 179–200. doi: 10.1177/10454411980090020301

Kaneko, T., Okiji, T., Kaneko, R., and Suda, H. (2008). Characteristics of resident dendritic cells in various regions of rat periodontal ligament. *Cell Tissue Res.* 331, 413–421. doi: 10.1007/s00441-007-0539-7

Keller, L., Kökten, T., Kuchler-Bopp, S., and Lesot, H. (2015). "Tooth organ engineering," in *Stem Cell Biology and Tissue Engineering in Dental Sciences*, eds A. Vishwakarma, P. Sharpe, S. Shi, X.-P. Wang, and M. Ramalingam (Cambridge, MA: Academic Press), 359–368. doi: 10.1016/B978-0-12-397157-9.00032-1

Keller, L. V., Kuchler-Bopp, S., and Lesot, H. (2012). Restoring physiological cell heterogeneity in the mesenchyme during tooth engineering. *Int. J. Dev. Biol.* 56, 737–746. doi: 10.1387/ijdb.120076hl

Keller, L. V., Kuchler-Bopp, S., Mendoza, S. A., Poliard, A., and Lesot, H. (2011). Tooth engineering: searching for dental mesenchymal cells sources. *Front. Physiol.* 2:7. doi: 10.3389/fphys.2011.00007

Kenan, S., Onur, ÖD., Solakoðlu, S., Kotil, T., Ramazanoðlu, M., Çelik, H. H., et al. (2019). Investigation of the effects of semaphorin 3A on new bone formation in a rat calvarial defect model. *J. Craniomaxillofac. Surg.* 47, 473–483. doi: 10.1016/j.jcms.2018.12.010

Kerschnitzki, M., Wagermaier, W., Roschger, P., Seto, J., Shahar, R., Duda, G. N., et al. (2011). The organization of the osteocyte network mirrors the extracellular matrix orientation in bone. *J. Struct. Biol.* 173, 303–311. doi: 10.1016/j.jsb.2010.11.014

Kjaer, I. (1990). Correlated appearance of ossification and nerve tissue in human fetal jaws. *J. Craniofac. Genet. Dev. Biol.* 10, 329–336.

Kokten, T., Bécavin, T., Keller, L., Weickert, J. L., Kuchler-Bopp, S., and Lesot, H. (2014a). Immunomodulation stimulates the innervation of engineered tooth organ. *PLoS One* 9:e86011. doi: 10.1371/journal.pone.0086011

Kokten, T., Lesot, H., and Kuchler-Bopp, S. (2014b). "Experimental design for the innervation of tooth forming from implanted cell re-associations," in *Cells and Biomaterials in Regenerative Medicine*, ed. D. Eberli (Rijeka: InTech Open Access Publisher), 345–373.

Komatsu, N., Kajiya, M., Motoike, S., Takewaki, M., Horikoshi, S., Iwata, T., et al. (2018). Type I collagen deposition via osteoinduction ameliorates YAP/TAZ activity in 3D floating culture clumps of mesenchymal stem cell/extracellular matrix complexes. *Stem Cell Res. Ther.* 9:342. doi: 10.1186/s13287-018-1085-9

Krivanek, J., Adameyko, I., and Fried, K. (2017). Heterogeneity and developmental connections between cell types inhabiting teeth. *Front. Physiol.* 8:376. doi: 10.3389/fphys.2017.00376

Kuchler-Bopp, S., Keller, L., Poliard, A., and Lesot, H. (2011). "Tooth organ engineering: biological constraints specifying experimental approaches," in *Tissue Engineering for Tissue and Organ Regeneration*, ed. D. Eberli (London: InTech), 317–346. doi: 10.5772/23483

Ladoux, B., and Mège, R. M. (2017). Mechanobiology of collective cell behaviours. *Nat. Rev. Mol. Cell Biol.* 18, 743–757. doi: 10.1038/nrm.2017.98

Lausch, A. J., Quan, B. D., Miklas, J. W., and Sone, E. D. (2013). Extracellular matrix control of collagen mineralization in vitro. *Adv. Funct. Mater.* 23, 4906–4912. doi: 10.1002/adfm.201203760

Lecanda, F., Warlow, P. M., Sheikh, S., Furlan, F., Steinberg, T. H., and Civitelli, R. (2000). Connexin43 deficiency causes delayed ossification, craniofacial abnormalities, and osteoblast dysfunction. *J. Cell Biol.* 151, 931–944. doi: 10.1083/jcb.151.4.931

Ledesma-Martínez, E., Mendoza-Núñez, V. M., and Santiago-Osorio, E. (2016). Mesenchymal stem cells derived from dental pulp: a review. *Stem Cells Int.* 2016:4709572. doi: 10.1155/2016/4709572

Lee, J. H., Pryce, B. A., Schweitzer, R., Ryder, M. I, and Ho, S. P. (2015). Differentiating zones at periodontal ligament-bone and periodontal ligament-cementum entheses. *J. Periodontal Res.* 50, 870–880. doi: 10.1111/jre.12281

Lekic, P., and McCulloch, C. A. (1996). Relationship of cellular proliferation to expression of osteopontin and bone sialoprotein in regenerating rat periodontium. *Cell Tissue Res.* 285, 491–500. doi: 10.1007/s004410050665

Leong, N. L., Hurng, J. M., Djomehri, S. I., Gansky, S. A., Ryder, M. I., and Ho, S. P. (2012). Age-related adaptation of bone-PDL-tooth complex: rattus-norvegicus as a model system. *PLoS One* 7:e35980. doi: 10.1371/journal.pone.0035980

Lin, H., Liu, H., Sun, Q., Yuan, G., Zhang, L., and Chen, Z. (2013). KLF4 promoted odontoblastic differentiation of mouse dental papilla cells via regulation of DMP1. *J. Cell. Physiol.* 228, 2076–2085. doi: 10.1002/jcp.24377

Lin, H., Xu, L., Liu, H., Sun, Q., Chen, Z., Yuan, G., et al. (2011). KLF4 promotes the odontoblastic differentiation of human dental pulp cells. *J Endod.* 37, 948–954. doi: 10.1016/j.joen.2011.03.030

Linde, A. (1995). Dentin mineralization and the role of odontoblasts in calcium transport. *Connect. Tissue Res.* 33, 163–170. doi: 10.3109/03008209509016997

Liu, Y. S., Liu, Y. A., Huang, C. J., Yen, M. H., Tseng, C. T., Chien, S., et al. (2015). Mechanosensitive TRPM7 mediates shear stress and modulates osteogenic differentiation of mesenchymal stromal cells through Osterix pathway. *Sci. Rep.* 5:16522. doi: 10.1038/srep16522

Luan, X., Ito, Y., Dangaria, S., and Diekwisch, T. G. (2006). Dental follicle progenitor cell heterogeneity in the developing mouse periodontium. *Stem Cells Dev.* 15, 595–608. doi: 10.1089/scd.2006.15.595

Lumsden, A. G. (1988). Spatial organization of the epithelium and the role of neural crest cells in the initiation of the mammalian tooth germ. *Development* 103(Suppl.), 155–169.

Lungova, V., Radlanski, R. J., Tucker, A. S., Renz, H., Misek, I., and Matalova, E. (2011). Tooth-bone morphogenesis during postnatal stages of mouse first molar development. *J. Anat.* 218, 699–716. doi: 10.1111/j.1469-7580.2011.01367.x

Luukko, K., and Kettunen, P. (2014). Coordination of tooth morphogenesis and neuronal development through tissue interactions: lessons from mouse models. *Exp. Cell Res.* 325, 72–77. doi: 10.1016/j.yexcr.2014.02.029

Luukko, K., and Kettunen, P. (2016). Integration of tooth morphogenesis and innervation by local tissue interactions, signaling networks, and semaphorin 3A. *Cell Adh. Migr.* 10, 618–626. doi: 10.1080/19336918.2016.1216746

MacDonald, M. E., and Hall, B. K. (2001). Altered timing of the extracellular-matrix-mediated epithelial-mesenchymal interaction that initiates mandibular skeletogenesis in three inbred strains of mice: development, heterochrony, and evolutionary change in morphology. *J. Exp. Zool.* 291, 258–273. doi: 10.1002/jez.1102.abs

MacNeil, R. L., and Thomas, H. F. (1993). Development of the murine periodontium. II. Role of the epithelial root sheath in formation of the periodontal attachment. *J. Periodontol.* 64, 285–291. doi: 10.1902/jop.1993.64.4.285

Maeda, Y., Miwa, Y., and Sato, I. (2017). Expression of CGRP, vasculogenesis and osteogenesis associated mRNAs in the developing mouse mandible and tibia. *Ann. Anat.* 221, 38–47. doi: 10.4081/ejh.2017.2750

Magloire, H., Couble, M. L., Thivichon-Prince, B., Maurin, J. C., and Bleicher, F. (2009). Odontoblast: a mechano-sensory cell. *J. Exp. Zool. B Mol. Dev. Evol.* 312B, 416–424. doi: 10.1002/jez.b.21264

Magloire, H., Maurin, J. C., Couble, M. L., Shibukawa, Y., Tsumura, M., Thivichon-Prince, B., et al. (2010). Topical review. Dental pain and odontoblasts: facts and hypotheses. *J. Orofac. Pain* 24, 335–349.

Mammoto, T., Mammoto, A., and Ingber, D. E. (2013). Mechanobiology and developmental control. *Annu. Rev. Cell Dev. Biol.* 29, 27–61. doi: 10.1146/annurev-cellbio-101512-122340

Mammoto, T., Mammoto, A., Jiang, A., Jiang, E., Hashmi, B., and Ingber, D. E. (2015). Mesenchymal condensation-dependent accumulation of collagen VI stabilizes organ-specific cell fates during embryonic tooth formation. *Dev. Dyn.* 244, 713–723. doi: 10.1002/dvdy.24264

Mammoto, T., Mammoto, A., Torisawa, Y. S., Tat, T., Gibbs, A., Derda, R., et al. (2011). Mechanochemical control of mesenchymal condensation and embryonic tooth organ formation. *Dev. Cell* 21, 758–769. doi: 10.1016/j.devcel.2011.07.006

Martin, T. J. (2005). Osteoblast-derived PTHrP is a physiological regulator of bone formation. *J. Clin. Invest.* 115, 2322–2324. doi: 10.1172/JCI26239

Matheson, S., Larjava, H., and Häkkinen, L. (2005). Distinctive localization and function for lumican, fibromodulin and decorin to regulate collagen fibril organization in periodontal tissues. *J. Periodontal Res.* 40, 312–324. doi: 10.1111/j.1600-0765.2005.00800.x

McKee, M. D., Hoac, B., Addison, W. N., Barros, N. M., Millán, J. L., and Chaussain, C. (2013). Extracellular matrix mineralization in periodontal tissues: noncollagenous matrix proteins, enzymes, and relationship to hypophosphatasia and X-linked hypophosphatemia. *Periodontol. 2000* 63, 102–122. doi: 10.1111/prd.12029

McKee, M. D., and Nanci, A. (1996). Osteopontin at mineralized tissue interfaces in bone, teeth, and osseointegrated implants: ultrastructural distribution and implications for mineralized tissue formation, turnover, and repair. *Microsc. Res. Tech.* 3, 141–164. doi: 10.1002/(sici)1097-0029(19960201)33:2<141::aid-jemt5>3.0.co;2-w

McKeown, S. J., Newgreen, D. F., and Farlie, P. G. (2005). Dlx2 over-expression regulates cell adhesion and mesenchymal condensation in ectomesenchyme. *Dev. Biol.* 281, 22–37. doi: 10.1016/j.ydbio.2005.02.004

Miletich, I., and Sharpe, P. T. (2003). Normal and abnormal dental development. *Hum. Mol. Genet.* 12, R69–R73. doi: 10.1093/hmg/ddg085

Mina, M., and Kollar, E. J. (1987). The induction of odontogenesis in non-dental mesenchyme combined with early murine mandibular arch epithelium. *Arch. Oral. Biol.* 32, 123–127. doi: 10.1016/0003-9969(87)90055-0

Minkoff, R., Rundus, V. R., Parker, S. B., Hertzberg, E. L., Laing, J. G., and Beyer, E. C. (1994). Gap junction proteins exhibit early and specific expression during intramembranous bone formation in the developing chick mandible. *Anat. Embryol.* 190, 231–241. doi: 10.1007/BF00234301

Moe, K., Kettunen, P., Kvinnsland, I. H., and Luukko, K. (2008). Development of the pioneer sympathetic innervation into the dental pulp of the mouse mandibular first molar. *Arch. Oral. Biol.* 53, 865–873. doi: 10.1016/j.archoralbio.2008.03.004

Moe, K., Sijaona, A., Shrestha, A., Kettunen, P., Taniguchi, M., and Luukko, K. (2012). Semaphorin 3A controls timing and patterning of the dental pulp innervation. *Differentiation* 84, 371–379. doi: 10.1016/j.diff.2012.09.003

Moorer, M. C., Hebert, C., Tomlinson, R. E., Iyer, S. R., Chason, M., and Stains, J. P. (2017). Defective signaling, osteoblastogenesis and bone remodeling in a mouse model of connexin 43 C-terminal truncation. *J. Cell Sci.* 130, 531–540. doi: 10.1242/jcs.197285

Nait Lechguer, A., Kuchler-Bopp, S., Hu, B., Haïkel, Y., and Lesot, H. (2008). Vascularization of engineered teeth. *J. Dent. Res.* 87, 1138–1143. doi: 10.1177/154405910808701216

Nakagawa, N., Kinosaki, M., Yamaguchi, K., Shima, N., Yasuda, H., Yano, K., et al. (1998). RANK is the essential signaling receptor for osteoclast differentiation factor in osteoclastogenesis. *Biochem. Biophys. Res. Commun.* 253, 395–400. doi: 10.1006/bbrc.1998.9788

Nakamura, H., Nakashima, T., Hayashi, M., Izawa, N., Yasui, T., Aburatani, H., et al. (2014). Global epigenomic analysis indicates protocadherin-7 activates osteoclastogenesis by promoting cell-cell fusion. *Biochem. Biophys. Res. Commun.* 455, 305–311. doi: 10.1016/j.bbrc.2014.11.009

Nakatomi, M., Hovorakova, M., Gritli-Linde, A., Blair, H. J., MacArthur, K., Peterka, M., et al. (2013). Evc regulates a symmetrical response to Shh signaling in molar development. *J. Dent. Res.* 92, 222–228. doi: 10.1177/0022034512471826

Nanci, A., Wazen, R., Nishio, C., and Zalzal, S. F. (2008). Immunocytochemistry of matrix proteins in calcified tissues: functional biochemistry on section. *Eur. J. Histochem.* 52, 201–214. doi: 10.4081/1218

Nava, M. M., Raimondi, M. T., and Pietrabissa, R. (2012). Controlling self-renewal and differentiation of stem cells via mechanical cues. *J. Biomed. Biotechnol.* 2012:797410. doi: 10.1155/2012/797410

Ng, T. K., Yang, Q., Fortino, V. R., Lai, N. Y., Carballosa, C. M., Greenberg, J. M., et al. (2019). MicroRNA-132 directs human periodontal ligament-derived neural crest stem cell neural differentiation. *J. Tissue Eng. Regen. Med.* 13, 12–24. doi: 10.1002/term.2759

Obara, N., and Lesot, H. (2007). Asymmetrical growth, differential cell proliferation, and dynamic cell rearrangement underlie epithelial morphogenesis in mouse molar development. *Cell Tissue Res.* 330, 461–473. doi: 10.1007/s00441-007-0502-7

Okiji, T., Jontell, M., Belichenko, P., Bergenholtz, G., and Dahlström, A. (1997). Perivascular dendritic cells of the human dental pulp. *Acta Physiol. Scand.* 159, 163–169. doi: 10.1046/j.1365-201X.1997.584337000.x

Okiji, T., Kawashima, N., Kosaka, T., Matsumoto, A., Kobayashi, C., and Suda, H. (1992). An immunohistochemical study of the distribution of immunocompetent cells, especially macrophages and Ia antigen-expressing cells of heterogeneous populations, in normal rat molar pulp. *J. Dent. Res* 71, 1196–1202. doi: 10.1177/00220345920710051201

Orsini, G., Ruggeri, A. Jr., Mazzoni, A., Papa, V., Mazzotti, G., Di Lenarda, R., et al. (2007). Immunohistochemical identification of decorin and biglycan in human dentin: a correlative field emission scanning electron microscopy/transmission electron microscopy study. *Calcif. Tissue Int.* 81, 39–45. doi: 10.1007/s00223-007-9027-z

Osborn, J. W., and Price, D. G. (1988). An autoradiographic study of periodontal development in the mouse. *J. Dent. Res.* 67, 455–461. doi: 10.1177/00220345880670020401

Oster, G. F., Murray, J. D., and Harris, A. K. (1983). Mechanical aspects of mesenchymal morphogenesis. *J. Embryol. Exp. Morphol.* 78, 83–125.

Paris, M., Götz, A., Hettrich, I., Bidan, C. M., Dunlop, J. W. C., Razi, H., et al. (2017). Scaffold curvature-mediated novel biomineralization process originates a continuous soft tissue-to-bone interface. *Acta Biomater.* 60, 64–80. doi: 10.1016/j.actbio.2017.07.029

Radlanski, R. J., Renz, H., Zimmermann, C. A., Mey, R., and Matalova, E. (2015). Morphogenesis of the compartmentalizing bone around the molar primordia in the mouse mandible during dental developmental stages between lamina, bell-stage, and root formation (E13-P20). *Ann. Anat.* 200, 1–14. doi: 10.1016/j.aanat.2015.01.003

Ray, P., and Chapman, S. C. (2015). Cytoskeletal reorganization drives mesenchymal condensation and regulates downstream molecular signaling. *PLoS One* 10:e0134702. doi: 10.1371/journal.pone.0134702

Reichenberger, E., Baur, S., Sukotjo, C., Olsen, B. R., Karimbux, N. Y., and Nishimura, I. (2000). Collagen XII mutation disrupts matrix structure of periodontal ligament and skin. *J. Dent. Res.* 79, 1962–1968. doi: 10.1177/00220345000790120701

Ricard-Blum, S. (2011). The collagen family. *Cold Spring Harb. Perspect. Biol.* 3:a004978. doi: 10.1101/cshperspect.a004978

Roguljic, H., Matthews, B. G., Yang, W., Cvija, H., Mina, M., and Kalajzic, I. (2013). In vivo identification of periodontal progenitor cells. *J. Dent. Res.* 92, 709–715. doi: 10.1177/0022034513493434

Rothova, M., Feng, J., Sharpe, P. T., Peterkova, R., and Tucker, A. S. (2011). Contribution of mesoderm to the developing dental papilla. *Int. J. Dev. Biol.* 55, 59–64. doi: 10.1387/ijdb.103083mr

Rothova, M., Peterkova, R., and Tucker, A. S. (2012). Fate map of the dental mesenchyme: dynamic development of the dental papilla and follicle. *Dev. Biol.* 366, 244–254. doi: 10.1016/j.ydbio.2012.03.018

Ruch, J. V. (1998). Odontoblast commitment and differentiation. *Biochem. Cell Biol.* 76, 923–938. doi: 10.1139/o99-008

Ruch, J. V., Lesot, H., and Bègue-Kirn, C. (1995). Odontoblast differentiation. *Int. J. Dev. Biol.* 39, 51–68.

Ruch, J. V., Lesot, H., Karcher-Djuricic, V., Meyer, J. M., and Olive, M. (1982). Facts and hypotheses concerning the control of odontoblast differentiation. *Differentiation* 21, 7–12. doi: 10.1111/j.1432-0436.1982.tb01187.x

Saghiri, M. A., Asatourian, A., Sorenson, C. M., and Sheibani, N. (2018). Mice dental pulp and periodontal ligament endothelial cells exhibit different proangiogenic properties. *Tissue Cell.* 50, 31–36. doi: 10.1016/j.tice.2017.11.004

Santagati, F., and Rijli, F. M. (2003). Cranial neural crest and the building of the vertebrate head. *Nat. Rev. Neurosci.* 4, 806–818. doi: 10.1038/nrn1221

Sawakami, K., Robling, A. G., Ai, M., Pitner, N. D., Liu, D., Warden, S. J., et al. (2006). The Wnt co-receptor LRP5 is essential for skeletal mechanotransduction but not for the anabolic bone response to parathyroid hormone treatment. *J. Biol. Chem.* 281, 23698–23711. doi: 10.1074/jbc.M601000200

Seo, B. M., Miura, M., Gronthos, S., Bartold, P. M., Batouli, S., Brahim, J., et al. (2004). Investigation of multipotent postnatal stem cells from human periodontal ligament. *Lancet* 364, 149–155. doi: 10.1016/S0140-6736(04)16627-0

Shahar, R., and Weiner, S. (2018). Open questions on the 3D structures of collagen containing vertebrate mineralized tissues: a perspective. *J. Struct. Biol.* 201, 187–198. doi: 10.1016/j.jsb.2017.11.008

Sharpe, P. T. (2016). Dental mesenchymal stem cells. *Development* 143, 2273–2280. doi: 10.1242/dev.134189

Shi, S., Bartold, P. M., Miura, M., Seo, B. M., Robey, P. G., and Gronthos, S. (2005). The efficacy of mesenchymal stem cells to regenerate and repair dental structures. *Orthod. Craniofac. Res.* 8, 191–199. doi: 10.1111/j.1601-6343.2005.00331.x

Shinagawa-Ohama, R., Mochizuki, M., Tamaki, Y., Suda, N., and Nakahara, T. (2017). Heterogeneous human periodontal ligament-committed progenitor and stem cell populations exhibit a unique cementogenic property under in vitro and in vivo conditions. *Stem Cells Dev.* 26, 632–645. doi: 10.1089/scd.2016.0330

Shyer, A. E., Rodrigues, A. R., Schroeder, G. G., Kassianidou, E., Kumar, S., and Harland, R. M. (2017). Emergent cellular self-organization and mechanosensation initiate follicle pattern in the avian skin. *Science* 357, 811–815. doi: 10.1126/science.aai7868

Silver, F. H., Horvath, I., and Foran, D. J. (2002). Mechanical implications of the domain structure of fiber-forming collagens: comparison of the molecular and fibrillar flexibilities of the alpha1-chains found in types I-III collagen. *J. Theor. Biol.* 216, 243–254. doi: 10.1006/jtbi.2002.2542

Steitz, S. A., Speer, M. Y., McKee, M. D., Liaw, L., Almeida, M., Yang, H., et al. (2002). Osteopontin inhibits mineral deposition and promotes regression of ectopic calcification. *Am. J. Pathol.* 161, 2035–2046. doi: 10.1016/S0002-9440(10)64482-3

Sun, Y., Chen, C. S., and Fu, J. (2012). Forcing stem cells to behave: a biophysical perspective of the cellular microenvironment. *Annu. Rev. Biophys.* 41, 519–542. doi: 10.1146/annurev-biophys-042910-155306

Suphasiriroj, W., Mikami, M., and Sato, S. (2013). Comparative studies on microvascular endothelial cells isolated from periodontal tissue. *J. Periodontol.* 84, 1002–1009. doi: 10.1902/jop.2012.120453

Tabata, S., Ozaki, H. S., Nakashima, M., Uemura, M., and Iwamoto, H. (1998). Innervation of blood vessels in the rat incisor pulp: a scanning electron microscopic and immunoelectron microscopic study. *Anat. Rec.* 251, 384–391. doi: 10.1002/(sici)1097-0185(199807)251:3<384::aid-ar14>3.0.co;2-k

Takebe, T., Enomura, M., Yoshizawa, E., Kimura, M., Koike, H., Ueno, Y., et al. (2015). Vascularized and complex organ buds from diverse tissues via mesenchymal cell-driven condensation. *Cell Stem Cell.* 16, 556–565. doi: 10.1016/j.stem.2015.03.004

Ten Cate, A. R. (1997). The development of the periodontium–a largely ectomesenchymally derived unit. *Periodontol. 2000* 13, 9–19. doi: 10.1111/j.1600-0757.1997.tb00093.x

Thesleff, I., Vaahtokari, A., Kettunen, P., and Aberg, T. (1995). Epithelial-mesenchymal signaling during tooth development. *Connect. Tissue Res.* 32, 9–15. doi: 10.3109/03008209509013700

Thesleff, I., Vaahtokari, A., Vainio, S., and Jowett, A. (1996). Molecular mechanisms of cell and tissue interactions during early tooth development. *Anat. Rec.* 245, 151–161. doi: 10.1002/(sici)1097-0185(199606)245:2<151::aid-ar4>3.0.co;2-#

Tomokiyo, A., Wada, N., and Maeda, H. (2019). Periodontal ligament stem cells: regenerative potency in periodontium. *Stem Cells Dev.* 28, 974–985. doi: 10.1089/scd.2019.0031

Tomokiyo, A., Yoshida, S., Hamano, S., Hasegawa, D., Sugii, H., and Maeda, H. (2018). Detection, characterization, and clinical application of mesenchymal stem cells in periodontal ligament tissue. *Stem Cells Int.* 2018:5450768. doi: 10.1155/2018/5450768

Trubiani, O., Pizzicannella, J., Caputi, S., Marchisio, M., Mazzon, E., Paganelli, R., et al. (2019). Periodontal ligament stem cells: current knowledge and future perspectives. *Stem Cells Dev.* 28, 995–1003. doi: 10.1089/scd.2019.0025

Vainio, S., and Thesleff, I. (1992). Sequential induction of syndecan, tenascin and cell proliferation associated with mesenchymal cell condensation during early tooth development. *Differentiation* 50, 97–105. doi: 10.1111/j.1432-0436.1992.tb00490.x

Vesela, B., Svandova, E., Bobek, J., Lesot, H., and Matalova, E. (2019). Osteogenic and angiogenic profiles of mandibular bone-forming cells. *Front. Physiol.* 10:124. doi: 10.3389/fphys.2019.00124

Volponi, A. A., and Sharpe, P. T. (2013). The tooth – a treasure chest of stem cells. *Br. Dent. J.* 215, 353–358. doi: 10.1038/sj.bdj.2013.959

Wada, N., Maeda, H., Hasegawa, D., Gronthos, S., Bartold, P. M., Menicanin, D., et al. (2014). Semaphorin 3A induces mesenchymal-stem-like properties in human periodontal, ligament cells. *Stem Cells Dev.* 23, 2225–2236. doi: 10.1089/scd.2013.0405

Wada, N., Menicanin, D., Shi, S., Bartold, P. M., and Gronthos, S. (2009). Immunomodulatory properties of human periodontal ligament stem cells. *J. Cell. Physiol.* 219, 667–676. doi: 10.1002/jcp.21710

Wang, L., Foster, B. L., Kram, V., Nociti, F. H. Jr., Zerfas, P. M., Tran, A. B., et al. (2014). Fibromodulin and biglycan modulate periodontium through TGFβ/BMP signaling. *J. Dent. Res.* 93, 780–787. doi: 10.1177/0022034514541126

Wang, Y., Wan, C., Deng, L., Liu, X., Cao, X., Gilbert, S. R., et al. (2007). The hypoxia-inducible factor alpha pathway couples angiogenesis to osteogenesis during skeletal development. *J. Clin. Invest.* 117, 1616–1626. doi: 10.1172/JCI31581

Wu, X., Shi, W., and Cao, X. (2007). Multiplicity of BMP signaling in skeletal development. *Ann. N. Y. Acad. Sci.* 1116, 29–49. doi: 10.1196/annals.1402.053

Xu, R. (2014). Semaphorin 3A: a new player in bone remodeling. *Cell Adh. Migr.* 8, 5–10. doi: 10.4161/cam.27752

Yamada, S., Tomoeda, M., Ozawa, Y., Yoneda, S., Terashima, Y., Ikezawa, K., et al. (2007). PLAP-1/asporin, a novel negative regulator of periodontal ligament mineralization. *J. Biol. Chem.* 282, 23070–23080. doi: 10.1074/jbc.M611181200

Yamamoto, N., Maeda, H., Tomokiyo, A., Fujii, S., Wada, N., Monnouchi, S., et al. (2012). Expression and effects of glial cell line-derived neurotrophic factor on periodontal ligament cells. *J. Clin. Periodontol.* 39, 556–564. doi: 10.1111/j.1600-051X.2012.01881.x

Yamaza, T., Ren, G., Akiyama, K., Chen, C., Shi, Y., and Shi, S. (2011). Mouse mandible contains distinctive mesenchymal stem cells. *J. Dent. Res.* 90, 317–324. doi: 10.1177/0022034510387796

Yang, N., Li, Y., Wang, G., Ding, Y., Jin, Y., and Xu, Y. (2017). Tumor necrosis factor-α suppresses adipogenic and osteogenic differentiation of human periodontal ligament stem cell by inhibiting miR-21/Spry1 functional axis. *Differentiation* 97, 33–43. doi: 10.1016/j.diff.2017.08.004

Yavropoulou, M. P., and Yovos, J. G. (2016). The molecular basis of bone mechanotransduction. *J. Musculoskelet. Neuronal. Interact.* 16, 221–236.

Yeasmin, S., Ceccarelli, J., Vigen, M., Carrion, B., Putnam, A. J., Tarle, S. A., et al. (2014). Stem cells derived from tooth periodontal ligament enhance functional angiogenesis by endothelial cells. *Tissue Eng. Part A* 20, 1188–1196. doi: 10.1089/ten.TEA.2013.0512

Yegutkin, G. G. (2008). Nucleotide- and nucleoside-converting ectoenzymes: important modulators of purinergic signalling cascade. *Biochim. Biophys. Acta* 1783, 673–694. doi: 10.1016/j.bbamcr.2008.01.024

Yen, A. H., and Sharpe, P. T. (2008). Stem cells and tooth tissue engineering. *Cell Tissue Res.* 331, 359–372. doi: 10.1007/s00441-007-0467-6

Yu, T., Volponi, A. A., Babb, R., An, Z., and Sharpe, P. T. (2015). Stem cells in tooth development, growth, repair, and regeneration. *Curr. Top. Dev. Biol.* 115, 187–212. doi: 10.1016/bs.ctdb.2015.07.010

Yuan, Y., and Chai, Y. (2019). Chapter Four - Regulatory mechanisms of jaw bone and tooth development. *Curr. Top. Dev. Biol.* 133, 91–118. doi: 10.1016/bs.ctdb.2018.12.013

Zhang, J., Kawashima, N., Suda, H., Nakano, Y., Takano, Y., and Azuma, M. (2006). The existence of CD11c+ sentinel and F4/80+ interstitial dendritic cells in dental pulp and their dynamics and functional properties. *Int. Immunol.* 18, 1375–1384. doi: 10.1093/intimm/dxl070

Zhao, Y., Bower, A. J., Graf, B. W., Boppart, M. D., and Boppart, S. A. (2013). Imaging and tracking of bone marrow-derived immune and stem cells. *Methods Mol. Biol.* 1052, 57–76. doi: 10.1007/7651_2013_28

Zhou, T., Pan, J., Wu, P., Huang, R., Du, W., Zhou, Y., et al. (2019). Dental follicle cells: roles in development and beyond. *Stem Cells Int.* 2019:9159605. doi: 10.1155/2019/9159605

Zvackova, I., Matalova, E., and Lesot, H. (2017). Regulators of collagen fibrillogenesis during molar development in the mouse. *Front. Physiol.* 8:554. doi: 10.3389/fphys.2017.00554

16

A Living Cell Repository of the Cranio-/Orofacial Region to Advance Research and Promote Personalized Medicine

*Ludovica Parisi[1], Patrick O. Knapp[1], Eleftheria Girousi[1], Silvia Rihs[1], Giorgio C. La Scala[2], Isabelle Schnyder[3], Alexandra Stähli[4], Anton Sculean[4], Dieter D. Bosshardt[4,5], Christos Katsaros[1] and Martin Degen[1]**

[1] Laboratory for Oral Molecular Biology, Dental Research Center, Department of Orthodontics and Dentofacial Orthopedics, University of Bern, Bern, Switzerland, [2] Division of Pediatric Surgery, Department of Pediatrics, University Hospital of Geneva, Geneva, Switzerland, [3] University Clinic for Pediatric Surgery, Bern University Hospital, Bern, Switzerland, [4] Department of Periodontology, School of Dental Medicine, University of Bern, Bern, Switzerland, [5] Robert K. Schenk Laboratory of Oral Histology, Dental Research Center, University of Bern, Bern, Switzerland

***Correspondence:**
Martin Degen
martin.degen@zmk.unibe.ch

The prevalence of congenital anomalies in newborns is estimated to be as high as 6%, many of which involving the cranio-/orofacial region. Such malformations, including several syndromes, are usually identified prenatally, at birth, or rarely later in life. The lack of clinically relevant human cell models of these often very rare conditions, the societal pressure to avoid the use of animal models and the fact that the biological mechanisms between rodents and human are not necessarily identical, makes studying cranio-/orofacial anomalies challenging. To overcome these limitations, we are developing a living cell repository of healthy and diseased cells derived from the cranio-/orofacial region. Ultimately, we aim to make patient-derived cells, which retain the molecular and genetic characteristics of the original anomaly or disease *in vitro*, available for the scientific community. We report our efforts in establishing a human living cell bank derived from the cranio-/orofacial region of otherwise discarded tissue samples, detail our strategy, processes and quality checks. Such specific cell models have a great potential for discovery and translational research and might lead to a better understanding and management of craniofacial anomalies for the benefit of all affected individuals.

Keywords: patient-derived cells, craniofacial anomalies, cell bank, quality control, rare diseases, personalized medicine

INTRODUCTION

Craniofacial development is a complex process that requires orchestrated interactions of multiple cell types derived from all germ layers (Kindberg and Bush, 2019). Among them, the neural crest cells (NCCs) are the most critical population. NCCs arise at the neural plate border, undergo an epithelial-mesenchymal transition (EMT), and then are guided to the periphery where they form the structures of the head and the face (Hall, 2000; Cordero et al., 2011; Green et al., 2015; Siismets and Hatch, 2020). All these intricate steps rely on precise spatio-temporally regulated networks of signaling cues, which, due to their complexity, are error prone, and may result in a diversity of craniofacial anomalies (CFAs) (Gorlin et al., 1990). In fact, it is estimated that CFAs occur in approximately 0.2% of all newborns (Shaw, 2004). Some, like cleft lip/palate (CLP), are among the most common congenital abnormalities affecting around 1 in 750 newborns (Kousa and Schutte, 2016), while others, such as Goldenhar syndrome (GH) are rarer with an estimated prevalence of 1 in 3000–5000 births (Bogusiak et al., 2017). CFAs can appear in isolation, as part of a syndrome with defects due to mutations in single genes or chromosomal abnormalities, or in combination with other defects without an identified genetic background.

CFA-affected children usually require surgery in order to repair the most debilitating defects, which is routinely followed by personalized treatment throughout childhood and adolescence. Although the surgical procedures have been optimized during the last decades, a number of common complications in CFA-affected children may still persist even after surgery, such as difficulties in feeding, speech and hearing, impaired dentition and wound healing complications (van Beurden et al., 2005; Aizenbud et al., 2011; Hortis-Dzierzbicka et al., 2012). These problems might require additional surgeries, which can be challenging as often not enough tissue is available to correct the anomaly (i.e., alveolar bone defects in CLP patients) (Zhang and Yelick, 2018). In addition, CFAs are still associated with an increased mortality as well as with a negative impact on a child's self-perception and social integration due to esthetical concerns. Consequently, CFAs represent a high economic, social, and psychological burden for affected individuals, their families, and the society as a whole. Therefore, there is an urgent need for a better understanding of CFAs, which could allow to optimize treatment options tailoring it to the specific patient needs.

Discovery molecular and cellular research on human CFAs is challenging due to the lack of proper models. At the moment knowledge is mostly based on animal studies. Fortunately, craniofacial development is a highly conserved process across many species (Hu et al., 2003) and mice and humans share the majority of protein-coding genes (Yue et al., 2014). However, certain discrepancies exist between humans and animals in regard to facial morphogenesis. For instance, disruption of genes in mice, which have been linked to CLP in humans, often do not perturb the formation of the primary palate and the lip in the animal and hence, produce only a cleft palate (CP) phenotype (Gritli-Linde, 2008; Van Otterloo et al., 2016). As not every finding in animal models can be transferred to humans, and considering the strong urge from the society to minimize animal experimentation by using other studies modalities, CFA patient-derived cells might represent an alternative *in vitro* study tool. However, working with primary cells is often experienced as cumbersome, since they require an established isolation protocol, unique growth media, more care in general, and they exhibit a limited lifespan. The use of postnatal tissues to study CFAs that arise early in development also comes with challenges and assumptions regarding the retention of the original tissue characteristics. However, increasing evidence shows the persistence of various cellular properties postnatally in tissues as well as in patient-derived cells (Beyeler et al., 2014; Hixon et al., 2017; Degen et al., 2018, 2020). In this regard, it is also noteworthy to mention that often it is very ambitious and difficult to have access to proper healthy control tissue and/or cells, which ideally should be age- and anatomically matched to the studied condition (Degen et al., 2020).

To facilitate the use of patient-derived cells as clinically relevant cell models to study CFAs, we have initiated a project to establish a living cell repository of the cranio-/orofacial region starting from routinely discarded tissue biopsies. To this purpose, we collaborate with the Pediatric Surgery Division, Children's Hospital, Bern, which is responsible for the surgical treatment of CLP-affected infants. In CLP patients, the cleft lip is closed at the age of about 4 months, after removing a small piece of superfluous lip tissue reaching into the cleft. We collect this excessive CLP lip tissue as well as healthy pediatric tissue remnants, obtained from the surgical management of minor injuries (i.e., lip lacerations) often requiring debridement. Similarly, numerous clinical samples are obtained during routine dental treatments, which take place on a daily basis at the Dental School, University of Bern, to which our laboratory is affiliated. Such samples include small tissue biopsies from the gingiva, the periodontal ligament (PDL) and the dental pulp from extracted healthy wisdom teeth, and the hard/soft palate. All these excised tissues are usually discarded since most of these conditions do not require any further diagnostic analyses. Such tissue remnants serve as optimal and easily accessible sources for the isolation of primary cells and for the establishment of a high-quality and readily available cell repository of the cranio-/orofacial region for discovery and translational research.

The aim of this report is to present our proof-of-concept study in creating a robust and high-quality cell bank and in exploiting its full potential for translational applications. Such a unique effort holds great promises in fostering scientific collaborations in the field of cranio-/orofacial development, thereby advancing and promoting personalized precision medicine for unmet medical needs.

MATERIALS AND METHODS

Cell Isolation and Culture

Tissue biopsies were collected in 50 ml conical tubes containing $\approx$ 25 ml of Dulbecco's modified Eagle's medium (DMEM) (Gibco/Life Technologies; Thermo Fisher Scientific, Lucerne, Switzerland) containing 10% fetal calf serum (FCS) (Sigma-Aldrich, St. Louis, MO, United States), 1× Pen/Strep (PS) solution (Gibco), and 1× Amphotericin B (AmphB) (Gibco) [=Collection Medium (CM)]. Samples were transferred to the research laboratory within 2 h (average time) after biopsy collection for further processing. In rare case, when urgent unplanned surgeries/treatments occurred on weekends or during the night, samples were stored overnight at 4°C. We did not notice any negative impact on cell isolation from such samples. Under sterile conditions, the CM was aspirated, and the tissues washed for an additional 5 min in CM. Using sterile tweezers and scalpels, the specimens were minced into small pieces (<1 mm^3), which were then transferred into six-well plates containing 800 μl of CM and placed in a humidified incubator at 37°C/5% CO_2. Two pieces were incubated per well of a six-well plate. The explant cultures were carefully washed with CM and re-fed with fresh medium every other day. Cellular outgrowths were daily observed under a light microscope and the cell types growing out of each tissue piece annotated (e.g., fibroblasts only, keratinocytes only, mixed populations). Cells were allowed to grow out to colonies of approximately 0.4 cm diameter before subculturing (passage 1) them into p60 or p100 culture dishes using trypsin/EDTA (TE) solution (Gibco). Pure fibroblast outgrowths were trypsinized using 0.05% TE and pure keratinocyte outgrowths using 0.25% TE. For mixed populations a differential TE approach was used: fibroblasts were detached first, followed by the dissociation of the keratinocytes. Keratinocytes were cultured in Keratinocyte serum-free medium (KSFM) (Gibco/Life Technologies), supplemented with 25 μg/ml bovine pituitary extract, 0.2 ng/ml epidermal growth factor and $CaCl_2$ to a final Ca^{2+} concentration of 0.4 mM and 1× PS (Gibco), as previously described (Degen et al., 2012). Fibroblasts were cultured in complete DMEM (Gibco) supplemented with 10% FCS and 1× PS. Cells were expanded in p100 culture dishes, quality-checked, and frozen at passage 2 (2×10^5–1×10^6 keratinocytes/vial and 1×10^5–5×10^5 fibroblasts/vial) in 2× freezing medium (DMEM, 20% FCS, 25 mM HEPES, 20% DMSO) diluted 1:1 in their respective culture medium and stored in liquid nitrogen. For all experiments cells at passage 3 have been used.

For mycoplasma detection, cells were grown for at least 5 days in their specific growth media in the absence of any antibiotics. Afterward cells were fixed in 4% paraformaldehyde (PFA) and the nuclei stained with DAPI using the Vectashield Mounting Medium containing DAPI (Vector Laboratories, Burlingame, CA, United States). In parallel, conditioned medium was collected from the cells, which was used as template for a PCR-based mycoplasma detection analysis as described (Praetorius, 2015).

Bone marrow-derived Mesenchymal Stem Cells (MSCs) (ScienCell, Carlsbad, CA, United States) were cultured in MSC medium (ScienCell).

RNA Extraction, cDNA Synthesis, and Quantitative Real-Time PCR (qPCR) Analysis

Total RNA was isolated using the innuPREP RNA Mini kit (Analytik Jena AG, Jena, Germany) according to the standard protocol for eukaryotic cells. RNA concentration was subsequently measured with a NanoDrop 2000c (Thermo Fisher Scientific) and stored at −80°C until use.

A 500 ng of total RNA were used as a template to synthetize cDNA using the M-MLV Reverse Transcriptase (Promega, Dübendorf, Switzerland) and Oligo$(dT)_{15}$ Primer (Promega). Gene expression was detected by quantitative real-time polymerase chain reaction (qPCR). qPCR was performed using a GoTaq® qPCR Master Mix (Promega) on a QuantStudio 3 instrument (Applied Biosystems, Thermo Fisher Scientific). Data analysis was performed using the dC_T method when absolute mRNA normalized to *GAPDH* levels were reported, or by ddC_T method when absolute mRNA normalized to *GAPDH* were further referenced to a control sample set to 1.

Sequences of the qPCR primers (**Supplementary Table 1**) were either taken from the PrimerBank database[1] or from the NCBI primer designing tool[2]. All qPCR primer pairs were tested for specificity and efficiency using cDNA standard curves.

Immunoblotting

Whole cell extracts were prepared in 1× RIPA buffer (10 mM Tris–HCl pH 8.0, 1 mM EDTA, 0.1% sodium deoxycholate, 0.1% SDS, 1% NP40, 140 mM NaCl) supplemented with cOmplete Mini™ Protease Inhibitor cocktail and PhosSTOP EASYpack (both from Sigma-Aldrich). Protein concentrations were measured using the BCA Protein Assay kit (Pierce, Thermo Fisher Scientific) following the manufacturer's recommendation. 10 μg of total protein were diluted in sample loading buffer (62.6 mM Tris–HCl pH 6.8, 2% SDS, 10% glycerol, 0.01% bromophenol blue) containing 100 mM dithiothreitol (DTT) (Sigma-Aldrich), boiled for 5 min at 95°C and separated under reducing conditions by SDS-PAGE. Proteins were subsequently blotted onto nitrocellulose membranes (Sigma-Aldrich). Membranes were stained with 0.1% amido black solution (Merck, Burlington, MA, United States) to control for equal protein loading and blotting efficiency. Afterward, membranes were washed in Tris-buffered saline (TBS-Tween) (pH 7.4) containing 0.05% Tween-20, blocked in 3.5% skim milk powder, incubated over-night with primary antibody at 4°C, washed three times in TBS-Tween buffer and incubated with horseradish peroxidase-conjugated anti mouse or rabbit IgG. Blots were developed using the SuperSignal West Dura kit (Pierce, Thermo Fisher Scientific). Data were acquired by scanning membranes with an Imager Chemi Premium Instrument (VWR, Darmstadt, Germany). Primary antibodies used are reported in **Supplementary Table 2.**

Some immunoblots were analyzed densitometrically using the ImageJ software, version 1.53g (NIH; Bethesda, MA, United States). Briefly, the intensity of each protein band was normalized to the β-actin or vinculin band intensity of the same extract in the same experiment.

Lifespan Analysis

For replicative lifespan analysis, cells were plated at a density of 10^4/p60 dish for keratinocytes and 10^5/p100 for fibroblasts in their standard growth media. Cells were re-fed every other day and subcultured when reaching 80% of confluency. The day of subculturing, cells were counted using a Countess 2 automated cell counter (Thermo Fisher Scientific) and re-seeded at the same initial cell density. Population doublings (PD) were calculated as log2 (# cells at the time for subculturing/# cells plated), while cumulative PDs were plotted against the total days in culture.

[1]https://pga.mgh.harvard.edu/primerbank/
[2]www.ncbi.nlm.nih.gov/tools/primer-blast

Immunofluorescence

For stainings, cells were grown in 35 mm dishes containing four separate wells (Greiner Bio-One, Frickenhausen, Germany). Fixation occurred in 4% paraformaldehyde at room temperature (RT) for 20 min when keratinocytes formed colonies of 8–10 cells and fibroblasts reached 50% of confluency. Afterward, cells were rinsed 3 times in Phosphate Buffer Saline (PBS), permeabilized with 0.1% Triton-X-100 for 5 min, blocked in 3% Bovine Serum Albumin (BSA) (Sigma-Aldrich) for 15 min and incubated with primary antibody at RT for 2 h. Cultures were washed three more times in PBS and incubated with a fluorescent-labeled secondary antibody (Molecular Probes, Thermo Fisher Scientific) with or without tetramethylrhodamine (TRITC)-phalloidin (Sigma-Aldrich) for 1 h protected from the light, washed with PBS and ddH_2O, and coverslip mounted with Vectashield Mounting Medium containing DAPI (Vector Laboratories). All the samples were examined under an Olympus BX-51 phase/fluorescence microscope (Olympus Life Science Solution Tokyo, Japan) equipped with a xenon lamp (X-Cite, series 120PC Q, Lumen Dynamics, Mississauga, Canada), and fluorescence filters U-MWIBA3 for Alexa Fluor 488, U-MWIGA3 for Alexa Fluor 568 and TRITC, and U-MNUA2 for DAPI (Olympus Life Science Solutions). Images were captured by a ProgRes CT3 camera with ProgRes Capture Pro software (Jenoptik, Jena, Germany). Primary antibodies used are reported in **Supplementary Table 2**.

All samples were examined under an Axio Imager M2 microscope (Carl Zeiss, Oberkochen, Germany) and images taken using a digital AxioCam MRc camera (Carl Zeiss).

Histology

In order to prepare formalin-fixed and paraffin-embedded (FFPE) blocks, tissue specimens were fixed in 10% formalin, which is roughly equivalent to 4% formaldehyde, for 48 h at RT. Samples were then dehydrated with increasing alcohol concentrations, followed by changes in xylene, before embedding in paraffin. Five to six-µm sections were finally cut on a Reichert-Jung microtome (Leica Microsystems, Wetzlar, Germany), deparaffinized and stained with hematoxylin-eosin (H&E). Alternatively, after fixation, samples were embedded in acrylic resin (LR White resin, Sigma-Aldrich), cut into 1 µm sections with a diamond knife and stained with Toluidine Blue.

All immunohistochemical (IHC) staining reactions were performed by automated staining using a BOND RX autostainer (Leica Microsystems). Sections were deparaffinized and antigen was retrieved using 1mM Tris solution (pH 9.0) for 30 min at 95°C. Sections were stained with primary antibodies (**Supplementary Table 2**), followed with secondary antibodies, and specific binding of primary antibodies was visualized using a polymer-based visualizing system with horseradish peroxidase as the enzyme and 3,3-diaminobenzidine (DAB) as a brown chromogen (Leica Microsystems). Finally, the samples were counterstained with hematoxylin and mounted with Aquatex (Merck, Burlington, MA, United States). To reveal cartilage, sections from the GH patient were stained with Safranin-O. Briefly, sections were deparaffinized and stained with 0.1% Safranin-O solution (Sigma-Aldrich) for 5 min at RT, followed by rinses with ddH_2O and nuclei counterstaining using hematoxylin. After extensive washes under running tap water, samples were mounted using resinous medium.

3D-Skin Models

To generate 3D-skin models using patient-derived keratinocytes, the protocol from CELLnTEC (CELLnTEC advanced cells systems AG, Bern, Switzerland) was used. Briefly, cells were seeded in 400 µl KSFM into polycarbonate inserts (0.4 µm pore size, 12 mm diameter, Nunc, Thermo Fisher Scientific) placed in 60 mm tissue culture dishes, immediately followed by the addition of 11 ml of KSFM outside the inserts. Confluent monolayer formation was confirmed with the staining kit (CnT-ST-100, CELLnTEC). If confluent, keratinocyte differentiation was induced in parallel cultures by the replacement of KSFM with 3D Barrier Medium (CnT-PR-3D, CELLnTEC) inside and outside of the insert (equal medium level) overnight. The insert was then lifted to the air-liquid interface by carefully removing the medium inside the insert and replenishing the outside medium with fresh 3D Barrier Medium up to the level of the membrane (approximately 3.2 ml for a p60 culture dish). Keratinocytes were cultured for 15 days at 37°C and 5% CO_2 with medium change every other day. For full-thickness skin models, fibroblasts were cultured without any antibiotics and seeded into polyethylene terephthalate (PET) inserts at 5×10^4 cells per insert and grown for 10 days before adding keratinocytes on top in a fully defined co-culture medium for culture at the air liquid-interface (CnT-PR-FTAL, CELLnTEC). Three days after seeding the keratinocytes on top of the dermal layer, the models were air-lifted and grown for further 12 days with medium changes three times per week.

To analyze the skin models, 3D-cultures were fixed overnight at 4°C in 4% PFA. Membranes were cut out of the inserts, placed between two biopsy pads in embedding cassettes, and stored in 0.1 M sodium cacodylate buffer at 4°C before proceeding for paraffin embedding and sectioning on a Reichert-Jung microtome (Leica Microsystems). Slides containing 5 µm thick paraffin sections were deparaffinized and rehydrated through xylene, ethanol, and ddH_2O, stained with H&E or primary antibodies as described in section Histology. Primary antibodies used are reported in **Supplementary Table 2**.

MTT-Assay

To evaluate the cytotoxic effects of a commercially available oral rinse (OR) on gingival fibroblasts and keratinocytes, an MTT (3-(4,5-dimethylthiazol-2-yl)-2,5-diphenyltetrazolium bromide) assay was performed (Sigma-Aldrich). Briefly, cells were seeded in triplicates at a density of 300 cells/mm^3 in 96-well plates. 24 h after seeding, they were rinsed twice in PBS and exposed to different concentrations of the OR for 2 min. Subsequently, cells were incubated with MTT solution at a final concentration of 0.5 mg/ml for 4 h to allow MTT conversion into formazan in metabolically active cells. After two PBS washes, converted MTT was solubilized with 4N HCl and the absorbance read at 570 nm on an EL808 BioTek microplate reader (BioTek, Winooski, VT, United States).

In vitro Differentiation

For *in vitro* differentiation, MSCs and PDL fibroblasts at a density of 10^5 cells/well of a six-well plate were seeded in their respective growth medium. 24 h afterward, medium was replaced with osteogenic medium [αMEM (Thermo Fisher Scientific) supplemented with 0.05 mg/ml L-Ascorbic acid, 0.01 M β-Glycerol Phosphate, and 0.1 mM Dexamethasone (all from Sigma-Aldrich)] for 21 days with medium change every third day. At the end of the culturing time, cells were fixed in 4% PFA for 20 min at RT, rinsed with ddH_2O and finally incubated with Alizarin Red S solution [68.45 mg Alizarin Red S (Sigma-Aldrich) in 5 ml ddH_2O, pH 4.1–4.5] for 45 min at 4°C protected from light. After extensive washing in ddH_2O, samples were air-dried and analyzed with a light microscope.

Statistical Analysis

Experiments were performed at least three times in multiple replicates. Data were analyzed using Prism 7 (GraphPad; La Jolla, CA, United States). Data are represented as means ± standard deviation (SD). Multiple comparisons were performed using one-way analysis of variance (ANOVA) with Tukey's *post hoc* test. Values of $p \leq 0.05$ were considered significant.

RESULTS

Establishment of a Solid and Reproducible Method for Keratinocyte and Fibroblast Isolations From Routinely Discarded Tissues of the Cranio-/Orofacial Region

To advance and promote discovery and translational research on CFAs we initiated a long-term project in establishing a living cell repository of the cranio-/orofacial region. The initial aim was to collect routinely discarded tissues made available by the Pediatric Surgery Division, Children's Hospital, Bern, and the Dental School, University of Bern. While we put our priority on the establishment of a highly robust and reproducible process for the isolation of patient-derived cells, our strategy also allowed us to collect and biobank corresponding tissues for histological analyses and snap frozen tissues for RNA and DNA extractions (**Figure 1**).

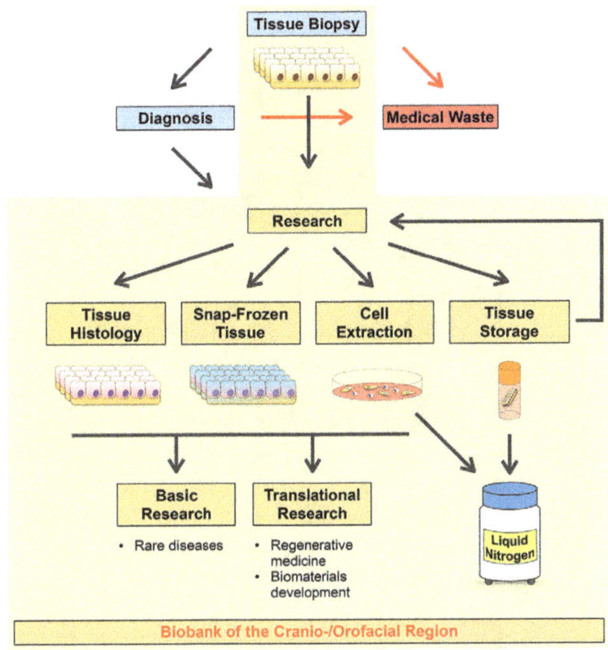

FIGURE 1 | Schematic diagram summarizing the strategy of our CFA biobank. The Pediatric Surgery Division, Children's Hospital, Bern, and the Dental School, University of Bern are responsible for tissue excisions and, if required, for further diagnostic analyses of the biopsies (blue boxes). Usually, tissues from the cranio-/orofacial region are discarded after their initial excision (no diagnosis required) or after their diagnostic analysis (medical waste, red box). The research laboratory (Laboratory for Oral Molecular Biology, University of Bern) collects such specimens and processes them in order to create a living cell repository of patient-derived cells (Cell Extraction). After isolation of the cells, if the tissue size allows it, the remaining tissue remnants are (1) stored in freezing medium in the liquid nitrogen tank for future processing and new cell extractions (Tissue Storage), (2) formalin-fixed and paraffin-embedded (FFPE) for histological analyses (Tissue Histology), and (3) snap-frozen for future tissue RNA and/or DNA extractions (Snap-Frozen Tissue). These patient-derived resources can be used for several downstream applications in discovery and translational research projects. Our workflow is highlighted in yellow.

The core of our biobank is represented by a collection of patient-derived cells of the cranio-/orofacial region. Our main goal is to specifically collect epithelial cells (keratinocytes) and the corresponding mesenchymal cells (fibroblasts) from the same tissue donor by the explant culture approach (**Figure 2A**). The opportunity to collect both cell types from the same individual will allow the establishment of relevant 3D-co-culture systems that closely mimic the *in vivo* situation, or the analysis of the preferred individual cell type in line with specific research interests in the future (see section "Our Cell Bank Offers Novel Tools and Models for Personalized Precision Medicine").

To successfully biobank all materials as described in our strategy, the tissue biopsy we receive should ideally have a minimal size of 0.1 cm^3. With this specimen size we are able to isolate keratinocytes and fibroblasts, prepare FFPE blocks, snap-freeze the sample, and store some of the tissue biopsy in liquid nitrogen for future use (**Figure 1**). When we receive tissues <0.1 cm^3, we prioritize our work and focus on cell isolations and storage of the tissue in freezing medium in the liquid nitrogen.

Tissue samples are collected in sterile 50 ml tubes containing 25 ml of Collection Medium (CM). Within less than 1 h after biopsy, tissue samples are processed (**Figure 2A-2**). For cell isolations we apply the explant culture technique, which is extensively described in section "Cell Isolation and Culture." First cells usually emerge within 4 days at 37°C, and colonies are ready for subculturing after approximately 10 days in culture (**Figure 2A-3a**). Pure cells are expanded (**Figure 2A-4**), checked for quality (**Figure 2A-5**, also see section "Cell Isolation and Culture") and finally frozen (usually 11 cryovials) for long-term storage in liquid nitrogen (**Figure 2A-6**).

If required, tissue pieces with successful cell outgrowths can be carefully transferred into a new well of a six-well plate containing 800 μl of CM allowing a 2nd round of explant cultures from

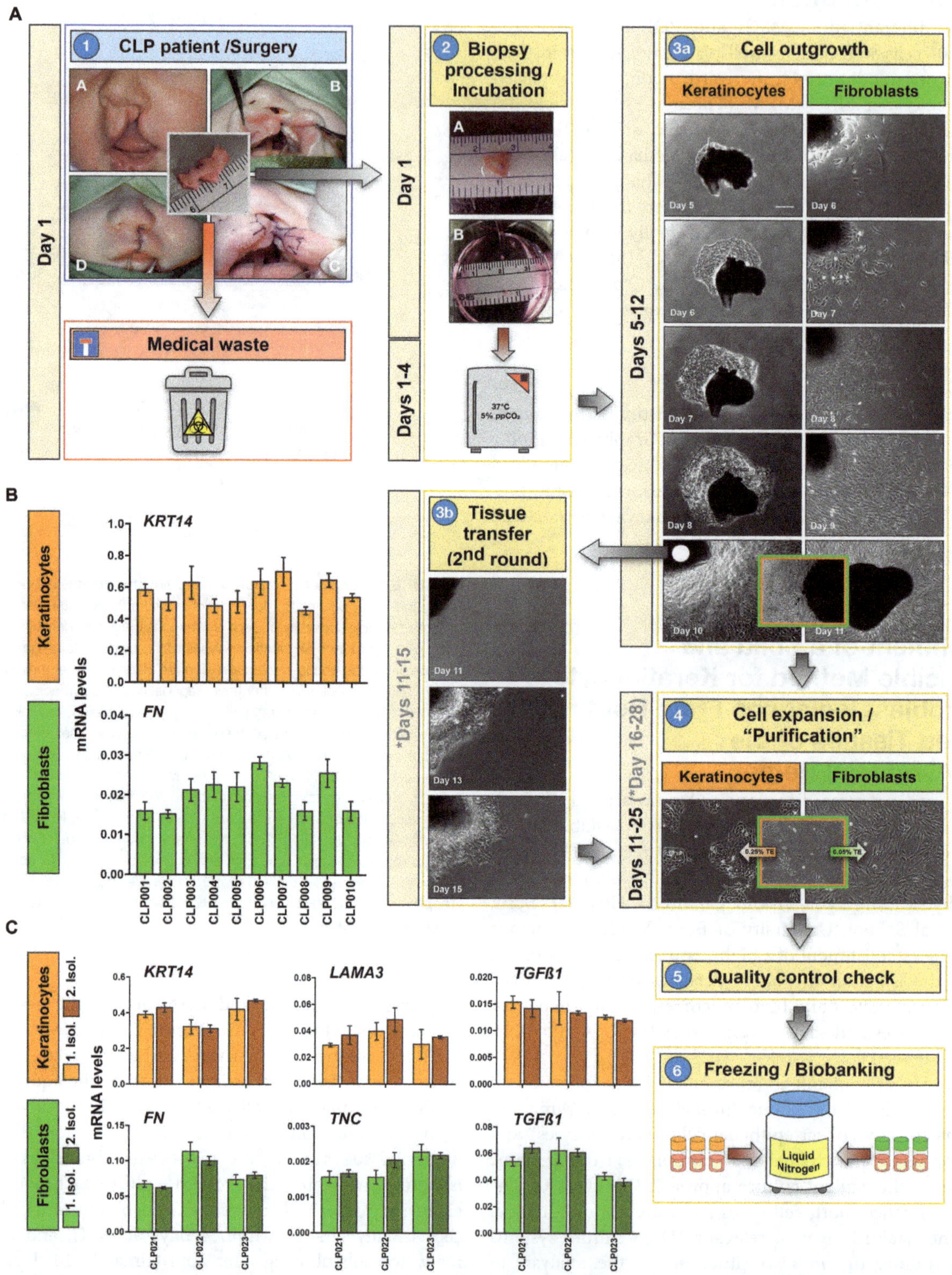

FIGURE 2 | Establishment of a robust and reproducible method for the isolation of keratinocytes and fibroblasts. **(A)** Illustration of the process we follow for the isolation of patient-derived cells from tissue biopsies. A representative example for a CLP biopsy is shown. Briefly, lip tissue from a corrective CLP surgery, which would be routinely discarded (medical waste), is collected in Collection Medium (CM) and transferred to the laboratory (1). After mincing the tissue biopsy, two small tissue fragments of about 0.1 mm^3 are put in one well of a six-well culture plate containing 800 µl of CM (2). These six-well plates are then incubated at 37°C/5% CO_2, re-fed every other day, and observed under the microscope for cellular outgrowths (3a). After approximately 10 days, outgrowths are usually ready for

(Continued)

FIGURE 2 | Continued
subculturing (3a). Cells are trypsinized, expanded in their respective medium, quality checked, and finally frozen (at passage 2) in freezing medium and stored in a liquid nitrogen tank (4–6). Note that in case of mixed keratinocyte/fibroblast cultures, differential trypsinization using 0.05% trypsin-EDTA (TE) solution for detaching fibroblasts, followed by 0.25% TE to dissociate keratinocyte is applied (4). Also note that tissue pieces can be re-used for another round of cell isolation if required (3b). Approximate incubation times (depends on cell type and tissue biopsies) are indicated in days. If a second round of cell isolation is required from an initial tissue piece, the days are indicated in gray. Scale bar: 100 μm. **(B)** qPCR analyses of ten individual non-syndromic CLP cell cultures for the epithelial marker *Keratin14* (*KRT14*) and the mesenchymal marker *Fibronectin* (*FN*). Although cells have been isolated from 10 different tissue donors, keratinocytes (orange) and fibroblasts (green) express similar levels of *KRT14* and *FN*, respectively among the cohort. $n = 3$ (biological replicates). **(C)** Analyses of CLP cells derived from three individual donors (CLP021-CLP023) from two distinct cell isolations to show reproducibility of our cell isolation protocol. In between the first and the second cell isolation (light vs. dark orange for keratinocytes, and light vs. dark green for fibroblasts), the tissue remnants have been stored in freezing medium in the liquid nitrogen tank for at least 3 years. qPCR shows comparable expression of *KRT14*, *Laminin* α3 (*LAMA3*), and *Transforming Growth Factor* β*1* (*TGF*β1) in keratinocytes (orange), and of *FN*, *Tenascin-C* (*TNC*) and *TGF*β1 in fibroblasts (green) derived from two consecutive cell isolations (Isol. 1: Isolation 1; Isol. 2: Isolation 2). $n = 3$ (technical replicates).

the same tissue (**Figure 2A-3b**). This possibility is especially useful when the initial biopsy is rather small. Note that each of the fibroblast and keratinocyte primary cell cultures originating from individual donors represent a mixture of fibroblasts and keratinocytes that grew out of multiple explants.

In our experience, we do get successful cellular outgrowths from approximately 75% of the small tissue pieces. Emergence of the first cells is usually observed 3–4 days after initiation of the explant cultures. Keratinocytes are often growing out of the tissues faster than fibroblasts, which is beneficial as the keratinocytes help to attach the tissue pieces to the culture dish.

In order to minimize the risk of inter-experimental variations during cell isolation, which would hamper any future comparative studies, we follow a highly reproducible workflow. Here, our main rules for cell isolations are detailed. First of all, tissues are all processed in the research laboratory within 1 h after collection. In rare cases, if this is not possible, tissues are stored at 4°C for longer times, and this is properly annotated in the digital databank platform. Secondly, only a team of three well-trained laboratory scientists is in charge of the practical performance of the explant cultures. Thirdly, a strict adherence to Standard Operating Procedures (SOPs) is maintained. SOPs rigorously define the outline of the practical work as well the responsibilities along the cell isolation process, starting from the tissue collection until the final inclusion of the sample into the biobank database. To test whether following these rules was enough to establish a highly robust and reproducible cell isolation process, we tested ten cell strains that have been isolated from ten different non-syndromic, age-matched CLP lip tissue donors for the variability in mRNA levels of some genes. We assumed that patient-derived keratinocytes as well as fibroblasts from the same passage and cultured to the same cell density should display similar levels of the genes *Keratin14* (*KRT14*) and *Fibronectin* (*FN*), respectively. **Figure 2B** clearly indicates that *KRT14* and *FN* are very evenly expressed within the group of tissue donors tested (CLP001-CLP010 $p > 0.05$). Our biobank strategy also includes the storage of tissue remnants in freezing medium in liquid nitrogen for potential cell re-isolation (secondary isolation). Robustness and reproducibility of our cell isolation protocol should result in identical cells after initial and secondary isolation from the same tissue donor. Therefore, we re-isolated cells from three individual tissue biopsies (CLP021-CLP023) that have been stored in freezing medium in the liquid nitrogen tank for more than 3 years (initial cell isolations: 2016–2017; secondary cell isolations: 2020–2021) according to our established SOP (**Figure 2A**). Keratinocytes and fibroblasts from secondary isolations were indistinguishable from the initially isolated cells in regard to cell growth and morphology (data not shown). Moreover, we used a qPCR approach to determine gene levels of the two independent isolations. Cells of the same passage (passage 3) and at the same density (60%) were compared. In keratinocytes (orange), *KRT14*, *Laminin*α*3* (*LAMA3*), and *Transforming Growth Factor* β1 (*TGF*β1) levels were indistinguishable in the original (light orange) and the "secondary" cells (dark orange) isolated from the same tissue donor (**Figure 2C**). Similarly, we did not detect any significant differences in the levels of *FN*, *Tenascin-C* (*TNC*), and *TGF*β1 in the fibroblasts from the primary (light green) vs. secondary (dark green) cell isolations (**Figure 2C**). The robustness of our explant assay guarantees that variations among individual patient-derived cell strains in regard to gene expression are only minimal as long as cell density, donor age, and anatomical site are comparable. Therefore, whenever a significant difference in gene or protein level is detected, this change might be real and relevant for the condition studied. In summary, we show that we have established a highly robust and reproducible explant culture protocol for the isolation of patient-derived fibroblasts and keratinocytes, which allows comparative studies as well.

Patient-Derived Cells Have to Successfully Pass a Quality Control Analysis Before Being Biobanked

Problems associated with the establishment of new cell strains, such as misidentification or mycoplasma contamination, are often ignored by the research community and may lead to unreliable research data (Drexler and Uphoff, 2002). Therefore, prior to biobanking, our newly isolated cells are submitted to a standardized quality control procedure (**Figure 3**).

Morphology and Gene Expression

To gain pure fibroblast and keratinocyte cultures, we have to avoid possible contaminations with the counterpart cell type. The morphologies of fibroblasts and keratinocytes allow the simple monitoring of cross-contaminations by brightfield microscopy and, if required, the two cell types are purified by the differential trypsinization approach as described above. Pure keratinocyte cell cultures suitable for biobanking should form regularly shaped and cohesive colonies (**Figure 3A**, first column), while

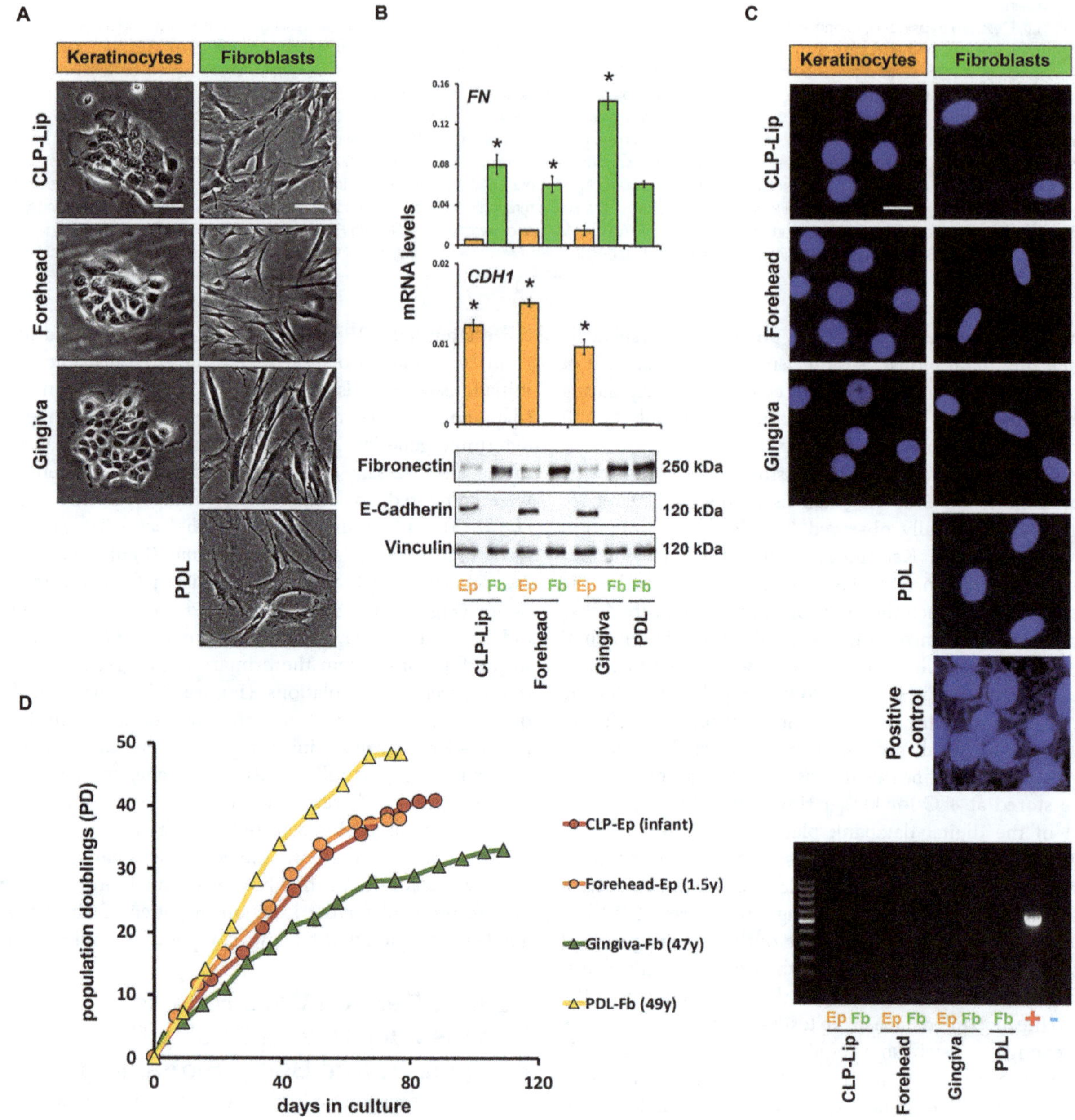

FIGURE 3 | Before biobanking, newly isolated cell cultures undergo a standardized quality control check. **(A)** In a representative set of primary cells (CLP-Lip, Forehead, Gingiva, and PDL) live imaging pictures show typical cell morphologies of the patient-derived keratinocytes (orange) and fibroblasts (green). While keratinocytes form tightly packed and cohesive colonies, fibroblasts appear with an elongated and spindle-like shape. Scale bar: 50 μm. **(B)** The same set of primary cells was used for qPCR (top) and immunoblot analysis (bottom) confirming E-Cadherin (*CDH1*) and fibronectin (*FN*) expression in keratinocytes (orange bars) and fibroblasts (green bars), respectively. Data are expressed as mean ± SD. $n = 3$. **(C)** Mycoplasma contamination of the new cell cultures is tested by DAPI staining of the nuclei and a PCR-based mycoplasma detection analysis. DAPI staining and PCR amplifications are shown to confirm absence of mycoplasma contamination in the same representative set of newly isolated primary cell cultures. Scale bars: 25 μm (Live Imaging keratinocytes), 50 μm (Live Imaging fibroblasts), 10 μm (DAPI). +positive control; −negative control; PDL: periodontal ligament. $^{*}p < 0.05$ Ep vs. Fb. **(D)** Lifespan analysis of two representative keratinocyte (CLP lip, red, and forehead, orange) and two fibroblast strains (gingiva, green, and PDL, yellow) reveals that all cell cultures tested have a replicative potential of at least 35 population doublings (PD). The age of the tissue donors is indicated in the brackets. Y: year; Ep: epithelial cells; Fb: fibroblasts.

fibroblast cultures should appear as homogenous monolayers of flat, elongated and spindle-shaped cells (**Figure 3A**, second column). However, cell purity and identity are not only assessed by visual examinations of their morphologies, but also by qPCR and immunoblots for epithelial and mesenchymal markers (epithelial markers: E-Cadherin, Laminin γ2 and Keratin14; mesenchymal markers: Fibronectin, Vimentin and Tenascin-C). **Figure 3B** shows that the epithelial cells (Ep, orange bars) only express E-Cadherin, but not Fibronectin, and *vice versa* for the mesenchymal cells (Fb, green bars).

Mycoplasma Contamination Detection

Although we strictly follow the rules of good laboratory practice, there is always the risk of mycoplasma contamination when working with primary cell cultures. The original source of tissue serves as the most probable source of mycoplasma in primary cell cultures, but contamination can also occur from exogenous factors (Barile and Rottem, 1993; Rottem et al., 2012). Testing for potential mycoplasma contaminations is a prerequisite for setting up a living cell repository. We routinely test all our newly isolated cell cultures for mycoplasma contamination by a DAPI- and PCR-based detection approach (Praetorius, 2015). **Figure 3C** shows examples of nuclei stained by DAPI without any signs of mycoplasma contamination in combination with the corresponding PCR-based mycoplasma detection test. A primary cell culture that is found to be contaminated is discarded so that only mycoplasma-negative cells are finally biobanked. So far, only one cell strain derived from a CLP patient was found to be mycoplasma-positive and hence excluded from the biobank.

Lifespan Assessment

Primary cell cultures have a finite lifespan. In order to promote them as promising cell models to study human CFAs, the patient-derived cells must possess a replicative potential allowing successful experimental manipulations. To assess this requirement, we regularly perform lifespan analyses with our newly isolated fibroblast and keratinocyte cultures. **Figure 3D** indicates that our patient-derived cells can be consistently propagated beyond 35 population doublings (PDs). This is substantially shorter than what has been reported for infant foreskin epidermal keratinocyte primary lines such as strain N, but similar to the lifespan of other p63-positive human epithelial cell types (Dabelsteen et al., 2009). It is evident that the replicative lifespan depends on cell types, cell origin, and donor age, which makes such comparisons difficult. Still, we are able to routinely grow our cells for more than 80 days and keep them healthy growing up to passage 11, which makes them highly suitable for standard research activities.

CFA BIOBANK – State of Our Living Cell Repository

Since April 2016, we received a total of 92 tissue biopsies from the cranio-/orofacial region of 71 different donors (**Table 1**). Samples can be grossly classified into four distinct groups in respect to their origin: (1) skin-derived specimens (n = 12; forehead, eyebrow, ear, nose and facial skin); (2) mucosa-derived specimens (n = 14; palate, oral mucosa, "lip pits" and gingiva); (3) mucocutaneous junction area-derived specimens (n = 53; CLP lip, upper lip, lower lip and lip scar); (4) tooth-derived specimens (n = 13; PDL and dental pulp) (**Figure 4A**).

The majority of our biopsy collection (60/92–65%) is represented by discarded tissue excised during corrective surgeries of CFAs. In addition, we biobanked four pediatric healthy facial skin specimens (4/92–4.3%) and 3 healthy lip samples (3/92–3.3%) obtained during surgeries for minor injuries (i.e., lip laceration, accidental cuts). The remaining samples were collected as tissue remnants after routine dental treatments (21/92–22.8%) performed at the Dental School, University of Bern or after secondary surgeries at the Pediatric

TABLE 1 | Total status of our cell bank, including the tissue category, number of samples, cell types that have been successfully isolated, donor sex and age as well as disease status (specifics).

	Category	# Samples	Cells		Donor Sex			Donor Age	Specifics			
			Ep	Fb	M	F	n.a.		healthy	diseased	CFA	
											ns	s
Skin	**Forehead**	1	X	X	1	0	0	2–4 years	1			
	Eyebrow	1	X		0	0	1	2–4 years	1			
	Ear	1	X	X	0	0	1	n.a.	1			
	Nose	1	X	X	1	0	0	2–4 years	1			
	Facial skin	8	X	X	5	3	0	3–5 months			7	1× GH (F)
Mucocutaneous junction area	**CLP Lip**	48	X	X	30	18	0	3–5 months			46	1× VWS (M) 1× T13 (F)
	Upper Lip	3	X	X	1	1	1	3–5 years	3			0
	Lower Lip	1	X	X	1	0	0	19 years				1× VWS (M)
	Scar (lip)	1		X	1	0	0	19 years				1× VWS (M)
Mucosa	**Palate**	2		X	1	1	0	>18 years	2			
	Oral Mucosa	4	X	X	2	2	0	3–5 months			4	
	"Lip Pits"	1	X	X	1	0	0	19 years				1× VWS (M)
	Gingiva	7	X	X	4	2	1	>18 years	4	2		1× VWS (M)
Teeth	**Periodontal Ligament**	10		X	5	3	2	>18 years	10			
	Dental Pulp	3		X	2	1	0	>18 years	3			

Diseased gingiva samples were received from periodontitis-affected patients. Ep: epithelial cells; Fb: fibroblasts; M: male; F: female; n.a.: not available; ns: non-syndromic; s: syndromic; CFA: craniofacial anomaly; GH: Goldenhar syndrome; VWS: Van der Woude syndrome; T13: Trisomy 13. Cells that have been used in this study, including cell name, donor sex, donor age, and characteristics are indicated.

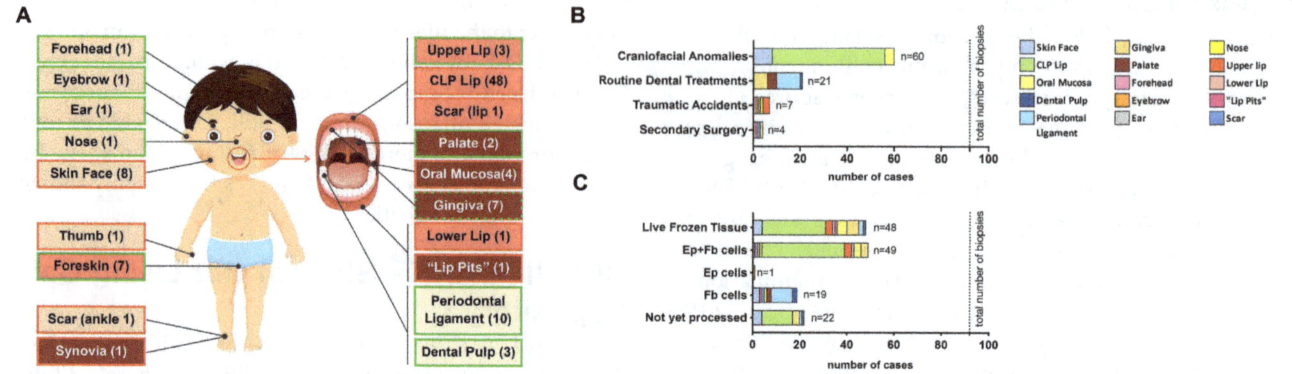

FIGURE 4 | Overall description of our living cranio-/orofacial cell repository. **(A)** Graphical illustration indicating the anatomical origin of stored tissue biopsies (including non-cranio-/orofacial-derived specimens). Light pink indicates skin-derived specimens; pink indicates mucocutaneous junction area-derived specimens; red indicates mucosal-derived specimens; while light yellow indicates tooth-derived specimens. Furthermore, a green border depicts healthy tissue while a red border represents tissue with anomalies. For the gingiva, we have both healthy and diseased tissues (green and red border). The number in the boxes in brackets represents the amount of tissues available. **(B)** Bar chart reporting the source of the specimens that were obtained for the generation of the living cell biobank. Total number of cranio-/orofacial region biopsies: 92 biopsies. **(C)** Bar chart of the outcome after tissue biopsy processing. The color code is shown in the legend. Total number of biopsies: 92.

Surgery Division, Children's Hospital, Bern (4/92–4.3%) (**Figure 4B**).

From this cohort of tissue biopsies, we so far processed 70 biopsies (70/92–76%) and were able to isolate cells from 69 samples (success rate 99%). The only tissue we were not able to obtain cellular outgrowths was a gingiva sample. We successfully isolated and purified 49 pairs of matching keratinocytes and fibroblasts (49/69–71%), while for 7 (7/69–10%) biopsies we could extract either only keratinocytes (eyebrow) or only fibroblasts (3 facial skin, 2 palate, and 1 oral mucosa biopsies). For additional 13 (13/69–19%) specimens (PDL, dental pulp, "lip pits" and scar) the tissue origin did not allow the isolation of keratinocytes. We did not yet perform cell extractions from 22 biopsies. Notably, we have remaining tissues of successful cell outgrowths for 48 samples (48/69–69%), which are stored in freezing medium in the liquid nitrogen tank for potential cell re-isolation in the future (**Figure 4C**).

Additionally, our biobank contains cells isolated from 10 more samples independent from the cranio-/orofacial region (**Supplementary Table 3**). This cohort resulted in eight successful matching keratinocyte/fibroblast pairs (seven foreskins, one thumb derived from polydactyly), while for two biopsies we only could get fibroblasts (synovia and ankle scar from a pigmented villonodular synovitis). The complete state of our biobank (CFA and other sources) is shown in **Supplementary Figure 1**.

Our Cell Bank Offers Novel Tools and Models for Personalized Precision Medicine

Establishing Cell Models for the Study of Rare Human Conditions *in vitro*

In 5–7% of all CLP cases, orofacial clefting can be part of rare syndromes that present with additional anomalies outside of the region of clefting and that are usually caused by a single gene mutation, chromosomal abnormalities or exposure to teratogens during pregnancy (Mossey and Modell, 2012; Leslie and Marazita, 2013). In fact, at least 275 syndromes have been identified, which are associated with a clefting phenotype (Leslie and Marazita, 2013). As such, primary cells isolated from syndromic CLP-affected individuals are also very appealing for the establishment of clinically relevant cell models for the study of rare conditions, as exemplified below. Among our cohort, there are cells isolated from four individual patients affected by rare human diseases/syndromes, Van der Woude syndrome (VWS) (two patients) (Van Der Woude, 1954), Patau syndrome (Trisomy 13) (Miryounesi et al., 2016) and GH (Bogusiak et al., 2017). Short descriptions of the main features associated with these syndromes are reported in **Figure 5** (Overview).

Regarding VWS, we have tissues and the corresponding cells from 2 affected patients: an infant (VWS1), who underwent primary corrective cleft lip surgery (CLP lip biopsy) and a 19 year old individual (VWS2), who had secondary surgery for functional as well as esthetical reasons (biopsies of the gingiva, lower lip, connective tissue of the lip pits, and the scar tissue from the primary corrective surgery to close the upper lip) (**Figure 5A**, Biopsies). While we were able to isolate both fibroblasts and keratinocytes from the lip and the gingiva tissues, we only managed to obtain fibroblasts from the scar and the "lip pits" connective tissue. We analyzed all cells for their morphologies as well as epithelial (E-Cadherin)- and mesenchymal-(FN)specific markers (**Figure 5A**, patient-derived cells). In addition, we prepared FFPE blocks and tissue sections from all four VWS2-derived biopsies. H&E and Toluidine Blue staining allow a preliminary descriptive appreciation of the tissue architecture, which could be further investigated by immunohistochemistry (IHC) (**Figure 5A**, Histology). By IHC staining of some sections, we were able to highlight the epidermis of the lip by E-Cadherin expression at adherent junctions between epithelial cells, scar tissue by strong positivity for α-smooth muscle actin (αSMA) in

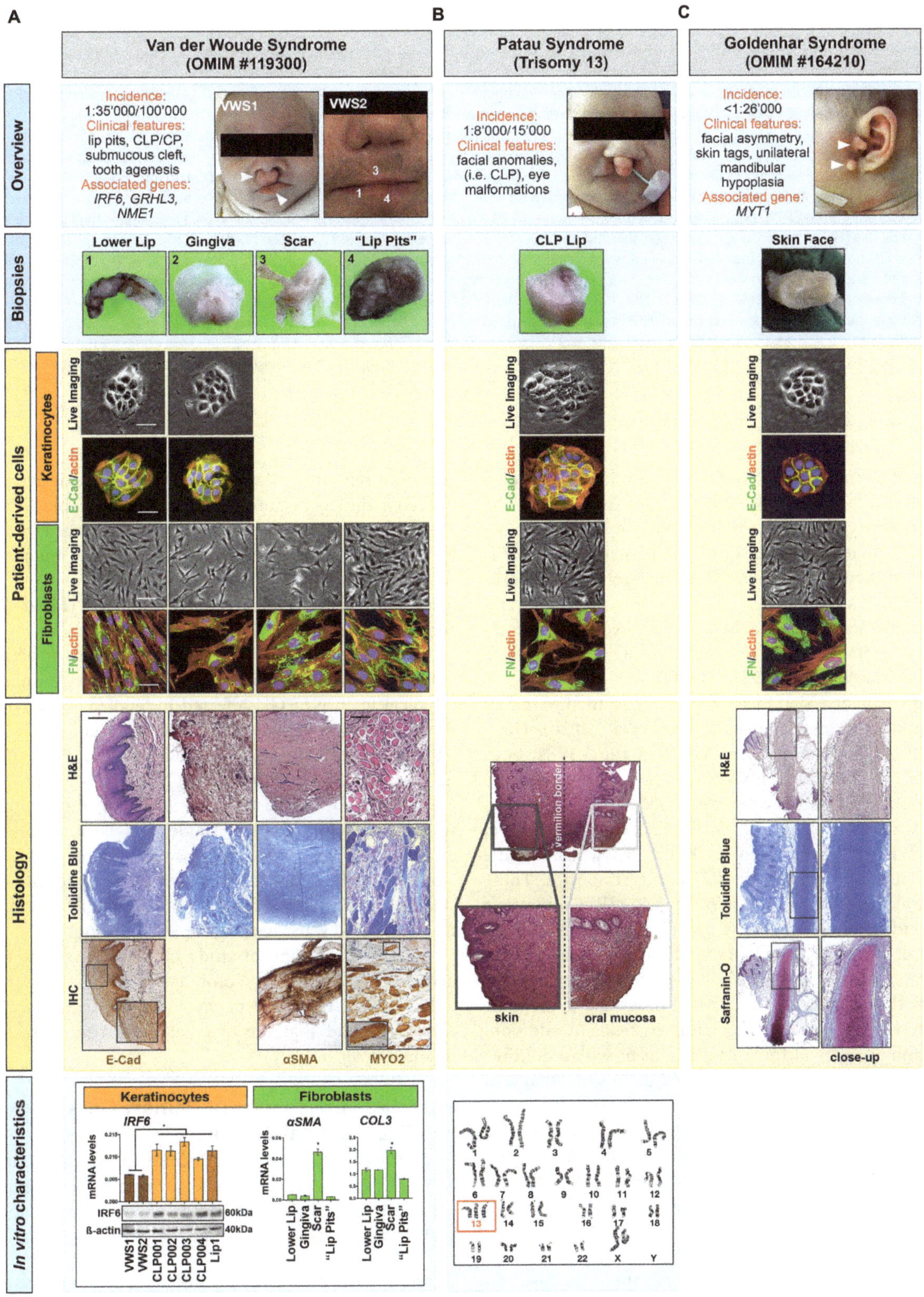

FIGURE 5 | Patient-derived cells can serve as promising research tools for studying rare human diseases. Our cohort of tissue donors encompasses individuals affected by **(A)** Van der Woude syndrome (VWS), **(B)** Patau syndrome, and **(C)** Goldenhar syndrome (GH). *Overview*: A brief description of the rare human diseases is shown as well as the clinical appearance of the tissue donors. Arrowheads indicate typical phenotypes such as bilateral lip pits and orofacial clefts (VWS1, **A**), and

(Continued)

FIGURE 5 | Continued
pathological skin tags in the GH-affected individual **(C)**. *Biopsies*: High magnification images of the tissue biopsies taken for histological analysis are depicted. Note that the biopsies shown for the VWS were all derived from a secondary surgery of a 19 years old individual (VWS2) and are indicated by numbers (1, 3, 4) in the "Overview" **(A)**. *Patient-derived cells*: Explant cultures allowed the isolation of patient-derived cells of the biopsies shown, which were thoroughly characterized by morphological as well as immunofluorescent analyses. All keratinocytes (orange) show the typical colony-forming morphology (Live Imaging) and are all positive for the epithelial marker E-Cadherin (E-Cad), while fibroblasts (green) present as elongated cells (Live Imaging) positive for the mesenchymal marker Fibronectin (FN). Note that explant cultures from the scar and the "lip pits" of the VWS2 individual **(A)** only resulted in fibroblasts. Scale bars: 25 μm (Live Imaging keratinocytes), 50 μm (Live Imaging fibroblasts), 25 μm (IF). *Histology*: Representative Toluidine Blue and/or H&E stainings of the tissues, with some close-ups are shown. For the VWS2-derived samples additional immunohistochemical analyses (IHC) were performed **(A)**. The expression of E-Cad indicating the skin epithelium was revealed in the lower lip sample. Similarly, the scar tissue revealed excessive staining for α-smooth muscle actin (α-SMA). Note also the abundant amount of striated muscles in the biopsy derived from the VWS2 "lip pits" connective tissue [anti-myosin II (MYOII) immunoreactivity and H&E/Toluidine Blue staining]. In the H&E staining of the Patau syndrome biopsy **(B)** the transition zone between skin and mucosa of the lip can be appreciated (Vermillion border). Finally, Safranin-O staining of the skin tag biopsied from the GH patient identifies the presence of pathological cartilage formation **(C)**. Scale bar: 0.1 mm. *In vitro characteristics*: **(A)** qPCR and immunoblot analyses show that the levels of IRF6 in VWS1 and VWS2 keratinocytes are significantly decreased compared to the levels in 4 non-syndromic [wild-type for the VWS-associated genes *IRF6* (NM_006147.4), *GRHL3* (NM_198173), and *NME1* (NM_198175)] CLP and one healthy lip keratinocyte cell cultures. These results strongly suggest that the VWS2 individual harbors an *IRF6* variant [this has been confirmed for VWS1 by genetic analysis (Degen et al., 2020)] (left). Additionally, fibroblasts isolated from the scar tissue of VWS2 showed higher expression of *α-SMA and Collagen type III (COL3)* mRNA levels compared to fibroblasts isolated from the same donor but from different origins (gingiva, lower lip, and "lip pits," right). Thus, the original characteristics are retained in the patient-derived cells. Data are expressed as mean ± SD. $n = 3$. * = $p < 0.05$. **(B)** Presence of three chromosomes 13 in the patient affected by the Patau syndrome is shown by karyotype analysis (red box).

the stroma, and to confirm presence of high amounts of striated muscles in the "lip pit" tissue, which were already visible in the H&E sections, by Myosin fast II (MYO2) (**Figure 5A**, Histology).

Cellular and molecular analyses of the patient-derived cells clearly demonstrated proof-of-concept: the original hallmarks of the syndrome are retained in the cells *in vitro* and represent promising study tools. Using the isolated keratinocytes (VWS1) we were able to confirm and thoroughly characterize a novel *IRF6* variant (c961_965delGTGTAinsC), which has been initially sequence-identified by the Division of Human Genetics, Children's Hospital Bern (Degen et al., 2020). Here, we show that in keratinocytes derived from the VWS2, both IRF6 protein as well as mRNA levels are comparable to VWS1, but robustly decreased when compared to non-syndromic (pathogenic variants in the known VWS-associated genes *IRF6*, *GRHL3*, and *NME1* have been excluded by whole exome sequencing) CLP- and healthy lip-derived keratinocytes. These data fit to the assumed notion that VWS-causing IRF6 mutations often result in haploinsufficiency of IRF6 (de Lima et al., 2009; Degen et al., 2020). Therefore, without knowledge of the underlying gene defect causing VWS in the second individual, we can speculate that the affected individual harbors a pathogenic IRF6 variant (**Figure 5A**, *In vitro* characteristics). In addition, gene expression analyses of the four different fibroblast cultures derived from the VWS2 individual allowed us to show that also fibroblasts retain their *in vivo* characteristics *in vitro*. Indeed, the scar-derived fibroblasts significantly present higher levels of the scar markers (Ehrlich et al., 1994; Tsou et al., 2000; Shinde et al., 2017) αSMA, *Collagen I* (*Col1*) (data not shown) and *Collagen III* (*Col3*) compared to the fibroblasts derived from other tissues (**Figure 5A**, *In vitro* characteristics), fitting to our IHC observations.

Among our cohort of tissue donors, there is also an individual affected by Trisomy 13 (**Figure 5B**), who underwent corrective surgery of the condition-associated orofacial cleft lip. Successful isolation of both keratinocytes and fibroblasts will allow scientists to study specific aspects of Trisomy 13 using clinically relevant cells (**Figure 5B**, Patient-derived cells). We collected the corresponding tissue as FFPE blocks. The initial H&E staining shows the complex anatomical structure of the lip as it represents a transition zone between mucosal and skin tissue (**Figure 5B**, Histology). In addition, we show presence of three chromosomes 13 by karyotype analysis (**Figure 5B**, *In vitro* characteristics).

Finally, we received a biopsy from a patient who presented with preauricular skin tags (**Figure 5C**, Overview and Biopsies), a typical feature of GH-affected individuals (Dole et al., 2017). From the biopsy, we were able to isolate and characterize patient-derived keratinocytes and fibroblasts (**Figure 5C**, Patient-derived cells). Such cells could represent an unprecedent research opportunity for scientists interested in this rare syndrome, since so far only one zebrafish model has been successful (Lopez et al., 2016). Next to the cells, we also biobanked FFPE blocks. Notably, H&E, Toluidine Blue and cartilage-specific Safranin-O staining confirmed the presence of pathological cartilage in these GH-associated skin tags (**Figure 5C**, Histology).

Our proof-of-concept study clearly shows that the patient-derived cells, often in combination with the corresponding FFPE blocks, represent promising tools to study rare human conditions and that the original cell/tissue characteristics are retained *in vitro*.

Potential Applications of Primary Cells in Preclinical and Translational Research

Finally, we would like to illustrate the translational potential of our living CFA cell bank in regard to regenerative and personalized medicine as well as to pharmaceutical, cosmetic, oral health and dental material industry.

Three-dimensional (3D) personalized skin models

Our approach of isolating keratinocytes as well as fibroblasts from the same tissue donor is very promising for the development of personalized 3D organotypic skin models, which mimic the *in vivo* skin as much as possible (Ravi et al., 2015). In **Figure 6A**

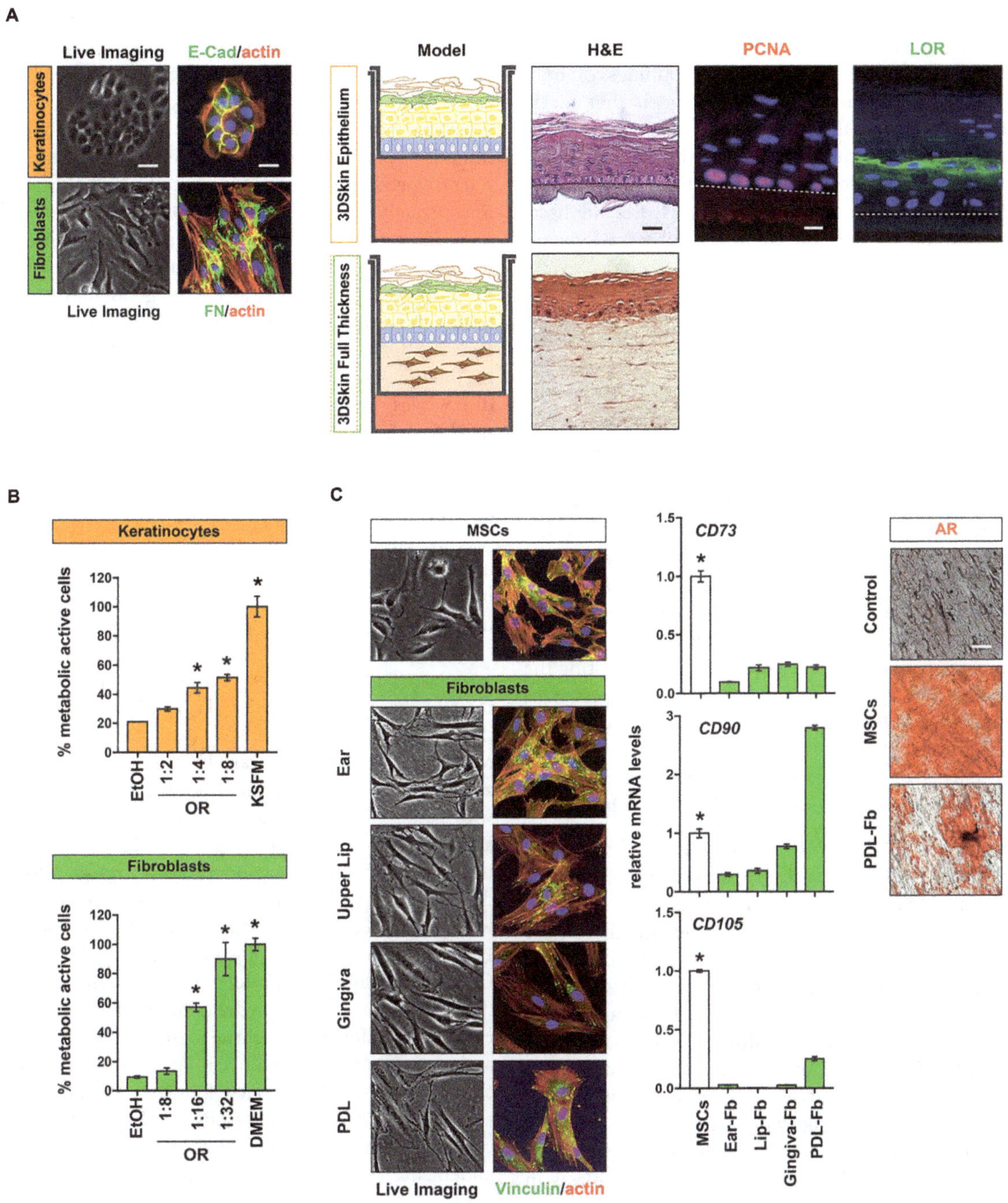

FIGURE 6 | Potential outlook for the use of patient-derived cells from the cranio-/orofacial region. **(A)** CLP patient-derived keratinocytes (orange) and fibroblasts (green) were isolated from CLP patients and characterized by staining for E-Cad (keratinocytes) and FN (fibroblasts). Scale bars: 50 μm (Live Imaging), 25 μm (IF). These cells were used to obtain 3D skin differentiation models (top) that can be stained for H&E, the proliferation marker PCNA (red) and Loricrin (LOR, green). Note that PCNA is only detectable in basal keratinocytes, whereas LOR is present in more superficial keratinocyte layers confirming the *in vivo* situation. Dotted line indicates the membrane. Scale bars: 50 μm (Live Imaging), 25 μm (IF). Alternatively, the isolation of both keratinocytes and fibroblasts from the same tissue donor allows the establishment of full-thickness 3D-skin models, in which CLP keratinocytes are plated on a dermis created by the corresponding fibroblasts that also can be stained (H&E, bottom). $^{*}p < 0.05$ EtOH vs. oral rinse or KSFM or DMEM. **(B)** Healthy gingival keratinocytes (orange) and fibroblasts (green) were used to determine cytotoxicity of a commercially available oral rinse (OR) at different dilutions after a 2 min exposure by MTT assay. Metabolic active cells are plotted as percentage of the initial cell population. **(C)** Cranio-/orofacial derived fibroblasts share similar characteristics with MSCs and may have a potential in personalized regenerative therapeutic approaches. Like MSCs, fibroblasts have a spindle-like morphology and are plastic-adherent, as revealed by live imaging and vinculin staining (green). Furthermore, qPCR analyses revealed that our patient-derived fibroblasts also express the typical MSC markers *CD73*, *CD90*, and *CD105*. $^{*}p < 0.05$ MSC vs. Fbs. Alizarin Red S (AR) staining indicates the potential of PDL fibroblasts to be differentiated into bone forming cells. Scale bar: 20 μm. Data are expressed as mean ± SD. $n = 3$.

we present preliminary data on the establishment of 3D-skin differentiation models (keratinocytes only) as well as on full thickness skin models (fibroblasts and keratinocytes) using non-syndromic CLP patient-derived cells. H&E stainings of both models indicate that both assays result in models that nicely resemble the *in vivo* skin with multiple superficial keratinocyte layers. Loricrin, a differentiation marker of the granular layer of epithelial cells can be detected in superficial keratinocyte layers (green), while PCNA (red) is only expressed in the basal proliferating keratinocytes (**Figure 6A**). Both observations are identical to the *in vivo* situation.

Modern dentistry and biomaterials

Our provision of cells isolated from most of the tissues represented in the oral cavity could be highly beneficial for dental material companies, in order to improve and advance the development of their products. For instance, primary gingival fibroblasts could represent an optimal model for studying the adhesion of soft tissues to the dental implant abutment or to dental composites for the treatment of submucosal lesion, while PDL and dental pulp fibroblasts may represent models for studying the efficacy of treatment for periodontal and dental regeneration, respectively. In addition, also the oral health industry (e.g., companies interested in the development of oral rinses or toothpastes) may benefit from clinically relevant cells available in our cell bank. Such cells could be used for testing the cytotoxic effects of new compounds in newly developed products. Using keratinocytes and fibroblasts isolated from healthy gingiva donors, we established straight-forward MTT assays to analyze the cytotoxic effects of commercially available oral rinses on paired gingiva-derived fibroblasts and keratinocytes (**Figure 6B**).

Tissue engineering and regenerative medicine

Our cohort of primary fibroblasts also shows certain criteria that have been attributed to MSCs: they are plastic-adherent and show a spindle-like morphology and express variable amounts of the MSC surface markers *CD73*, *CD90*, and *CD105*. Furthermore, our preliminary *in vitro* differentiation experiments revealed that similar to MSCs, PDL fibroblasts could be induced into bone forming cells as assessed by staining for Ca^{2+} deposits by Alizarin Red S (**Figure 6C**). These initial observations let us speculate that our patient-derived cells may represent a viable and easily accessible source of cells likely offering some regenerative potential. Clearly, further experimental evidence is warranted. However, we are encouraged to believe that the fibroblasts in our cell bank could be beneficial for the tissue donors themselves later in life if they might benefit from autologous, regenerative therapeutic options.

DISCUSSION

Discovery biomedical research is the foundation for an ever-increasing gain of knowledge concerning the biological processes underlying physiological as well as pathological craniofacial development. In the past years, significant progress has been made by using various model organisms to study genes required for proper face morphogenesis. More recently, this approach has been complemented by the availability of novel, state-of-the-art technologies allowing the identification of disease-causing gene mutations or chromosomal aberrations driving various anomalies. Thanks to these approaches, hundreds of genes and variants have been found to be linked to specific CFAs. However, scientific activities also envision to understand how certain gene mutations affect the behavior of cells and to establish genotype-phenotype correlations (Degen et al., 2020). Immortalized cell lines usually are used in such studies. However, nowadays, the scientific community is aware that often immortalized cells fail to recapitulate the *in vivo* situation as they often markedly differ in their phenotypes as well as genotypes from the original tissues. In addition, there are several reports about contaminated and misidentified cell lines (Masters, 2010; Lorsch et al., 2014), producing irreproducible results, on which many scientific discoveries and publications rely on. Therefore, there is urgent need for the availability of clinically relevant cell models that retain their original characteristics and that can be used as *in vitro* tools to further solidify the understanding of how genes affect cellular behavior in studying CFAs.

Our effort in establishing a cell biobank represents an unprecedented tool for the scientific community, who is interested in studying CFAs or periodontal/dental-related investigations. Such a project is only possible in a collaborative effort with the clinical counterparts, which provide all clinical samples. The availability of optimal cell models that retain their original characteristics (**Figure 5**) should help to advance discovery research on CFAs (see section "Establishing Cell Models for the Study of Rare Human Conditions *in vitro*"), but also could be of great benefit for the tissue donors themselves, who can rely on a personal repository of autologous cells at any moment of their life (**Figure 6**). In this regard, it is worth noting that in the literature cranio-/orofacial tissues have been described as very rich sources of progenitor cells or MSCs, with potential application for regenerative therapies (Sanz et al., 2015; Ebrahimi and Botelho, 2017). The International Society for Cellular Therapy (ISCT) defined a set of three minimal criteria that a cell has to fulfill in order to be viewed as an MSC (Dominici et al., 2006). However, the true identity of MSCs is still debatable as there is increasing evidence in the literature annotating similar characteristics to fibroblasts (Ichim et al., 2018; Soundararajan and Kannan, 2018). In this study, we show that some of the main characteristics defined for MSC are present also in our set of patient-derived fibroblasts (**Figure 6**). Clearly, more basic and functional studies are required to assess the clinical potential of patient-derived fibroblasts as alternatives to MSCs. However, our preliminary investigations let us believe that our cell bank might be beneficial for the tissue donors themselves for personalized regenerative therapies in their future.

To be successful and relevant for the economy and society, biomedical research increasingly relies on the existence and usage of data and samples stored in human biobanks (Hewitt, 2011; Coppola et al., 2019). Biobanks are organized collections of human biological samples and associated patient data, which are stored over lengthy periods allowing the availability of resources for research efforts. However, the establishment and the maintenance of human biobanks raises multiple ethical and juridical questions, which need to be addressed (Ashcroft and Macpherson, 2019). The acquisition, storage, and use of patient-derived specimens is indeed subject to stringent ethical as well as legal regulations. The protection of the privacy and identity of the research participants should be the top priority in all biobanking efforts. Unfortunately, there is not yet a harmonized legislative framework available within European countries regulating biobanking activities (Kaye et al., 2016). For the establishment of our CFA biobank, we included measures according to the https://www.wma.net/policies-post/wma-declaration-of-helsinki-ethical-principles-for-medical-research-involving-human-subjects/ and to the Swiss Human Act (HRA), which regulate the protection of the privacy and identity of participants on a global level and in Switzerland, respectively. First of all, all the projects involving the use of our cell models have to be approved by the regional research ethical committee. In addition to this, external investigators interested in using our cells are required to undersign a Material Transfer Agreement (MTA), a contract governing the transfer, intended use and rights of the research material. Secondly, all study participants or their legal representative in case of minors, are informed about the research and gave an informed consent, which allows individuals to decide whether and how their tissues samples can be used for research purposes. In both cases, patients have always the right to decide whether their personal data and tissue samples can or cannot be used in an encoded way for future biomedical research. Participants are also informed about the possibility to withdraw their consent at any time, which further exemplifies the protection and respect toward each individual. Notably, all the samples stored in our collection, are derived from planned and necessary surgical interventions, and all the biospecimens would have been otherwise discarded. Therefore, none of the participants experiences any supplemental consultation time, harm or any other disadvantages by donating their tissue for research purposes. Finally, we implemented various technological data security measures including the appropriate IT infrastructure in order to securely store patient data in a protected database.

In our workflow, the improvement of the protection of the patient's privacy has been obtained by defining clear and strict responsibilities shared between the Children's Hospital/Dental School and the research laboratory for the collection and encoding of the samples. All the clinically related data and work, such as the written consents, consultation and the diagnosis, are securely stored at the hospital/dental clinic. The laboratory receives the tissue sample in a pre-labeled tube (e.g., 001) in combination with minimal patient information (such as date of the surgery, age and gender) and the origin of the sample (e.g., bilateral cleft, gingiva). If applicable, the laboratory is also informed about the presence of any syndromes associated with the patient. This system does not allow the identification and tracking of patients and hence protects their privacy. If future research projects require more information about the tissue sample donor (e.g., patients requiring regenerative therapies using their own cells), this can only be achieved in consultation with the involved and trained personnel of the clinics. Clearly, it is our responsibility to regularly train all people involved in the biobanking process and to audit all our activities to ensure correct adherence to our guidelines.

We strongly believe that our approach in setting up a living cell repository for the cranio-/orofacial region derived from otherwise discarded tissues is unique and will represent an important asset for discovery and translational research on cranio-/orofacial anomalies as well as an essential tool to be combined with animal studies. 3D skin models established from patient-derived cells can be used as personalized organotypic cultures for drug screenings (e.g., to obtain better wound healing using CLP cells), cosmetics (facial skin cells), toxicity tests (oral cavity cells), bacterial infections related to periodontitis (gingiva cells) as well as for clinically relevant discovery research trying to elucidate specific molecular mechanisms. For instance, we applied such models in the understanding of how specific gene variants causing CLP and/or VWS affected the differentiation potential of skin and mucosa cells (Degen et al., 2018, 2020). Another research area that might benefit from such clinically relevant primary cells is dentistry. For the long-term success of regenerative procedures in dentistry, the integration of biomaterials within the oral cavity is of great clinical importance (van Steenberghe et al., 1991; Tayebi and Moharamzadeh, 2018). This largely depends on the behavior of cells at their interface and, particularly, on their initial attachment, adhesion and spreading (Anselme, 2000). However, these events can also be affected by the characteristics of the material itself, and this is the reason for why the development of more and more performant materials is currently a trend on the market. In spite of this, most of the available materials used in the daily clinical practices lack *in vitro* data, which could support and explain their clinical performance on a cellular level regulating biological events at the biomaterial interface (Parisi et al., 2020; Toffoli et al., 2020). Our primary dental-related cells could fill this gap and provide an optimal source for clinically relevant and tissue-specific cells. We are well aware that such a biobanking effort is time-consuming and requires a financial investment (e.g., infrastructure, IT support, trained personnel). Nevertheless, we are convinced that such a cell bank might be required in the pursuit of a complete understanding of specific CFAs, from which patients may benefit in the future.

In summary, here we presented our proof-of-concept study that patient-derived cells from the cranio-/orofacial region have great potential in discovery and translational research. We detailed our workflow and the main processes that we apply for the ongoing generation of our biobank to (1) promote, boost, and advance biomedical research on CFAs with high-quality primary cells, (2) have healthy primary control cells available from various cranio-/orofacial tissues, (3) establish patient-derived cell models for translational research such as drug testing using clinically relevant cells, (4) store patient-derived cells that could be used at a later time as an autologous source for personalized regenerative applications, and (5) gain more and urgently needed knowledge on the biological processes underlying various CFAs, which will be of great benefit to CFA-affected patients.

ETHICS STATEMENT

This work was performed according to the Ethical Principles for Medical Research Involving Human Subjects as defined by the World Medical Association (WMA Declaration of Helsinki-Ethical principles for medical research involving human subjects. Available at: https://www.wma.net/policies-post/wma-declaration-of-helsinki-ethical-principles-for-medical-research-involving-human-subjects). Isolation of human cleft lip- as well as control tissue-derived cells and their analyses for this study had been approved by the Regional Research Ethic Board (Kantonale Ethikkommission of Bern, Switzerland, protocol number: 2017-01394). Informed written consent was obtained from the patient or their legal representatives.

AUTHOR CONTRIBUTIONS

LP, PK, EG, SR, and MD performed the experiments and analyzed the data. LP and MD wrote the manuscript. LP, MD, and CK initiated the project and planned, coordinated, and designed the experiments. DB was responsible for the histological analyses. MD and CK critically revised the manuscript and provided support throughout the project. IS and GL performed the clinical work (CLP and other CFAs). ASt and ASc performed the clinical work (dental-related biopsies). All authors critically reviewed the manuscript.

ACKNOWLEDGMENTS

We truly wish to thank all the individuals and their legal representatives, who agreed to donate tissue for the advancement of discovery and translational research in the field of CFAs. We would also like to thank Julia Feldmann for her excellent technical assistance, Monika Aeberhard for her help with tissue processing for histology and histological analyses, Aliu Nijas, from the Division of Human Genetics, Children's Hospital Bern for the Trisomy 13 karyotyping, Andrea Roccuzzo from the Department of Periodontology, ZMK Bern, for kindly providing us with tissue biopsies obtained during routine dental treatments, and Albino Triaca, Zentrum für Kiefer- und Gesichtschirurgie, Klinik Pyramide am See, Zurich, Switzerland, for the VWS2 biopsies.

REFERENCES

Aizenbud, D., Coval, M., Hazan-Molina, H., and Harari, D. (2011). Isolated soft tissue cleft lip: epidemiology and associated dental anomalies. *Oral Dis.* 17, 221–231. doi: 10.1111/j.1601-0825.2010.01729.x

Anselme, K. (2000). Osteoblast adhesion on biomaterials. *Biomaterials* 21, 667–681. doi: 10.1016/s0142-9612(99)00242-2

Ashcroft, J. W., and Macpherson, C. C. (2019). The complex ethical landscape of biobanking. *Lancet Public Health* 4, E274–E275.

Barile, M. F., and Rottem, S. (1993). "Mycoplasmas in Cell Culture," in *Rapid Diagnosis of Mycoplasmas*, eds I. Kahane and A. Adoni (New York, USA: Plenum Press).

Beyeler, J., Schnyder, I., Katsaros, C., and Chiquet, M. (2014). Accelerated wound closure in vitro by fibroblasts from a subgroup of cleft lip/palate patients: role of transforming growth factor-α. *PLoS One* 9:e111752. doi: doi: 10.1371/journal.pone.0111752

Bogusiak, K., Puch, A., and Arkuszewski, P. (2017). Goldenhar syndrome: current perspectives. *World J. Pediatr.* 13, 405–415. doi: 10.1007/s12519-017-0048-z

Coppola, L., Cianflone, A., Grimaldi, A. M., Incoronato, M., Bevilacqua, P., Messina, F., et al. (2019). Biobanking in health care: evolution and future directions. *J. Transl. Med.* 17:172.

Cordero, D. R., Brugmann, S., Chu, Y., Bajpai, R., Jame, M., and Helms, J. A. (2011). Cranial neural crest cells on the move: their roles in craniofacial development. *Am. J. Med. Genet A* 155A, 270–279. doi: 10.1002/ajmg.a.33702

Dabelsteen, S., Hercule, P., Barron, P., Rice, M., Dorsainville, G., and Rheinwald, J. G. (2009). Epithelial cells derived from human embryonic stem cells display p16INK4A senescence, hypermotility, and differentiation properties shared by many P63+ somatic cell types. *Stem Cells* 27, 1388–1399. doi: 10.1002/stem.64

de Lima, R. L., Hoper, S. A., Ghassibe, M., Cooper, M. E., Rorick, N. K., Kondo, S., et al. (2009). Prevalence and nonrandom distribution of exonic mutations in interferon regulatory factor 6 in 307 families with Van der Woude syndrome and 37 families with popliteal pterygium syndrome. *Genet Med.* 11, 241–247. doi: 10.1097/gim.0b013e318197a49a

Degen, M., Girousi, E., Feldmann, J., Parisi, L., La Scala, G. C., Schnyder, I., et al. (2020). A Novel Van der Woude Syndrome-Causing IRF6 Variant Is Subject to Incomplete Non-sense-Mediated mRNA Decay Affecting the Phenotype of Keratinocytes. *Front. Cell Devel. Biol.* 8:583115. doi: 10.3389/fcell.2020.583115

Degen, M., Natarajan, E., Barron, P., Widlund, H. R., and Rheinwald, J. G. (2012). MAPK/ERK-Dependent Translation Factor Hyperactivation and Dysregulated Laminin gamma 2 Expression in Oral Dysplasia and Squamous Cell Carcinoma. *Am. J. Pathol.* 180, 2462–2478. doi: 10.1016/j.ajpath.2012.02.028

Degen, M., Wiederkehr, A., La Scala, G. C., Carmann, C., Schnyder, I., and Katsaros, C. (2018). Keratinocytes Isolated From Individual Cleft Lip/Palate Patients Display Variations in Their Differentiation Potential in vitro. *Front. Physiol.* 9:1703. doi: 10.3389/fphys.2018.01703

Dole, N. S., Mazur, C. M., Acevedo, C., Lopez, J. P., Monteiro, D. A., Fowler, T. W., et al. (2017). Osteocyte-Intrinsic TGF-beta Signaling Regulates Bone Quality through Perilacunar/Canalicular Remodeling. *Cell Rep.* 21, 2585–2596. doi: 10.1016/j.celrep.2017.10.115

Dominici, M., Le Blanc, K., Mueller, I., Slaper-Cortenbach, I., Marini, F. C., Krause, D. S., et al. (2006). Minimal criteria for defining multipotent mesenchymal stromal cells. The International Society for Cellular Therapy position statement. *Cytotherapy* 8, 315–317. doi: 10.1080/14653240600855905

Drexler, H. G., and Uphoff, C. C. (2002). Mycoplasma contamination of cell cultures: Incidence, sources, effects, detection, elimination, prevention. *Cytotechnology* 39, 75–90.

Ebrahimi, M., and Botelho, M. (2017). Adult Stem Cells of Orofacial Origin: Current Knowledge and Limitation and Future Trend in Regenerative Medicine. *Tissue Engin. Regener. Med.* 14, 719–733. doi: 10.1007/s13770-017-0078-6

Ehrlich, H. P., Desmouliere, A., Diegelmann, R. F., Cohen, I. K., Compton, C. C., Garner, W. L., et al. (1994). Morphological and immunochemical differences between keloid and hypertrophic scar. *Am. J. Pathol.* 145, 105–113.

Gorlin, R., Cohen, M., and Levin, L. (1990). *Syndromes of the Head and Neck*. Oxford, UK: Oxford University Press.

Green, S. A., Simoes-Costa, M., and Bronner, M. E. (2015). Evolution of vertebrates as viewed from the crest. *Nature* 520, 474–482. doi: 10.1038/nature14436

Gritli-Linde, A. (2008). The Etiopathogenesis of Cleft and Cleft Palate: Usefulness and Caveats of Mouse Models. *Curr. Top. Devel. Biol.* 84, 37–138. doi: 10.1016/s0070-2153(08)00602-9

Hall, B. K. (2000). The neural crest as a fourth germ layer and vertebrates as quadroblastic not triploblastic. *Evol. Dev.* 2, 3–5. doi: 10.1046/j.1525-142x.2000.00032.x

Hewitt, R. E. (2011). Biobanking: the foundation of personalized medicine. *Curr. Opin. Oncol.* 23, 112–119. doi: 10.1097/cco.0b013e32834161b8

Hixon, K., Rhea, L., Standley, J., Canady, F. J., Canady, J. W., and Dunnwald, M. (2017). Interferon Regulatory Factor 6 Controls Proliferation of Keratinocytes From Children With Van der Woude Syndrome. *Cleft Palate Craniofac. J.* 54, 281–286. doi: 10.1597/15-275

Hortis-Dzierzbicka, M., Radkowska, E., and Fudalej, P. S. (2012). Speech outcomes in 10-year-old children with complete unilateral cleft lip and palate after one-stage lip and palate repair in the first year of life. *J. Plast. Reconstr. Aesthet Surg.* 65, 175–181. doi: 10.1016/j.bjps.2011.09.015

Hu, D., Marcucio, R. S., and Helms, J. A. (2003). A zone of frontonasal ectoderm regulates patterning and growth in the face. *Development* 130, 1749–1758. doi: 10.1242/dev.00397

Ichim, T. E., O'heeron, P., and Kesari, S. (2018). Fibroblasts as a practical alternative to mesenchymal stem cells. *J. Transl. Med.* 16:212. doi: 10.1186/s12967-018-1536-1

Kaye, J., Briceño Moraia, L., Curren, L., Bell, J., Mitchell, C., Soini, S., et al. (2016). Consent for Biobanking: The Legal Frameworks of Countries in the BioSHaRE-EU Project. *Biopreserv. Biobank* 14, 195–200. doi: 10.1089/bio.2015.0123

Kindberg, A. A., and Bush, J. O. (2019). Cellular organization and boundary formation in craniofacial development. *Genesis* 57:e23271. doi: 10.1002/dvg.23271

Kousa, Y. A., and Schutte, B. C. (2016). Toward an orofacial gene regulatory network. *Devel. Dynam.* 245, 220–232. doi: 10.1002/dvdy.24341

Leslie, E. J., and Marazita, M. L. (2013). Genetics of Cleft Lip and Cleft Palate. *Am. J. Med. Genet. Part C* 163C, 246–258.

Lopez, E., Berenguer, M., Tingaud-Sequeira, A., Marlin, S., Toutain, A., Denoyelle, F., et al. (2016). Mutations in MYT1, encoding the myelin transcription factor 1, are a rare cause of OAVS. *J. Med. Genet.* 53, 752–760. doi: 10.1136/jmedgenet-2016-103774

Lorsch, J. R., Collins, F. S., and Lippincott-Schwartz, J. (2014). Cell Biology. Fixing problems with cell lines. *Science* 346, 1452–1453. doi: 10.1126/science.1259110

Masters, J. R. W. (2010). Cell line misidentification: the beginning of the end. *Nat. Rev. Cancer* 10, 441–448. doi: 10.1038/nrc2852

Miryounesi, M., Diantpour, M., Motevaseli, E., and Ghafouri-Fard, S. (2016). Homozygosity for a Robertsonian Translocation (13q;14q) in a Phenotypically Normal 44, XX Female with a History of Recurrent Abortion and a Normal Pregnancy Outcome. *J. Reprod. Infertil* 17, 184–187.

Mossey, P., and Modell, B. (2012). Epidemiology of oral clefts 2012: an international perspective. *Front. Oral Biol.* 16, 1–18. doi: 10.1159/000337464

Parisi, L., Ghezzi, B., Bianchi, M. G., Toffoli, A., Rossi, F., Bussolati, O., et al. (2020). Titanium dental implants hydrophilicity promotes preferential serum fibronectin over albumin competitive adsorption modulating early cell response. *Mater. Sci. Eng. C Mater. Biol. Appl.* 117:111307. doi: 10.1016/j.msec.2020.111307

Praetorius (2015). *Homemade PCR TEST for Mycoplasma Contamination* [Online]. Available online at: https://bitesizebio.com/23682/homemade-pcr-test-for-mycoplasma-contamination/. (accessed Jan 29, 2021).

Ravi, M., Paramesh, V., Kaviya, S. R., Anuradha, E., and Solomon, F. D. P. (2015). 3D Cell Culture Systems: Advantages and Applications. *J. Cell. Physiol.* 230, 16–26. doi: 10.1002/jcp.24683

Rottem, S., Kosower, N. S., and Kornspan, J. D. (2012). *Contamination of Tissue Cultures by Mycoplasma.* Available online at: https://www.intechopen.com/books/biomedical-tissue-culture/contamination-of-tissue-cultures-by-mycoplasmas (accessed Oct 17, 2012).

Sanz, A. R., Carrion, F. S., and Chaparro, A. P. (2015). Mesenchymal stem cells from the oral cavity and their potential value in tissue engineering. *Periodontology* 2000, 251–267. doi: 10.1111/prd.12070

Shaw, W. C. (2004). Global Strategies to Reduce the Health Care Burden of Craniofacial Anomalies: Report of WHO Meetings on International Collaborative Research on Craniofacial Anomalies. *Cleft Palate Craniofac. J.* 41, 238–43. doi: 10.1597/03-214.1

Shinde, A. V., Humeres, C., and Frangogiannis, N. G. (2017). The role of alpha-smooth muscle actin in fibroblast-mediated matrix contraction and remodeling. *Biochim. Biophys. Acta Mol. Basis Dis.* 1863, 298–309. doi: 10.1016/j.bbadis.2016.11.006

Siismets, E. M., and Hatch, N. E. (2020). Cranial Neural Crest Cells and Their Role in the Pathogenesis of Craniofacial Anomalies and Coronal Craniosynostosis. *J. Dev. Biol.* 8:18. doi: 10.3390/jdb8030018

Soundararajan, M., and Kannan, S. (2018). Fibroblasts and mesenchymal stem cells: Two sides of the same coin? *J. Cell. Physiol.* 233, 9099–9109. doi: 10.1002/jcp.26860

Tayebi, L., and Moharamzadeh, K. (2018). *Biomaterials for Oral and Dental Tissue Engineering.* New York: Elsevier.

Toffoli, A., Parisi, L., Bianchi, M. G., Lumetti, S., Bussolati, O., and Macaluso, G. M. (2020). Thermal treatment to increase titanium wettability induces selective proteins adsorption from blood serum thus affecting osteoblasts adhesion. *Mater. Sci. Engin. C Mater. Biol. Appl.* 107:110250. doi: 10.1016/j.msec.2019.110250

Tsou, R., Cole, J. K., Nathens, A. B., Isik, F. F., Heimbach, D. M., Engrav, L. H., et al. (2000). Analysis of hypertrophic and normal scar gene expression with cDNA microarrays. *J. Burn. Care Rehabil.* 21, 541–550. doi: 10.1097/00004630-200021060-00012

van Beurden, H. E., Von Den, Hoff, J. W., Torensma, R., Maltha, J. C., and Kuijpers-Jagtman, A. M. (2005). Myofibroblasts in palatal wound healing: prospects for the reduction of wound contraction after cleft palate repair. *J. Dent. Res.* 84, 871–880. doi: 10.1177/154405910508401002

Van Der Woude, A. (1954). Fistula labii inferioris congenita and its association with cleft lip and palate. *Am. J. Hum. Genet.* 2, 244–256.

Van Otterloo, E., Williams, T., and Artinger, K. B. (2016). The old and new face of craniofacial research: How animal models inform human craniofacial genetic and clinical data. *Dev. Biol.* 415, 171–187. doi: 10.1016/j.ydbio.2016.01.017

van Steenberghe, D., Branemark, P. I., Quirynen, M., De Mars, G., and Naert, I. (1991). The rehabilitation of oral defects by osseointegrated implants. *J. Clin. Periodontol.* 18, 488–493. doi: 10.1111/j.1600-051x.1991.tb02321.x

Yue, F., Cheng, Y., Breschi, A., Vierstra, J., Wu, W., Ryba, T., et al. (2014). A comparative encyclopedia of DNA elements in the mouse genome. *Nature* 515, 355–364.

Zhang, W., and Yelick, P. C. (2018). Craniofacial Tissue Engineering. *Cold Spring Harb. Perspect Med.* 8:a025775. doi: 10.1101/cshperspect.a025775

17

Centriolar Protein C2cd3 is Required for Craniofacial Development

*Ching-Fang Chang[1,2], Kari M. Brown[1,2], Yanfen Yang[1,2] and Samantha A. Brugmann[1,2,3,4]**

[1] Division of Developmental Biology, Department of Pediatrics, Cincinnati Children's Hospital Medical Center, Cincinnati, OH, United States, [2] Department of Pediatrics, University of Cincinnati College of Medicine, Cincinnati, OH, United States, [3] Division of Plastic Surgery, Department of Surgery, Cincinnati Children's Hospital Medical Center, Cincinnati, OH, United States, [4] Shriners Children's Hospital, Cincinnati, OH, United States

***Correspondence:**
Samantha A. Brugmann
samantha.brugmann@cchmc.org

The primary cilium is a ubiquitous, microtubule-based cellular organelle. Primary cilia dysfunction results in a group of disorders termed ciliopathies. C2 domain containing 3 centriole elongation regulator (C2cd3), encodes a centriolar protein essential for ciliogenesis. Mutations in human C2CD3 are associated with the human ciliopathy Oral-Facial-Digital syndrome type 14 (OFD14). In order to better understand the etiology of ciliopathies including OFD14, we generated numerous murine models targeting C2cd3. Initial analysis revealed several tissue-specific isoforms of C2cd3, and while the loss of C2cd3 has previously been reported to result in exencephaly, tight mesencephalic flexure, pericardial edema, abnormal heart looping and a twisted body axis, further analysis revealed that genetic background may also contribute to phenotypic variation. Additional analyses of a conditional allelic series targeting C-terminal PKC-C2 domains or the N-terminal C2CD3N-C2 domain of C2cd3 revealed a variable degree of phenotypic severity, suggesting that while the N-terminal C2CD3N-C2 domain was critical for early embryonic development as a whole, there was also a craniofacial specific role for the C2CD3N-C2 domains. Together, through generation of novel models and evaluation of C2cd3 expression, these data provide valuable insight into mechanisms of pathology for craniofacial ciliopathies that can be further explored in the future.

Keywords: primary cilia, ciliopathies, C2cd3, craniofacial development, neural crest

INTRODUCTION

The primary cilium is a cellular organelle comprised of a microtubule-based axoneme extending from the cell surface, and a basal body that resides internally at the base of axoneme. Defects in the structure or function of the ciliary complex result in a class of diseases called ciliopathies. Ciliopathies affect as many as 1 in 800 people. Currently, there are 26 known ciliopathies, 25 predicted ciliopathies and another 400 human diseases considered possible ciliopathies that have yet to be classified (Schock and Brugmann, 2017). Although ciliopathies often present with pleiotropic phenotypes including renal disease, retinal degeneration, obesity, skeletal dysplasia, and craniofacial anomalies (Reiter and Leroux, 2017), 30% of ciliopathies are primarily classified by their craniofacial phenotypes. Craniofacial ciliopathies are most frequently defined by the combinatorial presentation of cleft lip/palate, craniosynostosis, hypertelorism, and micrognathia (Schock and Brugmann, 2017). Interestingly, among the 187 genes that are associated with known ciliopathies, 50 genes encode proteins that localize to basal bodies or centrosomes, and an additional five genes encode proteins that localize to centriolar satellites (Reiter and Leroux, 2017). Thus, understanding formation and function of the basal body is essential for gaining insights for therapeutic treatment of ciliopathies.

The basal body is a modified mother centriole within the centrosome. During G1-S phase of the cell cycle, the daughter centriole gradually loses its daughter centriole-specific proteins and acquires distal and subdistal appendages in late G2 phase. The acquisition of distal appendages and subdistal appendages marks the maturation of the mother centriole and distinguishes the mother centriole from the daughter centriole. During intracellular cilium assembly, Golgi-derived ciliary vesicles dock and fuse at the distal end of the mother centriole, a step called centriole-to-basal body transition. The ciliary axoneme is then assembled by extension of centriolar microtubules underneath the ciliary vesicular cap, while the basal body migrates to the plasma membrane. This basal body/nascent cilium complex then docks and fuses to the plasma membrane through vesicular fusion, a process mediated by distal appendages, which is followed by the further growth and maintenance of the axoneme at the cell surface (Wang and Dynlacht, 2018). The mother centriole within the basal body, the daughter centriole, pericentriolar material (PCM), and centriolar satellites comprise the centrosome, the major microtubule organizing center (MTOC) of the cell. Components localized to the cilium and/or centrosome play essential roles in the dynamics between both organelles; therefore, regulation of the two organelles are tightly linked (Joukov and De Nicolo, 2019).

Recent studies have uncovered several key regulators of centriole maturation and subsequent ciliogenesis. For example, several distal centriolar proteins including C2 domain containing 3 centriole elongation regulator (C2cd3), Oral-Facial-Digital Syndrome 1 Protein (Ofd1) and others are required for the recruitment of distal appendage proteins to the distal end of mother centriole (Singla et al., 2010; Ye et al., 2014; Kazatskaya et al., 2017). C2cd3 and Ofd1 colocalize and physically interact at the distal end of centriole to control centriolar length. Ofd1 acts as a negative regulator of centriole elongation, constraining centriole elongation (Singla et al., 2010). Conversely, C2cd3 is a positive regulator of centriole elongation, as loss of C2cd3 results in shorter centrioles and overexpression of C2cd3 produces hyper-elongated centrioles. More intriguingly, this hyper-elongated centriole can be suppressed by Ofd1 (Thauvin-Robinet et al., 2014). While several other centriolar proteins are required for centriole maturation, elongation, and uncapping (Hsiao et al., 2009; Schmidt et al., 2012; Burke et al., 2014; Kobayashi et al., 2014; Lu et al., 2015; Bhattacharyya et al., 2016), C2cd3 and Ofd1 have been a focus of study because of their association with the human ciliopathy Oral-facial-digital syndrome (OFD).

Oral-facial-digital syndromes represent a group of human ciliopathies caused by mutations to various ciliary proteins. OFDs can be characterized by facial, oral and digital malformations. To date, there are approximately 18 subtypes of OFD syndromes,[1] and each subtype is classified according to the associated gene. Although affected individuals in each subtype present with largely overlapping phenotypes, they do have distinct and unique clinical features. For example, whereas patients with OFD IV display severe tibial dysplasia, patients with OFD VI display cerebellar abnormalities, and patients with OFD IX are characterized by retinal coloboma, in addition to oral, facial and digital defects. Among the subtypes in which causative genes have been identified, almost all genes express proteins which localize to the basal body (Cortes et al., 2016; Franco and Thauvin-Robinet, 2016; Bruel et al., 2017). For example, the most frequent OFD subtype, OFD I, is associated with mutations in *OFD1*, which encodes a protein localized to the basal body. Mutations in *NEK1*, a centrosomal protein responsible for centriole elongation, are associated with OFD II.

Mutations in C2CD3 are associated with OFD14. C2CD3 contains a tandem array of five classical Protein Kinase C C2 domains (PKC-C2) and a novel, divergent C2CD3 N-terminal C2 (C2CD3N-C2) domain (Zhang and Aravind, 2012). C2 domains are present in many proteins and were first discovered as calcium-dependent membrane-targeting domains in the conventional (or Ca^{2+}-activated) PKC isoforms (α, β, γ) (Steinberg, 2008; Farah and Sossin, 2012); however, a variety of C2 domains that have Ca^{2+}-independent membrane-targeting abilities have also been identified (Lee et al., 1999; Djordjevic and Driscoll, 2002). While the PKC-C2 domain predicts membrane-anchoring function of C2CD3, the function of the divergent C2CD3N-C2 domain remains unknown (Zhang and Aravind, 2012). Over 70% of identified OFD14 causing C2CD3 mutations are located within PKC-C2 or C2CD3N-C2 domains, further suggesting the importance for understanding the role of each domain (Boczek et al., 2018).

More recently murine and avian models for OFD14 have been used to examine C2CD3 function. *Hearty* (*Hty*), a recessive lethal mouse mutant identified by forward genetic screening, showed severe developmental defects including those of the neural tube, heart and limb (Hoover et al., 2008). The *Hty* mutation resulted in a largely truncated protein, which contained the divergent C2CD3N-C2 domain but none of the more C-terminal PKC-C2 domains. *talpid*^{2} (*ta*^{2}), a naturally occurring avian mutant, was recently identified as being caused by a 19 bp deletion in exon 32 of *C2CD3* (Chang et al., 2014). Long gestational survival of *ta*^{2} has allowed for additional analyses and determination that it is a bona fide model for OFD14. Mutations in C2cd3 impair the formation and function of primary cilia, and perhaps most notably the transduction of cilia-dependent Hedgehog signaling (Hoover et al., 2008; Chang et al., 2014). Moreover, migration and differentiation of cranial neural crest cells were affected in *ta*^{2}, suggesting a possible cellular etiology of OFD14 (Chang et al., 2014; Schock et al., 2015). Although *ta*^{2} is a model for human OFD14, the lack of avian genetic techniques necessitates murine models for further mechanistic and tissue-dependent study.

[1]https://www.omim.org

Here we report and characterize several novel C2cd3 mouse models, including a publicly available conditional knockout line and two novel CRISPR-targeted lines, targeting regions in the divergent C2CD3N-C2 domain or PKC-C2 domains. We identified the predominant C2cd3 isoforms in a tissue-specific manner and propose that phenotypic variability is a consequence of both tissue-specific isoforms and genetic background. In sum, data presented herein can be used not only to study the etiology of ciliopathic pathologies, but also to address the specific roles of various C2-domains during development.

RESULTS

C2cd3 Is Dynamically Expressed During Embryonic and Craniofacial Development

Despite an accepted role in ciliogenesis, *C2cd3* expression has not been well documented during embryogenesis or craniofacial development. To comprehensively characterize *C2cd3* expression, $C2cd3^{TM1a(EUCOMM)Wtsi}$ mouse ES cells were injected into mouse blastocysts. Recovered transgenic mice (hereafter referred to as $C2cd3^{LacZ}$) expressed a *LacZ*-expression cassette after exon 3 of *C2cd3*, as well as LoxP sites flanking exon 4/5 for the option of tissue-specific gene deletion using Cre-LoxP system (**Figure 1A**). Heterozygous $C2cd3^{LacZ/+}$ mice were viable and morphologically normal, while homozygous $C2cd3^{LacZ/LacZ}$ mice died at approximately E10.5 (data not shown). Whole mount X-gal staining revealed that *C2cd3* was expressed ubiquitously at E10.5 (**Figure 1B**). At E11.5, however, *C2cd3* expression was more spatially distinct with the most robust expression in the neural epithelium, optic cup, oral epithelium, and tongue mesenchyme (**Figure 1C**). Ubiquitous, but variable levels of C2cd3 protein isoforms (255, 232, and 205 kDa) were detected in various embryonic tissues at E11.5 via Western blot analysis (**Figure 1D** asterisks and **Supplementary Figure 1**). The 255 kDa isoform was expressed at varible levels across all isolated tissues (brain, face, heart, limb, and liver) (**Figure 1D**, top asterisk). The 232 kDa isoform was also detected across all tissues, albiet at much lower levels (**Figure 1D**, middle asterisk). The 205 kDa isoform was distinct from other isoforms, as it was robustly expressed in heart tissue (**Figure 1D**, bottom asterisk). While protein prediction tools predicted an additional 214 kDa isoform, we were unable to detect it due to the lack of the C-terminal epitope which the antibody recognizes (**Supplementary Figure 1**). *C2cd3* expression was maintained later in development in both epithelial and mesenchymal tissues, including the lateral ganglionic eminence and ventricular zone of developing neocortex, perichondrium of developing cranial bones, palatal epithelium, oral epithelium, and mesenchyme surrounding Meckel's cartilage at E14.5 (**Figure 1E**). Together, these results suggested that *C2cd3* expression was dynamic throughout embryonic and craniofacial development. We next sought to examine the consequences of impaired *C2cd3* expression.

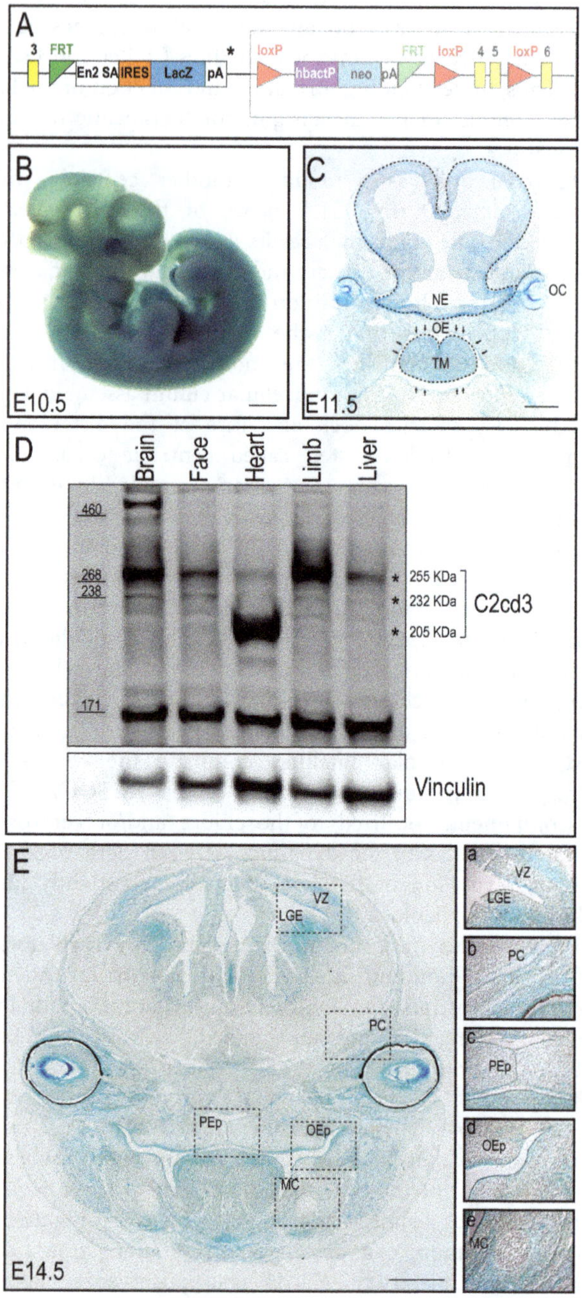

FIGURE 1 | C2cd3 expression in developing mouse embryos. **(A)** Schematic of $C2cd3^{LacZ}$ targeted allele. LacZ expression cassette containing a stop codon (*) was inserted after exon (yellow box) 3. The remaining, unexpressed part of the construct designed for conditional knockout is indicated in the shaded box. **(B)** Whole mount X-gal staining indicates ubiquitous C2cd3 expression in E10.5 embryos. **(C)** Frontal section of an E11.5 embryo showing robust C2cd3 expression in neural epithelium (NE, dotted line), otic cup (OC), oral epithelium (OE, arrows) and tongue mesenchyme (TM, dotted line). **(D)** Western blot of C2cd3 expression in different tissues of E11.5 wild type embryos, showing three C2cd3 isoforms (asterisks). **(E)** Frontal section of E14.5 embryo, revealing robust C2cd3 expression in the lateral ganglionic eminence (LGE) and ventricle zone (VZ) of developing neocortex, perichondrium (PC) of developing cranial bones, palatal epithelium (PEp), oral epithelium (OEp) and mesenchyme surrounding Meckel's cartilage (MC). All scale bars: 0.5 mm.

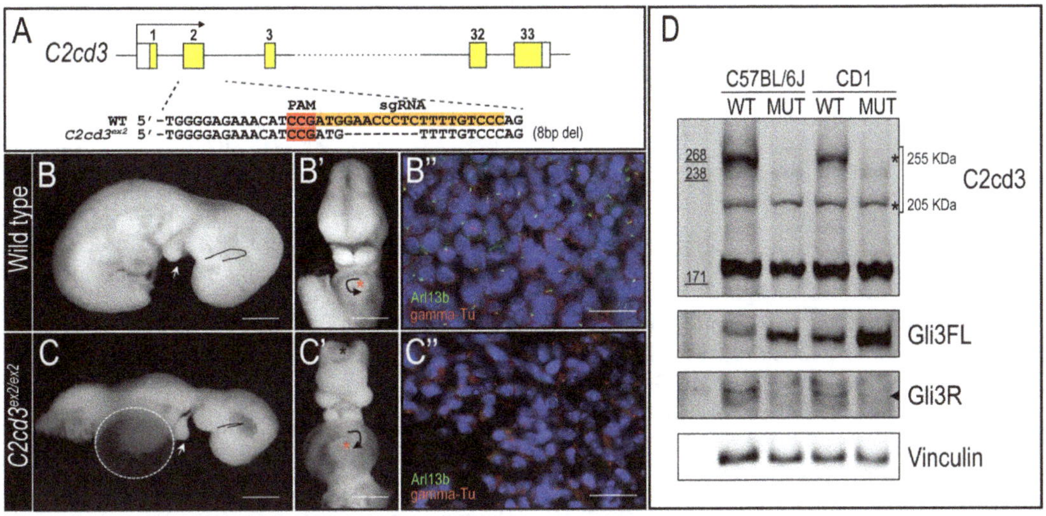

FIGURE 2 | *C2cd3*$^{ex2/ex2}$ mutants present with phenotypes indicative of a ciliopathy. **(A)** Schematic of CRISPR-targeted 8 bp deletion in *C2cd3* at exon 2 which results in a premature stop codon. **(B,C)** Lateral and **(B′,C′)** frontal views of E9.5 wild-type and *C2cd3*$^{ex2/ex2}$ embryos. *C2cd3*$^{ex2/ex2}$ embryos exhibit pericardial edema (white dashed line), tight mesencephalic flexure (black line), mandibular hypoplasia (white arrowhead), abnormal heart looping (black arrow), and exencephaly (black asterisk). The heart is labeled with red asterisks. **(B′′,C′′)** Axonemal (Arl13b) and basal body (gamma-tubulin) immunostaining of E9.5 embryos in wild-type and *C2cd3*$^{ex2/ex2}$ embryos. Scale bars for panels **(B–C′)**: 0.5 mm; **(B′′–C′′)**: 50 μm. **(D)** Western blot of E9.5 wild-type and *C2cd3*$^{ex2/ex2}$ whole embryos showing deletion of the 255 kDa isoform in both C57BL/6J and CD1 backgrounds. The ratio of Gli3FL/Gli3R is increased in *C2cd3*$^{ex2/ex2}$ compared to wild-type.

C2cd3 Mutants Present With Multiple Embryonic Defects

To better understand the biological function of *C2cd3*, we utilized CRISPR-mediated genome editing to generate an 8 bp deletion in exon 2 that resulted in a premature stop codon (henceforth referred to as *C2cd3*^{ex2}) (**Figure 2A**). *C2cd3*$^{ex2/ex2}$ mutants were embryonic lethal at approximately E10.5 and presented with phenotypes similar to those previously reported in *Hty* mutants (Hoover et al., 2008). Mutants were present in Mendelian ratios (**Table 1A**) and 90% of mutants exhibited exencephaly and a twisted body axis (**Figures 2B–C** and **Table 1B**). In addition, 30% of *C2cd3*$^{ex2/ex2}$ mutants presented with pericardial edema, abnormal heart looping, and a tight mesencephalic flexure (**Figures 2B–C′** and **Table 1B**). Compared to the previously reported *C2cd3 Hty* mutants, which commonly presented with twisted body axis, pericardial edema, and tight mesencephalic flexure, the most common phenotypes in *C2cd3*$^{ex2/ex2}$ mutants were exencephaly and twisted body axis. Although polydactyly was also observed in *Hty* mutants at E12.5, we were unable to assess this phenotype in *C2cd3*$^{ex2/ex2}$ mutants because they did not survive past E10.5. To confirm that *C2cd3*$^{ex2/ex2}$ mutants failed to extend primary cilia, immunostaining for Arl13b (ciliary axoneme) and gamma-tubulin (basal body) was performed. Relative to the facial mesenchyme of wild-type embryos, *C2cd3*$^{ex2/ex2}$ mutants lacked Arl13b while maintaining gamma-tubulin staining, indicating that the extension of primary cilia was abolished but the basal body remained intact (**Figure 2B′′,C′′**). Thus, *C2cd3*$^{ex2/ex2}$ mutants lacked cilia and presented with phenotypes indicative of a ciliopathic model.

Genetic modifiers have been hypothesized to alter phenotypic presentation associated with mutations in ciliary genes (Reiter and Leroux, 2017). Given the variation in phenotypic penetrance between *Hty* (C3H/HeN background) and *C2cd3*$^{ex2/ex2}$ mutants, we examined if background strain contributed to severity and degree of penetrance in *C2cd3*$^{ex2/ex2}$ mutants. The *C2cd3*^{ex2} line was generated on an outbred CD1 background, and backcrossed over seven generations onto the inbred C57BL/6J background. We observed that embryos with abnormal heart looping, pericardial edema, and tight mesencephalic flexure

TABLE 1 | Phenotypic presentations of C2cd3 mutants. **(A)** Total number of wild-type, *C2cd3*$^{ex2/+}$, and *C2cd3*$^{ex2/ex2}$ embryos, *n* = number of litters on CD1 and C57BL/6J backgrounds. **(B)** Percentages of phenotypes present in *C2cd3*$^{ex2/ex2}$ mutant embryos.

TABLE 1A | Number of wild-type, *C2cd3* $^{ex2/+}$, and *C2cd3* $^{ex2/ex2}$ embryos on CD1 and C57BL/6J backgrounds.

Background	Total	*n*	Wild-type	Het	Mutant
Outcrossed CD1	52	4	13 (25%)	29 (56%)	10 (19%)
Backcrossed C57BL/6J F4	48	6	13 (27%)	26 (54%)	9 (19%)

TABLE 1B | Observed phenotypic penetrance of *C2cd3*$^{ex2/ex2}$ mutants on CD1 and C57BL/6J backgrounds.

Phenotype	Outcrossed	Backcrossed
	CD1 (*n* = 10)	**C57BL/6J F4 (*n* = 9)**
Exencephaly	9 (90%)	6 (67%)
Tight mesencephalic flexure	3 (30%)	3 (33%)
Abnormal heart looping	3 (30%)	5 (56%)
Twisted body axis	9 (90%)	7 (78%)
Pericardial edema	3 (30%)	4 (44%)

TABLE 2 | Percentage of diagnostic alleles present in *C2cd3*$^{ex2/+}$ mice on CD1 and C57BL/6J backgrounds.

Background	C57BL/6J substrain, %
CD1	28.6
CD1;C57BL/6J, F2	97.4
CD1;C57BL/6J, F7	98.1

increased from 30% on a CD1 background to 56, 44, and 33%, respectively on a C57BL/6J:CD1 mixed background, whereas the percentage of embryos showing exencephaly and twisted body phenotypes was reduced (**Table 1B**, C57BL/6J, F4). The purity of genetic background was examined by miniMUGA (Mouse Universal Genotyping Array) analysis. *C2cd3*$^{ex2/+}$ embyros on an outbred CD1 background possessed 28.6% of the potential diagnostic alleles for C57BL/6J (**Table 2**). In subsequent crosses on the C57BL/6J background, approximately 97% of the potential diagnostic alleles were observed in F2 mice and 98% in F7 mice.

In light of these variable phenotypic presentations, we examined C2CD3 protein expression in both control and *C2cd3*$^{ex2/ex2}$ mutants on C57BL/6J and CD1 backgrounds. Lysates from E9.5 whole embryos of C57BL/6J or CD1 background revealed that the expression of the 255 kDa isoform was lost in mutant embryos on both genetic backgrounds, while the 205 kDa isoform was maintained (**Figure 2D**, top and bottom asterisks, respectively). Interestingly, 232 kDa isoform was undetectable likely because the lysate was collected from whole embryos instead of specific tissue. As deletion of primary cilia often results in aberrant Gli protein processing, we also assayed for Gli3 full length (Gli3FL) and Gli3 repressor (Gli3R) expression in *C2cd3*$^{ex2/ex2}$ mutants. While *C2cd3*$^{ex2/ex2}$ mutants on either background exhibited impaired Gli3 processing, the total amount of Gli3 protein was more robust in embryos on the CD1 background and the ratio between Gli3FL and Gli3R was higher on C57BL/6J background (**Figure 2D** and **Supplementary Figure 2**). Thus, variation in Gli3 protein expression and the Gli3FL/R ratio could contribute to changes in expressivity of phenotypes as the mutation was backcrossed onto a C57BL/6J background.

C2cd3 Is Required for Craniofacial Development

The majority of craniofacial malformations associated with mutations in C2cd3 and OFD14 stem from neural crest derived tissues. Early embryonic lethality in *C2cd3*$^{ex2/ex2}$ mutants prevented an indepth examination of neural crest and craniofacial development. To better understand the function and processing of *C2cd3* relative to craniofacial development, we generated two conditional murine mutants targeting distinct protein domains, and crossed them to neural crest specific drivers.

As the name implies, C2cd3 contains an array of five classical PKC-C2 domains which are predicted to be involved in targeting proteins to the cell membrane. Despite the presence of these domains, there has been very little exploration into their distinct role relative to C2CD3 function, specifically during craniofacial development. To examine the role of PKC-C2 domains, we generated a conditional mouse line in which LoxP sequences flanked exon 9 (*C2cd3*$^{ex9-flox}$, **Figures 3A,A′**). Exon 9 was chosen because upon Cre recombination, all PKC-C2 domains would be excised, generating a 445 aa truncated protein. Moreover, all the *C2cd3* splice variants containing exon 9 were recombined when Cre was expressed. Western blot analysis in wild-type and *C2cd3*$^{ex9fl/fl}$;*Wnt1-Cre* embryos confirmed the loss of the 255 and 232 kDa isoforms in E11.5 mutant facial prominences (**Figure 3B**). Mutant facial prominences also exhibited increased Gli3FL/Gli3R ratio (**Figure 3B**), indicating the cilia were functionally impaired. *C2cd3*$^{ex9fl/fl}$;*Wnt1-Cre* mutant mice survived until late gestation (E18.5) and presented with phenotypes common in OFD14, including cleft palate and a dysmorphic tongue (**Figures 3C–D′**). Whole mount skeletal staining as well as microCT analysis of E17.5 embryos did not show defects in frontal bone or frontal suture formation (**Figures 3E–F′** and **Supplementary Figure 4**), but revealed delayed ossification of palatine bone in *C2cd3*$^{ex9fl/fl}$;*Wnt1-Cre* mutant embryos (**Figures 3G–H′**).

In addition to the array of PKC-C2 domains, C2cd3 also contains a divergent C2CD3N-C2 domain at the N-terminus of the protein. While this domain is conserved among various species (Zhang and Aravind, 2012), the function of C2CD3N-C2 domain remains completely unknown. To determine the role of the C2CD3N-C2 domain, *C2cd3*^{LacZ} mice were bred to FLPeR mice (Farley et al., 2000) to excise the LacZ expression cassette (**Figure 4A**). The resulting progeny (*C2cd3*$^{ex4-5-flox}$), in which LoxP sequences flanked exon 4 and 5, generated a protein with a truncated C2CD3N-C2 domain (**Figure 4A′**). To assess the C2CD3N-C2 domain in neural crest cells, we utilized the *Wnt1-Cre2* driver (Lewis et al., 2013) and assayed protein expression in facial prominences of E11.5 embryos via Western Blot analysis. Relative to wild-type embryos, the 255 kDa isoform of C2cd3 was lost in *C2cd3*$^{ex4-5fl/fl}$;*Wnt1-Cre2* facial prominences. Interestingly, the 232 kDa isoform remained detectable in mutants (**Figure 4B**), suggesting that the 255 kDa isoform is required craniofacial development. Typical of many ciliopathic mutants, *C2cd3*$^{ex4-5fl/fl}$;*Wnt1-Cre2* embryos also displayed an increased Gli3FL/Gli3R ratio (**Figure 4B**). *C2cd3*$^{ex4-5fl/fl}$;*Wnt1-Cre2* mutants survived until late gestation (E18.5). Contrary to *C2cd3*$^{ex9fl/fl}$;*Wnt1-Cre* mutants which didn't reveal a phenotype until approximately E15.5, *C2cd3*$^{ex4-5fl/fl}$;*Wnt1-Cre2* phenotypes were detected as early as E11.5, with characteristic midline widening (**Figures 4C,C′**, dotted line), which was exacerbated by E15.5 (**Figures 4D,D′**, dotted line). *C2cd3*$^{ex4-5fl/fl}$;*Wnt1-Cre2* mutants also presented with cleft palate (**Figures 4E,E′**, dotted line) and a hypoplastic tongue (**Figures 4F,F′**, asterisk). Thus, relative to *C2cd3*$^{ex9fl/fl}$;*Wnt1-Cre*, *C2cd3*$^{ex4-5fl/fl}$;*Wnt1-Cre2* mutants had an earlier onset of craniofacial phenotypes that were more severe in nature. Whole mount skeletal staining of E18.5 *C2cd3*$^{ex4-5fl/fl}$;*Wnt1-Cre2* mutants did not reveal defects in frontal bones or frontal suture (**Figures 4G–H′**), but exhibited delayed ossifications in sphenoid (**Figures 4J,J′**, black arrowhead) and palatine bones (**Figures 4J,J′**, white arrowhead) near the cranial base (**Figures 4I–J′**). These results

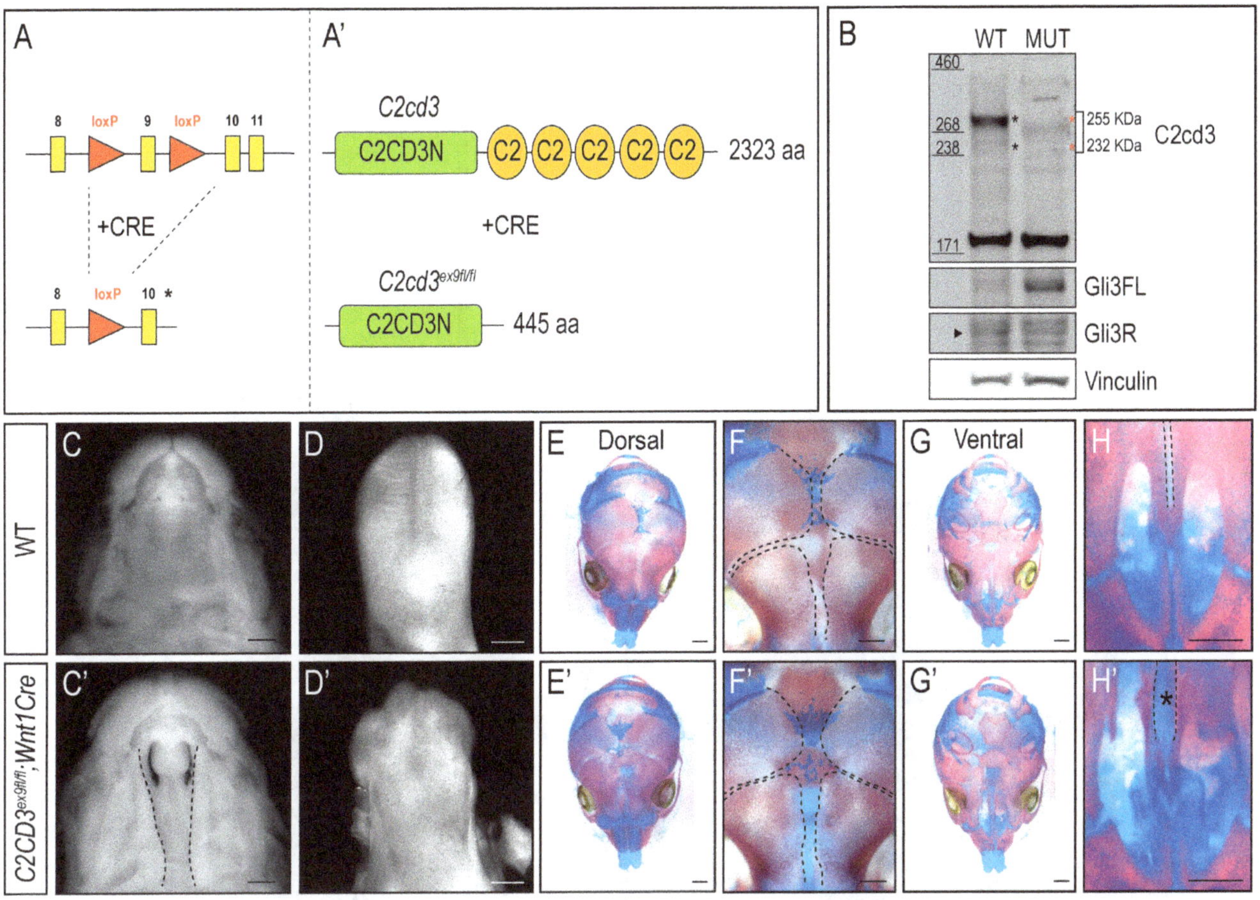

FIGURE 3 | Conditional loss of PKC-C2 domains of C2cd3 results in craniofacial phenotypes. **(A,A′)** Schematic of conditional mouse line generated by CRISPR-targeting with LoxP sequences flanking exon 9. **(B)** Western blot of C2cd3 expression in E11.5 facial prominences showing deletion of the 255 and 232 kDa isoforms in and $C2cd3^{ex9fl/fl}$;*Wnt1-Cre* embryos (red asterisks, $n = 4$ for both wild type and mutant, not shown). **(C,C′)** Palatal and **(D,D′)** glossal views of wild-type and $C2cd3^{ex9fl/fl}$;*Wnt1-Cre* E15.5 embryos. Cleft palate [**(C′)**, dotted lines] and dysmorphic tongue are present in $C2cd3^{ex9fl/fl}$;*Wnt1-Cre* embryos. **(E–H′)** Dorsal and ventral views of whole mount skeletal staining reveals delayed ossification of palatine bone in $C2cd3^{ex9fl/fl}$;*Wnt1-Cre* embryos [**(H,H′)**, asterisk]. Scale bars: 0.5 mm.

suggested that the C2CD3N-C2 domain also plays a functional role during neural crest and craniofacial development, distinct from PKC-C2 domains.

DISCUSSION

Ciliopathies represent a growing disease class with a significant impact on craniofacial development. As no treatments are currently available for these disorders, gaining increased mechanistic understanding of their etiology through model systems is vitally important. Herein, we report three novel animal model systems to allow for future mechanistic studies regarding the onset of ciliopathic phenotypes. Our initial analyses revealed that *C2cd3* was expressed ubiquitously during early embryonic development, and heterogeneously later in development. Robust knockdown of *C2cd3* expression via CRISPR genome editing resulted in severe developmental defects culminating in early embryonic lethality. Moreover, the phenotypic penetrance and severity varied according to genetic background. We also demonstrated that the N-terminal C2CD3N-C2 domain was functionally more critical compared to C-terminal PKC-C2 domains during craniofacial development, by examining conditional alleles with two neural crest-specific drivers. These studies not only generate several new resources for the craniofacial community, but also suggest several factors that contribute to the onset of craniofacial phenotypes in ciliopathic conditions.

Variation in Ciliopathic Phenotypes Is Likely Due to Genetic Modifiers

Variable penetrance and lack of genotype-phenotype concordance has long been a challenge for definitive diagnoses of many genetic diseases. Ciliopathies often exhibit multiple and overlapping clinical features owing to the fact that cilia extend from almost all types of cells in the body. For example, Oral-facial-digital syndrome 1-18 (OFD1-18), short-rib polydactyly syndromes (SRPS), Jeune asphyxiating thoracic

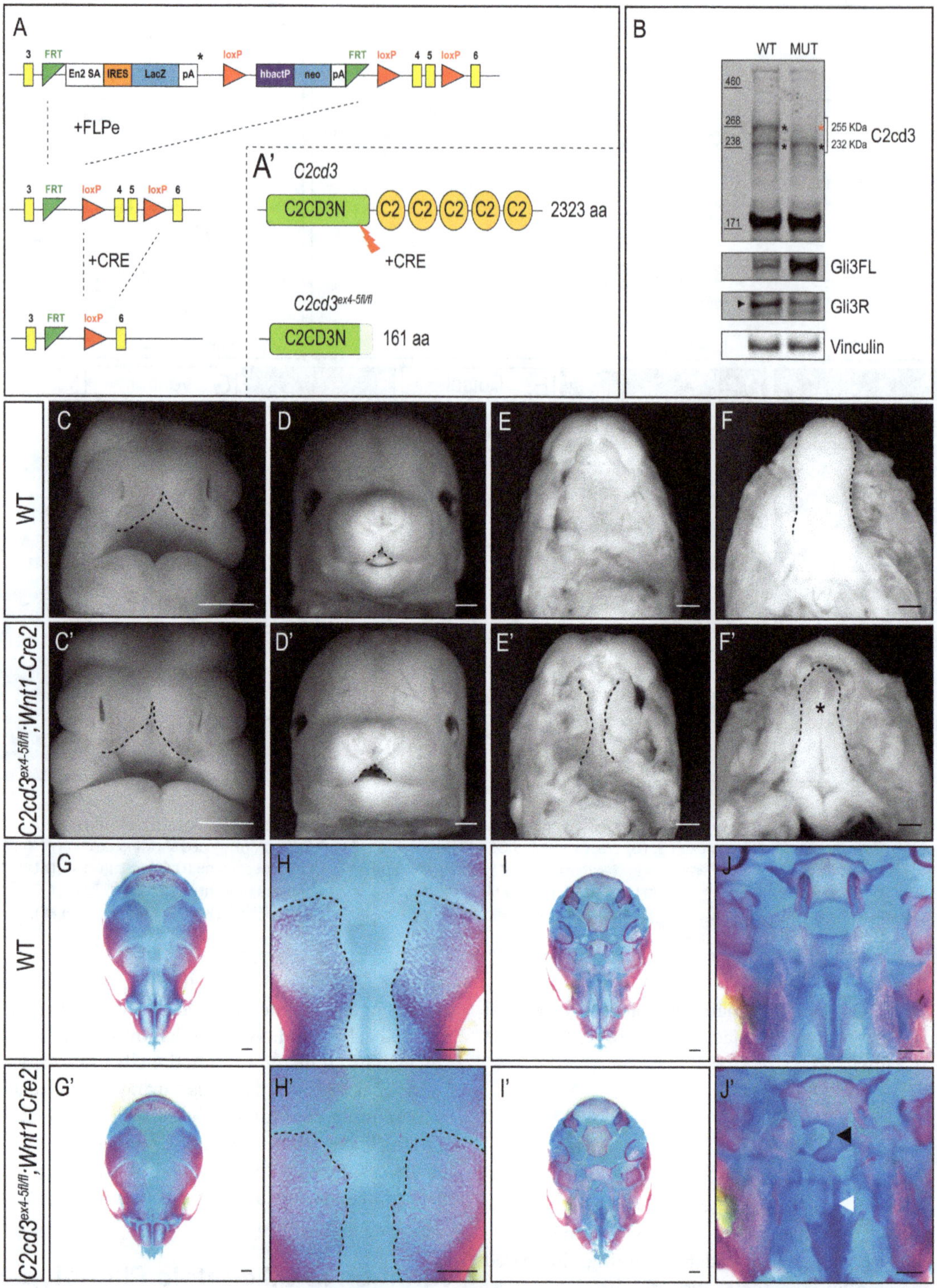

FIGURE 4 | Conditional loss of C2CD3N-C2 domain results in craniofacial phenotypes. **(A,A′)** *C2cd3*^{LacZ} mice were bred to FLPeR mice to excise the LacZ expression cassette, resulting in *C2cd3*$^{ex4-5flox}$ progeny with LoxP sequences flanking exon 4 and 5 and generating a protein with a truncated C2CD3N-C2 domain. **(B)** Western blot of C2cd3 expression in E11.5 facial prominences showing deletion of the longest C2cd3 isoform 255 kDa in and *C2cd3*$^{ex4-5fl/fl}$; *Wnt1-Cre* (red asterisk, $n = 4$ for both wild type and mutant, not shown). **(C,C′)** *C2cd3*$^{ex4-5fl/fl}$;*Wnt1-Cre2* embryos have characteristic midline widening (dotted line) at E11.5 compared to wild-type, which is exacerbated at E15.5 [**(D,D′)**, dotted lines], as well as cleft palate [**(E,E′)**, dotted line] and a hypoplastic tongue [**(F,F′)**, asterisk]. **(G,G′)** Dorsal views of skull. E18.5 *C2cd3*$^{ex4-5fl/fl}$;*Wnt1-Cre2* embryos have normal frontal bone and frontal suture **(H,H′)** development. **(I,I′)** Ventral views of skull. E18.5 *C2cd3*$^{ex4-5fl/fl}$;*Wnt1-Cre2* embryos present with abnormal bone growth of the sphenoid [**(J,J′)**, black arrowhead] and palatine bone [**(J,J′)**, white arrowhead]. Scale bars: 0.5 mm.

dystrophy (JATD), Ellis van Creveld syndrome (EVC), and Cranioectodermal dysplasia (CED) all present with varied and overlapping phenotypes making diagnosis difficult. Yet, despite this understanding, the factors that contribute to variable and overlapping phenotypic presentation remain nebulous.

Studies using murine models on inbred background have provided valuable information as to the factors that contribute to phenotypic variability (Nadeau, 2001; Hamilton and Yu, 2012; Kousi and Katsanis, 2015). Numerous studies have reported different levels of phenotypic severity on various inbred backgrounds (Jones et al., 2008), as utilization of these strains can more readily identify genetic modifiers via SNP array, GigaMuga and quantitative trait locus (QTL) analysis (Morgan et al., 2015; Snedeker et al., 2019). Studies such as these have been instrumental in identifying genetic modifiers that can contribute to increasing the variability of phenotypic presentations in ciliopathies. One example of evidence of such modifiers was the report demonstrating that a 430C to T transition in *MGC1203* gene (a pericentriolar protein CCDC28B that interacts with several Bardet–Biedl syndrome, BBS proteins) has an epistatic effect on *BBS* patients (Badano et al., 2006). While mutations in *MGC1203* were insufficient to cause BBS, individual BBS patients who carry the 430T variant of *MGC1203* were more severely affected and have early onset retinitis pigmentosa. Another example of genetic modifiers impacting ciliopathic phenotypes was demonstrated via the relationship between *AHI1* and *NPHP1*. Both *AHI1* and *NPHP1* encode ciliary proteins that physically interact, and mutations found in these two genes are associated with Joubert syndrome. Interestingly, specific variants in these genes significantly increased the risk for onset of tissue-specific phenotypes in patients (Louie et al., 2010).

Although it remains a challenge to identify genetic modifiers for disease-linked genes in humans, murine models may provide useful insight into origins of phenotypic variation. Our data indicated that the severity of phenotypic presentations in $C2cd3^{ex2/ex2}$ mutant mice is variable on different genetic background (**Table 1B**), suggesting there are potential genetic modifiers for C2cd3. As C2cd3 localizes to the distal end of the mother centriole and interacts with other centriolar proteins in a hierarchical manner, it is possible that any variant within proteins that localize to that area could impact phenotypic severity of C2cd3 mutations. Furthermore, hypotheses such as these could also apply to variation in human OFD patients, in terms of phenotypic presentation, diagnostic assessment and clinical outcome.

Functional Roles of *C2cd3* Splice Variants and Isoforms

Most genes have multiple exons, which can contribute to specific isoforms via alternative splicing. Exons are defined by the 5′ splice site, the 3′ splice site and the branch point. These sequence elements can be recognized by the spliceosome complex, which undergoes serial events to remove the introns of pre-mRNA and to form mature mRNA. In general, exons that are used and included alternatively in the mature mRNA, have splice sites and branch point that deviate moreso than the consensus sequences present in constitutively used exons; hence, they have lower binding affinity for the spliceosome. From an evolutionary point of view, alternative splicing is used to increase diversity under different physiological conditions to affect function, binding affinity, and localizations of the protein products (Kelemen et al., 2013). Murine *C2cd3* has 33 exons and 8 splice variants.[2] Among these variants, seven are protein-coding, producing four distinct protein isoforms (255, 232, 214, and 205 kDa), while one is a non-coding mRNA (**Supplementary Figure 1**). Our data revealed that while *C2cd3* was expressed ubiquitously in early developmental stages, the level of expression and the prevalence of distinct isoforms varied between different tissues. Given the variable temporal and spatial expression of *C2cd3* during craniofacial development, it will be important to understand the distribution and spatial expression of individual splice variants/protein isoforms over time. Our data herein suggested that the N-terminal C2CD3N-C2 domain was more critical during craniofacial development than C-terminal PKC-C2 domain. Interestingly, within the four C2cd3 protein isoforms there are two isoforms that contain a C2CD3N-C2 domain (255 and 214 kDa; **Supplementary Figures 1A,C**). We hypothesize that these two isoforms are expressed in tissues most affected in $C2cd3^{ex2/ex2}$ or $C2cd3^{ex4-5fl/fl}$;*Wnt1Cre2* mutants, in which the targeted mutations disrupt C2CD3N-C2 domain. Alternatively, we hypothesize that isoforms without a C2CD3N-C2 domain (232 and 205 kDa; **Supplementary Figures 1B,D**) are dispensable for craniofacial development, as the 232 kDa isoform is still expressed $C2cd3^{ex4-5fl/fl}$;*Wnt1Cre2* facial mesenchyme. Our future studies will focus on the spatial expressions and specialized functions for each C2cd3 isoform expressed in craniofacial tissues.

A Role for the C2CD3N-C2 Domain During Ciliogenesis and Protein–Protein Interaction

Many ciliary proteins in the transition zone contain both classical PKC-C2 and novel C2-domains. These domains have been hypothesized to serve as a functional interaction module within the transition zone (Zhang and Aravind, 2010, 2012; Remans et al., 2014). Although the classical PKC-C2 domain contains a Ca^{2+}-binding pocket, which makes contact with the plasma membrane, all other C2 domains within the superfamily do not bind Ca^{2+} (Zhang and Aravind, 2010). Moreover, novel C2 domains, including the C2CD3N-C2 domain, have a unique sequence and are highly conserved among different orthologs, yet share little sequence homology to other known C2 domains. For example, a recent study reported that centriolar protein CEP120 possessed three Ca^{2+}-independent, novel C2 domains that potentially played a role in mediating microtubule-binding (Sharma et al., 2018). Our data provide further evidence for the functional importance of a non-classical C2 domain, specifically within craniofacial development. Disruption of C2CD3N-C2 domain in $C2cd3^{ex4-5fl/fl}$;*Wnt1Cre2* mice resulted

[2]https://www.ncbi.nlm.nih.gov/gene/277939

in severe craniofacial phenotypes including midfacial widening, palatal clefting and hypoglossia; while deletion of all PKC-C2 domains in *C2cd3*$^{ex9fl/fl}$*;Wnt1Cre* mice produced only mild craniofacial phenotypes. Interestingly, it has been shown that C2CD3 ortholog SAS-1 in *C. elegans* contains a unique N-terminal, non-classical C2 domain (von Tobel et al., 2014). SAS-1 also localizes to the centriole and has the ability to bind to and stabilize microtubules. Based on these results, we hypothesize that the C2CD3N-C2 domain may have a distinct and required function when compared to the five PKC-C2 domains, specifically in microtubule binding/stabilization, in addition to the known functions in membrane targeting and vesicle docking. Our future studies will address the specific role of the C2CD3N-C2 domain within tissues of the craniofacial complex.

Functional Importance of Ciliary Proteins in Skeletogenesis

In addition to axial skeletal defects, patients with ciliopathies also frequently present with malformation of the craniofacial skeleton (Baker and Beales, 2009; Schock and Brugmann, 2017). The importance of cilia in skeletal development has been demonstrated in many animal models (Yuan and Yang, 2015). Here we show that deletion of *C2cd3* within the progenitors of the craniofacial skeleton (neural crest cells) affected the development of intramembranous skeletal elements. With deletion of all PKC-C2 domains in C2cd3, we observed delayed ossifications in the cranial base (palatine bones). Moreover, deletion of N-terminal C2CD3N-C2 domains in addition to all PKC-C2 domains extended the delayed ossifications further to the sphenoid bone. This result was consistent with the previous findings that deletion of ciliary genes *Kif3a* or *Ift88* using *Wnt1-Cre* resulted in reduced neural crest cell-derived cranial bones (Kolpakova-Hart et al., 2007; Tian et al., 2017). As the majority of the craniofacial skeleton is derived from cranial neural crest cells and differentiates through intramembranous ossification, it will be important to understand how deletion of C2cd3 impacts the sequential steps of intramembranous ossification including neural crest condensation, osteoblast/osteocyte differentiation, and matrix/periosteum formation. Our future work will specifically address this question and examine the molecular basis for the onset of these phenotypes.

Mouse models established here can serve as powerful tools to study the function of C2cd3 and primary cilia during development of the craniofacial skeleton. Ciliopathy patients with craniofacial anomalies often have abnormal skeletogenesis and require surgical reconstructions using autologous grafts from mesodermal-derived bones like the rib or iliac crest. The surgical process is painful and often the tissue fails to engraft. Using tools like those described herein, we are able to begin understanding cellular and molecular mechanisms necessary for skeletogenesis within the craniofacial complex and potentially apply this knowledge toward the application of alternative surgical repair for OFD, as well as ciliopathy patients, in general.

MATERIALS AND METHODS

Mice

Mouse ES cell line *C2cd3*$^{TM1a(EUCOMM)Wtsi}$ was purchased from EuMMCR.[3] ES cell microinjection was performed by Transgenic Animal and Genome Editing (TAGE) Core facility of Cincinnati Children's Hospital Medical Center (CCHMC). The resulting chimeric mice were bred to wild type to obtain heterozygous (*C2cd3*$^{LacZ/+}$) animals. CRISPR-targeted *C2cd3* knockout mice were designed and generated by TAGE Core facility of CCHMC. All animals were maintained by Veterinary Services of CCHMC with IACUC approval.

Analysis of Mutant Embryos

C2cd3 mice were maintained on a CD1 background or serially backcrossed to C57BL/6J. Genotyping for the 8 bp deletion was performed by PCR and Sanger Sequencing. Embryos were harvested via Caesarian section, dissected, and examined. Embryos were fixed in Bouin's fixative overnight at room temperature, washed 3 times with PBS, and imaged on the Leica M165FC microscope.

X-Gal Staining

C2cd3$^{LacZ/+}$ embryos at various time points were dissected in cold PBS (pH 7.4) and fixed with 2% Paraformaldehyde (PFA) plus 0.25% Glutaraldehyde, 0.02% NP-40, 0.1% Sodium Deoxycholate in PBS at 4°C with gentle shaking for 1-2 hours. The samples were then switched to X-gal staining solution (5 mM $K_3Fe(CN)_6$, 5 mM $K_4Fe(CN)_6*3H_2O$, 2 mM $MgCl_2$, and 1 mg/mL X-gal in PBS) at 37°C with gentle shaking for 12-16 hours. The staining was terminated with 3% DMSO in PBS and post-fixed by 4% PFA in PBS. Whole mount images were taken before obtaining microtome sections.

Western Blot

Protein lysate was prepared from E9.5 mouse embryos or E11.5 facial prominences (epithelium was removed by treating the samples with 3 mg/mL Dispase/PBS at 37°C for 30 min) in RIPA buffer with protease and phosphatase inhibitors and 20 μg of sample was loaded onto 3–8% NuPAGE Tris-Acetate gels (ThermoFisher) for Western blot. C2cd3 (1:500; Antibodies-online.com ABIN2591132), Gli3 (1:1,000; R&D Systems, AF3690), and Vinculin (1:2,000; Santa Cruz, sc-73614) antibodies were used. Blots were imaged on LICOR Odyssey imager.

Immunofluorescence Staining

Cryosections of E9.5 embryos were fixed in 4% PFA for 5 min, washed three times with PBS. The sections were then blocked in 5% normal goat serum in PBS for 30 min and then incubated with Arl13b (1:1,000; Proteintech, 17711-1-AP) and gamma-Tubulin (1:1,000; Sigma, T6557) in blocking buffer at 4°C overnight. Goat anti-rabbit Alexa 488 and goat anti-mouse Alexa 594 were used for secondary antibodies at 1:1,000 in blocking buffer, room temperature, 1–2 h. DAPI (1:10,000) was used for nuclear staining.

[3]https://www.eummcr.org

MiniMUGA Genotyping

MiniMUGA (Mouse Universal Genotyping Array genotyping, Neogen Genomics Co.) genotyping was performed by GeneSeek (Neogen; Lincoln, NE, United States). Genomic DNA was isolated using ThermoFisher PureLink gDNA kit. Approximately 10,800 markers were analyzed with MiniMUGA.

ETHICS STATEMENT

The animal study was reviewed and approved by Veterinary Services of CCHMC with IACUC approval.

AUTHOR CONTRIBUTIONS

C-FC performed all embryonic and expression analysis. KB and YY performed all backcrossing studies and genetic background analysis. SB conceived and funded project. SB, C-FC, and KB wrote and edited manuscript. All authors contributed to the article and approved the submitted version.

ACKNOWLEDGMENTS

We would like to thank Lisa Lemen for assistance in microCT acquisition and analysis (Preclinical Imaging Core - University of Cincinnati) and Yueh-Chiang Hu (The Transgenic Animal and Genome Editing Core—CCHMC). We would also like to thank members of the Brugmann lab for helpful comments and feedback.

SUPPLEMENTARY MATERIAL

Supplementary Figure 1 | Reported splice variants in murine C2cd3. Seven protein-coding variants (NCBI accession number NM or XM) produce four protein isoforms (one non-coding mRNA is also predicted (XR_003946487.1, not shown)). Two isoforms contain C2CD3N-C2 domain **(A,C)** while two isoforms contain only PKC-C2 domains **(B,D)**.

Supplementary Figure 2 | (A) Western blot of Gli3FL and Gli3R in CD1 and C57BL/6J backgrounds. **(B)** Densitometry of Gli3FL and Gli3R in each lane was measured by ImageJ. Gli3FL/Gli3R ratio is higher on C57BL/6J background ($n = 4$, *t*-test, * indicates $P < 0.05$).

Supplementary Figure 3 | Exon expression in *C2cd3* mutants. **(A)** RT-qPCR of exon 8-9 and 32-33 in wild-type ($n = 5$), *C2cd3*$^{ex2/+}$ ($n = 6$), and *C2cd3*$^{ex2/ex2}$ ($n = 4$) embryos shows significantly reduced, but detectable levels of *C2cd3* downstream of exon 2 (*t*-test, * indicates $P < 0.05$; ** indicates $P < 0.01$; NS: not significant).

Supplementary Figure 4 | MicroCT analysis of E17.5 mouse embryos. Snapshots of microCT 3D images of **(A,A′)** wild type and **(B,B′)** *C2cd3*$^{ex9fl/fl}$;*Wnt1Cre* mutant embryos. The frontal bones **(A,B)** and mandibular bones **(A′,B′)** are marked by blue. The bone volume of **(C)** frontal bones and mandibular bones **(D)** was measured by Inveon Workstation Software (Siemens Medical Inc), the results indicates that there is no significant difference between wild type and mutant ($n = 4$ for wild type or mutant, *t*-test, NS: not significant).

REFERENCES

Badano, J. L., Leitch, C. C., Ansley, S. J., May-Simera, H., Lawson, S., Lewis, R. A., et al. (2006). Dissection of epistasis in oligogenic Bardet-Biedl syndrome. *Nature* 439, 326–330. doi: 10.1038/nature04370

Baker, K., and Beales, P. L. (2009). Making sense of cilia in disease: the human ciliopathies. *Am. J. Med. Genet. C Semin. Med. Genet.* 151C, 281–295. doi: 10.1002/ajmg.c.30231

Bhattacharyya, S., Rainey, M. A., Arya, P., Mohapatra, B. C., Mushtaq, I., Dutta, S., et al. (2016). Endocytic recycling protein EHD1 regulates primary cilia morphogenesis and SHH signaling during neural tube development. *Sci. Rep.* 6:20727.

Boczek, N. J., Hopp, K., Benoit, L., Kraft, D., Cousin, M. A., Blackburn, P. R., et al. (2018). Characterization of three ciliopathy pedigrees expands the phenotype associated with biallelic C2CD3 variants. *Eur. J. Hum. Genet.* 26, 1797–1809. doi: 10.1038/s41431-018-0222-3

Bruel, A. L., Franco, B., Duffourd, Y., Thevenon, J., Jego, L., Lopez, E., et al. (2017). Fifteen years of research on oral-facial-digital syndromes: from 1 to 16 causal genes. *J. Med. Genet.* 54, 371–380.

Burke, M. C., Li, F. Q., Cyge, B., Arashiro, T., Brechbuhl, H. M., Chen, X., et al. (2014). Chibby promotes ciliary vesicle formation and basal body docking during airway cell differentiation. *J. Cell Biol.* 207, 123–137. doi: 10.1083/jcb.201406140

Chang, C. F., Schock, E. N., O'Hare, E. A., Dodgson, J., Cheng, H. H., Muir, W. M., et al. (2014). The cellular and molecular etiology of the craniofacial defects in the avian ciliopathic mutant talpid2. *Development* 141, 3003–3012. doi: 10.1242/dev.105924

Cortes, C. R., McInerney-Leo, A. M., Vogel, I., Rondon Galeano, M. C., Leo, P. J., Harris, J. E., et al. (2016). Mutations in human C2CD3 cause skeletal dysplasia and provide new insights into phenotypic and cellular consequences of altered C2CD3 function. *Sci. Rep.* 6:24083.

Djordjevic, S., and Driscoll, P. C. (2002). Structural insight into substrate specificity and regulatory mechanisms of phosphoinositide 3-kinases. *Trends Biochem. Sci.* 27, 426–432. doi: 10.1016/s0968-0004(02)02136-9

Farah, C. A., and Sossin, W. S. (2012). The role of C2 domains in PKC signaling. *Adv. Exp. Med. Biol.* 740, 663–683. doi: 10.1007/978-94-007-2888-2_29

Farley, F. W., Soriano, P., Steffen, L. S., and Dymecki, S. M. (2000). Widespread recombinase expression using FLPeR (flipper) mice. *Genesis* 28, 106–110. doi: 10.1002/1526-968x(200011/12)28:3/4<106::aid-gene30>3.0.co;2-t

Franco, B., and Thauvin-Robinet, C. (2016). Update on oral-facial-digital syndromes (OFDS). *Cilia* 5:12.

Hamilton, B. A., and Yu, B. D. (2012). Modifier genes and the plasticity of genetic networks in mice. *PLoS Genet.* 8:e1002644. doi: 10.1371/journal.pgen.1002644

Hoover, A. N., Wynkoop, A., Zeng, H., Jia, J., Niswander, L. A., and Liu, A. (2008). C2cd3 is required for cilia formation and Hedgehog signaling in mouse. *Development* 135, 4049–4058. doi: 10.1242/dev.029835

Hsiao, Y. C., Tong, Z. J., Westfall, J. E., Ault, J. G., Page-McCaw, P. S., and Ferland, R. J. (2009). Ahi1, whose human ortholog is mutated in Joubert syndrome, is required for Rab8a localization, ciliogenesis and vesicle trafficking. *Hum. Mol. Genet.* 18, 3926–3941. doi: 10.1093/hmg/ddp335

Jones, N. C., Lynn, M. L., Gaudenz, K., Sakai, D., Aoto, K., Rey, J. P., et al. (2008). Prevention of the neurocristopathy Treacher Collins syndrome through inhibition of p53 function. *Nat. Med.* 14, 125–133. doi: 10.1038/nm1725

Joukov, V., and De Nicolo, A. (2019). The centrosome and the primary cilium: the yin and yang of a hybrid organelle. *Cells* 8:701. doi: 10.3390/cells8070701

Kazatskaya, A., Kuhns, S., Lambacher, N. J., Kennedy, J. E., Brear, A. G., McManus, G. J., et al. (2017). Primary cilium formation and ciliary protein trafficking is regulated by the atypical MAP Kinase MAPK15 in *Caenorhabditis elegans* and human cells. *Genetics* 207, 1423–1440. doi: 10.1534/genetics.117.300383

Kelemen, O., Convertini, P., Zhang, Z., Wen, Y., Shen, M., Falaleeva, M., et al. (2013). Function of alternative splicing. *Gene* 514, 1–30. doi: 10.1002/9783527678679.dg00350

Kobayashi, T., Kim, S., Lin, Y. C., Inoue, T., and Dynlacht, B. D. (2014). The CP110-interacting proteins Talpid3 and Cep290 play overlapping and distinct roles in cilia assembly. *J. Cell Biol.* 204, 215–229. doi: 10.1083/jcb.201304153

Kolpakova-Hart, E., Jinnin, M., Hou, B., Fukai, N., and Olsen, B. R. (2007). Kinesin-2 controls development and patterning of the vertebrate skeleton by Hedgehog- and Gli3-dependent mechanisms. *Dev. Biol.* 309, 273–284. doi: 10.1016/j.ydbio.2007.07.018

Kousi, M., and Katsanis, N. (2015). Genetic modifiers and oligogenic inheritance. *Cold Spring Harb. Perspect. Med.* 5:a017145. doi: 10.1101/cshperspect.a017145

Lee, J. O., Yang, H., Georgescu, M. M., Di Cristofano, A., Maehama, T., Shi, Y., et al. (1999). Crystal structure of the PTEN tumor suppressor: implications for its phosphoinositide phosphatase activity and membrane association. *Cell* 99, 323–334.

Lewis, A. E., Vasudevan, H. N., O'Neill, A. K., Soriano, P., and Bush, J. O. (2013). The widely used Wnt1-Cre transgene causes developmental phenotypes by ectopic activation of Wnt signaling. *Dev. Biol.* 379, 229–234. doi: 10.1016/j.ydbio.2013.04.026

Louie, C. M., Caridi, G., Lopes, V. S., Brancati, F., Kispert, A., Lancaster, M. A., et al. (2010). AHI1 is required for photoreceptor outer segment development and is a modifier for retinal degeneration in nephronophthisis. *Nat. Genet.* 42, 175–180. doi: 10.1038/ng.519

Lu, Q., Insinna, C., Ott, C., Stauffer, J., Pintado, P. A., Rahajeng, J., et al. (2015). Early steps in primary cilium assembly require EHD1/EHD3-dependent ciliary vesicle formation. *Nat. Cell Biol.* 17, 228–240. doi: 10.1038/ncb3109

Morgan, A. P., Fu, C. P., Kao, C. Y., Welsh, C. E., Didion, J. P., Yadgary, L., et al. (2015). The mouse universal genotyping array: from substrains to subspecies. *G3 (Bethesda)* 6, 263–279. doi: 10.1534/g3.115.022087

Nadeau, J. H. (2001). Modifier genes in mice and humans. *Nat. Rev. Genet.* 2, 165–174. doi: 10.1038/35056009

Reiter, J. F., and Leroux, M. R. (2017). Genes and molecular pathways underpinning ciliopathies. *Nat. Rev. Mol. Cell Biol.* 18, 533–547. doi: 10.1038/nrm.2017.60

Remans, K., Burger, M., Vetter, I. R., and Wittinghofer, A. (2014). C2 domains as protein-protein interaction modules in the ciliary transition zone. *Cell Rep.* 8, 1–9. doi: 10.1016/j.celrep.2014.05.049

Schmidt, K. N., Kuhns, S., Neuner, A., Hub, B., Zentgraf, H., and Pereira, G. (2012). Cep164 mediates vesicular docking to the mother centriole during early steps of ciliogenesis. *J. Cell Biol.* 199, 1083–1101. doi: 10.1083/jcb.201202126

Schock, E. N., and Brugmann, S. A. (2017). Discovery, diagnosis, and etiology of craniofacial ciliopathies. *Cold Spring Harb. Perspect. Biol.* 9:a028258. doi: 10.1101/cshperspect.a028258

Schock, E. N., Chang, C. F., Struve, J. N., Chang, Y. T., Chang, J., Delany, M. E., et al. (2015). Using the avian mutant talpid2 as a disease model for understanding the oral-facial phenotypes of oral-facial-digital syndrome. *Dis. Model. Mech.* 8, 855–866.

Sharma, A., Gerard, S. F., Olieric, N., and Steinmetz, M. O. (2018). Cep120 promotes microtubule formation through a unique tubulin binding C2 domain. *J. Struct. Biol.* 203, 62–70. doi: 10.1016/j.jsb.2018.01.009

Singla, V., Romaguera-Ros, M., Garcia-Verdugo, J. M., and Reiter, J. F. (2010). Ofd1, a human disease gene, regulates the length and distal structure of centrioles. *Dev. Cell* 18, 410–424. doi: 10.1016/j.devcel.2009.12.022

Snedeker, J., Gibbons, W. J. Jr., Paulding, D. F., Abdelhamed, Z., Prows, D. R., and Stottmann, R. W. (2019). Gpr63 is a modifier of microcephaly in Ttc21b mouse mutants. *PLoS Genet.* 15:e1008467. doi: 10.1371/journal.pgen.1008467

Steinberg, S. F. (2008). Structural basis of protein kinase C isoform function. *Physiol. Rev.* 88, 1341–1378. doi: 10.1152/physrev.00034.2007

Thauvin-Robinet, C., Lee, J. S., Lopez, E., Herranz-Perez, V., Shida, T., Franco, B., et al. (2014). The oral-facial-digital syndrome gene C2CD3 encodes a positive regulator of centriole elongation. *Nat. Genet.* 46, 905–911. doi: 10.1038/ng.3031

Tian, H., Feng, J., Li, J., Ho, T. V., Yuan, Y., Liu, Y., et al. (2017). Intraflagellar transport 88 (IFT88) is crucial for craniofacial development in mice and is a candidate gene for human cleft lip and palate. *Hum. Mol. Genet.* 26, 860–872.

von Tobel, L., Mikeladze-Dvali, T., Delattre, M., Balestra, F. R., Blanchoud, S., Finger, S., et al. (2014). SAS-1 is a C2 domain protein critical for centriole integrity in *C. elegans*. *PLoS Genet.* 10:e1004777. doi: 10.1371/journal.pgen.1004777

Wang, L., and Dynlacht, B. D. (2018). The regulation of cilium assembly and disassembly in development and disease. *Development* 145:dev151407.

Ye, X., Zeng, H., Ning, G., Reiter, J. F., and Liu, A. (2014). C2cd3 is critical for centriolar distal appendage assembly and ciliary vesicle docking in mammals. *Proc. Natl. Acad. Sci. U.S.A.* 111, 2164–2169. doi: 10.1073/pnas.1318737111

Yuan, X., and Yang, S. (2015). Cilia/Ift protein and motor -related bone diseases and mouse models. *Front. Biosci.* 20:515–555. doi: 10.2741/4323

Zhang, D., and Aravind, L. (2010). Identification of novel families and classification of the C2 domain superfamily elucidate the origin and evolution of membrane targeting activities in eukaryotes. *Gene* 469, 18–30. doi: 10.1016/j.gene.2010.08.006

Zhang, D., and Aravind, L. (2012). Novel transglutaminase-like peptidase and C2 domains elucidate the structure, biogenesis and evolution of the ciliary compartment. *Cell Cycle* 11, 3861–3875. doi: 10.4161/cc.22068

18

The Chromatin Regulator *Ankrd11* Controls Palate and Cranial Bone Development

Daniela Marta Roth[1†], Pranidhi Baddam[1†], Haiming Lin[1†], Marta Vidal-García[2†], Jose David Aponte[2†], Sarah-Thea De Souza[1†], Devyn Godziuk[3], Adrianne Eve Scovil Watson[3], Tim Footz[3], Nathan F. Schachter[4,5], Sean E. Egan[4,5†], Benedikt Hallgrímsson[2†], Daniel Graf[1,3†] and Anastassia Voronova[3,6*†]*

[1] School of Dentistry, Faculty of Medicine and Dentistry, University of Alberta, Edmonton, AB, Canada, [2] Department of Cell Biology & Anatomy, Alberta Children's Hospital Research Institute, University of Calgary, Calgary, AB, Canada, [3] Department of Medical Genetics, Faculty of Medicine and Dentistry, University of Alberta, Edmonton, AB, Canada, [4] Cell Biology Program, Hospital for Sick Children, Toronto, ON, Canada, [5] Department of Molecular Genetics, University of Toronto, Toronto, ON, Canada, [6] Department of Cell Biology, Faculty of Medicine and Dentistry, University of Alberta, Edmonton, AB, Canada

***Correspondence:**
Daniel Graf
dgraf@ualberta.ca
Anastassia Voronova
voronova@ualberta.ca

Epigenetic and chromatin regulation of craniofacial development remains poorly understood. Ankyrin Repeat Domain 11 (*ANKRD11*) is a chromatin regulator that has previously been shown to control neural stem cell fates via modulation of histone acetylation. *ANKRD11* gene variants, or microdeletions of the 16q24.3 chromosomal region encompassing the *ANKRD11* gene, cause KBG syndrome, a rare autosomal dominant congenital disorder with variable neurodevelopmental and craniofacial involvement. Craniofacial abnormalities include a distinct facial gestalt, delayed bone age, tooth abnormalities, delayed fontanelle closure, and frequently cleft or submucosal palate. Despite this, the dramatic phenotype and precise role of *ANKRD11* in embryonic craniofacial development remain unexplored. Quantitative analysis of 3D images of KBG syndromic subjects shows an overall reduction in the size of the middle and lower face. Here, we report that mice with heterozygous deletion of *Ankrd11* in neural crest cells ($Ankrd11^{nchet}$) display a mild midfacial hypoplasia including reduced midfacial width and a persistent open fontanelle, both of which mirror KBG syndrome patient facial phenotypes. Mice with a homozygous *Ankrd11* deletion in neural crest cells ($Ankrd11^{ncko}$) die at birth. They show increased severity of several clinical manifestations described for KBG syndrome, such as cleft palate, retrognathia, midfacial hypoplasia, and reduced calvarial growth. At E14.5, *Ankrd11* expression in the craniofacial complex is closely associated with developing bony structures, while expression at birth is markedly decreased. Conditional deletion of *Ankrd11* leads to a reduction in ossification of midfacial bones, with several ossification centers failing to expand and/or fuse. Intramembranous bones show features of delayed maturation, with bone remodeling severely curtailed at birth. Palatal shelves remain hypoplastic at all developmental stages, with a local reduction in proliferation at E13.5. Our study identifies *Ankrd11* as a critical regulator of intramembranous ossification and palate development and suggests that Ankrd11^{nchet} and Ankrd11^{ncko} mice may serve as pre-clinical models for KBG syndrome in humans.

Keywords: KBG syndrome, epigenetic regulation, craniofacial development and malformations, intramembranous ossification, bone remodeling, cleft palate, neurodevelopmental disorders, chromatin regulation

INTRODUCTION

Molecular studies in developmental biology have been instrumental in defining gene regulatory and signaling networks that control cell and tissue differentiation to a considerable extent. These studies have revealed that throughout tissue development, specific transcription factors or signaling molecules are often used in a reiterated fashion to elicit discrete, developmental stage-specific cellular responses. Epigenetic mechanisms, defined here as external modifications of chromatin, facilitate these stage-specific responses. Through control of global regulation of gene expression at the various developmental stages (Bannister and Kouzarides, 2011; Budhavarapu et al., 2013), they control cell identity and facilitate stage-specific molecular responses (Barrero et al., 2010; Mirabella et al., 2016). A fitting example for complex tissue development is craniofacial development, which involves the coordinated but often asynchronous development, growth, and maturation of initially independent bone and cartilage structures. Epigenetic control mechanisms help facilitate different bone-related processes: bone development, bone mass accumulation and growth, maintenance and remodeling, and bone loss at different stages (Strobl-Mazzulla et al., 2012; Hu et al., 2014; Marini et al., 2016). The complexity of chromatin regulation controlling DNA accessibility to transcriptional machinery during craniofacial morphogenesis is still poorly understood, although dysregulation of epigenetic mechanisms has been implicated in a number of musculoskeletal and rheumatic diseases (Jeffries and Sawalha, 2015).

The entry point for this study was the association of the chromatin regulator *ANKRD11* (Ankyrin Repeat Domain 11; previously named ANCO-1) with KBG syndrome (OMIM #148050), a rare, autosomal dominant, congenital disorder characterized by a distinct craniofacial gestalt (Morel Swols and Tekin, 2018). *ANKRD11* contains an Ankyrin domain consisting of five Ankyrin repeats, two repression domains, and one activation domain (Zhang et al., 2007), and regulates global gene expression (Gallagher et al., 2015) by interacting with a variety of histone acetylation modifying proteins, such as HDAC3 (histone deacetylase 3) (Zhang et al., 2004; Gallagher et al., 2015) and components of the P/CAF (p300/CBP-associated factor) acetyltransferase complex (Li et al., 2008). While the full-length *ANKRD11* protein acts as a transcriptional repressor, the activation domain elicits transcriptional activation (Zhang et al., 2004, 2007; Li et al., 2008). Moreover, *ANKRD11* interacts with and increases acetylation of p53, potentiating the ability of p53 to act as a transcription factor (Neilsen et al., 2008), which itself is involved in many aspects of craniofacial development (Bowen and Attardi, 2019).

KBG syndrome is associated with heterozygous mutations in *ANKRD11* or micro-deletions of 16q24.3 encompassing *ANKRD11*. While patients with KBG syndrome display a range of phenotypes, a consistent feature is the distinct craniofacial gestalt (Morel Swols and Tekin, 2018). KBG syndrome diagnosis is typically suspected in an individual that displays macrodontia and/or characteristic facial appearance along with two additional criteria, such as palatal abnormalities, hearing loss, short stature, delayed bone age, scoliosis, learning difficulty, etc. (Morel Swols and Tekin, 2018). Delayed closure of a large anterior fontanelle is also frequently observed (Low et al., 2016).

The facial skeleton is mainly formed by neural crest cell-derived intramembranous bones, which develop from mesenchymal condensations at defined ossification centers (Berendsen and Olsen, 2015). During this process, osteochondroprogenitor cells sequentially differentiate into osteoblasts to form intramembranous bone. Osteoblasts deposit initially unmineralized osteoid that subsequently mineralizes (Berendsen and Olsen, 2015). As bone matures, osteoblasts become trapped within and terminally differentiate into osteocytes (St John et al., 2014). Maturation of osteocytes involves loss of organelles and changes in molecular properties (Irie et al., 2000). Newly formed bone matures through a process termed bone remodeling. This term describes the continuous process of bone resorption and bone formation that allows bone to attain its mature shape and optimal mechanical strength (Hadjidakis and Androulakis, 2006). These events require coordinated function of bone-resorbing osteoclasts, bone-depositing osteoblasts, and mature osteocytes. During this process, trabecular bone matures, and many osteocytes are resorbed.

Mineralization of the craniofacial complex begins in the mouse embryo around embryonic day 14 (Flaherty and Richtsmeier, 2018). While the involvement of epigenetics in the components of the ossification process is well documented

---

Abbreviations: *Ankrd11,* Ankyrin Repeat Domain 11; *ncko,* neural crest knockout; *nchet,* neural crest heterozygous deletion; E__, embryonic day __; *36B4,* acidic ribosomal phosphoprotein P0; *Alpl,* alkaline phosphatase; CBP, CREB-associated factor; *CC3,* cleaved caspase 3; CREB, cAMP-response element-binding protein; EDTA, ethylenediaminetetraacetic acid; ENU, *N*-ethyl-*N*-nitrosourea mutagenesis; Flp, flippase; HBSS, Hanks' Balanced Salt Solution; HDAC3/5, histone deacetylase 3/5; *Hh,* Hedgehog; *Ibsp,* integrin-binding sialoprotein; Ki67, Marker of Proliferation Ki-67; *Ocn,* osteocalcin; *Opn,* osteopontin; P/CAF, p300/CBP-associated acetyltransferase complex; P0, postnatal day 0; PFA, paraformaldehyde; *Prickle1,* Prickle Planar Cell Polarity Protein 1; RT-qPCR, reverse transcriptase quantitative polymerase chain reaction; *Runx2,* Runt-related transcription factor 2; *Sost,* sclerostin; *Sp7,* osterix; TRAP, tartrate-resistant acid phosphatase; *Wnt1,* Wnt family member 1; *Wnt*/PCP, Wnt planar cell polarity; αMEM, minimum essential medium α; μCT, micro-computed tomography.

(Schroeder et al., 2004; Li et al., 2009; Wein et al., 2015), there is little known about the overall contribution of chromatin regulators to craniofacial development.

Palate development describes the process by which the initially vertically growing maxillary appendages, termed palatal shelves, reorient to move above the tongue, grow horizontally and fuse to separate oral and nasal cavities (Kouskoura et al., 2011). The proliferation and differentiation of the palatal mesenchyme are regulated by intricate epithelial-mesenchymal interactions along the anterior-posterior axis. Palatal abnormalities, which occur when any of these required developmental events are disturbed, are relatively frequent and can present as complete, partial, or submucosal clefts. There is good evidence from the mouse for the involvement of epigenetic regulation during palate development (Kuriyama et al., 2008; Seelan et al., 2013; Juriloff et al., 2014) although direct evidence from humans is largely missing (Sharp et al., 2018).

Craniofacial and palate anomalies associated with KBG syndrome patients suggest a direct role for *ANKRD11* during craniofacial development. A homozygous *Ankrd11* missense mutation in mice is lethal in early embryonic stages (E9), preventing studies on craniofacial development with complete loss of *Ankrd11* (Barbaric et al., 2008). As neural crest cells contribute significantly to development of the anterior craniofacial complex, we used a neural crest-specific Wnt1Cre2 Cre-*lox* mouse line (Lewis et al., 2013) to delete *Ankrd11* in the developing neural crest.

We found that homozygous deletion of *Ankrd11* in neural crest (conditional knockout; Ankrd11^{ncko}) is perinatal lethal, while mice lacking one copy of *Ankrd11* (conditional heterozygote; Ankrd11^{nchet}) survive into adulthood. Adult heterozygous mice recapitulate some of the overall craniofacial phenotypes seen in KBG patients, whereas knockout embryos and pups display increased severity of numerous craniofacial anomalies commonly reported for patients with KBG syndrome (delayed ossification, cleft palate, midfacial hypoplasia, persistent anterior fontanelle, retrognathia). Our study identifies *Ankrd11* as a critical regulator of intramembranous ossification and palate development and suggests that Ankrd11^{nchet} and Ankrd11^{ncko} mice may serve as novel pre-clinical models for KBG syndrome.

MATERIALS AND METHODS

Mice

Animal experiments were approved by the Research Ethics Office at the University of Alberta (Animal Care and Use Committee, AUP1149, AUP2527) in compliance with guidelines set by the Canadian Council of Animal Care. Mice on a C57Bl/6 background were housed in the animal facility at the University of Alberta. Ankrd11$^{TM1a(EUCOMM)Wtsi//}$IcsOrl mice, in which exon 7 was floxed, were rederived from sperm (EM:07651, the European Mouse Mutant Archive – Infrafrontier) and crossed with Flp recombinase expressing (Jackson Labs) mice to generate Ankrd11^{TM1c} conditional ready mice (Ankrd11$^{fl/fl}$) as described (Skarnes et al., 2011). Exon 7 is located within the Ankyrin repeat domain. Ankrd11$^{fl/fl}$ mice were crossed with B6.Cg-E2f1Tg(Wnt1-cre)$^{2Sor/J}$ (Jackson Labs) (Lewis et al., 2013) mice for neural crest-specific deletion of *Ankrd11* (Ankrd11^{ncko}). Deletion of exon 7 results in out-of-frame splicing of exon 6 to exon 8, leading to a pre-mature stop and truncation of *Ankrd11*. Genotyping of mice was performed using Taq DNA Polymerase 2x Master Mix RED (Ampliqon, Denmark) from ear-notch or tissue biopsies. The following primers and PCR conditions were used: (1) for *Ankrd11*: forward, 5′-CTGTCTCAGAGAGGAGAGTGAGGAGGAC-3′; reverse, 5′-TACCTTACACCCTGAGACGGCGTC-3′; 34 cycles of: 94°C-30 s, 62°C-45s, 72°C-60s; (2) for the Cre transgene: forward, 5′-TTCCCGCAGAACCTGAAGATG-3′; reverse, 5′-CCCCAGAAATGCCAGATTACG-3′; Twsg1 internal control forward, 5′-AACAACAATGGCACAACCTAAT-3′, Twsg1 reverse, 5′-ACTTTCTCCCCACCCGTCTA-3′; 35 cycles of: 94°C-15s, 60°C-30s, 72°C-90s.

Micro-Computed Tomography

Mice were imaged using a MILabs μCT scanner at the School of Dentistry at the University of Alberta. Heads were fixed in 4% paraformaldehyde (PFA) for 24 h, then scanned at the following parameters: voltage = 50 kV, current = 0.24 mA, exposure time = 75 ms, 1600 exposures/full rotation. Scans were reconstructed at a voxel size of 25–35 μm, and the volumes were exported as NifTI-1 files. NifTI-1 files were directly analyzed using Amira software (version 2019.2, Life Technologies). NifTI-1 files were batch-converted to MINC-2 format using a custom made bash script and the MINC toolkit (Vincent et al., 2016).

Morphometric Analysis

Human Morphometrics

We acquired four three-dimensional (3D) scans of confirmed KBG syndrome patients from FaceBase (Samuels et al., 2020). All human subjects provided informed consent for the use of facial image data as approved by Institutional Review Boards at the University of Calgary, University of Colorado, Denver and the University of California, San Francisco. Each scan was non-linearly registered to a dense atlas (27,000 vertices) using the non-rigid iterative closest point method described in Bannister et al. (2020). We used a linear model with the first 400 principal components of facial shape to adjust the dense registered meshes for the effects of age and sex as described in Hallgrímsson et al. (2020). We then compared the mean age and sex-adjusted KBG mesh to the mean non-syndromic mesh. We visualized the differences between means as a heatmap using the meshDist() function in the Morpho package for R (Schlager, 2017).

Mouse Morphometrics

We used the MINC toolkit (Vincent et al., 2016) to gather 3D coordinates of 68 anatomical landmarks, from x-ray micro-CT volumes of the cranium of *Ankrd11* and control mice (**Supplementary Figure 1**). We also placed landmarks on a mouse skull atlas (average) and extracted a surface mesh of its segmented cranium, using marching cubes in VTK (Schroeder et al., 1998) and the MINC toolkit (Vincent et al., 2016).

We imported the specimen landmark files and the atlas landmark data into R (R Core Team, 2020) using the functions tag2array() and tag2lm(), respectively (Vidal-García, 2021). We performed a Generalized Procrustes Analysis (GPA) using the function gpagen() in geomorph (Adams et al., 2020), in order to obtain shape coordinates and remove effects due to size, rotations, and translations in the 3D landmark data. We then calculated group means on the shape coordinates for *Ankrd11* and control specimens, using the function mshape() in geomorph (Adams et al., 2020).

We mapped these 3D shape coordinate means to the atlas mesh and landmark coordinates using the function tps3d() in Morpho (Schlager, 2017). This function uses a thin plate spline method (Bookstein, 1989) to interpolate a target set of landmarks to the reference landmark set (atlas), which then warps the atlas mesh to fit the target landmark data. We visualized morphological differences between the *Ankrd11* and control mean meshes with heatmaps, using the function meshDist() in Morpho (Schlager, 2017).

Three-dimensional segmentation was performed using 3D slicer software. Automated segmentation function was used utilizing island and scissor functions to isolate individual bones. Bone volume was determined using statistics functions.

Tissue Preparation and Histology

Embryos were dissected from uterus at embryonic days (E) 13.5, 14.5, and 15.5 and collected at birth at postnatal day (P) 0. Embryos were decapitated and heads were fixed overnight at 4°C in 4% PFA. P0 heads were decalcified in 0.5M EDTA overnight before processing. Heads were processed and sectioned as previously described (Baddam et al., 2020). Before further analysis, slides were warmed in a 60°C oven, deparaffinized with xylene, and rehydrated through graded ethanol washes.

Histological Analysis

Rehydrated slides were stained with hematoxylin & eosin (H&E) (Harris modified hematoxylin Fisher SH30, eosin Sigma E4382), Alcian blue (1% Alcian blue solution, pH 1, 0.1N hydrochloric acid rinse, nuclear fast red counterstain), picrosirius red (Direct red 80 Fisher B21693, picric acid ACPchem P-2095), or Tartrate-Resistant Acid Phosphatase (TRAP). Briefly, TRAP staining was performed by incubating slides in pre-warmed enzymatic TRAP Staining Solution containing Fast Red Violet LB salt (Sigma F-331) at 37°C for 40 min, or until the control slide is slightly overstained. Slides were then counterstained with 0.02% Fast Green (Sigma F-7252). After staining, slides were dehydrated, cleared with xylene, and mounted with Permount (Fisher SP-15).

Immunofluorescent Analysis

Immunofluorescent staining was performed as described previously (Malik et al., 2020). Details of primary and secondary antibodies and dilutions used are summarized in **Supplementary Table 1**. Images were either taken on an Olympus IX73 microscope using 10x, 20x, or 40x objectives to photograph in a single plane and images were captured using the included cellSens Dimension program. Analysis was performed on at least three independent biological replicates; a representative image is shown. Polarized light images were acquired using a polarizer and analyzer cube (Olympus).

Image and Statistical Analysis

Density of cells forming the palatal shelves was quantified at E13.5 using DAPI nuclear stain (not shown). Semi-automated cell counting was performed in ImageJ on spatially defined regions within the palatal shelves (oral or nasal domains).

The number of immunostained Ki67-positive cells were counted on a minimum of six separate images per age and genotype from a palatal shelf. Sections were from a minimum of five different embryos from at least three different litters. The region counted is indicated in **Figure 5** with white dotted lines. Counting was automated in ImageJ using thresholding, watershed and particle analysis functions. Values presented in the graph are number of Ki67 positive cells divided over DAPI positive cells to normalize for hypoplasticity of shelves. Quantification of Runx2 and Sp7 domains at E12.5/13.5 was performed similarly, with values reported as percent of a defined field of view occupied by the stain and/or number of positive cells within the field of view. At least 3 (E14.5) or 6 (P0) sections were analyzed from 3 to 5 mice per genotype from at least three different litters. Statistical significance was determined via an unpaired two-tailed *t*-test.

In vitro Culture

Primary osteoblast cultures were established from calvaria for the gene expression time-course experiment. Calvaria were dissected and cut into small fragments, discarding cranial suture tissue. Calvarial bones were dissected into HBSS (Sigma H-9394) and used for osteoblast isolation using a modified protocol (Bakker and Klein-Nulend, 2012; Perpétuo et al., 2019). HBSS was replaced with 0.25% trypsin for 10-min digestion at 37°C, washed in αMEM (Gibco 12561-056), and digested twice with 0.2% Collagenase Type II solution (Worthington 4176) for 30 min each. Final digestion product was collected. Remaining bone pieces were washed with αMEM – solution was added to final digest and bone pieces were rinsed three times with cCM (complete culture medium: αMEM supplemented with Penicillin-Streptomycin [Gibco 15240-062], ascorbate [100 μg/mL, Sigma, A-8960], 10% Fetal Bovine Serum [Sigma F-1051]), then transferred to 75 cm^2 flasks containing cCM. Final digest was centrifuged for 5 min at 1500 *g* and the pellet was resuspended in 1 mL αMEM per calvarium. Cell suspension was combined with bone pieces in flask and incubated at 37°C and 5% CO_2 in air until confluent. cCM media changed every 3 days.

Once confluent, cells were trypsinized and seeded in a 12-well plate at 5–10 $\times$ 10^4 cells per well. Osteogenic medium (αMEM supplemented with ascorbate [50 μg/mL] and 2 mM β-glycerophosphate [Sigma G-5422]) was added when cells reached 80–90% confluency. Medium was changed every 3 days. Cells from three wells were harvested using Trizol (Invitrogen

15596026) at days 0, 3, 6, 9, 12, 15 for mRNA isolation and RT-qPCR quantification. Three independent experiments with two mice each were performed with three wells/time-point/experiment. For mRNA isolation, wells from within an experiment were combined. A representative result is shown.

RT-qPCR

RNA extraction, cDNA synthesis, and quantitative RT-qPCR were performed as previously described (Malik et al., 2020) using appropriate primer pairs normalized to *36B4* as a reference gene (see **Supplementary Table 2**). Fold change was calculated using $2^{-\Delta\Delta\ \text{Ct method}}$ (Livak and Schmittgen, 2001). MIQE guidelines were followed (Bustin et al., 2009).

RESULTS

KBG Syndrome Patients and Heterozygous Neural Crest-Specific *Ankrd11*-Mutant Mice (Ankrd11^{nchet}) Share Craniofacial Features

Three-dimensional facial images from four genetically confirmed KBG syndrome patients were combined and mapped against a reference face (**Figure 1A**) (Hallgrímsson et al., 2020). The resulting mesh heatmaps revealed a consensus hypoplastic mid- and lower faces, with an expansion of the upper third of the craniofacial complex. The *Ankrd11* neural crest-specific haploinsufficient deletion was generated by crossing *Ankrd11* floxed mice with Wnt1Cre2^{+} mice (Ankrd11^{nchet}) (**Figure 1B**). Analysis of μCT scans from mice Ankrd11^{nchet} mice revealed distinct changes to several craniofacial structures (**Figure 1C**): a persistent open fontanelle, a unique ossification defect in the posterior frontal suture, a slight change in pterygoid bone morphology evident from coronal ortho-slices anterior to the coronal suture (**Figure 1C**, lower panels). The angle of medial aspect of the pterygoid bone relative to ventrolateral was altered in Ankrd11^{nchet} mice. Comparative mesh heatmaps of Ankrd11^{nchet} and control scans revealed growth alterations in comparable regions as described for the human faces: reduced facial width, hypoplasia of midface, nasal region, and an expanded cranial vault (**Figure 1D**). Note: mandibles were omitted from analysis because of their variable position with respect to the skull.

Neural Crest Specific Deletion of *Ankrd11* (Ankrd11^{ncko}) Results in Severe Craniofacial Phenotypes

While pups lacking both copies of *Ankrd11* in the neural crest (Ankrd11^{ncko}) died at birth, precluding our analysis at the postnatal and adult stage, visual inspection of the neonatal head at postnatal day 0 (P0) revealed partially open eyelids, variable midfacial hypoplasia, reduction of calvarial growth (evident as reduction in calvarial microvasculature), loss of pigment on the nose, fully penetrant cleft palate, and a smaller tongue relative to control mice (**Supplementary Figure 2**).

Ankrd11^{ncko} Mice Exhibit Severe Bone Growth Defects

Skeletal preparations of P0 neonates demonstrated an underdeveloped midface and severe micrognathia in Ankrd11^{ncko} mice when compared to littermate controls (**Figure 2A**). A cleft palate was evident, as was the reduced ossification of the palatine bones and the anterior cranial base (presphenoid and sphenoid) (**Figure 2A**). Micro-computed tomography (μCT) showed that all intramembranously formed orofacial bones were reduced in size, resulting in underdeveloped midface and mandible (**Figure 2B**). Ossification of the anterior cranial bones was similarly severely stunted, and bones failed to cover the majority of the cranium at birth when compared to control mice (**Figure 2B**). Ossification of the anterior cranial base (presphenoid and basisphenoid) was similarly reduced. Several of the primary ossification centers failed to expand and formation of the pterygoid wings was largely missing. In contrast, more posterior, mesoderm-derived components of the cranial base (basioccipital bone) appeared unaffected. Quantification of the volumes of isolated craniofacial bones confirmed 39% reduction of the mandible ($p < 0.001$), 83% reduction of the frontal bone ($p < 0.001$), and 76% reduction of parietal bone ($p < 0.05$), with interparietal, occipital and basioccipital bones being not significantly different (**Figure 2C**).

Ankrd11^{ncko} Mice Display Hypoplastic Palatal Shelves and Cleft Palate

Histological analysis confirmed the notable size difference of the head and the cleft palate phenotype (**Figure 3A**). All major structures were present and developed to a recognizable stage, with exception of the tongue and palatal shelves that remained hypoplastic (**Figure 3A**). Note that due to retrognathia, mandibular structures on the sections appear more anterior. The developing palatal shelves were hypoplastic and dysmorphic already at embryonic day 12.5 (E12.5) (**Figure 3B**). Hypoplasia of the tip of the palatal shelf remained evident at later developmental stages. Elevation of palatal shelves appeared normal, but hypoplastic shelves did not meet to fuse, resulting in failure to separate oral and nasal cavities (**Figure 3B**). Analysis of cell density in the oral and nasal domains of the palatal shelves at E13.5 revealed a 15% increase in cell density in the nasal domain only ($p < 0.05$), with no differences observed in the oral domain (**Figure 3C**).

Ankrd11 Expression Is Associated With Early Bone Development and Bone-Lining Cells

To gauge when and how *Ankrd11* could cause the above-described phenotypes, we performed expression analysis for *Ankrd11* at E13.5, E14.5, and P0 (**Figure 4A**). At E13.5, Ankrd11 expression was discrete in orofacial regions with clear expression in a mesenchymal condensation in the developing maxillary region (sphenoid wing). Some expression was noted

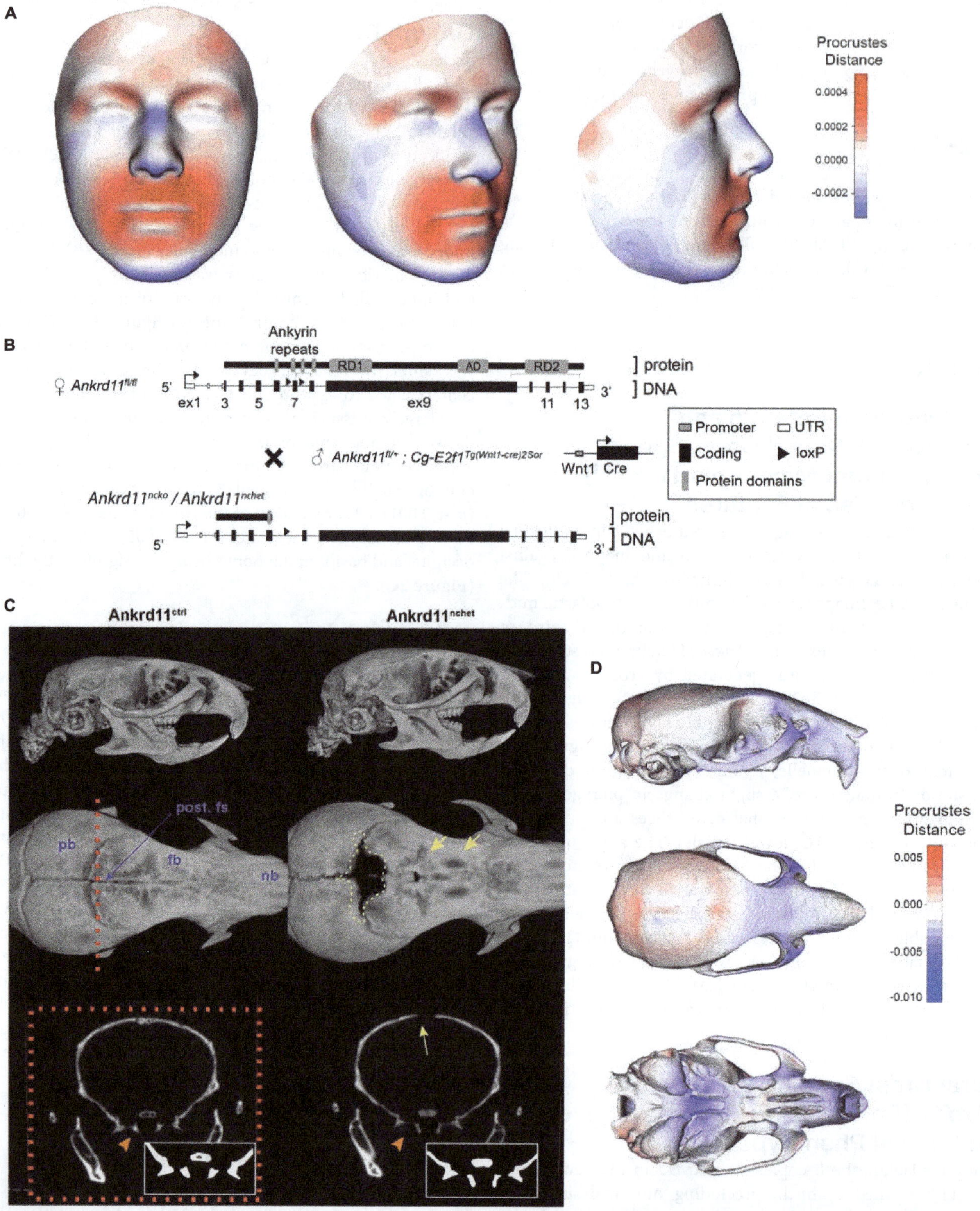

FIGURE 1 | KBG syndrome patients and Ankrd11^{nchet} mice share craniofacial similarities. **(A)** Mesh morphometric analysis of 4 KBG syndrome patient 3D images. Images shown are a mean representation of craniofacial changes on a reference face. Heat map representation in Procrustes distance (relative to superimposition). Red color indicates positive change in size relative to reference mesh and blue indicates negative size difference. White color indicates no change in highlighted region. **(B)** Brief summary of gene targeting and breeding strategy to produce Ankrd11^{nchet} mice, shown in panels **(C,D)**, and Ankrd11^{ncko} mice. **(C)** Reconstructions

(Continued)

FIGURE 1 | Continued
of μCT scans of Ankrd11^{ctrl} (Ankrd11$^{wt/fl}$) and Ankrd11^{nchet} mice. Top panel: lateral view of whole skull. Middle panel: Superior view of frontal bone; mandible and cranial base are clipped out of plane. Red dotted line indicates plane of sectioning for lower row of panels. Yellow dotted line highlights calvarial defect surrounding posterior frontal suture in Ankrd11^{nchet} mice. Yellow arrows point to regions of hard tissue anomalies in Ankrd11^{nchet} frontal bone. Lower panels: orthogonal slice through posterior frontal suture indicating pterygoid abnormalities (orange arrow) and open posterior frontal suture (yellow arrow). Inset in lower right corner of images is high contrast representation of cranial base structures affected in image. pb, parietal bone; fb, frontal bone; nb, nasal bone; post. fs, posterior frontal suture. **(D)** Mesh morphometric analysis of three Ankrd11^{nchet} mouse skulls. Images shown are a mean mesh of three Ankrd11^{nchet} skulls relative to a mean mesh of five Ankrd11^{ctrl} skulls. Note: mandibles were excluded from analysis due to the variable position with respect to the skull. Colors depict Procrustes distances between Ankrd11^{ctrl} and Ankrd11^{nchet} mean meshes, with blue indicating negative values (Ankrd11^{nchet} values fall within Ankrd11^{ctrl} mesh) and red indicating positive values (Ankrd11^{nchet} values fall outside of Ankrd11^{ctrl} mesh). White values indicate no changes, meaning the vertices for these anatomical regions in both mice are very close.

in the developing palatal shelves and lining oral epithelium. Note the distinct expression in the developing forebrain at this stage. At E14.5, Ankrd11 expression was overall stronger, more widely expressed, and could be observed in several developing mesenchymal structures. Distinct expression was observed in ossification centers and at sites of bone development in the mandible and maxilla, as well as in pre-odontoblasts in the developing molars. Ankrd11 was also present in some cartilaginous structures (nasal septum, developing turbinates), parts of the tongue, and the midline epithelial seam of the fusing palate. In the eye, expression was prominent in the developing lens as well as in the anterior segment (**Figure 4A**). Extent and intensity of Ankrd11 expression waned by P0, with the majority of Ankrd11 at this point restricted to the oral epithelium. Expression in the mandibular and maxillary bones was strongly reduced or absent, as was expression in teeth. In the eye, expression was now restricted to the posterior segment (**Figure 4A**). This indicates dynamic, but discrete, expression of Ankrd11 throughout development of craniofacial structures.

This dynamic expression is nicely illustrated in the developing mandibular bone (**Figure 4B**), one of the earliest bones to mature in the craniofacial complex (Flaherty and Richtsmeier, 2018). While at E14.5, at the onset of ossification, Ankrd11 signal lined the forming mandibular bone, expression was negligible in the comparable region at P0 (**Figure 4B**). Similarly, in the cranial vault, Ankrd11 was localized to the forming ossification centers at E14.5, whereas at P0 weak expression was observed in cells lining the calvarial bone, but not in osteocytes within the mature bone (**Figure 4B**).

In comparison, Ankrd11 expression in the developing palatal shelves and the developing maxilla was more discrete. At E12.5, a mostly epithelial expression pattern was observed in palatal shelves (**Figure 4C**). A few Ankrd11-positive mesenchymal cells were evident in the buccal aspect toward its tip, as well as in its upper, dorsal aspects (**Figure 4C**). At E13.5 and E14.5, the epithelial and mesenchymal expression largely remained comparable to E12.5. Overall, at E14.5, Ankrd11 expression was strongest in epithelium of the newly forming nasal cavity, the oral epithelium, the developing maxillary bones, as well as in the fusing palatal shelf, restricted to the midline epithelial seam. With the exception of some epithelial structures, Ankrd11 expression at P0 was reduced in all of these places. Residual weak expression in presumptive bone-lining cells was noted (**Figure 4C**).

Ankrd11 Controls Proliferation in the Buccal Half of the Palatal Shelf

To assess the cause for the hypoplastic palatal shelves in Ankrd11^{ncko} embryos, we assessed apoptosis and proliferation. No significant apoptosis was observed at any of the time points between E12.5–E13.5 (**Supplementary Figure 3**). The overall ratio of Ki67-positive cells to DAPI-positive nuclei was comparable at E12.5 and E13.5 in Ankrd11^{ncko} palatal shelves when compared to Ankrd11^{ctrl} (**Figures 5A,B**). When shelves were separated into oral and nasal domains and a spatially restricted quantitative analysis was performed (**Figure 5A**, right panels), a 40% decrease in mesenchymal proliferation became obvious in the E13.5 oral domain ($n \geq 5$ each, $p < 0.05$) (**Figure 5B**). To test for changes to cellular and extracellular organization, E13.5 palatal sections were stained with Alcian blue to identify distribution of glycosaminoglycans (GAGs). The overall organization and direction of cell orientation differs between Ankrd11^{ncko} and control shelves (**Figure 5C**). In addition, a disorganization of the mesenchymal cells lining the shelf epithelium was noticed (**Figure 5C**). These findings indicate that loss of *Ankrd11* has multiple subtle effects on palatal shelf organization and maturation, which likely underlie the cleft palate phenotype.

Ankrd11 Is Required for Normal Ossification of Intramembranous Bones

To better understand the reduction in intramembranous ossification observed in **Figure 2**, protein expression of two master regulators of ossification, Runx2 and Sp7 (Hojo et al., 2016; Komori, 2017) was assessed within the field of view indicated in **Figure 6A**. At E14.5, expression of Runx2 and Sp7 quite homogenously outlined the growing maxillary bones in control embryos (**Figure 6A**, top row). In contrast, in Ankrd11^{ncko} mutant embryos, Runx2 and Sp7 expression was only strong in the center, becoming more diffuse toward the periphery. Sp7 expression was more contained in comparison to Runx2 (**Figure 6A**). Quantification of the respective expression domains indicated that expression of both Runx2 and Sp7 was more contained, however the differences in the area occupied did not reach statistical significance (**Figure 6B**).

Differences in expression became even more striking at P0, a time-point of significant maxillary bone growth and remodeling. Expression of Runx2 and Sp7 could be observed in osteoblasts lining the newly formed trabeculae in control

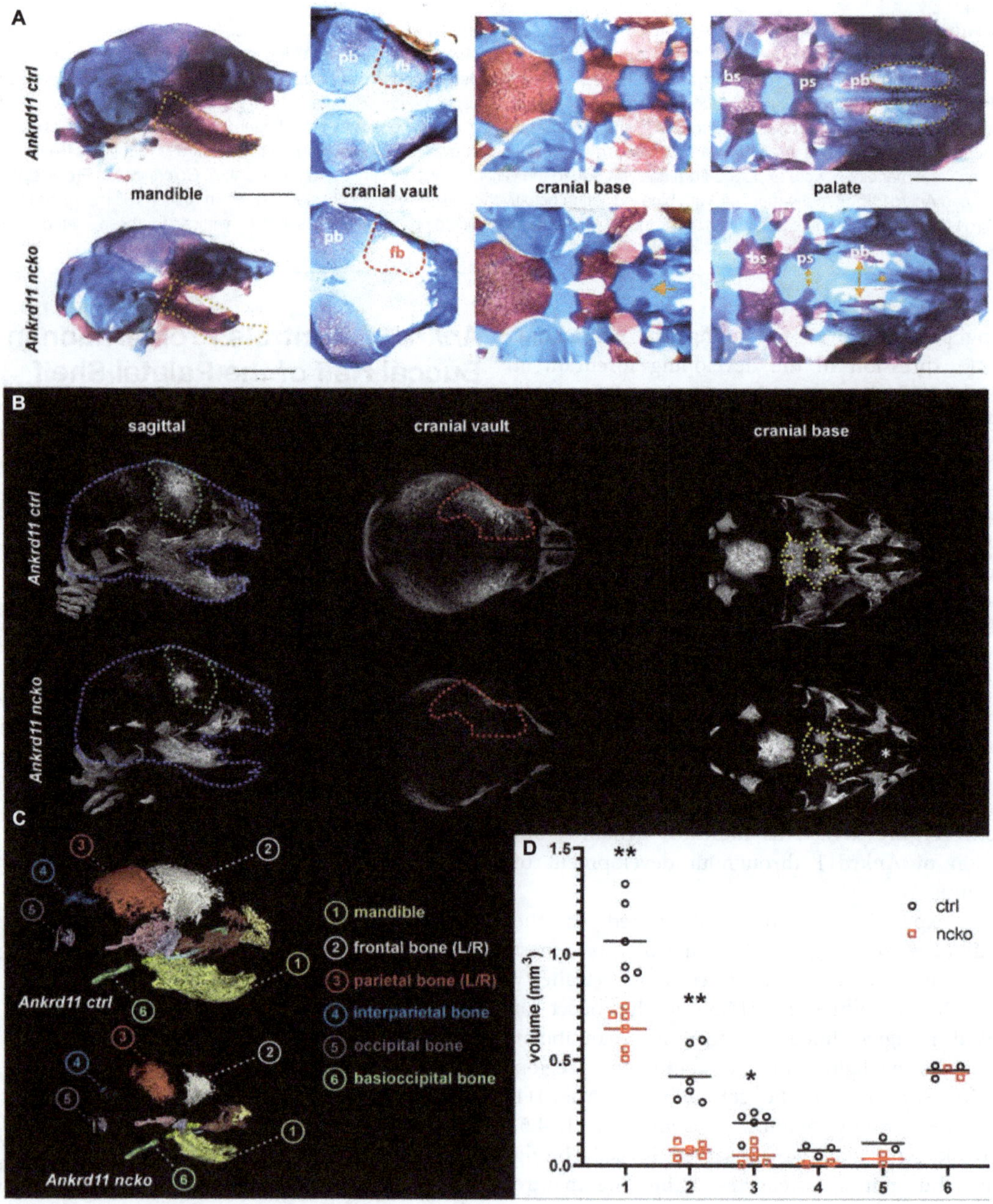

FIGURE 2 | Ankrd11^{ncko} mice have compromised ossification in craniofacial structures at birth. **(A)** Wholemount images of postnatal day 0 (P0) skull skeletal preparations, stained with Alizarin red and Alcian blue. Left panels: Orange dotted lines outline Ankrd11^{ctrl} (Ankrd11$^{fl/fl}$) mandible to indicate micrognathia in the mutant. Middle left panels: Red dotted lines outline Ankrd11^{ctrl} (Ankrd11$^{fl/fl}$) frontal bone to indicate its smaller size in the mutant. Middle right panels: Yellow arrows indicate extra space between presphenoid and palatine bones of the cranial base. Yellow asterisk to the right highlights clefting of hard palate in Ankrd11^{ncko} mouse. Right panels: magnified view of palate. bs, basisphenoid bone; ps, presphenoid bone; pb, palatine bone. Scale bar represents 2 mm, third column represents 1 mm. **(B)** μCT scans of P0 Ankrd11^{ncko} and Ankrd11^{ctrl} skulls reconstructed in Amira. Blue dotted lines: Ankrd11^{ctrl} skull outline. Green dotted lines: control frontal bone outline. Tan dotted fill in Ankrd11^{ncko}: negative space between control mouse and mutant. Red dotted lines: control frontal bone outline. Yellow dotted lines: control basisphenoid and presphenoid hard tissue outline. White asterisk indicates reduction in palatine bone ossification in the mutant mouse. **(C)** representative segmentation of individual bones from μCT scans of P0 Ankrd11^{ncko} and Ankrd11^{ctrl} skulls. **(D)** Quantification of segmented bone volumes (mm^3) from Ankrd11^{ncko} and Ankrd11^{ctrl} pups (independent two-sample *t*-test assuming unequal variances, $^{**}p < 0.001$, $^{*}p < 0.05$, $n = 6$). Segmentation and volume analysis performed using 3D Slicer.

neonates (**Figure 6C**, top row). In Ankrd11^{ncko}, this trabecular pattern appeared disturbed. Expression of both Runx2 and Sp7 appeared patchy and locally more restricted to the small, sparse trabeculae in maxillary bone (**Figure 6C**, bottom row). Tracing the outlines of cells expressing Runx2 and Sp7 revealed the presence of extended, Runx2-positive cellular assemblies

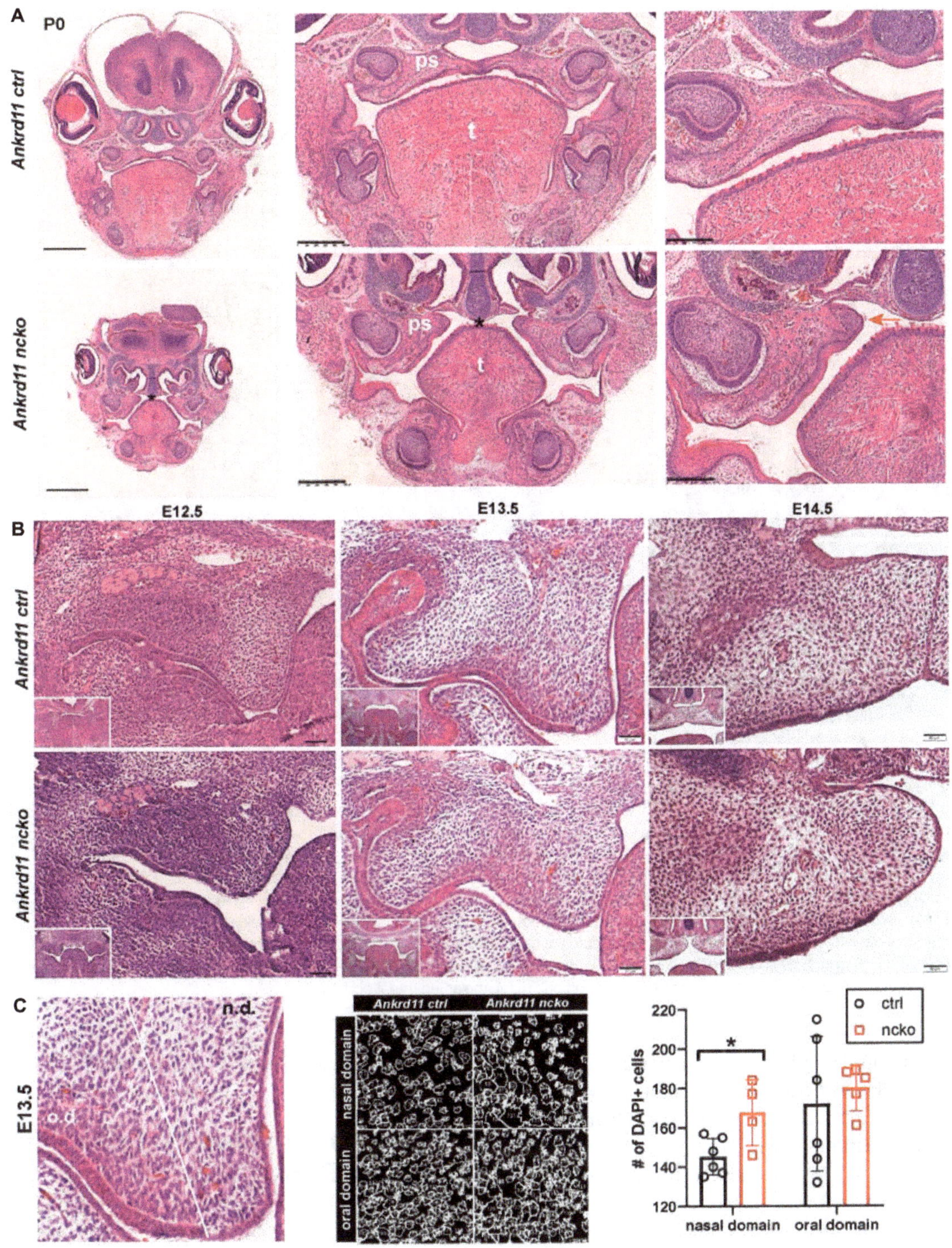

FIGURE 3 | Ankrd11^{ncko} mice display craniofacial changes early in development. Hematoxylin and eosin (H&E) stain. **(A)** Representative images of P0 coronal sections of Ankrd11^{ctrl} (top) and Ankrd11^{ncko} (bottom) skulls. Note relative size difference between heads. Black asterisk indicates absence of complete palatine boundary separating oral and nasal cavities in Ankrd11^{ncko} image. Second column images demonstrate overall differences in oral cavity, including smaller tongue and cleft palate. Differences in plane of section in mandible are due to retrognathia in Ankrd11^{ncko} mice. Right panels focus on palatal shelves, with red arrow indicating unfused advancing medial edge of palatal shelf in mutant mouse. t, tongue; ps, palatal shelf; *cleft palate. Scale bar indicates: 1 mm (first column), 500 μm (second column), and 250 μm (third column). **(B)** Coronal sections of palatal shelves at E12.5, E13.5, and E14.5. Inset in lower right corner of each view is lower magnification image of same mouse, showing overall organization of oral cavity in each mouse. $n = 3$ from 3 litters. Scale bar represents 50 μm. **(C)** Analysis of cell density based on DAPI stain in E13.5 palatal shelves separated into oral and nasal domains. Left: representative H&E stain. Middle: ImageJ-generated density profile showing individual cells. Right: Statistical representation of analysis showing increased cell density in the nasal domain of Ankrd11^{ncko} palatal shelves (independent two-sample T-test assuming unequal variances, $^*p < 0.05$). n.d., nasal domain; o.d., oral domain.

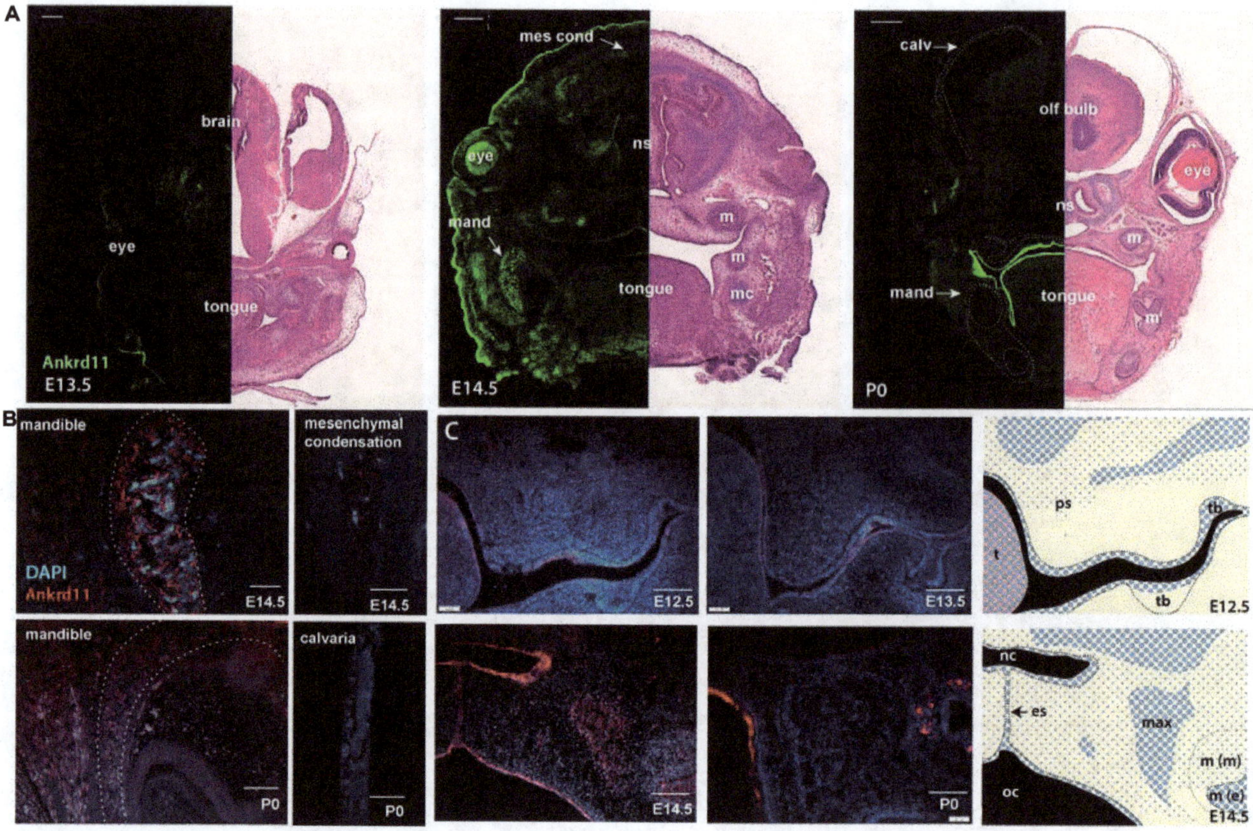

FIGURE 4 | Ankrd11 is expressed in embryonic craniofacial tissues. Expression pattern of Ankrd11 on immunofluorescent staining of Ankrd11^{ctrl} coronal paraffin sections. **(A)** Split view of coronal sections of C57/BL6 mice immunostained for Ankrd11 (left, green) or processed for H&E for morphological orientation (purple, right) at ages E13.5, E14.5 and P0. ns, nasal septum; mand, mandible; m, molar; mc, Meckel's cartilage; olf bulb, olfactory bulb of brain; calv, calvaria. White dotted lines on P0 immunofluorescent panel outline bony structures of the craniofacial complex including calvaria, maxillary/palatine bones, and mandibular bone shown in **(B)**. Scale bars represent 200 μm (left) and 500 μm (right). **(B,C)** High magnification representative images from coronal sections immunostained for Ankrd11 (red), with DAPI nuclear counterstain in blue from mandible and calvaria **(B)** as well as palatal shelves **(C)**. White dotted lines in **(B)** (mandible panels) indicate boundaries of mandibular bone indicated in **(A)**. Cranial/calvarial images are taken from comparable anatomic locations indicated in **(A)**. Images in **(B,C)** are presented from E14.5 and P0. Images in **(C)** are presented from E12.5, E13.5, E14.5, and P0. Graphic representation of Ankrd11 expression at E12.5 and E14.5 in right panels created in Adobe Illustrator. Blue represents Ankrd11 expression, with larger dots indicating relatively brighter regions. $n = 3$ from 3 litters. Scale bars in **(B)** represent 50 μm, except for E14.5 calvaria (200 μm). Scale bars in **(C)** represent 100 μm. ps, palatal shelf; t, tongue; tb, tooth bud; nc, nasal cavity; oc, oral cavity; es, epithelial seam; max, developing maxillary bone; m(m), molar (mesenchymal portion); m (e), molar (epithelial portion).

reminiscent of developing trabecula (**Figure 6D**, red dotted line), while the cellular structures in the mutant were more self-contained (**Figure 6D**, yellow arrowheads). Quantification indicated an 85% reduction of the Runx2-expression domain ($p < 0.001$) as well as 76% reduction in the number of Runx2-positive cells ($p < 0.001$). In contrast, despite a trend toward lower values, neither the number nor area of Sp7-positive cells were significantly different (**Figure 6E**).To test whether *Ankrd11* is indeed expressed and changes during osteoblast differentiation, we performed an *in vitro* time course of calvarial osteoblast differentiation. RT-qPCR analysis revealed that expression of *Ankrd11* changes dynamically over the course of osteogenic differentiation (**Figure 7A**). For reference, expression of several markers of osteoblast differentiation is shown: osteocalcin (*Ocn*), integrin binding sialoprotein *(Ibsp)*, Osteopontin (*Opn*), alkaline phosphatase 1 (*Alpl*). This co-expression was mirrored *in vivo*, where Ankrd11, albeit more discrete, largely aligned with expression of Sp7 at E14.5, but not at P0 (**Figure 7B**).

Ankrd11 Is Required for Bone Maturation and Bone Remodeling

The altered appearance of maxillary bones in **Figure 7** prompted us to analyze maxilla, mandible, and calvaria trabeculae in more detail. In control mice, discrete trabeculae with widely interspaced osteocytes of mostly elongated appearance were readily identified (**Figure 8A**, top row). In contrast, trabeculae appeared less refined with a higher number of poorly aligned osteocytes evident in all bones from Ankrd11^{ncko} mice (**Figure 8A**, bottom row). Staining for the Wnt antagonist Sclerostin (Sost), a marker for mature osteocytes and an important regulator of bone remodeling (Winkler et al., 2003; Husain and Jeffries, 2017), revealed a strong reduction in Ankrd11^{ncko} mice (**Figure 8A**, right column), suggesting that

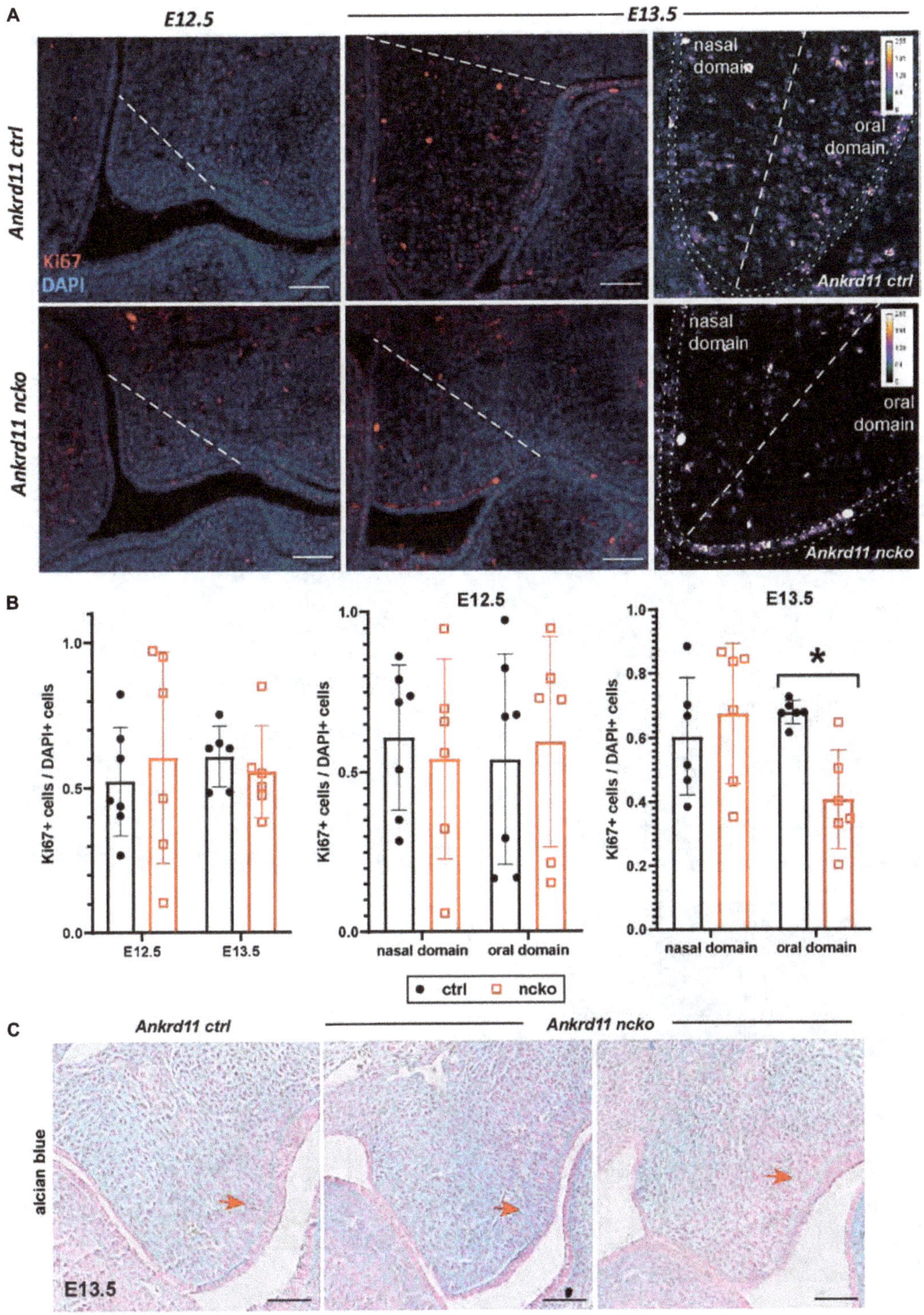

FIGURE 5 | Palatal shelf proliferation is locally affected in Ankrd11^{ncko} embryos. **(A)** Representative images of palatal shelves at each age and timepoint immunostained for Ki67 (red). DAPI-labeled nuclei are in blue. White dotted line delineates region counted for quantification shown in **(B)**. White scale bars represent 50 μm. Right panels: Magnification of E13.5 palatal shelf showing heatmap of Ki67 expression using ImageJ. White dotted line separates the nasal and oral domains of the palatal shelf. Scale bars represent 50 μm. **(B)** Left panel: Quantification of Ki67-positive cells relative to DAPI-positive nuclei plotted for each genotype (Ankrd11^{ctrl} depicted in black and Ankrd11^{ncko} depicted in red at E12.5 and E13.5). Middle and right panel: Cell proliferation in nasal and oral domains respectively (independent two-sample *T*-test assuming unequal variances, minimum of six sections/genotype from minimum of five embryos per genotype, $^{*}p < 0.05$, $n = 6$). **(C)** Alcian blue/nuclear fast red staining of E13.5 palatal shelves. Red arrow indicates mesenchymal cells lining epithelium on buccal side of shelf. $n = 3$/genotype, representative images shown. Scale bars represent 50 μm.

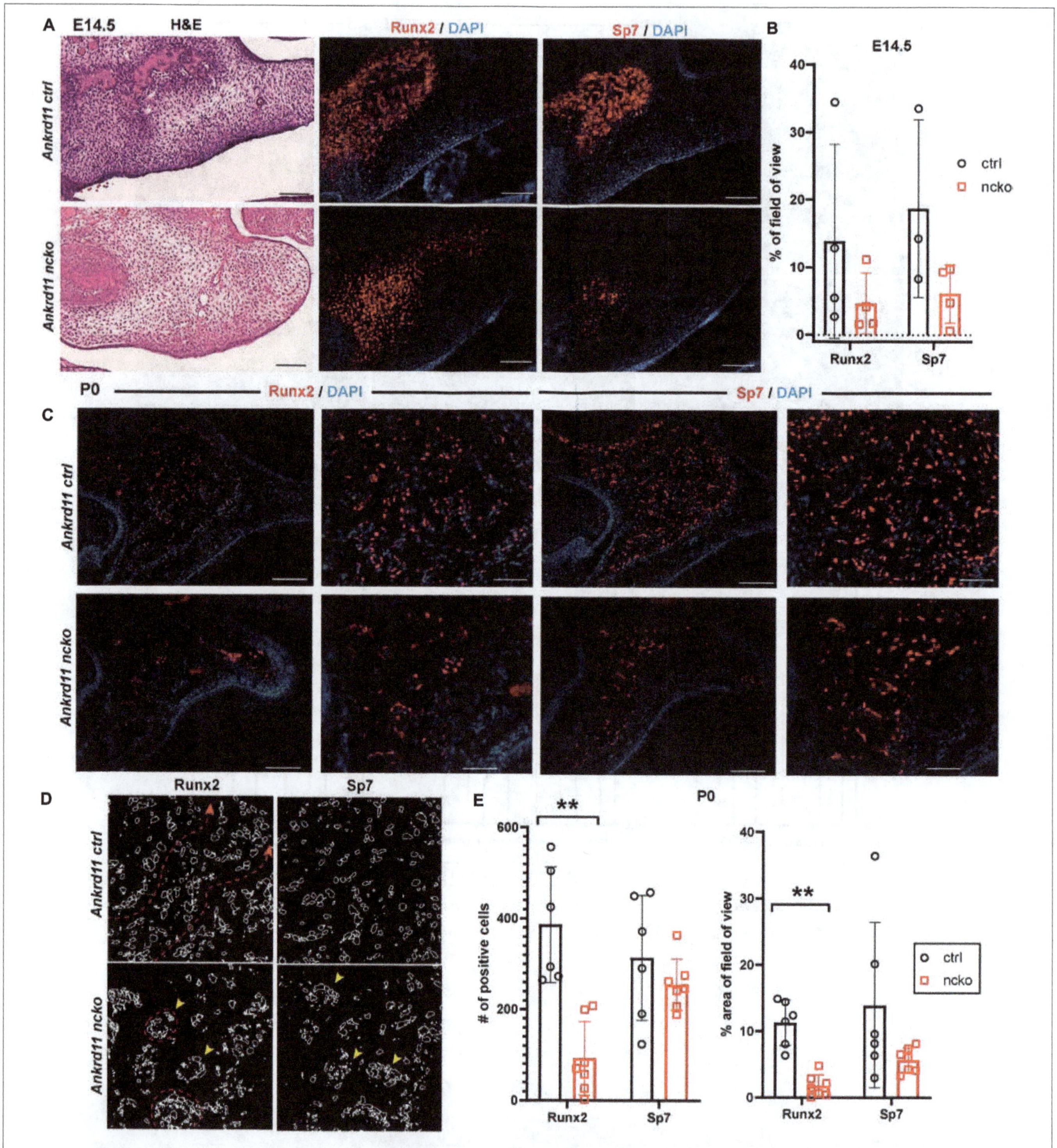

FIGURE 6 | Bone formation in Ankrd11^{ncko} mice is dysregulated in late embryonic development. **(A)** Palatal region in E14.5 Ankrd11^{ctrl} (upper row) and Ankrd11^{ncko} (lower row) embryos H&E stained for orientation (left column) and immunostained for runt-related transcription factor 2 (Runx2) and Osterix (Sp7) (middle and right columns). Scale bars indicate 100 μm. **(B)** Quantification of % occupancy of field of view stained for Runx2 and Sp7 (independent two-sample *T*-test assuming unequal variances). **(C)** Low and high magnification images of palatal bone in P0 Ankrd11^{ctrl} (upper row) and Ankrd11^{ncko} (lower row) pups immunostained for Runx2 (left two columns) and Sp7 (right two columns). DAPI (blue) was used to counterstain nuclei. **(D)** Representation of individual cells expressing Runx2 and Sp7 generated using ImageJ showing altered cell distribution in the mutant. Red dotted line and arrowhead indicates extended trabeculae in control, whereas red circles and yellow arrowheads indicate more contained cellular clusters in the mutant. Scale bars in first and third columns represent 100 μm, and second and fourth represent 50 μm. **(E)** Quantification of Runx2 and Sp7 expression at P0 (left: number of positive cells; right: percent area per field of view) showing significant reduction of the area of Runx2 expression, whereas Sp7 expression domain was more contained but not statistically different at P0 (n = minimum of six sections form 3–5 pups/genotype, independent two-sample *T*-test assuming unequal variances, $^{**}p < 0.001$).

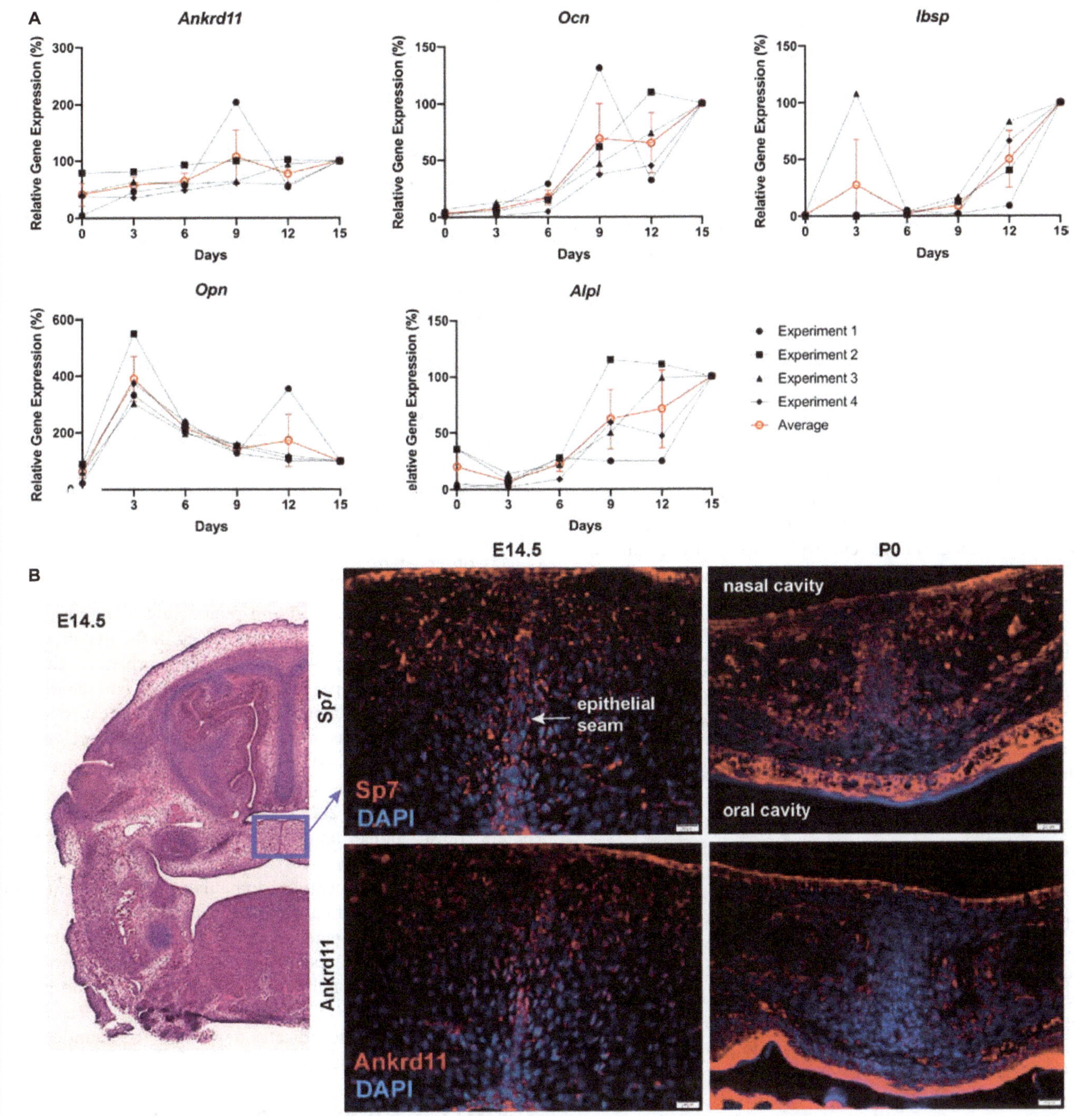

FIGURE 7 | Ankrd11 is upregulated with bone induction. **(A)** RT-qPCR analysis of *Ankrd11, Ocn, Ibsp, Opn, and Alp1* mRNA expression during *in vitro* osteogenic differentiation of P6 calvarial osteoblast precursor cells from wild-type mice. Data was normalized to *36B4* housekeeping gene. Results are relative to d15 expression from four independent biological replicates with d15 values equated to 100%. **(B)** Low magnification of approximate location (blue box, H&E stain) of panels showing immunostaining for Osterix (Sp7, red, top row) and Ankrd11 (red, bottom row) in E14.5 and P0 Ankrd11^{ctrl} mice. Images indicate similar expression domains of Sp7 and Ankrd11 at embryonic stages with expression pattern varying at birth. DAPI (blue) was used to counterstain nuclei. *n* = 3. D, days; E, embryonic; P, postnatal.

osteocyte maturation is delayed and bone remodeling might be compromised. To better illustrate this, we stained coronal sections of the craniofacial complex with Picrosirius red to reveal collagen fiber networks and osteoclast-specific tartrate resistant alkaline phosphatase (TRAP). An overall reduction in trabeculation was seen in the maxilla, calvaria (**Figure 8B**), and mandible (**Figure 8C**). This was mirrored by a 99% reduction in TRAP-positive regions in the maxilla, 85% reduction in the mandible, and 99.5% reduction in the calvaria (**Figure 8D** bottom graph; $p < 0.05$) despite presence of comparable amounts of bone within the region of interest (**Figure 8D** top graph; n.s.). In the calvaria (**Figure 8B**, bottom panels), a single-layered bone was observed in Ankrd11^{ncko} mice indicative of reduced or defective bone remodeling. TRAP staining revealed an almost complete lack of bone resorption and, by extension, remodeling. Birefringent imaging under polarized light of picrosirius red-stained sections confirmed changes in trabeculation, interconnectivity, and crosslinking of collagen fibrils (**Figure 8E**). Thus, *Ankrd11* appears to be comparatively more important in bone growth and remodeling than the initial induction of intramembranous bone, despite its prominent expression in ossification centers.

DISCUSSION

Neural crest-specific deletion of *Ankrd11* reveals direct roles for *Ankrd11* in various aspects of craniofacial development. Our study focused on intramembranous bone formation of facial bones and the skull, as well as palate formation, as these structures are commonly affected in patients with KBG syndrome. Similarly to KBG syndrome, adult Ankrd11^{nchet} mice present with discrete phenotypic changes that match the descriptions of 'triangular' face, persistent anterior fontanelle, and palatal abnormalities in humans. These observations complement the phenotypic description of heterozygous "Yoda" mice, in which an ENU-induced point-mutation in the C-terminus of *Ankrd11* leads to a shorter and wider face, decreased bone mineral density, incomplete closure of the interfrontal suture, and persistent opening of the anterior fontanelle (Barbaric et al., 2008). While both heterozygous Yoda and Ankrd11^{nchet} mutants are valuable to relate effects of *Ankrd11* mutations on development, they do not allow for attribution of systemic consequences and overall developmental delay to discrete roles of *Ankrd11*. In contrast, relating phenotypic consequences of homozygous, cell-specific deletion of *Ankrd11* to cellular expression of *Ankrd11* elucidates the involvement of *Ankrd11* in a precise and applicable manner. In this study, we focused on neural crest and craniofacial development. Ankrd11^{ncko} neonates exhibit a triangular shape face, cleft palate, midfacial hypoplasia, retrognathia, bone defects including an expanded anterior fontanelle, hypoplastic frontal bones, and a delay in bone maturation. Ankrd11^{ncko} die at birth, which underscores the overall importance of *Ankrd11* in neural crest-derived structures. Our findings on intramembranous ossification and palate development indicate that *Ankrd11* controls neural crest-derived cell progenitor proliferation or differentiation in a spatio-temporal manner, without affecting apoptosis. These data support and extend previous reports, where knockdown of *Ankrd11* in neural precursors decreases their proliferation and resulting number of differentiated neurons during murine cortical development (Gallagher et al., 2015). Our findings that *Ankrd11* impinges on intramembranous bone formation and maturation allow comparison to 3D morphometric analysis in both mice and humans to make precise conclusions on functional impact. Thus, the homozygous deletion of *Ankrd11* in a tissue-specific manner provides a powerful approach to model the KBG syndrome phenotypes in mice. Furthermore, this approach highlights how discrete perturbations in chromatin and epigenetic control can compromise tissue development and function long-term.

Ankrd11 Is Expressed Discretely in a Variety of Craniofacial Tissues

Neural crest-specific deletion reveals the broad involvement of *Ankrd11* during craniofacial development. In line with this, Ankrd11 shows restricted and dynamic expression in many craniofacial tissues. At E13.5 and E14.5, Ankrd11 is localized to discrete parts of the eye, bones, teeth, cartilage, and several muscular components. At a later developmental stage, expression in these regions is comparatively low and is primarily restricted to oral epithelium. Some expression in muscular compartments and olfactory bulb was noted in line with Gallagher et al. (2015). Relating expression to phenotypic manifestations allows strong predictions on the involvement of *Ankrd11* in the development of these different structures. For instance, Ankrd11 expression is noted from E13.5 onward in mesenchymal condensations and at E14.5 in ossification centers. This implies that the bony defects observed in Ankrd11^{ncko} mice might precipitate from differences during bone induction, although some of the defects such as osteocyte maturation and remodeling manifest only at much later stages. A similar pattern is seen in the maxillary and calvarial bones, where Ankrd11 is strongly expressed early in development, yet the impact on bone maturation and remodeling is noted only in much later stages when Ankrd11 expression is markedly reduced. It was previously suggested that development of bone involves epigenetic mechanisms, which might in part be controlled by lineage-specific transcription factors such as Sp7/Osterix (Park-Min, 2017). Whereas induction of ossification centers appears not to be compromised, significant differences are observed with respect to growth and maturation of these ossification centers. Expression domains of Runx2 and Sp7 are differentially affected. Thus, our study illustrates how expression of these two master genes are variably affected by loss of *Ankrd11*. At present, it is unclear if the weak expression of Ankrd11 seen in more mature bone indicates a continuing requirement for *Ankrd11* to maintain established epigenetic signatures, or whether it indicates ongoing, not-yet-understood *de novo* genomic fine-tuning.

Ankrd11 Is Required for Expansion of Intramembranous Ossification Centers

Both 3D morphological as well as phenotypic analysis indicate that *Ankrd11* is particularly important for intramembranous ossification. Establishment of ossification centers appears not to be compromised in the Ankrd11^{ncko} embryos; however, they universally fail to fully expand. This was not due to changes in proliferation or apoptosis (**Supplementary Figure 3**) but rather appeared to be the consequence of other, not fully understood mechanisms affecting specification, maturation, cell orientation, or migration of the induced bone-forming cells. In this light, Yoda mice or mice with *Ankrd11* knockdown in cortical

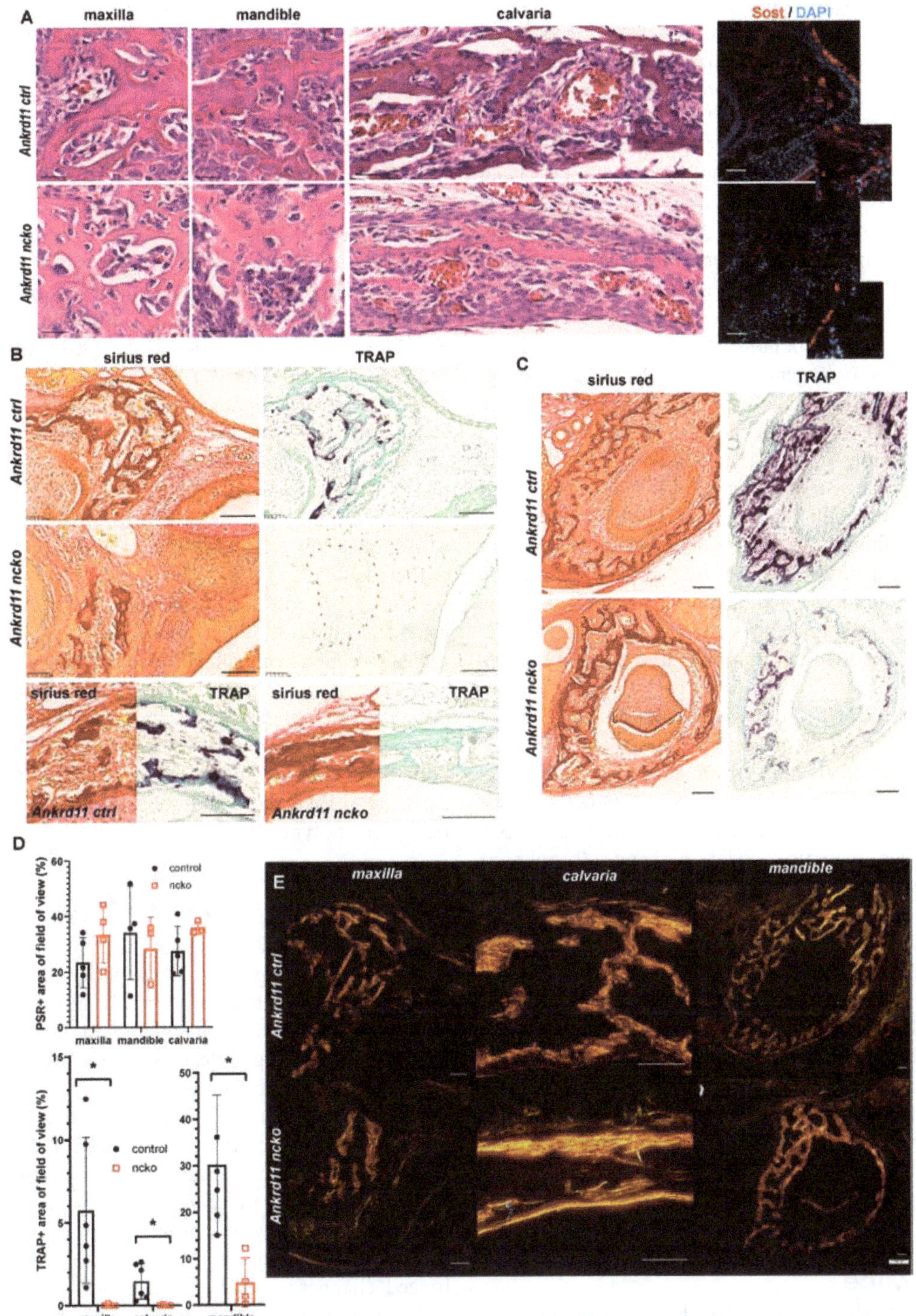

FIGURE 8 | Bone maturation is delayed in Ankrd11^{ncko} mice. **(A)** Representative sections of maxillary, mandibular, and calvarial bone from Ankrd11^{ctrl} (top row) and Ankrd11^{ncko} (bottom row) mice at P0. Sections were stained simultaneously for H&E to reveal cell morphology and bone organization. Images were taken at anatomically matching locations. Images in right column depict sections immunostained for sclerostin (Sost, red) in the P0 maxillary bone, demonstrating a reduction in Sost^{+} cells in Ankrd11^{ncko} maxillary bone. DAPI (blue) was used to counterstain nuclei. Scale bars in first two columns represent 25 μm, and last two represent 50 μm. **(B)** Sirius red and tartrate-resistant acid phosphatase (TRAP) staining of maxilla and calvaria of Ankrd11^{ctrl} and Ankrd11^{ncko} mice at P0 on neighboring sections. Red dotted line outlines region of bone in Ankrd11^{ncko} maxilla with no TRAP-positive cells, indicating a reduction in remodeling. Calvarial images are taken at the same point midway between the eye and fontanelle. Scale bars represent 100 μm. **(C)** Sirius red and TRAP staining of the mandible in Ankrd11^{ctrl} and Ankrd11^{ncko} mice at P0 showing a decrease in TRAP-positive cells in the mandibular bone. Scale bars represent 100 μm. **(D)** Quantification of images shown in **(B,C)** (independent two-sample *T*-test assuming unequal variances, $^{*}p < 0.05$, $n = 5$). **(E)** Polarized light images of sirius red stained maxilla, calvaria, and mandible in control and Ankrd11^{ncko} mice at P0 showing differences in extent of collagen fibril interconnection and orientation. Scale bars represent 50 μm.

progenitors display aberrant positioning of neurons in the developing cortex linked to dysregulated epigenetic mechanisms (Gallagher et al., 2015). Together with our craniofacial data, this could underscore that control of cell migration may be a common mechanism.

Intramembranous calvarial bone development generally occurs in two stages: (1) development of bone primordia from mesenchymal condensations, e.g. anterior-superior of eye for the frontal bone (beginning at E12.5), and (2) expansion, e.g. of the frontal bone front to cover the top of the skull (Yoshida et al., 2008). Defects in either or both of these stages result in insufficient bone formation. Our results suggest that loss of *Ankrd11* predominantly affects extension of the bone via growth at the osteogenic front and bone remodeling. The frontal bone insufficiency seen in Ankrd11^{ncko} mice mirrors the phenotype observed in the Beetlejuice mouse, which carries a mutation in *Prickle1* (Prickle1$^{bj/bj}$) (Wan et al., 2018). Prickle1$^{bj/bj}$ mice also have hypoplastic frontal bones, an expanded anterior fontanelle, and frequently cleft palate. The Prickle1 mutation is thought to affect a *Wnt*/Planar cell polarity (*Wnt*/PCP) signaling pathway. Apoptosis and proliferation are not affected, but unlike the *Ankrd11* mutant, a notable decrease in Sp7 alongside minimal changes to Runx2 expression is observed (Wan et al., 2018). Mutations in core components of the *Wnt*/PCP pathway cause Robinow syndrome which, like KBG syndrome, results in a wider midface and shorter stature. Notwithstanding these phenotypic similarities, changes in Ankrd11^{ncko} mice are likely caused by inappropriate epigenetic regulation in differentiating osteoblasts. Histones associated with several gene loci for key osteogenic factors including Runx2, Sp7, and Alp undergo dynamic acetylation changes throughout the ossification process (Zhang et al., 2015). Of interest, Runx2 interacts directly with HDAC3, a histone deacetylase previously shown to directly interact with Ankrd11 (Schroeder et al., 2004; Zhang et al., 2004; Gallagher et al., 2015). It is thus possible that *Ankrd11* and *Runx2* participate in common gene regulatory networks to set up osteoblast differentiation during craniofacial bone development. Potential changes in epigenetic signatures were not investigated as part of this study, because craniofacial structures are too heterogeneous following different developmental kinetics, posing significant challenges for the analysis of subtle epigenetic changes.

Delayed Maturation of Bone in Ankrd11^{ncko} Mice

Bone remodeling begins soon after bone formation. In Ankrd11^{ncko} mice, bone remodeling was severely compromised. The only notable remodeling occurred in the mandible, but even there it was dramatically reduced. Osteocytes appeared to retain an immature phenotype, evidenced by their increased numbers, plump morphology, apparent failure to align along stress/force lines, and lack of Sclerostin (Sost) expression, a characteristic of immature osteocytes. This could be the consequence of a delay in bone formation or an intrinsic defect in osteocyte differentiation. As Ankrd11 is not expressed in osteocytes (**Figure 4B**), this phenotype is likely caused by abnormal osteoblast differentiation, possibly involving inappropriate epigenetic osteoblast programming or specification as discussed earlier.

Immature osteocytes lack the exquisite mechanosensory properties of mature osteocytes. The primary cilium has been suggested to play an important role in bone mechanotransduction (Temiyasathit and Jacobs, 2010). Inability to sense or respond to mechanical cues would manifest as failure to align along stress lines, increased cell number, and failure to induce bone remodeling (exemplified by loss of TRAP staining). On the other hand, osteocyte maturation is dependent on mineralization, as the transition to mature osteocytes is triggered by differences in mechanosensing of mineralized and unmineralized matrix (Irie et al., 2008). Changes to ordered mineralization in Ankrd11^{ncko} bones could equally explain the failure in osteocyte maturation and associated bone remodeling. Osteoclasts are related to monocytes and are of hematopoietic origin. Neural crest-specific *Ankrd11* deletion would not directly affect these cells. The defect in remodeling is therefore most likely due to defective mechanosensing or defective communication with osteoclasts, underlining interconnection of these systems.

While lack of Sost expression could reflect a failure of osteocyte maturation, it must be noted that *Sost* itself is under epigenetic control. HDAC5 deficiency results in increased Sost expression, impaired osteogenesis, and low bone density (Wein et al., 2015). Sost activity-blocking antibodies are an approved treatment modality for osteoporosis aiming to reduce bone resorption. A more detailed analysis will be required to carefully dissect the cause and consequence of these bone-related phenotypes.

A Role for *Ankrd11* in Palate Development

In contrast to bone primordia, the pattern of Ankrd11 expression in the palate is relatively discrete. It also differs from the often broad expression domains described for many transcription factors and signaling molecules in the developing palatal shelves (He et al., 2011; Danescu et al., 2015). This restricted Ankrd11 expression was seen at all stages from E12.5-E14.5 and could be attributed to discrete cells organizing palate development, or a tight window of expression governing reprogramming. Thus, Ankrd11 might be involved in the spatial organization of the palatal shelf, possibly regulating the expression of a growth factor or its receptors, facilitating growth of the palatal shelf secondarily. Indeed, changes in cellular distribution were observed.

Furthermore, an asymmetric pattern of proliferation was observed at E13.5, with a decrease in the buccal half of the shelf. The affected region roughly corresponds to the gene expression domain of the Hedgehog signaling receptor Patched (Ptch) (Xiong et al., 2009), raising the possibility that Ankrd11 somehow intersects with Hh signaling and cilia. Hedgehog and Wnt signaling are indeed both critical for cilia maturation, and functional cilia are required for normal palatal development (Brugmann et al., 2010; Nakaniwa et al., 2019). Recently, *Ankrd11* was directly associated with ciliopathies (Breslow et al., 2018). The interplay between Hedgehog and Wnt signaling and chromatin remodeling by Ankrd11 may provide important clues for understanding both palate and bone phenotypes and will be investigated in future studies.

Clinical Implications

Mesh analysis of four patients with KBG syndrome revealed hypoplastic mid- and lower face and enlarged upper face. This is largely mimicked in Ankrd11^{nchet} and Ankrd11^{ncko} mice (**Figures 1, 2**). Given the stunted intramembranous ossification in the Ankrd11^{ncko} mouse, we propose that the expansion of the upper 1/3 of the face is a consequence of underdeveloped midfacial bones as well as intramembranously formed extensions of the cranial base – the pterygoid wings. The resultant narrower cranial base and midface would necessitate increased cranial bone growth to accommodate the expanding brain, leading to a triangular face. The calvaria would not be able to meet the increased demand in bone growth (as they are compromised in bone formation themselves) resulting in a persistent anterior fontanelle.

Patients with KBG syndrome show various accompanying craniofacial anomalies. Macrodontia, dental crowding, and hypo/oligodontia are often observed, necessitating invasive jaw surgery (Ockeloen et al., 2015; Low et al., 2016; Morel Swols and Tekin, 2018). Our results and expression analysis suggest that these malformations may be due to abnormal tooth and jaw development. Moreover, speech and feeding difficulties are frequently observed in KBG syndrome patients (Ockeloen et al., 2015; Low et al., 2016; Morel Swols and Tekin, 2018). The anomalies in palate development, more severe in Ankrd11^{ncko} mice but evident also in Ankrd11^{nchet} mice, can provide a structural explanation for these observations. High-arched palate or submucosal cleft, considered milder variants of defective palate development, lead to similar problems. Thus, our results will precipitate further investigations into the underpinnings of the various phenotypic craniofacial anomalies associated with *ANKRD11*.

ANKRD11 is one of the most disrupted genes in monogenic neurodevelopmental disorders with *de novo* mutations (Wilfert et al., 2017; Satterstrom et al., 2020). Yet, most patients with KBG syndrome are not diagnosed until 20–30 years of age, if at all (personal communication with Drs. Charlotte Ockeloen, Tjitske Kleefstra, and Peter Kannu). The gold standard for diagnosis of KBG syndrome is genetic testing to detect *ANKRD11* variants or 16q24.3 deletion involving the gene. Specific craniofacial features such as persistent anterior fontanelle, submucosal or high-arched palate, macrodontia, and reduced bone mineral density are currently only suggestive of KBG syndrome and clinical phenotypic criteria for proper diagnosis remain poorly defined (Morel Swols and Tekin, 2018). This study confirms the power of 3D morphometric analysis to assist with syndrome diagnosis (Hallgrímsson et al., 2020) and illustrates the power of disease modeling in the mouse to unearth the underlying cellular basis for the malformation. Indeed, many craniofacial features observed in KBG syndrome (Ockeloen et al., 2015; Low et al., 2016; Morel Swols and Tekin, 2018) are recapitulated in the Ankrd11^{ncko} mouse. This study has begun to unravel some of the unknowns of *Ankrd11*-mediated regulation of craniofacial development and has allowed assessment of craniofacial malformations as a result of *Ankrd11* deletion or loss-of-function. Systematic assessment of cataloged craniofacial features in patients with KBG syndrome can potentially drive further understanding of clinical penetrance and future establishment of definitive phenotypic diagnostic criteria to achieve earlier differential diagnosis, as well as clarify the impact of *ANKRD11* variants of unknown significance (VUS). Similarly, studies in other organ systems often involved in KBG syndrome will further clarify the role of *Ankrd11* in epigenetic and genomic control of tissue and organ development.

Summary

Our phenotypic characterization of conditional ablation of *Ankrd11* in the murine neural crest revealed novel roles of *Ankrd11* in craniofacial development, specifically in intramembranous bone formation and palate development. Our results will help improve clinical assessment of patients with KBG syndrome based on craniofacial phenotypic diagnosis, particularly early in life. Ultimately, early diagnosis and better understanding of *ANKRD11* function will assist with genetic counseling for patients with KBG syndrome and their affected families.

ETHICS STATEMENT

The studies involving human participants were reviewed and approved by Institutional Review Boards at the University of Calgary, University of Colorado, Denver, and the University of California, San Francisco. Written informed consent to participate in this study was provided by the participants' legal guardian/next of kin. The animal study was reviewed and approved by Research Ethics Office at the University of Alberta (Animal Care and Use Committee) under AUP1149 and AUP2527.

AUTHOR CONTRIBUTIONS

DR performed the experiments, analyzed the results, and wrote the manuscript. PB performed the experiments, analyzed the results, and edited the manuscript. HL and MV-G performed the experiments and analyzed the results. S-TD and DGo performed the preliminary experiments. AW and TF performed the supporting experiments and mouse line management. NS and SE generated the Ankrd11$^{fl/fl}$ mice. MV-G, JA, and BH performed the morphometric analyses of human subjects and mice and edited the manuscript. DGr and AV conceived the study, analyzed the results, wrote and edited the manuscript, and provided funding. All the authors contributed to the article and approved the submitted version.

ACKNOWLEDGMENTS

We acknowledge the microCT facility of the School of Dentistry, University of Alberta and the Centre for Prions and Protein Folding Diseases for the use of their NanoZoomer equipment. We thank Dr. David Callen for his generous gift of the α-Ankrd11 polyclonal antibody. We would also like to acknowledge the generous support of trainees through the following scholarships: NSERC Postgraduate (Doctoral) Scholarship (PB), Alberta Graduate Excellence Scholarship (PB and AW), LiKaShing Foundation (HL), Medical Sciences Graduate Program (DR, PB, and AW), 75th Anniversary Award of the Faculty of Medicine (PB and AW), Violett Kilburn Scholarship (PB), School of Dentistry (DR), Alberta Children's Hospital Research Institute (ACHRI) PDF (MV-G) and Alberta Innovates PDF in Health Innovation (MV-G), Women and Children Research Institute (WCHRI) Graduate Studentship Award (AW), and the NSERC Undergraduate Student Research Award (S-TD).

SUPPLEMENTARY MATERIAL

Supplementary Figure 1 | Landmarks used for mesh morphometric analysis. Sixty-eight anatomical landmarks placed on micro-CT volumes of the cranium using the MINC toolkit.

Supplementary Figure 2 | Ankrd11^{ncko} mice are born with a macroscopically recognizable craniofacial phenotype. Left column: Ankrd11^{ctrl} P0 mice. Right column: Ankrd11^{ncko} P0 mice. **(A,B)** Lateral view of head, with a white arrow indicating layer of skin covering eye, incomplete in Ankrd11^{ncko} mice. Ankrd11^{ncko} mice also have a growth deficiency in the midface and retrognathia. **(C,D)** Superior view of head. Ankrd11^{ncko} appears paler, with a more domed head shape. **(E,F)** View of the snout from the front. White arrow indicates black pigment that is absent in Ankrd11^{ncko} mice. **(G,H)** View of dissected palate, viewed from below. Left side is anterior. Asterisk highlights cleft palate in Ankrd11^{ncko} mouse. **(I,J)** View of dissected mandible and tongue, viewed from above. Left side is anterior. Note tongue (central, spanning left to right in image) is thinner and shorter in Ankrd11^{ncko} mouse. Consistent amongst three mice from different litters.

Supplementary Figure 3 | Cleaved Caspase 3 (CC3) dependent apoptosis does not differ between Ankrd11^{ctrl} and Ankrd11^{ncko} palatal shelves. Representative immunofluorescent staining for cleaved caspase 3 (CC3) on coronal paraffin sections (green). Nuclei are counterstained with DAPI (red). $n = 3$ from 3 l. Scale bar represents 50 μm on all images.

Supplementary Table 1 | Antibodies used for immunofluorescent staining.

Supplementary Table 2 | Oligonucleotide primer pairs used for quantitative RT-PCR.

REFERENCES

Adams, D., Collyer, M., and Kaliontzopoulou, A. (2020). *geomorph: Geometric Morphometric Analyses of 2D/3D Landmark Data*. Available online at: https://CRAN.R-project.org/package=geomorph (accessed Decembaer 20, 2020).

Baddam, P., Kung, T., Adesida, A. B., and Graf, D. (2020). Histological and molecular characterization of the growing nasal septum in mice. *J. Anat.* 238, 751–764. doi: 10.1111/joa.13332

Bakker, A. D., and Klein-Nulend, J. (2012). "osteoblast isolation from murine calvaria and long bones," in *Bone Research Protocols Methods in Molecular Biology*, eds M. H. Helfrich and S. H. Ralston (Totowa, NJ: Humana Press), 19–29. doi: 10.1007/978-1-61779-415-5_2

Bannister, A. J., and Kouzarides, T. (2011). Regulation of chromatin by histone modifications. *Cell Res.* 21, 381–395. doi: 10.1038/cr.2011.22

Bannister, J. J., Crites, S. R., Aponte, J. D., Katz, D. C., Wilms, M., Klein, O. D., et al. (2020). Fully automatic landmarking of syndromic 3D facial surface scans using 2D Images. *Sensors* 20:3171. doi: 10.3390/s20113171

Barbaric, I., Perry, M. J., Dear, T. N., Rodrigues Da Costa, A., Salopek, D., Marusic, A., et al. (2008). An ENU-induced mutation in the *Ankrd11* gene results in an osteopenia-like phenotype in the mouse mutant Yoda. *Physiol. Genomics* 32, 311–321. doi: 10.1152/physiolgenomics.00116.2007

Barrero, M. J., Boué, S., and Izpisúa Belmonte, J. C. (2010). Epigenetic mechanisms that regulate cell identity. *Cell Stem Cell* 7, 565–570. doi: 10.1016/j.stem.2010.10.009

Berendsen, A. D., and Olsen, B. R. (2015). Bone development. *Bone* 80, 14–18. doi: 10.1016/j.bone.2015.04.035

Bookstein, F. L. (1989). Principal warps: thin-plate splines and the decomposition of deformations. *IEEE Trans. Pattern Anal. Mach. Intell.* 11, 567–585. doi: 10.1109/34.24792

Bowen, M. E., and Attardi, L. D. (2019). The role of p53 in developmental syndromes. *J. Mol. Cell Biol.* 11, 200–211. doi: 10.1093/jmcb/mjy087

Breslow, D. K., Hoogendoorn, S., Kopp, A. R., Morgens, D. W., Vu, B. K., Kennedy, M. C., et al. (2018). A CRISPR-based screen for Hedgehog signaling provides insights into ciliary function and ciliopathies. *Nat. Genet.* 50, 460–471. doi: 10.1038/s41588-018-0054-7

Brugmann, S. A., Cordero, D. R., and Helms, J. A. (2010). Craniofacial ciliopathies: a new classification for craniofacial disorders. *Am. J. Med. Gene.t A* 152A, 2995–3006. doi: 10.1002/ajmg.a.33727

Budhavarapu, V. N., Chavez, M., and Tyler, J. K. (2013). How is epigenetic information maintained through DNA replication? *Epigenet. Chromatin* 6:32. doi: 10.1186/1756-8935-6-32

Bustin, S. A., Benes, V., Garson, J. A., Hellemans, J., Huggett, J., Kubista, M., et al. (2009). The MIQE guidelines: minimum information for publication of quantitative real-time PCR experiments. *Clin. Chem.* 55, 611–622. doi: 10.1373/clinchem.2008.112797

Danescu, A., Mattson, M., Dool, C., Diewert, V. M., and Richman, J. M. (2015). Analysis of human soft palate morphogenesis supports regional regulation of palatal fusion. *J. Anat.* 227, 474–486. doi: 10.1111/joa.12365

Flaherty, K., and Richtsmeier, J. T. (2018). It's about time: ossification center formation in C57BL/6 mice from E12–E16. *J. Dev. Biol.* 6:31. doi: 10.3390/jdb6040031

Gallagher, D., Voronova, A., Zander, M. A., Cancino, G. I., Bramall, A., Krause, M. P., et al. (2015). Ankrd11 is a chromatin regulator involved in autism that is essential for neural development. *Dev. Cell* 32, 31–42. doi: 10.1016/j.devcel.2014.11.031

Hadjidakis, D. J., and Androulakis, I. I. (2006). Bone remodeling. *Ann. N. Y. Acad. Sci.* 1092, 385–396. doi: 10.1196/annals.1365.035

Hallgrímsson, B., Aponte, J. D., Katz, D. C., Bannister, J. J., Riccardi, S. L., Mahasuwan, N., et al. (2020). Automated syndrome diagnosis by three-dimensional facial imaging. *Genet. Med.* 22, 1682–1693. doi: 10.1038/s41436-020-0845-y

He, F., Xiong, W., Wang, Y., Li, L., Liu, C., Yamagami, T., et al. (2011). Epithelial Wnt/β-catenin signaling regulates palatal shelf fusion through regulation of Tgfβ3 expression. *Dev. Biol.* 350, 511–519. doi: 10.1016/j.ydbio.2010.12.021

Hojo, H., Ohba, S., He, X., Lai, L. P., and McMahon, A. P. (2016). Sp7/osterix is restricted to bone-forming vertebrates where it acts as a Dlx Co-factor in osteoblast specification. *Dev. Cell* 37, 238–253. doi: 10.1016/j.devcel.2016.04.002

Hu, N., Strobl-Mazzulla, P. H., and Bronner, M. E. (2014). Epigenetic regulation in neural crest development. *Dev. Biol.* 396, 159–168. doi: 10.1016/j.ydbio.2014.09.034

Husain, A., and Jeffries, M. A. (2017). Epigenetics and bone remodeling. *Curr. Osteoporos. Rep.* 15, 450–458. doi: 10.1007/s11914-017-0391-y

Irie, K., Ejiri, S., Sakakura, Y., Shibui, T., and Yajima, T. (2008). Matrix mineralization as a trigger for osteocyte maturation. *J. Histochem. Cytochem.* 56, 561–567. doi: 10.1369/jhc.2008.950527

Irie, K., Ozawa, H., and Yajima, T. (2000). The histochemical and cytochemical changes from formative to resorptive osteocytes. *Acta Histochem. Cytochem.* 33, 385–391. doi: 10.1267/ahc.33.385

Jeffries, M. A., and Sawalha, A. H. (2015). Autoimmune disease in the epigenetic era: how has epigenetics changed our understanding of disease and how can we expect the field to evolve? *Expert Rev. Clin. Immunol.* 11, 45–58. doi: 10.1586/1744666X.2015.994507

Juriloff, D. M., Harris, M. J., Mager, D. L., and Gagnier, L. (2014). Epigenetic mechanism causes Wnt9b deficiency and nonsyndromic cleft lip and palate in the A/WySn mouse strain. *Birth Defects Res. Part A Clin. Mol. Teratol.* 100, 772–788. doi: 10.1002/bdra.23320

Komori, T. (2017). "Roles of Runx2 in skeletal development," in *RUNX Proteins in Development and Cancer Advances in Experimental Medicine and Biology*, eds Y. Groner, Y. Ito, P. Liu, J. C. Neil, N. A. Speck, and A. van Wijnen (Singapore: Springer), 83–93. doi: 10.1007/978-981-10-3233-2_6

Kouskoura, T., Fragou, N., Alexiou, M., John, N., Sommer, L., Graf, D., et al. (2011). The genetic basis of craniofacial and dental abnormalities. *Schweiz Monatsschr Zahnmed* 121, 636–646.

Kuriyama, M., Udagawa, A., Yoshimoto, S., Ichinose, M., Sato, K., Yamazaki, K., et al. (2008). DNA methylation changes during cleft palate formation induced by retinoic acid in mice. *Cleft Palate Craniofac. J.* 45, 545–551. doi: 10.1597/07-134.1

Lewis, A. E., Vasudevan, H. N., O'Neill, A. K., Soriano, P., and Bush, J. O. (2013). The widely used Wnt1-Cre transgene causes developmental phenotypes by ectopic activation of Wnt signaling. *Dev. Biol.* 379, 229–234. doi: 10.1016/j.ydbio.2013.04.026

Li, C.-W., Dinh, G. K., Zhang, A., and Chen, J. D. (2008). Ankyrin repeats-containing cofactors interact with ADA3 and modulate its co-activator function. *Biochem. J.* 413, 349–357. doi: 10.1042/BJ20071484

Li, H., Xie, H., Liu, W., Hu, R., Huang, B., Tan, Y.-F., et al. (2009). A novel microRNA targeting HDAC5 regulates osteoblast differentiation in mice and contributes to primary osteoporosis in humans. *J. Clin. Invest.* 119, 3666–3677. doi: 10.1172/JCI39832

Livak, K. J., and Schmittgen, T. D. (2001). Analysis of relative gene expression data using real-time quantitative PCR and the 2(-Delta Delta C(T)) Method. *Methods* 25, 402–408. doi: 10.1006/meth.2001.1262

Low, K., Ashraf, T., Canham, N., Clayton-Smith, J., Deshpande, C., Donaldson, A., et al. (2016). Clinical and genetic aspects of KBG syndrome. *Am. J. Med. Genet. A* 170, 2835–2846. doi: 10.1002/ajmg.a.37842

Malik, Z., Roth, D. M., Eaton, F., Theodor, J. M., and Graf, D. (2020). Mesenchymal Bmp7 controls onset of tooth mineralization: a novel way to regulate molar cusp shape. *Front. Physiol.* 11:698. doi: 10.3389/fphys.2020.00698

Marini, F., Cianferotti, L., and Brandi, M. L. (2016). Epigenetic mechanisms in bone biology and osteoporosis: can they drive therapeutic choices? *Int. J. Mol. Sci.* 17:1329. doi: 10.3390/ijms17081329

Mirabella, A. C., Foster, B. M., and Bartke, T. (2016). Chromatin deregulation in disease. *Chromosoma* 125, 75–93. doi: 10.1007/s00412-015-0530-0

Morel Swols, D., and Tekin, M. (2018). "KBG Syndrome," in *Gene Reviews*, eds M. P. Adam, H. H. Ardinger, R. A. Pagon, S. E. Wallace, L. J. Bean, K. Stephens, et al. (Seattle, WA: University of Washington, Seattle).

Nakaniwa, M., Kawasaki, M., Kawasaki, K., Yamada, A., Meguro, F., Takeyasu, M., et al. (2019). Primary cilia in murine palatal rugae development. *Gene Expression Patterns* 34:119062. doi: 10.1016/j.gep.2019.119062

Neilsen, P., Cheney, K. M., Li, C.-W., Chen, J., Cawrse, J. E., Schulz, R. B., et al. (2008). Identification of ANKRD11 as a p53 coactivator. *J. Cell Sci.* 121(Pt 21), 3541–3552. doi: 10.1242/jcs.026351

Ockeloen, C. W., Willemsen, M. H., de Munnik, S., van Bon, B. W. M., de Leeuw, N., Verrips, A., et al. (2015). Further delineation of the KBG syndrome phenotype caused by ANKRD11 aberrations. *Eur. J. Hum. Genet.* 23, 1176–1185. doi: 10.1038/ejhg.2014.253

Park-Min, K. H. (2017). Epigenetic regulation of bone cells. *Connect Tissue Res.* 58, 76–89. doi: 10.1080/03008207.2016.1177037

Perpétuo, I. P., Bourne, L. E., and Orriss, I. R. (2019). Isolation and generation of osteoblasts. *Methods Mol Biol* 1914, 21–38. doi: 10.1007/978-1-4939-8997-3_2

R Core Team (2020). *R: A Language and Environment for Statistical Computing.* Available online at: https://www.R-project.org/ (accessed December 20, 2020).

Samuels, B. D., Aho, R., Brinkley, J. F., Bugacov, A., Feingold, E., Fisher, S., et al. (2020). FaceBase 3: analytical tools and FAIR resources for craniofacial and dental research. *Development* 147:dev191213. doi: 10.1242/dev.191213

Satterstrom, F. K., Kosmicki, J. A., Wang, J., Breen, M. S., De Rubeis, S., An, J.-Y., et al. (2020). Large-scale exome sequencing study implicates both developmental and functional changes in the neurobiology of autism. *Cell* 180, 568.e23–584.e23. doi: 10.1016/j.cell.2019.12.036

Schlager, S. (2017). "Chapter 9 - morpho and rvcg – shape analysis in R: R-Packages for geometric morphometrics, shape analysis and surface manipulations," in *Statistical Shape and Deformation Analysis*, eds G. Zheng, S. Li, and G. Székely (Cambridge, MA: Academic Press), 217–256. doi: 10.1016/B978-0-12-810493-4.00011-0

Schroeder, T. M., Kahler, R. A., Li, X., and Westendorf, J. J. (2004). Histone deacetylase 3 Interacts with Runx2 to repress the osteocalcin promoter and regulate osteoblast differentiation. *J. Biol. Chem.* 279, 41998–42007. doi: 10.1074/jbc.M403702200

Schroeder, W., Martin, K., and Lorensen, W. (1998). *The Visualization Toolkit : An Object-Oriented Approach to 3D Graphics*, 2nd Edn. Hoboken, NJ: Prentice Hall.

Seelan, R. S., Mukhopadhyay, P., Warner, D. R., Webb, C. L., Pisano, M., and Greene, R. M. (2013). Epigenetic regulation of Sox4 during palate development. *Epigenomics* 5, 131–146. doi: 10.2217/epi.13.1

Sharp, G., Stergiakouli, E., Sandy, J., and Relton, C. (2018). Epigenetics and orofacial clefts: a brief introduction. *Cleft Palate Craniofac. J.* 55, 795–797. doi: 10.1597/16-124

Skarnes, W. C., Rosen, B., West, A. P., Koutsourakis, M., Bushell, W., Iyer, V., et al. (2011). A conditional knockout resource for the genome-wide study of mouse gene function. *Nature* 474, 337–342. doi: 10.1038/nature10163

St John, H. C., Bishop, K. A., Meyer, M. B., Benkusky, N. A., Leng, N., Kendziorski, C., et al. (2014). The osteoblast to osteocyte transition: epigenetic changes and response to the vitamin D3 hormone. *Mol. Endocrinol.* 28, 1150–1165. doi: 10.1210/me.2014-1091

Strobl-Mazzulla, P. H., Marini, M., and Buzzi, A. (2012). Epigenetic landscape and miRNA involvement during neural crest development. *Dev. Dyn.* 241, 1849–1856. doi: 10.1002/dvdy.23868

Temiyasathit, S., and Jacobs, C. R. (2010). Osteocyte primary cilium and its role in bone mechanotransduction. *Ann. N. Y. Acad. Sci.* 1192, 422–428. doi: 10.1111/j.1749-6632.2009.05243.x

Vidal-García, M. (2021). *morpho. Tools. GM v1.0.0: A Set of R Tools to Help With Geometric Morphometric Analyses of 3D Data.* doi: 10.5281/zenodo.4673771

Vincent, R. D., Neelin, P., Khalili-Mahani, N., Janke, A. L., Fonov, V. S., Robbins, S. M., et al. (2016). MINC 2.0: a flexible format for multi-modal images. *Front. Neuroinform.* 10:35. doi: 10.3389/fninf.2016.00035

Wan, Y., Lantz, B., Cusack, B. J., and Szabo-Rogers, H. L. (2018). Prickle1 regulates differentiation of frontal bone osteoblasts. *Sci. Rep.* 8:18021. doi: 10.1038/s41598-018-36742-0

Wein, M. N., Spatz, J., Nishimori, S., Doench, J., Root, D., Babij, P., et al. (2015). HDAC5 controls MEF2C-driven sclerostin expression in osteocytes. *J. Bone Miner Res.* 30, 400–411. doi: 10.1002/jbmr.2381

Wilfert, A. B., Sulovari, A., Turner, T. N., Coe, B. P., and Eichler, E. E. (2017). Recurrent de novo mutations in neurodevelopmental disorders: properties and clinical implications. *Genome Med.* 9:101. doi: 10.1186/s13073-017-0498-x

Winkler, D. G., Sutherland, M. K., Geoghegan, J. C., Yu, C., Hayes, T., Skonier, J. E., et al. (2003). Osteocyte control of bone formation via sclerostin, a novel BMP antagonist. *EMBO J.* 22, 6267–6276. doi: 10.1093/emboj/cdg599

Xiong, W., He, F., Morikawa, Y., Yu, X., Zhang, Z., Lan, Y., et al. (2009). Hand2 is required in the epithelium for palatogenesis in mice. *Dev. Biol.* 330, 131–141. doi: 10.1016/j.ydbio.2009.03.021

Yoshida, T., Vivatbutsiri, P., Morriss-Kay, G., Saga, Y., and Iseki, S. (2008). Cell lineage in mammalian craniofacial mesenchyme. *Mech. Dev.* 125, 797–808. doi: 10.1016/j.mod.2008.06.007

Zhang, A., Li, C.-W., and Chen, J. D. (2007). Characterization of transcriptional regulatory domains of ankyrin repeat cofactor-1. *Biochem. Biophys. Res. Commun.* 358, 1034–1040. doi: 10.1016/j.bbrc.2007.05.017

Zhang, A., Yeung, P. L., Li, C.-W., Tsai, S.-C., Dinh, G. K., Wu, X., et al. (2004). Identification of a novel family of ankyrin repeats containing cofactors for p160 nuclear receptor coactivators. *J. Biol. Chem.* 279, 33799–33805. doi: 10.1074/jbc.M403997200

Zhang, Y.-X., Sun, H.-L., Liang, H., Li, K., Fan, Q.-M., and Zhao, Q.-H. (2015). Dynamic and distinct histone modifications of osteogenic genes during osteogenic differentiation. *J. Biochem.* 158, 445–457. doi: 10.1093/jb/mvv059

19

Insights into the Complexity of Craniofacial Development From a Cellular Perspective

*Andrea P. Murillo-Rincón and Marketa Kaucka**

Max Planck Research Group Craniofacial Biology, Max Planck Institute for Evolutionary Biology, Plön, Germany

***Correspondence:**
Marketa Kaucka
kaucka@evolbio.mpg.de

The head represents the most complex part of the body and a distinctive feature of the vertebrate body plan. This intricate structure is assembled during embryonic development in the four-dimensional process of morphogenesis. The head integrates components of the central and peripheral nervous system, sensory organs, muscles, joints, glands, and other specialized tissues in the framework of a complexly shaped skull. The anterior part of the head is referred to as the face, and a broad spectrum of facial shapes across vertebrate species enables different feeding strategies, communication styles, and diverse specialized functions. The face formation starts early during embryonic development and is an enormously complex, multi-step process regulated on a genomic, molecular, and cellular level. In this review, we will discuss recent discoveries that revealed new aspects of facial morphogenesis from the time of the neural crest cell emergence till the formation of the chondrocranium, the primary design of the individual facial shape. We will focus on molecular mechanisms of cell fate specification, the role of individual and collective cell migration, the importance of dynamic and continuous cellular interactions, responses of cells and tissues to generated physical forces, and their morphogenetic outcomes. In the end, we will examine the spatiotemporal activity of signaling centers tightly regulating the release of signals inducing the formation of craniofacial skeletal elements. The existence of these centers and their regulation by enhancers represent one of the core morphogenetic mechanisms and might lay the foundations for intra- and inter-species facial variability.

Keywords: craniofacial development, neural crest, mesenchymal condensations, chondrocranium, facial shape, signaling centers, cellular behavior

INTRODUCTION

The shape of the face possesses species-specific features that give each vertebrate group its unique facial appearance. In some species such as humans, the otherwise conserved shaping mechanism is flexible enough to allow for shape fine-tuning, resulting in an impressive facial variability (Liu et al., 2012; Adhikari et al., 2016; Cole et al., 2016; Xiong et al., 2019). The shape of the face strongly depends on the geometry of underlying skeletal elements, adipose tissue, and muscles. While the postnatal facial skeleton in the majority of vertebrates is formed by bony elements, the embryonic face is built up entirely from cartilage and is represented by a complex structure called the chondrocranium. Most of the chondrocranium is substituted by the bone postnatally (McBratney-Owen et al., 2008; Kawasaki and Richtsmeier, 2017) and the functional and evolutionary meaning of chondrocranium is not fully understood. However, changes in chondrocranium morphology or morphometry remain even after its replacement by the bone (Kaucka et al., 2017), therefore, the formation of chondrocranium can be considered a key process in the acquisition of facial shape.

The chondrocranium formation is an intricate, multi-step process utilizing cells derived from all three germ layers and driven by, for instance, complex cell and tissue interactions, specific cellular behavior, or by a multitude of spatiotemporally active morphogens. In this review, we will summarize the advancements in our understanding of its developmental complexity. In the first part, we will focus on mechanisms driving the specification, delamination, and migration of cranial neural crest cells to their respective destinations, and their interactions with surrounding cells that result in sensory placode formation. Next, we will pinpoint to mutual interactions between different cell and tissue types, the cellular response to changing physical forces, and specific clonal behavior such as oriented cell division. In the end, we will expose the importance of the spatiotemporally defined activity of signaling centers driving the early craniofacial morphogenesis and discuss the possible genetic basis of facial variability.

SPECIFICATION AND CELL FATE ACQUISITION OF THE NEURAL CREST CELL

A milestone in the process of head formation is the emergence and migration of the neural crest cells (NCCs). The NCCs are transient multipotent progenitors arising from the borders of the closing neural tube (**Figures 1IA,B**; Basch et al., 2006; Pla and Monsoro-Burq, 2018; Prasad et al., 2020). Depending on the location of their origin along the anterioposterior axis of the neural tube and their post-migratory target destination, the cells are classified as cranial (or cephalic), cardiac, vagal (including enteric), trunk, and sacral NCCs (Rothstein et al., 2018). After the NCCs specification, the cells undergo epithelial-to-mesenchymal transition (EMT), delaminate from the neural tube, and follow conserved stereotypical dorsolateral migratory streams (**Figures 1IC,D**; Minoux and Rijli, 2010; Theveneau and Mayor, 2012; Rothstein et al., 2018).

Interestingly, cranial and trunk NCCs utilize distinct migration strategies (Richardson et al., 2016). Trunk NCCs migrate as chains of single cells following the leader cells in the front of the streams. The leader cells manifest characteristic morphological properties that are observed already before the onset of migration and if ablated, the follower cells are unable to proceed ventrally pointing at the irreplaceable fixed role of the leader cell. Cranial NCCs move directionally as a whole and all the cells show similar migratory properties. All the cranial NCCs can serve as transient leaders and their ablation does not affect the migration of the following cells. Both cranial and trunk NCCs maintain continuous and dynamic cell-cell contact to keep migration and directionality (Richardson et al., 2016; Li et al., 2019). Analysis of the hierarchical clustering of NCCs in cyclostomes shed new light on the evolutionary origin of the cranial crest. The cranial subpopulation of lamprey NCCs showed transcriptional similarity to the gene signature of trunk NCCs in amniotes. These observations suggest that the NCCs underwent gradual acquisition of regulatory complexity during the evolution of vertebrates, leading to the existence of distinct NCC populations such as cranial and trunk, and likely affecting the vertebrate body plan (Martik et al., 2019).

The NCCs give rise to a broad spectrum of cell types such as neurons and glial cells of the peripheral nervous system, smooth muscles, endocrine cells, melanocytes, chondrocytes, odontoblasts, connective tissue, and bone (Bronner and LeDouarin, 2012; Baggiolini et al., 2015; Kaucka et al., 2016). In mouse, the analysis of the progenies (or clones) derived from genetically labeled single NCCs showed that each clone occupies a specific area in the forming head and has the potential to acquire diverse cell fates, therefore contributing to the formation of multiple structures in that particular location (Baggiolini et al., 2015; Kaucka et al., 2016). The impressive cell fate repertoire of the NCCs raised the question of how do NCCs generate and control their extraordinary multipotency and what are the molecular drivers of cell fate specification. Analysis of the pluripotency marker expression in cranial NCCs identified a neural crest stem cell niche located in the central-most portion of the dorsal neural tube (Lignell et al., 2017). Other NCC subpopulations positioned dorsolaterally to the stem cell niche expressed more canonical NCC markers or showed a typical migratory gene expression signature (Lignell et al., 2017). With increasing distance of NCCs from the central part of the neural tube, the effect of Wnt signaling coming from the neural tube decreases and results in the miRNA-mediated silencing of typical neural crest stem cell markers, leading to the loss of NCCs multipotency (Bhattacharya et al., 2018).

Epigenetic regulation is one of the further mechanisms controlling the cranial NCC plasticity, especially concerning their axial regional identity. The cranial NCCs maintain broad facial patterning competence and can contribute to different structures in the forming head. Cranial NCCs show similar chromatin accessibility patterns even though their transcriptional profile differs. The chromatin pattern is maintained until post-migratory stages when the cells commit to a specific fate in response to local cues (Minoux et al., 2017). In Xenopus, the activity of histone deacetylases (HDACs), enzymes regulating chromatin accessibility, was shown to be crucial in blastula cells for patterning the ectoderm and the establishment of NCCs, and in the NCCs to maintain their pluripotency (Rao and LaBonne, 2018).

The combination of the single-cell transcriptomics and bioinformatical analysis of branching trajectories of murine NCCs, revealed new aspects of NCC multipotency, EMT, and fate specification (La Manno et al., 2018; Soldatov et al., 2019). Recent findings disproved previous beliefs that these are abrupt events driven by the activation of a specific gene regulatory network or dependent on the expression of a master regulator gene. For instance, pre-migratory NCCs express both neural plate border-specific genes and several neural tube markers (Lignell et al., 2017; Soldatov et al., 2019; Williams et al., 2019). The expression of NCC-specific markers gradually outweighs the expression of

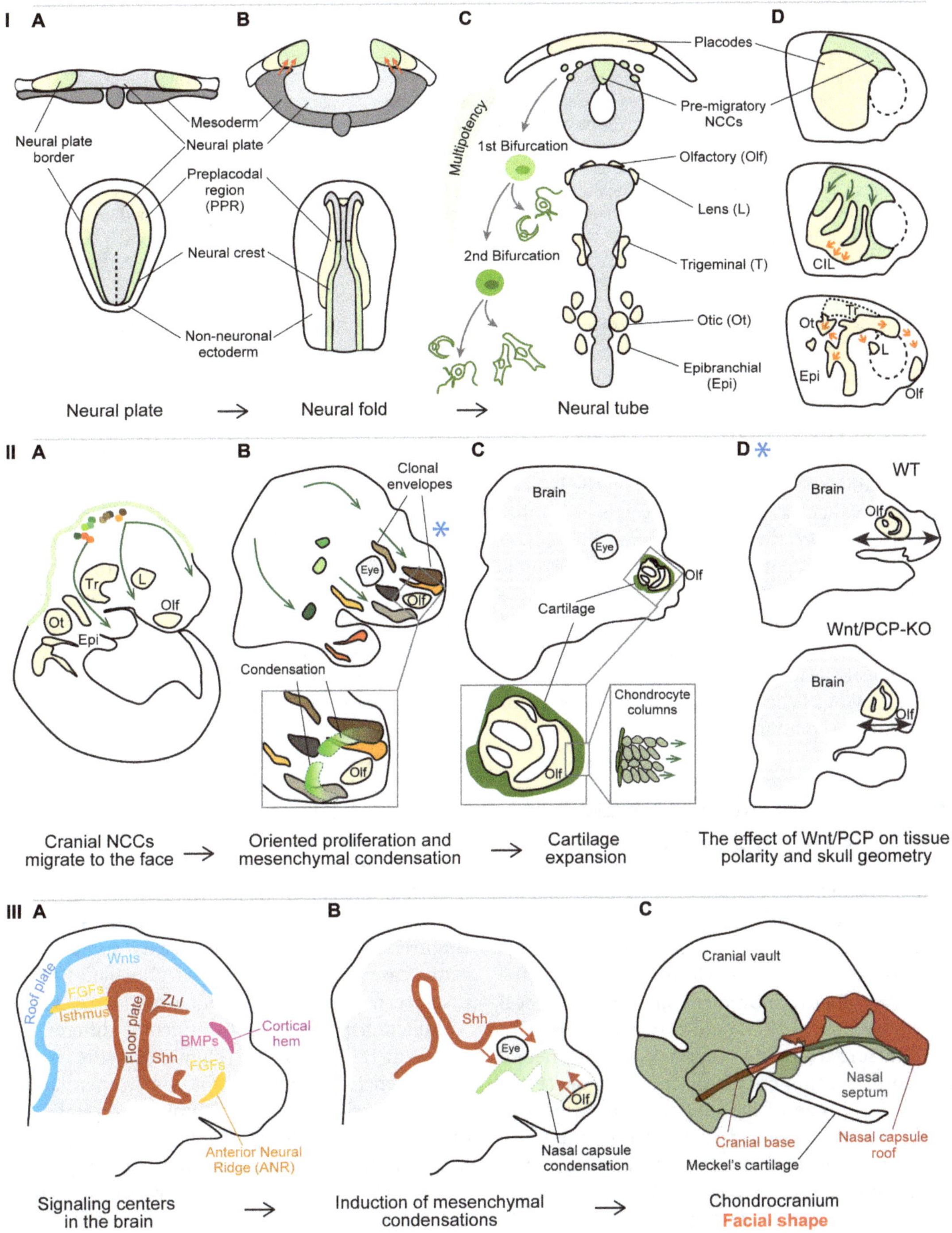

FIGURE 1 | Panel I: Specification and cell fate acquisition of the neural crest cells (NCCs). **(A)** NCCs and placode progenitor cells are localized adjacent to each other at the neural plate border. **(B)** When neural folds are brought together, the stiffened mesoderm underlying the cranial NCCs (red arrows) triggers NCC EMT and initiate NCC migration. **(C)** The migrating NCCs undergo a gradual process of cell fate acquisition, during which the NCCs pass through two main bifurcation points. The first separation leads to the split of sensory and autonomic/mesenchymal fates, and the second separation leads to the emergence of autonomic and mesenchymal fates. Placode progenitors are split from the common PPR into individual placodes to give rise to different sensory organs or cranial ganglia. **(D)** NCCs migration streams and placode separation are a result of the interaction between NCCs and placode cells (middle): NCCs are attracted by placode cells (green arrows), after their direct contact placode cells are repolarized and move away from the NCCs (orange arrows), in a process called contact inhibition locomotion (CIL). Due to their active directed cell migration (orange arrows, below), the individual placode territories are established and NCCs had along their stereotypical migratory pathways. **(A–C)** Upper row transversal view, lower row: dorsal view; **(D)** lateral view. **Panel II:** Cellular behavior during early craniofacial morphogenesis. **(A)** The cranial NCCs migrated into their respective destinations and proliferate generating facial ectomesenchyme. **(B)** The progeny of each cranial NCC occupies a

(Continued)

FIGURE 1 | Continued
3D area referred to as the clonal envelope. NCCs undergo cell divisions in an oriented manner, the shapes of clonal envelopes reflect the anisotropic growth of the head. The mesenchymal condensations originate from the local ectomesenchyme and represent the blueprint for chondrocranium and future facial shape. Extensive cell proliferation in quite distant locations results in collective cell movement translocating the whole micro-domains. **(C)** The mesenchymal condensations start differentiating into cartilage, the chondrocytes undergo a series of polarized cell divisions resulting in surface expansion of the chondrocranium. **(D)** Polarized cell division of NCC-derived ectomesenchyme is controlled by Wnt/Planar cell polarity (PCP) pathway and its disruption leads to shorter and wider facial proportions. The Blue asterisk shows the relevant time point of the Wnt/PCP signaling effect – during the proliferation of ectomesenchyme **(panel IIB)**. **Panel III:** Signaling centers establish facial geometry. **(A)** Signaling centers located in the developing brain instruct the formation of mesenchymal condensations from the ectomesenchyme. **(B)** Sonic hedgehog (Shh) from the floor plate induces the condensation leading to the formation of nasal septum as well some elements of the cranial base, while morphogenetic signals from the olfactory epithelium induce the formation of nasal capsule roof. **(C)** Removal of morphogenetic signals from distinct locations results in the absence or malformation of the respective cartilaginous structures.

neural tube-specific genes and the NCCs initiate delamination from the neural plate. The further existence of migrating NCCs is also defined by an extensive sequence of transcriptional events (Soldatov et al., 2019). Specifically, cell fate commitment is a result of co-activation of gene expression programs that would normally lead to mutually exclusive cell fates. Their competition is resolved after a bifurcation point, which is likely reached due to the effect of extrinsic signal such as WNT, BMP, Notch, or another signaling (**Figure 1IC**). Before the cell passes the bifurcation point, it can be perceived as bipotent progenitor. Interestingly, the first bifurcation point leads to division of progenitors into the sensory and autonomic neuronal/mesenchymal lineage, followed by the subsequent separation of autonomic neuronal progenitors from mesenchymal lineage (**Figure 1IC**; Soldatov et al., 2019), which is contrary to previous belief that each type of progenitor is directly derived from one common precursor.

CELL AND TISSUE DYNAMICS IN EARLY CRANIOFACIAL MORPHOGENESIS

Migration of single cells and large-scale collective cell movements represent important aspects of early facial morphogenesis. Such movements enable both mechanical and molecular interactions between cells and tissues, and their environment. One of the examples of such coordinated movement are the reciprocal interactions between the cranial NCCs and cranial placode cells. Cranial placode precursors arise at the anterior part of the neural plate border, and form a common pre-placodal region (PPR) characterized by the expression of the transcription factor Six1 (**Figure 1IA**). The PPR is positioned in close proximity and laterally to the emerging neural crest cells (Sato et al., 2010; Saint-Jeannet and Moody, 2014; Riddiford and Schlosser, 2016; Roellig et al., 2017). The cranial placodes together with the cranial NCCs form specialized sensory organs in the vertebrate head (**Figure 1IC**; Bouchard et al., 2010; Ladher et al., 2010; Huang et al., 2011; Cvekl and Ashery-Padan, 2014). The separation of common PPR into individual placodes is closely related to NCCs migration (**Figure 1ID**). Delaminating NCCs are attracted by the chemokine Sdf1 (CXCL12) produced by the placode cells (Shellard and Mayor, 2019). Once the NCCs get in direct contact with placodal cells, a transient junction complex is formed and Wnt/PCP components together with N-cadherin signaling trigger contact inhibition locomotion (CIL) (Theveneau et al., 2013). The cell protrusions and focal adhesions of placodal cells at the region of contact collapse, which leads to their repolarization and the directional migration away from the NCCs. Such "chase and run" behavior of NCCs following the Sdf1-producing placodal cells results in both the physical separation of future placodal regions and the establishment of the NCCs the migration streams (**Figure 1ID**; Szabó et al., 2019).

The cranial NCCs then follow stereotypical migratory streams and proliferate on their way to finally settle in various compartments of the head and produce ectomesenchyme (**Figure 1IIA**; Minoux and Rijli, 2010; Kaucka et al., 2016; Rothstein et al., 2018). While active and directional cell migration rather than cell proliferation drives the formation of the olfactory, lens, and otic placodes (Steventon et al., 2016; Breau et al., 2017), the ectomesenchyme expands by series of cell divisions and only very limited individual cell migration (Kaucka et al., 2016). A single NCC clone ultimately occupies a certain 3D space, referred to as a clonal envelop (**Figure 1IIB**). The shape and size of the clonal envelopes mirror the local directional cell behavior (the extent and the polarity of cell division), the level of mixing with other NCC clones, and reflect the anisotropic growth of different regions in the head. Each location is populated by several NCC-derived clones that extensively mix and jointly contribute to the formation of different structures in that area (**Figure 1IIB**). This might represent a compensation mechanism in the case that one or a few NCCs would be eliminated by, for instance, negative somatic mutations (Kaucka et al., 2016).

Functional experiments targeting different components of the Wnt/PCP signaling highlighted the importance of the ectomesenchyme polarity for the proper facial outgrowth in several developmental time-points. Overall, the rate of cell divisions in Wnt/PCP mutants does not appear to be affected, however, the impaired direction of daughter cell allocation during cell division results in a variety of pathologies, such as shorter and wider facial proportions, abnormal mesenchymal patterning during early palatogenesis or misoriented and misshaped chondrocytes affecting the facial morphometry (**Figures 1IIC,D**; Le Pabic et al., 2014; Brock et al., 2016; Kaucka et al., 2016). Oriented deposition of daughter cells also represents a core elongation mechanism driving the longitudinal growth of flat facial cartilage composing the mammalian chondrocranium (**Figure 1IIC**; Kaucka et al., 2017). Normal facial morphogenesis furthermore relies on coordinated collective cell movements, where the shift of large cell masses resembles the behavior of viscous fluids and allow large-scale cell rearrangements (David et al., 2014; Méhes and Vicsek, 2014;

Kaucka et al., 2016; Tao et al., 2019). These crowd movements are driven by extensive cell proliferation in relatively remote regions positioned laterally or posteriorly to the respective area and allow the preservation of cellular arrangements of the pushed microdomains (Kaucka et al., 2016).

Furthermore, physical forces generated by morphogenetic events contribute to various aspects of head formation. Cranial mesoderm stiffening was shown to be necessary and even sufficient to induce NCCs EMT and migration in *Xenopus* (**Figure 1IB**; Barriga et al., 2018). The stiffness of the cranial mesoderm, underlying the cranial NCCs at the time of neurulation, is generated by the increase in cell density in the process of convergent extension. The NCCs use their integrin-vinculin-talin mechanosensory complex to perceive the mechanical changes in the environment, and respond by switching the expression of E-cadherin to N-cadherin, gaining motility and responsiveness to chemotactic cues (Scarpa et al., 2015; Barriga et al., 2018). Mechanical forces also drive tooth morphogenesis (Mammoto et al., 2011; Panousopoulou and Green, 2016). The invagination of epithelial thickening into the mesenchyme is driven by the physical contraction of superficial layers of cells (i.e., suprabasal cells) (Panousopoulou and Green, 2016). The contraction is generated by the suprabasal cells intercalating and extending their cell shape apically and centripetally while remaining attached to the basal lamina. This process appears to be evolutionary conserved and may represent a fundamental morphogenetic mechanism driving the formation of multiple ectodermal organs such as a tooth, hair follicle, mammary gland, and sweat glands (Panousopoulou and Green, 2016). Subsequently, mesenchymal cells are attracted to underneath the early dental epithelium, which results in their physical compaction (Mammoto et al., 2011). Such mesenchymal cell condensation in turn triggers the induction of odontogenic expression programs and cell fate specification.

ESTABLISHING THE FACIAL GEOMETRY: THE MESENCHYMAL CONDENSATIONS

The first solid geometrical layout of the future facial shape is represented by the chondrocranium, the cartilaginous template of the future skull. The chondrocranium is induced when the ectomesenchyme formed the frontonasal outgrowth. A key step preceding the formation of cartilage is the induction of mesenchymal condensations (**Figure 1IIB**). These are defined areas of mesenchyme that are compacted due to local rapid cell division (Kaucka et al., 2017, 2018; Giffin et al., 2019), and differentiate into cartilage shortly after their emergence (**Figure 1IIC**). The spatially defined sources of morphogenetic signals, often represented by secreted ligands with long-range action potential (e.g., WNTs, FGFs, BMPs, and Hedgehogs), are referred to as signaling centers or organizers (**Figure 1IIIA**; Martinez Arias and Steventon, 2018; La Manno et al., 2020). The known signaling centers involved in craniofacial morphogenesis are located in the emerging nervous system, in the foregut endoderm and in spatially defined areas of the facial ectoderm (Marcucio et al., 2005; Wada et al., 2005; Brito et al., 2006; Eberhart et al., 2006; Foppiano et al., 2007; Szabo-Rogers et al., 2008, 2009; Gitton et al., 2011; Reid et al., 2011; Bhullar et al., 2015; Kaucka et al., 2018; Crane-Smith et al., 2019). Tissue- and/or time-specific ablation of morphogens or their sources, such as Sonic Hedgehog (Shh) or the olfactory placodes, showed that the condensations, and in turn the cartilage, are induced by different signaling centers at distinct time points as independent units, pointing at the composite character of the chondrocranium and the future skull (**Figures 1 – IIIB,C**; McBratney-Owen et al., 2008; Kaucka et al., 2018). Based on the association of the positions of both the signaling centers and skeletal structures induction points (Fabbri et al., 2017), it has been proposed that the species-specific localization of signaling centers located in the brain may represent a reliable criterion to assess skull bone homology (Teng et al., 2019). The Frontonasal Ectodermal Zone (FEZ) of birds and mammals represents a signaling center in the frontal facial ectoderm secreting SHH and FGF8, coordinating ectomesenchyme behavior and affecting the size, position, shape, and orientation of mesenchymal condensations (Abzhanov et al., 2007; Foppiano et al., 2007; Hu and Marcucio, 2009; Hu et al., 2015a,b).

Both the position of the signaling centers in the developing head and the expression levels of the inductive signals can be modified by several mechanisms. One of them is represented by the cis-regulatory elements (i.e., enhancers) that alter the levels of gene expression. Deletion of enhancers or changes in their sequence can result in a wide range of facial phenotypes (Attanasio et al., 2013; Kaucka et al., 2018). The sequence variation found in regulatory elements of genes associated with facial shape variability and identified epigenetic modifications controlling the enhancer activity in humans (Claes et al., 2018), show that enhancers represent an exceptionally flexible mechanism allowing facial shape fine-tuning (Kaucka et al., 2018) and may account for one of the mechanisms behind intra- and/or inter-species facial differences. Understanding the basis and regulation of mesenchymal condensation induction is further important for the comprehension and management of human craniofacial syndromes. More than 30% of all congenital abnormalities are represented by craniofacial malformation, ranging from subtle changes of facial features or symmetry to severe conditions affecting feeding, breathing, or other aspects of survival (Xavier et al., 2016; Abramyan, 2019). Interestingly, human craniofacial syndromes are often associated with disorders affecting the central nervous system or the sensory organs (Marcucio et al., 2011; Twigg and Wilkie, 2015), which further underlines the conserved link between the development of the nervous system and the formation of chondrocranium.

DISCUSSION

The development and availability of new techniques in the last decade have significantly advanced our understanding of the complexity of craniofacial development and opened new perspectives for future research. Single-cell omics analysis can be applied to uncover the gene regulatory networks driving the transitions from mesenchyme to cartilage or to reveal the enhancer-driven control of gene expression levels in different cellular populations. This approach, in combination with genetic tracing and live imaging, can further dissect the interactions between various cell or tissue types in detail and resolve, among others, the still enigmatic processes of placode specification and individualization. The precise spatiotemporal mapping of the signaling centers in the developing embryos of various model organisms and exploring their genomic regulation will advance our understanding of both the intra- and inter-species facial variability and the genetic basis of facial features heritability. Additionally, such investigation will allow us to better comprehend the nature of rare craniofacial pathologies. Further research of the conserved developmental link between the formation of the nervous system and the skull may identify new therapeutic targets to reduce the impact of severe congenital syndromes manifested with craniofacial deformities or offer new strategies to enhance cartilage regeneration in adulthood.

AUTHOR CONTRIBUTIONS

AM-R and MK wrote the manuscript and designed the figure. Both authors contributed to the article and approved the submitted version.

REFERENCES

Abramyan, J. (2019). Hedgehog signaling and embryonic craniofacial disorders. *J. Dev. Biol.* 7:9. doi: 10.3390/jdb7020009

Abzhanov, A., Cordero, D. R., Sen, J., Tabin, C. J., and Helms, J. A. (2007). Cross-regulatory interactions between Fgf8 and Shh in the avian frontonasal prominence. *Congenit. Anom.* 47, 136–148. doi: 10.1111/j.1741-4520.2007.00162.x

Adhikari, K., Fuentes-Guajardo, M., Quinto-Sánchez, M., Mendoza-Revilla, J., Camilo Chacón-Duque, J., Acuña-Alonzo, V., et al. (2016). A genome-wide association scan implicates DCHS2, RUNX2, GLI3, PAX1 and EDAR in human facial variation. *Nat. Commun.* 7:11616. doi: 10.1038/ncomms11616

Attanasio, C., Nord, A. S., Zhu, Y., Blow, M. J., Li, Z., Liberton, D. K., et al. (2013). Fine tuning of craniofacial morphology by distant-acting enhancers. *Science* 342:1241006. doi: 10.1126/science.1241006

Baggiolini, A., Varum, S., Mateos, J. M., Bettosini, D., John, N., Bonalli, M., et al. (2015). Premigratory and migratory neural crest cells are multipotent in vivo. *Cell Stem Cell* 16, 314–322. doi: 10.1016/j.stem.2015.02.017

Barriga, E. H., Franze, K., Charras, G., and Mayor, R. (2018). Tissue stiffening coordinates morphogenesis by triggering collective cell migration in vivo. *Nature* 554, 523–527. doi: 10.1038/nature25742

Basch, M. L., Bronner-Fraser, M. E., and García-Castro, M. I. (2006). Specification of the neural crest occurs during gastrulation and requires Pax7. *Nature* 441, 218–222. doi: 10.1038/nature04684

Bhattacharya, D., Rothstein, M., Azambuja, A. P., and Simoes-Costa, M. (2018). Control of neural crest multipotency by wnt signaling and the Lin28/let-7 axis. *Elife* 7:e40556. doi: 10.7554/eLife.40556

Bhullar, B.-A. S., Morris, Z. S., Sefton, E. M., Tok, A., Tokita, M., Namkoong, B., et al. (2015). A molecular mechanism for the origin of a key evolutionary innovation, the bird beak and palate, revealed by an integrative approach to major transitions in vertebrate history. *Evolution* 69, 1665–1677. doi: 10.1111/evo.12684

Bouchard, M., De Caprona, D., Busslinger, M., Xu, P., and Fritzsch, B. (2010). Pax2 and Pax8 cooperate in mouse inner ear morphogenesis and innervation. *BMC Dev. Biol.* 10:89. doi: 10.1186/1471-213X-10-89

Breau, M. A., Bonnet, I., Stoufflet, J., Xie, J., De Castro, S., and Schneider-Maunoury, S. (2017). Extrinsic mechanical forces mediate retrograde axon extension in a developing neuronal circuit. *Nat. Commun.* 8:282. doi: 10.1038/s41467-017-00283-283

Brito, J. M., Teillet, M.-A., and Le Douarin, N. M. (2006). An early role for sonic hedgehog from foregut endoderm in jaw development: ensuring neural crest cell survival. *Proc. Natl. Acad. Sci. U.S.A.* 103, 11607–11612. doi: 10.1073/pnas.0604751103

Brock, L. J., Economou, A. D., Cobourne, M. T., and Green, J. B. A. (2016). Mapping cellular processes in the mesenchyme during palatal development in the absence of Tbx1 reveals complex proliferation changes and perturbed cell packing and polarity. *J. Anat.* 228, 464–473. doi: 10.1111/joa.12425

Bronner, M. E., and LeDouarin, N. M. (2012). Development and evolution of the neural crest: an overview. *Dev. Biol.* 366, 2–9. doi: 10.1016/j.ydbio.2011.12.042

Claes, P., Roosenboom, J., White, J. D., Swigut, T., Sero, D., Li, J., et al. (2018). Genome-wide mapping of global-to-local genetic effects on human facial shape. *Nat. Genet.* 50, 414–423. doi: 10.1038/s41588-018-0057-4

Cole, J. B., Manyama, M., Kimwaga, E., Mathayo, J., Larson, J. R., Liberton, D. K., et al. (2016). genomewide association study of african children identifies association of SCHIP1 and PDE8A with facial size and shape. *PLoS Genet.* 12:e1006174. doi: 10.1371/journal.pgen.1006174

Crane-Smith, Z., Schoenebeck, J., Graham, K., Devenney, P., Rose, L., Ditzell, M., et al. (2019). A highly conserved Shh enhancer coordinates hypothalamic and craniofacial development. *bioRxiv* [Preprint]. doi: 10.1101/794198

Cvekl, A., and Ashery-Padan, R. (2014). The cellular and molecular mechanisms of vertebrate lens development. *Development* 141, 4432–4447. doi: 10.1242/dev.107953

David, R., Luu, O., Damm, E. W., Wen, J. W. H., Nagel, M., and Winklbauer, R. (2014). Tissue cohesion and the mechanics of cell rearrangement. *Development* 141, 3672–3682.

Eberhart, J. K., Swartz, M. E., Crump, J. G., and Kimmel, C. B. (2006). Early Hedgehog signaling from neural to oral epithelium organizes anterior craniofacial development. *Development* 133, 1069–1077. doi: 10.1242/dev.02281

Fabbri, M., Mongiardino Koch, N., Pritchard, A. C., Hanson, M., Hoffman, E., Bever, G. S., et al. (2017). The skull roof tracks the brain during the evolution and development of reptiles including birds. *Nat. Ecol. Evol.* 1, 1543–1550. doi: 10.1038/s41559-017-0288-2

Foppiano, S., Hu, D., and Marcucio, R. S. (2007). Signaling by bone morphogenetic proteins directs formation of an ectodermal signaling center that regulates craniofacial development. *Dev. Biol.* 312, 103–114. doi: 10.1016/j.ydbio.2007.09.016

Giffin, J. L., Gaitor, D., and Franz-Odendaal, T. A. (2019). The forgotten skeletogenic condensations: a comparison of early skeletal development amongst vertebrates. *J. Dev. Biol.* 7:4. doi: 10.3390/JDB7010004

Gitton, Y., Benouaiche, L., Vincent, C., Heude, E., Soulika, M., Bouhali, K., et al. (2011). Dlx5 and Dlx6 expression in the anterior neural fold is essential for patterning the dorsal nasal capsule. *Development* 138, 897–903. doi: 10.1242/dev.057505

Hu, D., and Marcucio, R. S. (2009). Unique organization of the frontonasal ectodermal zone in birds and mammals. *Dev. Biol.* 325, 200–210. doi: 10.1016/j.ydbio.2008.10.026

Hu, D., Young, N. M., Li, X., Xu, Y., Hallgrimsson, R. S., and Marcucio, R. S. (2015a). A dynamic shh expression pattern, regulated by SHH and BMP signaling, coordinates fusion of primordia in the amniote face. *Development* 142, 567–574.

Hu, D., Young, N. M., Xu, Q., Jamniczky, R. M., Green, R. M., Mio, R. S., et al. (2015b). Signals from the brain induce variation in avian facial shape. *Dev. Dyn.* 244, 1133–1143.

Huang, J., Rajagopal, R., Liu, Y., Dattilo, L. K., Shaham, O., Ashery-Padan, R., et al. (2011). The mechanism of lens placode formation: a case of matrix-mediated morphogenesis. *Dev. Biol.* 355, 32–42. doi: 10.1016/j.ydbio.2011.04.008

Kaucka, M., Ivashkin, E., Gyllborg, D., Zikmund, T., Tesarova, M., Kaiser, J., et al. (2016). Analysis of neural crest-derived clones reveals novel aspects of facial development. *Sci. Adv.* 2, 11–16. doi: 10.1126/sciadv.1600060

Kaucka, M., Petersen, J., Tesarova, M., Szarowska, B., Kastriti, M. E., Xie, M., et al. (2018). Signals from the brain and olfactory epithelium control shaping of the mammalian nasal capsule cartilage. *Elife* 7:e34465.

Kaucka, M., Zikmund, T., Tesarova, M., Gyllborg, D., Hellander, A., Jaros, J., et al. (2017). Oriented clonal cell dynamics enables accurate growth and shaping of vertebrate cartilage. *Elife* 6, e25902. doi: 10.7554/eLife.25902

Kawasaki, K., and Richtsmeier, J. T. (2017). "Association of the chondrocranium and dermatocranium in early skull formation," in *Building Bones: Bone Formation and Development in Anthropology*, eds C. Percival and J. Richtsmeier (Cambridge: Cambridge University Press), doi: 10.1017/9781316388907.004

La Manno, G., Soldatov, R., Zeisel, A., Braun, E., Hochgerner, H., Petukhov, V., et al. (2018). RNA velocity of single cells. *Nature* 560, 494–498. doi: 10.1038/s41586-018-0414-6

Ladher, R. K., O'Neill, P., and Begbie, J. (2010). From shared lineage to distinct functions: the development of the inner ear and epibranchial placodes. *Development* 137, 1777–1785. doi: 10.1242/dev.040055

Le Pabic, P., Ng, C., and Schilling, T. F. (2014). Fat-dachsous signaling coordinates cartilage differentiation and polarity during craniofacial development. *PLoS Genet.* 10:1004726. doi: 10.1371/journal.pgen.1004726

Li, Y., Vieceli, F. M., Gonzalez, W. G., Li, A., Tang, W., Lois, C., et al. (2019). In vivo quantitative imaging provides insights into trunk neural crest migration. *Cell Rep.* 26, 1489.e3–1500.e3. doi: 10.1016/j.celrep.2019.01.039

Lignell, A., Kerosuo, L., Streichan, S. J., Cai, L., and Bronner, M. E. (2017). Identification of a neural crest stem cell niche by Spatial Genomic Analysis. *Nat. Commun.* 8:1830. doi: 10.1038/s41467-017-01561-w

Liu, F., van der Lijn, F., Schurmann, C., Zhu, G., Chakravarty, M. M., Hysi, P. G., et al. (2012). A genome-wide association study identifies five loci influencing facial morphology in europeans. *PLoS Genet.* 8:1002932. doi: 10.1371/journal.pgen.1002932

Mammoto, T., Mammoto, A., Torisawa, Y., Tat, T., Gibbs, A., Derda, R., et al. (2011). Mechanochemical control of mesenchymal condensation and embryonic tooth organ formation. *Dev. Cell* 21, 758–769. doi: 10.1016/j.devcel.2011.07.006

La Manno, G., Siletti, K., Furlan, A., Gyllborg, D., Vinsland, E., et al. (2020). Molecular architecture of the developing mouse brain. *bioRxiv* [Preprint]. doi: 10.1101/2020.07.02.184051

Marcucio, R. S., Cordero, D. R., Hu, D., and Helms, J. A. (2005). Molecular interactions coordinating the development of the forebrain and face. *Dev. Biol.* 284, 48–61. doi: 10.1016/J.YDBIO.2005.04.030

Marcucio, R. S., Young, N. M., Hu, D., and Hallgrimsson, B. (2011). Mechanisms that underlie co-variation of the brain and face. *Genesis* 49, 177–189. doi: 10.1002/dvg.20710

Martik, M. L., Gandhi, S., Uy, B. R., Gillis, J. A., Green, S. A., Simoes-Costa, M., et al. (2019). Evolution of the new head by gradual acquisition of neural crest regulatory circuits. *Nature* 574, 675–678. doi: 10.1038/s41586-019-1691-4

Martinez Arias, A., and Steventon, B. (2018). On the nature and function of organizers. *Developemt* 145:dev159525. doi: 10.1242/dev.159525

McBratney-Owen, B., Iseki, S., Bamforth, S. D., Olsen, B. R., and Morriss-Kay, G. M. (2008). Development and tissue origins of the mammalian cranial base. *Dev. Biol.* 322, 121–132. doi: 10.1016/j.ydbio.2008.07.016

Méhes, E., and Vicsek, T. (2014). Collective motion of cells: from experiments to models. *Integr. Biol.* 6, 831–854.

Minoux, M., Holwerda, S., Vitobello, A., Kitazawa, T., Kohler, H., Stadler, M. B., et al. (2017). Gene bivalency at Polycomb domains regulates cranial neural crest positional identity. *Science* 355:eaal2913. doi: 10.1126/science.aal2913

Minoux, M., and Rijli, F. M. (2010). Molecular mechanisms of cranial neural crest cell migration and patterning in craniofacial development. *Development* 137, 2605–2621. doi: 10.1242/DEV.040048

Panousopoulou, E., and Green, J. B. A. (2016). Invagination of ectodermal placodes is driven by cell intercalation-mediated contraction of the suprabasal tissue canopy. *PLoS Biol.* 14:e1002405. doi: 10.1371/journal.pbio.1002405

Pla, P., and Monsoro-Burq, A. H. (2018). The neural border: induction, specification and maturation of the territory that generates neural crest cells. *Dev. Biol.* 444, S36–S46. doi: 10.1016/j.ydbio.2018.05.018

Prasad, M. S., Uribe-Querol, E., Marquez, J., Vadasz, S., Yardley, N., Shelar, P. B., et al. (2020). Blastula stage specification of avian neural crest. *Dev. Biol.* 458, 64–74. doi: 10.1016/j.ydbio.2019.10.007

Rao, A., and LaBonne, C. (2018). Histone deacetylase activity has an essential role in establishing and maintaining the vertebrate neural crest. *Developmet* 145:dev163386. doi: 10.1242/dev.163386

Reid, B. S., Yang, H., Melvin, V. S., Taketo, M. M., and Williams, T. (2011). Ectodermal Wnt/β-catenin signaling shapes the mouse face. *Dev. Biol.* 349, 261–299. doi: 10.1016/J.YDBIO.2010.11.012

Richardson, J., Gauert, A., Briones Montecinos, L., Fanlo, L., Alhashem, Z. M., Assar, R., et al. (2016). Leader cells define directionality of trunk, but not cranial, neural crest cell migration. *Cell Rep.* 15, 2076–2088. doi: 10.1016/j.celrep.2016.04.067

Riddiford, N., and Schlosser, G. (2016). Dissecting the pre-placodal transcriptome to reveal presumptive direct targets of Six1 and Eya1 in cranial placodes. *Elife* 5:e17666. doi: 10.7554/eLife.17666

Roellig, D., Tan-Cabugao, J., Esaian, S., and Bronner, M. E. (2017). Dynamic transcriptional signature and cell fate analysis reveals plasticity of individual neural plate border cells. *Elife* 6:e21620. doi: 10.7554/eLife.21620

Rothstein, M., Bhattacharya, D., and Simoes-Costa, M. (2018). The molecular basis of neural crest axial identity. *Dev. Biol.* 444, S170–S180. doi: 10.1016/j.ydbio.2018.07.026

Saint-Jeannet, J. P., and Moody, S. A. (2014). Establishing the pre-placodal region and breaking it into placodes with distinct identities. *Dev. Biol.* 389, 13–27. doi: 10.1016/j.ydbio.2014.02.011

Sato, S., Ikeda, K., Shioi, G., Ochi, H., Ogino, H., Yajima, H., et al. (2010). Conserved expression of mouse Six1 in the pre-placodal region (PPR) and identification of an enhancer for the rostral PPR. *Dev. Biol.* 344, 158–171. doi: 10.1016/j.ydbio.2010.04.029

Scarpa, E., Szabó, A., Bibonne, A., Theveneau, E., Parsons, M., and Mayor, R. (2015). Cadherin switch during EMT in neural crest cells leads to contact inhibition of locomotion via repolarization of forces. *Dev. Cell* 34, 421–434. doi: 10.1016/j.devcel.2015.06.012

Shellard, A., and Mayor, R. (2019). Integrating chemical and mechanical signals in neural crest cell migration. *Curr. Opin. Genet. Dev.* 57, 16–24. doi: 10.1016/j.gde.2019.06.004

Soldatov, R., Kaucka, M., Kastriti, M. E., Petersen, J., Chontorotzea, T., Englmaier, L., et al. (2019). Spatiotemporal structure of cell fate decisions in murine neural crest. *Science* 364:eaas9536. doi: 10.1126/science.aas9536

Steventon, B., Mayor, R., and Streit, A. (2016). Directional cell movements downstream of Gbx2 and Otx2 control the assembly of sensory placodes. *Biol. Open* 5, 1620–1624. doi: 10.1242/bio.020966

Szabó, A., Theveneau, E., Turan, M., and Mayor, R. (2019). Neural crest streaming as an emergent property of tissue interactions during morphogenesis. *PLoS Comput. Biol.* 15:e1007002. doi: 10.1371/journal.pcbi.1007002

Szabo-Rogers, H. L., Geetha-Loganathan, P., Nimmagadda, S., Fu, K. K., and Richman, J. M. (2008). FGF signals from the nasal pit are necessary for normal facial morphogenesis. *Dev. Biol.* 318, 289–302. doi: 10.1016/J.YDBIO.2008.03.027

Szabo-Rogers, H. L., Geetha-Loganathan, P., Whiting, C. J., Nimmagadda, S., Fu, K., and Richman, J. M. (2009). Novel skeletogenic patterning roles for the olfactory pit. *Development* 136, 219–229. doi: 10.1242/dev.023978

Tao, H., Zhu, M., Lau, K., Whitley, O. K. W., Samani, M., Xiao, X., et al. (2019). Oscillatory cortical forces promote three dimensional cell intercalations that shape the murine mandibular arch. *Nat. Commun.* 10:1703. doi: 10.1038/s41467-019-09540-z

Teng, C. S., Cavin, L., Maxson, R. E., Sánchez-Villagra, M. R., and Crump, J. G. (2019). Resolving homology in the face of shifting germ layer origins: lessons from a major skull vault boundary. *Elife* 8:e52814. doi: 10.7554/eLife.52814

Theveneau, E., and Mayor, R. (2012). Neural crest delamination and migration: from epithelium-to-mesenchyme transition to collective cell migration. *Dev. Biol.* 366, 34–54. doi: 10.1016/j.ydbio.2011.12.041

Theveneau, E., Steventon, B., Scarpa, E., Garcia, S., Trepat, X., Streit, A., et al. (2013). Chase-and-run between adjacent cell populations promotes directional collective migration. *Nat. Cell Biol.* 15, 763–772. doi: 10.1038/ncb2772

Twigg, S. R. F., and Wilkie, A. O. M. (2015). A genetic-pathophysiological framework for craniosynostosis. *Am. J. Hum. Genet.* 97, 359–377. doi: 10.1016/j.ajhg.2015.07.006

Wada, N., Javidan, Y., Nelson, S., Carney, T. J., Kelsh, R. N., and Schilling, T. F. (2005). Hedgehog signaling is required for cranial neural crest morphogenesis and chondrogenesis at the midline in the zebrafish skull. *Development* 132, 3977–3988. doi: 10.1242/dev.01943

Williams, R. M., Candido-Ferreira, I., Repapi, E., Gavriouchkina, D., Senanayake, U., Ling, I. T. C., et al. (2019). Reconstruction of the global neural crest gene regulatory network in vivo. *Dev. Cell* 51, 255.e7–276.e7. doi: 10.1016/j.devcel.2019.10.003

Xavier, G. M., Seppala, M., Barrell, W., Birjandi, A. A., Geoghegan, F., and Cobourne, M. T. (2016). Hedgehog receptor function during craniofacial development. *Dev. Biol.* 415, 198–215. doi: 10.1016/j.ydbio.2016.02.009

Xiong, Z., Dankova, G., Howe, L. J., Lee, M. K., Hysi, P. G., De Jong, M. A., et al. (2019). Novel genetic loci affecting facial shape variation in humans. *Elife* 8:e49898. doi: 10.7554/eLife.49898

Permissions

All chapters in this book were first published by Frontiers; hereby published with permission under the Creative Commons Attribution License or equivalent. Every chapter published in this book has been scrutinized by our experts. Their significance has been extensively debated. The topics covered herein carry significant findings which will fuel the growth of the discipline. They may even be implemented as practical applications or may be referred to as a beginning point for another development.

The contributors of this book come from diverse backgrounds, making this book a truly international effort. This book will bring forth new frontiers with its revolutionizing research information and detailed analysis of the nascent developments around the world.

We would like to thank all the contributing authors for lending their expertise to make the book truly unique. They have played a crucial role in the development of this book. Without their invaluable contributions this book wouldn't have been possible. They have made vital efforts to compile up to date information on the varied aspects of this subject to make this book a valuable addition to the collection of many professionals and students.

This book was conceptualized with the vision of imparting up-to-date information and advanced data in this field. To ensure the same, a matchless editorial board was set up. Every individual on the board went through rigorous rounds of assessment to prove their worth. After which they invested a large part of their time researching and compiling the most relevant data for our readers.

The editorial board has been involved in producing this book since its inception. They have spent rigorous hours researching and exploring the diverse topics which have resulted in the successful publishing of this book. They have passed on their knowledge of decades through this book. To expedite this challenging task, the publisher supported the team at every step. A small team of assistant editors was also appointed to further simplify the editing procedure and attain best results for the readers.

Apart from the editorial board, the designing team has also invested a significant amount of their time in understanding the subject and creating the most relevant covers. They scrutinized every image to scout for the most suitable representation of the subject and create an appropriate cover for the book.

The publishing team has been an ardent support to the editorial, designing and production team. Their endless efforts to recruit the best for this project, has resulted in the accomplishment of this book. They are a veteran in the field of academics and their pool of knowledge is as vast as their experience in printing. Their expertise and guidance has proved useful at every step. Their uncompromising quality standards have made this book an exceptional effort. Their encouragement from time to time has been an inspiration for everyone.

The publisher and the editorial board hope that this book will prove to be a valuable piece of knowledge for researchers, students, practitioners and scholars across the globe.

List of Contributors

Eva Svandova
Institute of Animal Physiology and Genetics, Academy of Sciences, Brno, Czechia

Neal Anthwal and Abigail S. Tucker
Centre for Craniofacial and Regenerative Biology, King's College London, Guy's Hospital, London, United Kingdom

Eva Matalova
Institute of Animal Physiology and Genetics, Academy of Sciences, Brno, Czechia
Department of Physiology, University of Veterinary and Pharmaceutical Sciences, Brno, Czechia

Marcella Martinelli, Annalisa Palmieri and Luca Scapoli
Department of Experimental, Diagnostic and Specialty Medicine, Alma Mater Studiorum – University of Bologna, Bologna, Italy

Francesco Carinci
Department of Morphology, Surgery and Experimental Medicine, University of Ferrara, Ferrara, Italy

Fuqiang Yuan, Huadong Fan, Yihong Li, Lanhai Lu, Jie Liu and Shao-yu Chen
Department of Pharmacology and Toxicology, University of Louisville Health Sciences Center, Louisville, KY, United States
University of Louisville Alcohol Research Center, Louisville, KY, United States

Yang Yun
Department of Pharmacology and Toxicology, University of Louisville Health Sciences Center, Louisville, KY, United States
University of Louisville Alcohol Research Center, Louisville, KY, United States
College of Environment and Resource, Research Center of Environment and Health, Shanxi University, Taiyuan, China

Wenke Feng
Department of Pharmacology and Toxicology, University of Louisville Health Sciences Center, Louisville, KY, United States
University of Louisville Alcohol Research Center, Louisville, KY, United States
Department of Medicine, University of Louisville, Louisville, KY, United States

S. T. Raterman
Radboud Institute of Molecular Life Sciences, Nijmegen, Netherlands
Department of Dentistry-Orthodontics and Craniofacial Biology, Radboud University Medical Center, Nijmegen, Netherlands
Department of Animal Ecology and Physiology, Institute for Water and Wetland Research, Radboud University, Nijmegen, Netherlands

J. R. Metz
Department of Animal Ecology and Physiology, Institute for Water and Wetland Research, Radboud University, Nijmegen, Netherlands

Frank A. D. T. G. Wagener and Johannes W. Von den Hoff
Radboud Institute of Molecular Life Sciences, Nijmegen, Netherlands
Department of Dentistry-Orthodontics and Craniofacial Biology, Radboud University Medical Center, Nijmegen, Netherlands

Marilisa Carneiro Leão Gabardo, Prescila Mota de Oliveira Kublitski, Isabela Rodrigues Sette, Thaís Lauschner, Mariana Martins Juglair, Flares Baratto-Filho and João Armando Brancher
School of Health Sciences, Universidade Positivo, Curitiba, Brazil

Edgard Michel-Crosato
Department of Dentistry, Universidade de São Paulo, São Paulo, Brazil

Benny S. Latief
Department of Oral and Maxillofacial Surgery, Faculty of Dentistry, Universitas Indonesia, Jakarta, Indonesia

Mette A. R. Kuijpers
Department of Dentistry – Orthodontics and Craniofacial Biology, Radboud University Medical Center, Radboud Institute for Health Sciences, Nijmegen, Netherlands

Adam Stebel
Department of Maxillofacial Surgery, F. D. Roosevelt University Hospital, Banská Bystrica, Slovakia
Department of Stomatology and Maxillofacial Surgery, Faculty of Medicine, Comenius University Bratislava, Slovakia

Anne Marie Kuijpers-Jagtman
Faculty of Dentistry, Universitas Indonesia, Jakarta, Indonesia
Department of Orthodontics, University Medical Center Groningen, Groningen, Netherlands
Department of Orthodontics and Dentofacial Orthopedics, University of Bern, Bern, Switzerland

Piotr S. Fudalej
Department of Orthodontics and Dentofacial Orthopedics, University of Bern, Bern, Switzerland
Department of Orthodontics, Jagiellonian University, Kraków, Poland
Department of Orthodontics, Institute of Dentistry and Oral Sciences, Palacký University Olomouc, Olomouc, Czechia

Mona Mozaffari
Centre for Craniofacial and Regenerative Biology, King's College London, Guy's Hospital, London, United Kingdom

Robert Nash
Department of Paediatric Otolaryngology, Cochlear Implants, Great Ormond Street Hospital for Children NHS Trust, London, United Kingdom

Barbora Vesela and Adela Kratochvilova
Laboratory of Odontogenesis and Osteogenesis, Institute of Animal Physiology and Genetics, Academy of Sciences, Brno, Czechia

Petr Benes and Kamila Rihova
Department of Experimental Biology, Faculty of Science, Masaryk University, Brno, Czechia

Anne Poliard
Laboratory of Orofacial Pathologies, Imaging and Biotherapies, UFR Odontology Montrouge, Paris University, Paris, France

Miranda R. Sun and Dustin M. Fink
Department of Comparative Biosciences, School of Veterinary Medicine, University of Wisconsin-Madison, Madison, WI, United States

Hannah M. Chung, Veronika Matsuk and Robert J. Lipinski
Department of Comparative Biosciences, School of Veterinary Medicine, University of Wisconsin-Madison, Madison, WI, United States
Molecular and Environmental Toxicology Center, University of Wisconsin-Madison, Madison, WI, United States

Matthew J. Stebbins and Sean P. Palecek
Department of Chemical and Biological Engineering, University of Wisconsin-Madison, Madison, WI, United States

Eric V. Shusta
Department of Chemical and Biological Engineering, University of Wisconsin-Madison, Madison, WI, United States
Department of Neurological Surgery, University of Wisconsin-Madison, Madison, WI, United States

Shu Lou, Shiyi Kan, Xin Yu, Yuting Wang, Fan Yang, Guirong Zhu, Liwen Fan, Dandan Li, Hua Wang, Wei Wang and Weibing Zhang
Jiangsu Key Laboratory of Oral Diseases, Nanjing Medical University, Nanjing, China
Department of Orthodontics, Affiliated Hospital of Stomatology, Nanjing Medical University, Nanjing, China

Lin Wang and Yongchu Pan
Jiangsu Key Laboratory of Oral Diseases, Nanjing Medical University, Nanjing, China
Department of Orthodontics, Affiliated Hospital of Stomatology, Nanjing Medical University, Nanjing, China
State Key Laboratory of Reproductive Medicine, Nanjing Medical University, Nanjing, China

Lan Ma
Jiangsu Key Laboratory of Oral Diseases, Nanjing Medical University, Nanjing, China
Department of Environmental Genomics, School of Public Health, Nanjing Medical University, Nanjing, China

Mohammad Khursheed Alam
Orthodontic Division, Department of Preventive Dental Science, College of Dentistry, Jouf University, Sakaka, Saudi Arabia

Ahmed Ali Alfawzan
Department of Preventive Dentistry, College of Dentistry in Ar Rass, Qassim University, Ar Rass, Saudi Arabia

Noriko Funato
Department of Signal Gene Regulation, Tokyo Medical and Dental University, Tokyo, Japan
Research Core, Tokyo Medical and Dental University, Tokyo, Japan

Luana Mordask Bonetto, Paola Fernanda Cotait de Lucas Corso, Gabrielle Grosko Kuchar, Jennifer Tsi Gerber, Leonardo Fernandes Cunha, João Cesar Zielak and Carla Castiglia Gonzaga
Department of Dentistry, Positivo University, Curitiba, Brazil

Mohammed Elsalanty
Department of Medical Anatomical Science, Western University of Health Sciences, Pomona, CA, Unioted States

Rafaela Scariot
Department of Dentistry, Federal University of Parana, Curitiba, Brazil

Herve Lesot
Laboratory of Odontogenesis and Osteogenesis, Institute of Animal Physiology and Genetics, Academy of Sciences, Brno, Czechia

Renata Peterkova
Department of Histology and Embryology, Third Faculty of Medicine, Charles University, Prague, Czechia

Ludovica Parisi, Patrick O. Knapp, Eleftheria Girousi, Silvia Rihs, Christos Katsaros and Martin Degen
Laboratory for Oral Molecular Biology, Dental Research Center, Department of Orthodontics and Dentofacial Orthopedics, University of Bern, Bern, Switzerland

Giorgio C. La Scala
Division of Pediatric Surgery, Department of Pediatrics, University Hospital of Geneva, Geneva, Switzerland

Isabelle Schnyder
University Clinic for Pediatric Surgery, Bern University Hospital, Bern, Switzerland

Alexandra Stähli and Anton Sculean
Department of Periodontology, School of Dental Medicine, University of Bern, Bern, Switzerland

Dieter D. Bosshardt
Department of Periodontology, School of Dental Medicine, University of Bern, Bern, Switzerland
Robert K. Schenk Laboratory of Oral Histology, Dental Research Center, University of Bern, Bern, Switzerland

Ching-Fang Chang, Kari M. Brown and Yanfen Yang
Division of Developmental Biology, Department of Pediatrics, Cincinnati Children's Hospital Medical Center, Cincinnati, OH, United States
Department of Pediatrics, University of Cincinnati College of Medicine, Cincinnati, OH, United States

Samantha A. Brugmann
Division of Developmental Biology, Department of Pediatrics, Cincinnati Children's Hospital Medical Center, Cincinnati, OH, United States
Department of Pediatrics, University of Cincinnati College of Medicine, Cincinnati, OH, United States
Division of Plastic Surgery, Department of Surgery, Cincinnati Children's Hospital Medical Center, Cincinnati, OH, United States
Shriners Children's Hospital, Cincinnati, OH, United States

Daniela Marta Roth, Pranidhi Baddam, Haiming Lin and Sarah-Thea De Souza
School of Dentistry, Faculty of Medicine and Dentistry, University of Alberta, Edmonton, AB, Canada,

Marta Vidal-García, Jose David Aponte and Benedikt Hallgrímsson
Department of Cell Biology & Anatomy, Alberta Children's Hospital Research Institute, University of Calgary, Calgary, AB, Canada

Devyn Godziuk, Adrianne Eve Scovil Watson and Tim Footz
Department of Medical Genetics, Faculty of Medicine and Dentistry, University of Alberta, Edmonton, AB, Canada,

Nathan F. Schachter and Sean E. Egan
Cell Biology Program, Hospital for Sick Children, Toronto, ON, Canada
Department of Molecular Genetics, University of Toronto, Toronto, ON, Canada

Daniel Graf
School of Dentistry, Faculty of Medicine and Dentistry, University of Alberta, Edmonton, AB, Canada
Department of Medical Genetics, Faculty of Medicine and Dentistry, University of Alberta, Edmonton, AB, Canada

Anastassia Voronova
Department of Medical Genetics, Faculty of Medicine and Dentistry, University of Alberta, Edmonton, AB, Canada
Department of Cell Biology, Faculty of Medicine and Dentistry, University of Alberta, Edmonton, AB, Canada

Andrea P. Murillo-Rincón and Marketa Kaucka
Max Planck Research Group Craniofacial Biology, Max Planck Institute for Evolutionary Biology, Plön, Germany

Index

www.ingramcontent.com/pod-product-compliance
Lightning Source LLC
LaVergne TN
LVHW082134200926
848484LV00008B/2055